Hepatic Arterial Infusion for Malignancy

Michael D'Angelica • Michael Lidsky
Editors

Hepatic Arterial Infusion for Malignancy

Springer

Editors
Michael D'Angelica
Department of Surgery
Memorial Sloan Kettering Cancer Center
New York, NY, USA

Michael Lidsky
Department of Surgery
Duke University
Durham, NC, USA

ISBN 978-3-031-74937-7 ISBN 978-3-031-74935-3 (eBook)
https://doi.org/10.1007/978-3-031-74935-3

This Springer imprint is published by the registered company Springer Nature Switzerland AG
The registered company address is: Gewerbestrasse 11, 6330 Cham, Switzerland

Foreword

When I began my career as a medical oncologist in 1974, patients with metastatic colorectal cancer had a poor prognosis, especially if they had liver metastases. The average survival was 12 months, and almost no one survived 3 years.

Hepatic metastasis is a significant problem for patients with colorectal cancer since it is present initially in 15–25% of patients, and another 50% develop liver metastases during the course of their disease. Researchers have long ago demonstrated that liver metastases are perfused by the hepatic artery, while the normal liver is perfused by both the artery and portal vein. Therefore, it was thought that therapy injected into the liver via the hepatic artery may lead to better control of liver metastases. Initially, hepatic arterial infusion (HAI) therapy was attempted with an external pump connected to a percutaneously placed catheter. There were some responses, but complications such as thrombosis and displacement of the catheter were common. In the 1980s, a totally implantable pump was developed which could be filled easily and was associated with fewer complications, such as catheter occlusion and infection. The original reports using this pump were with the drug floxuridine (FUDR), which has a short half-life and excellent hepatic extraction allowing for high concentrations to be delivered to the liver with minimal systemic exposure.

From 1970 to 1980, 5-flurouracil (5-FU) was the only useful drug for colorectal cancer with a response rate of 20% and a median survival of 12 months for patients with metastatic disease. The first randomized studies comparing HAI-FUDR versus systemic 5-FU showed excellent response rates and an improvement in hepatic progression-free survival, but many of the early studies did not show an improvement in overall survival because these randomized studies allowed for crossover from the systemic arm to HAI arm at the time of progression. I therefore led a CALGB study of HAI-FUDR versus systemic 5-FU, without a crossover design, to answer this question. The study showed an increase in overall survival and hepatic progression-free survival with HAI-FUDR pump therapy. After I presented this positive CALGB study at ASCO, reviewers were critical stating that the majority of the patients were from MSKCC. However, all cases were reviewed by CALGB investigators for inclusion, exclusion, and all clinical outcomes. We believed the results were real, but the reviewers put a negative connotation on the study.

In the 1990s, drugs such as irinotecan and oxaliplatin were developed and led to improved response rates of 40% and median survival of 20 months. Further improvement was observed in patients with KRAS wild-type tumors where survival of 30 months was accomplished with targeted therapy with agents such as cetuximab or panitumumab. Despite these important advances, I thought there was still a need for more effective therapy for this disease. As these new drugs came to the clinic at the time the randomized trial was completed, another criticism of the CALGB study was that the systemic arm used only 5-FU. Many oncologists at the time the study was completed (and today) felt that the same results obtained with HAI-FUDR in the CALGB study could be achieved with the new, more effective "modern" systemic drugs that have now become the cornerstones of therapy for advanced disease. Despite these criticisms, I believed in the study and we continued to investigate the use of HAI-FUDR at MSKCC.

The original trials were with HAI-FUDR therapy alone, without systemic therapy. We therefore conducted several trials testing HAI-FUDR combined with systemic 5-FU alone and then in combination with newer systemic drugs (irinotecan alone, irinotecan and 5-FU, oxaliplatin and irinotecan, oxaliplatin and 5-FU, irinotecan with 5-FU and panitumumab, oxaliplatin with 5-FU and Avastin). We studied the efficacy and toxicity of these combinations. These trials demonstrated excellent response rates and the ability to get patients to liver resection who originally were thought to be unresectable.

After many phase 1 and phase 2 studies demonstrated the benefit of HAI therapy in patients with unresectable colorectal liver metastases, we decided to work on trials using HAI-FUDR and systemic therapy after liver resection, as an adjuvant therapy. Since most recurrences occur in the liver after hepatic resection, we thought using HAI would prove to be particularly beneficial. First, we performed trials to test the safety of HAI pump therapy after resection. At this time, the administration at MSKCC demanded a randomized study to prove that it was worth paying the expense of the pump. I therefore led a randomized study of HAI plus systemic therapy versus systemic therapy alone in patients with colorectal cancer who underwent resection of hepatic metastases. When we started this adjuvant study, there were many naysayers in our own institution, and it was hard to get the patients to accept randomization. At first, I was the only physician randomizing patients. This became more difficult when I became pregnant, because patients did not want to sign up for a study where they thought the investigator would leave and not be there to take care of them. In fact, we demonstrated that there were significantly fewer patients randomized during the time I was pregnant compared to other time periods. We finally completed the study and published it in the *New England Journal of Medicine*, where we reported a significant increase in 2-year survival, a significant increase in hepatic disease-free survival, and overall disease-free survival, in patients who received HAI-FUDR and systemic 5-FU versus systemic 5-FU alone. Prior to that publication, I presented the results at ASCO where it was given a special press review, but again the reviewers of the study at the meeting put a negative twist on a positive study and said that the results in the systemic arm could have been better if we had used newer systemic agents which became available as we ran this study.

Despite this critique, three other randomized studies after this presentation have been published, which also demonstrated a significant increase in progression-free survival and especially hepatic progression-free survival in 3 of the 4 trials.

The surgeons at our institution had seen the results in their patients and they were impressed, so we continued our work at MSKCC, though it was still not accepted in many other institutions. However, a review of 2380 patients who had a liver resection at MSKCC showed a 2-year increase in survival in patients who received HAI therapy versus those who received systemic therapy (even with new agents), despite the fact that the HAI group had significantly poorer baseline characteristics. At this point, other institutions, often led by physicians who had trained at MSKCC and believed in this therapy, started HAI therapy programs in their institutions.

The promising results in colorectal cancer led us to investigate the use of HAI therapy in cholangiocarcinoma. We demonstrated a significant increase in response and survival in this disease as well. A new randomized trial of HAI with systemic agents versus systemic agents alone is currently being conducted.

Sometimes one believes in something that is not accepted by the majority but continues to work with the idea. Most investigators still feel that these results need to be duplicated in a larger multi-institutional randomized study. Now, with several institutions adopting HAI therapy, we can run such studies. We also may be able to persuade pharmaceutical companies to allow us to test new classes of drugs for delivery directly into the hepatic artery, or new systemic drugs in combination with HAI therapy, such as combining systemic immunotherapy and HAI.

This book will describe what we have achieved to date and will also discuss how best to use HAI therapy. We hope to inspire future investigators to continue to make progress in this field.

Emeritus at Memorial Sloan Kettering Cancer Center Nancy Kemeny
New York, NY, USA

Contents

Part VII The Future of Hepatic Arterial Infusion

Contributors

Peter Allen Department of Surgery, Duke University, Durham, NC, USA

Celina Ang Department of Medical Oncology, Mount Sinai Hospital, New York, NY, USA

Federico Aucejo Department of General Surgery, Digestive Disease and Surgery Institute, Cleveland Clinic, Cleveland, OH, USA

David Bartlett Surgical Oncology, Allegheny Health Network, Pittsburgh, PA, USA
Surgical Oncology, Allegheny Healthy Network Cancer Institute, Pittsburgh, PA, USA

Yael Berger Department of Surgery, Hepatobiliary and Pancreatic Surgery Unit, Beilinson Hospital, Rabin Medical Center, Petah-tikva, Israel
Tel Aviv University, Faculty of Medical & Health Sciences, Tel Aviv, Israel

Benjamin A. Bleiberg Department of Medicine, University of Pennsylvania Pearlman College of Medicine, Philadelphia, PA, USA

Hakan Bokhoven Department of Surgery, Erasmus University Medical Center, Rotterdam, The Netherlands

Lynn A. Brody Interventional Radiology Service, Department of Radiology, Memorial Sloan Kettering Cancer Center, New York, NY, USA

F. E. Buisman Department of Surgical Oncology, Erasmus University Medical Center, Rotterdam, the Netherlands

Jason Castellanos Department of Surgical Oncology, Fox Chase Cancer Center, Philadelphia, PA, USA

Michael J. Cavnar Department of Surgery, University of Kentucky College of Medicine, Lexington, KY, USA

Andrea Cercek Memorial Sloan Kettering Cancer Center, New York, NY, USA

Sree B. Chalasani Memorial Sloan Kettering Cancer Center, New York, NY, USA

Gloria Y. Chang Division of Surgical Oncology, Department of Surgery, University of Texas Southwestern Medical Center, Dallas, TX, USA

William C. Chapman Section of Abdominal Organ Transplant, Department of Surgery, Washington University School of Medicine, Washington University, St Louis, MO, USA

Thomas J. Chirichella III Department of Surgery, Mercy Health St. Elizabeth Youngstown Hospital, Youngstown, OH, USA

Noah A. Cohen Division of Surgical Oncology, Department of Surgery, Icahn School of Medicine at Mount Sinai, New York, NY, USA

Emilio Conde-Flores Centro Oncológico Diana Laura Riojas de Colosio, Médica Sur, Ciudad de México, México

Louise Connell Memorial Sloan Kettering Cancer Center, New York, NY, USA

Anne M. Covey Interventional Radiology Service, Department of Radiology, Memorial Sloan Kettering Cancer Center, New York, NY, USA

Andrew Crocker St. Elizabeth's Medical Center, Boston, MA, USA

Jashodeep Datta Department of Surgery, Sylvester Cancer Center/University of Miami/Jackson Memorial Hospital, Miami, FL, USA

Ronald P. DeMatteo Department of Surgery, Perelman School of Medicine, University of Pennsylvania, Philadelphia, PA, USA

Maria Diab Division of Hematology and Medical Oncology, Department of Internal Medicine, Henry Ford Health, Detroit, MI, USA

Bradley Digney Steward Surgical Specialists, Jordan Valley Medical Center, West Jordan, UT, USA

I. Dominguez-Rosado Department of Surgery, Instituto Nacional de Ciencias Medicas y Nutricion Salvador Zubiran, Mexico City, Mexico

Vikas Dudeja Division of Surgical Oncology, Department of Surgery, University of Alabama at Birmingham, Birmingham, AL, USA

Carleton Scott Ellis University of Kentucky College of Pharmacy, Lexington, KY, USA

Macie Enman Division of Surgical Oncology, Department of Surgery, University of Alabama at Birmingham, Birmingham, AL, USA

Marwan G. Fakih Department of Medicine, Hematology and Medical Oncology, City of Hope Helford Clinical Research Hospital, Duarte, CA, USA

Benjamin D. Ferguson Department of Surgery, University of Michigan, Ann Arbor, MI, USA

Ryan C. Fields Section of Surgical Oncology, Division of General Surgery, Department of Surgery, Washington University School of Medicine, St. Louis, MO, USA

Yuman Fong Department of Surgery, City of Hope Medical Center, Duarte, CA, USA

Lauren Gallegos University of Miami Sylvester Comprehensive Cancer Center, Miami, FL, USA

Sepideh Gholami Division of Surgical Oncology, Northwell Health Cancer Institute, Northwell Health, New Hyde Park, NY, USA

Ana L. Gleisner Division of Surgical Oncology, Department of Surgery, University of Colorado Anschutz Medical Campus, Aurora, CO, USA

Vikram C. Gorantla Division of Medical Oncology, University of Pittsburgh Medical Center, Pittsburgh, PA, USA

Patrick Grierson Division of Oncology, Department of Medicine, Washington University School of Medicine, St. Louis, MO, USA

Isabella Guajardo Department of Surgery, University of California San Diego, San Diego, CA, USA

Jane S. Han Department of Surgery, NYU Langone Hospital Brooklyn, Brooklyn, NY, USA

Emily C. Harrold Memorial Sloan Kettering Cancer Center, New York, NY, USA

Jonathan Hernandez Surgical Oncology Program, National Cancer Institute, National Institutes of Health, Bethesda, MD, USA

Angela L. Hill Division of General Surgery, Department of Surgery, Washington University School of Medicine, St. Louis, MO, USA

Marjolein Homs Erasmus Medical Center, Rotterdam, Netherlands

Lauren M. Janczewski Department of Surgery, Northwestern University Feinberg School of Medicine, Chicago, IL, USA

William R. Jarnagin Department of Surgery, Hepatopancreatobiliary Service, Memorial Sloan Kettering Cancer Center, New York, NY, USA
Cornell University, Weill Medical College, Memorial Sloan Kettering Cancer Center, New York, NY, USA

Georgios Karagkounis Department of Surgery, Hepatopancreatobiliary Service, Memorial Sloan Kettering Cancer Center, New York, NY, USA

P. J. Karanicolas Department of Hepatobiliary, Pancreatic, and GI Surgical Oncology, The Edmond Odette Cancer Centre @ Sunnybrook Health Sciences Centre, Toronto, ON, Canada

Adel Kardosh Division of Hematology/Medical Oncology, Knight Cancer Institute, Oregon Health and Science University, Portland, OR, USA

Jesse Kelley Corewell Health/Michigan State University College of Human Medicine, Grand Rapids, MI, USA

Margaret Kemeny Icahn School of Medicine at Mt Sinai, New York, NY, USA

Moh'd M. Khushman Department of Medicine, Washington University in St. Louis, St. Louis, MO, USA

Alex C. Kim Division of Surgical Oncology, University of Virginia Health Systems, Charlottesville, VA, USA
Division of Surgical Oncology, University of Texas Southwestern Medical Center, Charlottesville, Dallas, USA

T. Peter Kingham Department of Surgery, Memorial Sloan Kettering Cancer Center, New York, NY, USA

Kelly Koch Department of Surgical Oncology, Sylvester Cancer Center/ University of Miami/Jackson Memorial Hospital, Miami, FL, USA

Bas Groot Koerkamp Surgical Oncologist and Epidemiologist, Department of Surgery, Erasmus University Medical Center, Rotterdam, The Netherlands

John C. Krauss University of Michigan, Ann Arbor, MI, USA

K. F. D. Kuhlmann Department of Surgical Oncology, The Netherlands Cancer Institute, Amsterdam, the Netherlands

Kelly J. Lafaro Department of Surgery, Johns Hopkins University School of Medicine, Baltimore, MD, USA

Jacob Lambdin Surgical Oncology Program, National Cancer Institute, National Institutes of Health, Bethesda, MD, USA

Kristoffer Lassen Department of HPB-Surgery, Oslo University Hospital at Rikshospitalet, Oslo, Norway
Department of Clinical Medicine, UiT The Arctic University of Norway, Tromsø, Norway

Michael Lidsky Department of Surgery, Duke University, Durham, NC, USA

Kian-Huat Lim Division of Oncology, Department of Medicine, Washington University School of Medicine, St. Louis, MO, USA

Mengyuan Liu Department of Surgery, Memorial Sloan Kettering Cancer Center, New York, NY, USA

Kelly M. Mahuron Department of Surgery, City of Hope National Medical Center, Duarte, CA, USA

Ajay V. Maker Division of Surgical Oncology, University of California-San Francisco, San Francisco, CA, USA
UCSF Helen Diller Family Comprehensive Cancer Center, University of California San Francisco, San Francisco, CA, USA

Skye C. Mayo Division of Surgical Oncology, Oregon Health and Science University, Knight Cancer Institute, Portland, OR, USA

Hannah G. McDonald Department of Surgery, University of Kentucky College of Medicine, Lexington, KY, USA

Fidel David Huitzil-Meléndez Departamento de Hematología y Oncología, Instituto Nacional de Ciencias Médicas y Nutrición Salvador Zubirán, Ciudad de México, México

Laleh G. Melstrom Department of Surgery, City of Hope National Medical Center, Duarte, CA, USA

Humberto G. Mendoza Molecular Imaging and Therapy Service, Memorial Sloan Kettering Cancer Center, New York, NY, USA

Monica Isabel Meneses-Medina Departamento de Hematología y Oncología, Instituto Nacional de Ciencias Médicas y Nutrición Salvador Zubirán, Ciudad de México, México

Ryan P. Merkow Division of Surgical Oncology, Department of Surgery, University of Chicago, Chicago, IL, USA

Mary Mulcahy Northwestern University, Evanston, IL, USA

Hari Nathan Department of Surgery, University of Michigan, Ann Arbor, MI, USA

Daniel P. Nussbaum Department of Surgery, Duke University, Durham, NC, USA

Lee Ocuin Division of Surgical Oncology, Lehigh Valley Topper Cancer Institute, Allentown, PA, USA

Chandrasekhar Padmanabhan Department of Surgery, Vanderbilt University, Nashville, TN, USA

Maranda Pahlkotter Division of Surgical Oncology, Department of Surgery, Icahn School of Medicine at Mount Sinai, New York, NY, USA

Roheena Z. Panni Division of Hepatopancreatobiliary Surgery, Department of Surgery, Washington University School of Medicine, St. Louis, MO, USA

Reema Anil Patel Medical Oncology, Markey Cancer Center, University of Kentucky, Lexington, KY, USA

Sefali Patel Surgical Oncology, Allegheny Health Network, Pittsburgh, PA, USA

Gali Perl Department of Oncology, Petah-tikva, Israel

Tel Aviv University, Faculty of Medical & Health Sciences, Tel Aviv, Israel

Agustin Pimentel Sylvester Comprehensive Cancer Center, Division of Medical Oncology, University of Miami School of Medicine, Miami, FL, USA

James Pingpank Department of Surgery, University of Pittsburgh Medical Center, Pittsburgh, PA, USA

Alejandro Pita Department of General Surgery, Digestive Disease and Surgery Institute, Cleveland Clinic, Cleveland, OH, USA

Michael J. Raphael Odette Cancer Center, University of Toronto, Toronto, ON, Canada

Caio Max S. Rocha Lima Medical Oncology and Hematology, Atrium Health Wake Forest Baptist Comprehensive Cancer Center, Winston-Salem, NC, USA

Vanessa Rosas-Camargo Departamento de Hematología y Oncología, Instituto Nacional de Ciencias Médicas y Nutrición Salvador Zubirán, Ciudad de México, México

Robert E. Roses Department of Surgery, Hospital of the University of Pennsylvania, Philadelphia, PA, USA

Samantha M. Ruff Division of Surgical Oncology, University of Virginia Health Systems, Charlottesville, VA, USA

Eran Sadot Department of Surgery, Hepatobiliary and Pancreatic Surgery Unit, Beilinson Hospital, Rabin Medical Center, Petah-tikva, Israel
Tel Aviv University, Faculty of Medical & Health Sciences, Tel Aviv, Israel

Carl Schmidt Department of Surgery, West Virginia University, Morgantown, WV, USA

Charles J. Schneider Department of Medicine, University of Pennsylvania Pearlman College of Medicine, Philadelphia, PA, USA

Heiko Schöder Molecular Imaging and Therapy Service, Memorial Sloan Kettering Cancer Center, New York, NY, USA

Anthony Scholer Hackensack Meridian Medical Group, Jersey Shore University Medical Center, Neptune, NJ, USA

Issac R. Schwantes Division of Surgical Oncology, Oregon Health and Science University, Knight Cancer Institute, Portland, OR, USA

J. Eva Selfridge University Hospitals Seidman Cancer Center and Case Comprehensive Cancer Center, Case Western Reserve University, Cleveland, OH, USA

Jason K. Sicklick Department of Surgery, University of California San Diego, San Diego, CA, USA
Division of Surgical Oncology, University of California San Diego, San Diego, CA, USA
Moores Cancer Center, University of California San Diego, La Jolla, CA, USA
Department of Pharmacology, University of California San Diego, San Diego, CA, USA

Patrick Silveira Molecular Imaging and Therapy Service, Memorial Sloan Kettering Cancer Center, New York, NY, USA

Deborah Small Department of Nursing, University of California Davis, Sacramento, CA, USA

Ann E. Stevens Mayo Clinic, Rochester, MN, USA

Elwin Tham Department of Surgery, West Virginia University, Morgantown, WV, USA

Cornelius A. Thiels Mayo Clinic, Rochester, MN, USA

Hope E. Uronis Division of Medical Oncology, Department of Medicine, Duke Health, Durham, NC, USA

Namrata Vijayvergia Department of Hematology/Oncology, Fox Chase Cancer Center, Philadelphia, PA, USA

Lisa Vlastelica Duke Cancer Institute, Durham, NC, USA

Gregory Wilson Division of Surgical Oncology, Department of Surgery, University of Cincinnati Medical Center, Cincinnati, OH, USA

Paul Wong Division of Surgical Oncology, University of California-San Francisco, San Francisco, CA, USA

Terence Z. Wong Division of Nuclear Medicine and Radiotheranostics, Department of Radiology, Duke University, Durham, NC, USA

G. Paul Wright Corewell Health/Michigan State University College of Human Medicine, Grand Rapids, MI, USA

Adam C. Yopp Division of Surgical Oncology, Department of Surgery, University of Texas Southwestern Medical Center, Dallas, TX, USA

Mohammad Zaidi Department of Surgery, Duke University, Durham, NC, USA

Sabino Zani Jr Department of Surgery, Duke University, Durham, NC, USA

Part I

History of Hepatic Arterial Infusion

1 Philosophy and Rationale for Liver-Directed Therapy and Hepatic Arterial Infusion

Sefali Patel, Margaret Kemeny, and David Bartlett

Over 150,000 patients are diagnosed with colorectal cancer per year in the United States, and it is the second most common cause of cancer death worldwide. The liver is by far the most common site of metastasis and although surgical resection can be curative if the cancer is found early, once it has metastasized to the liver it can be very difficult to treat. Over the last 50 years there have been several advancements in treatment options including surgical excision as well as regionally infused chemotherapy and radiotherapy. Regional chemotherapy was popularized in the 1980s because of the invention of an implantable pump that was reliable and could deliver a continuous infusion of chemotherapy. Thus, the era of continuous hepatic artery infusion (HAI) began.

The ideology for liver-directed therapy came about due to the liver's dual blood supply by the portal vein and hepatic artery. The portal vein drains blood from all the gastrointestinal organs to the liver to be detoxified prior to entering the systemic circulation via the hepatic veins. Thus, hepatocytes responsible for detoxification receive 70% of their blood supply from the portal vein and this route has been shown to propagate the hepatic spread of gastrointestinal metastases. Interestingly, further studies to map the route of hepatic circulation and cancer metastasis have been performed using radioactive dye tracers. These studies went on to show that although these cancer cells reach the liver via the portal vein it is the hepatic artery that provides the cancer its nutrients for growth. Thus, the hepatic artery could be targeted to deliver chemotherapy agents specifically to cancer cells while limiting the concentration of chemotherapy reaching the normal hepatocytes and other organs by the liver's detoxification ability.

In this context the liver is the first capillary bed for colorectal metastasis and the cells grow in the liver prior to reaching other organs via hematogenous spread. With the advent of improved imaging as well as long-term natural history studies, we now know that the liver can be the sole site of metastatic spread making the liver best suited for the purpose of regionally infused chemotherapy.

When studying hepatic metabolism of chemotherapy agents, it was clear that some drugs were more potent than others. So, the tumors could receive significant exposure to the

S. Patel
Surgical Oncology, Allegheny Health Network, Pittsburgh, PA, USA
e-mail: sefali.patel@ahn.org

M. Kemeny
Icahn School of Medicine at Mt Sinai, New York, NY, USA
e-mail: KEMENYM@nychhc.org

D. Bartlett (✉)
Surgical Oncology, Allegheny Health Network, Pittsburgh, PA, USA

Surgical Oncology, Allegheny Healthy Network Cancer Institute, Pittsburgh, PA, USA
e-mail: david.bartlett@ahn.org

M. D'Angelica, M. Lidsky (eds.), *Hepatic Arterial Infusion for Malignancy*,
https://doi.org/10.1007/978-3-031-74935-3_1

agent while systemic exposure was minimal. 5-Fluoro-2deoxyuridine (FUDR) was the agent that was most efficiently extracted by the liver and had 100- to 400-fold increase in tumor exposure with 94–99% clearing of the agent via hepatic metabolism making it nearly a "one pass phenomenon," meaning that it is almost completely cleared from the blood by the liver before the blood is systemically distributed. 5-Fluorouracil (5-FU) is the most common chemotherapy for systemic use but only had a ten-fold increase in exposure thus limiting its dosage due to systemic toxicity.

The use of continuous infusion of chemotherapy has been shown to be more effective than IV bolus therapy. In a large meta-analysis continuous systemic IV infusion of 5-FU was found to have higher tumor response (22%) compared to IV bolus (14%) in patients with advanced colorectal cancer [1]. The implantable pump takes advantage of this phenomenon by delivering the chemotherapy continuously.

Continuous infusion via an implantable pump would ensure that the medication is always present and negate the need for patients to have frequent office visits and therapy infusion sessions. Compared to IV bolus injections, an implantable hepatic artery infusion pump can have several other advantages. No maintenance is required to care for the pump after surgical implantation and it has a very low infection rate. It would be refilled once every 2 weeks and allow for higher drug concentrations to improve effectiveness of treatment while minimizing the risk of systemic side effects.

When chemotherapy is administered through the hepatic artery there is a risk of artery thrombosis. This can limit the effectiveness of treatment and may result in liver damage. However, the use of an implantable pump allows for more targeted delivery of chemotherapy directly to the liver which minimizes the risk of hepatic artery thrombosis. As opposed to an implantable port, the pump is constantly delivering positive pressure with infusion of either chemotherapy or heparin-based fluid which prevents thrombosis of the catheter. The pump can also be periodically flushed with heparin or other anticoagulants to help prevent clot formation and maintain the patency. While the risk of hepatic artery thrombosis can never be eliminated the use of an implantable pump minimizes this risk.

The original infusion pumps were easy to implant and very reliable. They worked on a freon-based system which could give around 1.2 mL of chemotherapy per day, and with a reservoir of 30 mL this meant that 2 week infusions were practical. Only a few outside conditions could affect the flow including the patient's body temperature and air pressure around the pump. Fevers could also increase the flow but only minimally. Although patients had to be careful when going on airplanes, because of pressure changes, they usually did not have chemotherapy in their pumps at those times. Every time the pump was emptied the amount left in the reservoir would help recalculate the flow and readjust the dose needed in the pump. Because of the innovative design of a long-coiled wire tube and a diaphragm pushed by the freon there were amazingly few problems with drug delivery, less than 1 in a 1000. Early doses were generally in the 3 mg/kg/day range but because of liver toxicity they were reduced to approximately 1 mg/kg/day.

Modern day infusion pumps can be implanted laparoscopically or robotically and the drug is delivered from the reservoir through the catheter using an electrical or mechanical motor. The pump can also be designed to have safety features to help prevent over or under delivery. In some cases, the pump may have a mechanism that regulates the flow rate of the drug such as a piston or an electronic pump that can adjust the rate of infusion. And the pump may have a pressure sensor that measures the pressure in the catheter or an alarm that sounds if the pump malfunctions or the reservoir is empty.

Technical complications and durability of modern pumps has been evaluated in patients with unresectable colorectal liver metastases. A single institution study found that the overall technical complication rate was 18.1% [2]. The most common complication was related to the hepatic arterial system, being arterial occlusion occurring in 6% of patients overall. They also noted a very low rate of infectious complications in 2% of all patients. Even with these complications most patients discontinued treatment due to progression of disease rather than pump-related complications, showing that hepatic artery infusion pumps are a durable and relatively safe treatment option.

Several studies have also assessed the safety as well as the efficacy of hepatic artery infusion pumps and have found them to be reliable and well tolerated by patients. One such study was a multi-institutional randomized trial assessing the safety and effectiveness of hepatic artery infusion therapy in patients with unresectable liver metastasis from colorectal cancer. This study found that patients who underwent pump implantation had a median overall survival of 24.4 months vs. 20 months in patients who received systemic chemotherapy. There was also improved physical quality of life in patients who underwent pump implantation [3] presumably from limited systemic chemotherapy effects as well as reduced need for chemotherapy infusion sessions.

Moreover, hepatic artery infusion therapy has been able to convert patients who are diagnosed with unresectable cancer to resectable status after treatment. A prospective phase I clinical trial published in the *Journal of Clincal Oncology* in 2009 aimed to evaluate the efficacy of hepatic artery infusion (HAI) plus systemic chemotherapy with oxaliplatin and irinotecan in converting unresectable liver metastases from colorectal carcinoma to resectable disease. The primary endpoint of the study was the conversion rate to resectable disease. The secondary endpoints included progression-free survival, overall survival, and toxicity [4]. This study found that the combination of HAI and systemic chemotherapy resulted in a high conversion rate to resectable disease. Specifically, 92% of the 49 patients had complete (8%) or partial (84%) response and 47% were able to undergo resection. The entire cohort experienced a median overall survival of 39.8 months (50.8 months for chemo-naïve patients and 35 months for previously treated patients). Overall, the study suggests that the use of HAI plus systemic chemotherapy could be an effective treatment approach for patients with unresectable liver metastases from colorectal carcinoma, and that it could potentially increase the likelihood of achieving curative surgical resection. Similar results were seen in a more contemporary phase II single-arm trial evaluating conversion rates with HAI and modern chemotherapy. In that study, 52% of patients converted to resection which yielded a 5-year survival of 63% [5].

Despite technical improvements and short-term mortality benefit of hepatic resection, the long-term survival of resection of hepatic metastases in colorectal cancer remains below 30%, with most patients experiencing cancer recurrence in the liver. Because arterial chemotherapy regimens targeted to the liver have demonstrated high response rates, studies were performed evaluating adjuvant therapy for patients undergoing hepatic resection of liver metastases from colorectal cancer.

A randomized trial was performed where patients with resectable liver metastasis from colorectal cancer were assigned to receive either hepatic artery chemotherapy infusion with concurrent systemic chemotherapy vs. systemic chemotherapy infusion only after hepatic resection. This study found that median overall survival was 72.2 months in the patients who underwent pump implantation vs. 59.3 months in patients who underwent systemic chemotherapy. And after 2 years the rate of recurrence-free survival was 90% in pump implanted patients vs. 60% in the systemic chemotherapy group [6].

Another randomized clinical trial randomized patients with 1–3 potentially resectable tumors to receive either surgery alone or surgery plus continuous infusion of chemotherapy. The systemic chemotherapy used was a combination of fluorouracil and leucovorin. This study found that the combined-modality treatment approach was associated with a significant improvement in both disease-free survival and overall survival, compared to surgery alone. The 4-year recurrence-free survival rate and liver-specific recurrence-free survival was 45.7% and 66.9%, respectively, in the combined-modality treatment group compared to 25.2% and 43%, respectively, in the surgery alone group [7].

Overall, these studies demonstrate that the use of continuous infusion chemotherapy in combination with surgical resection of liver metastases can be an effective approach to improve long-term disease-free and overall survival.

Although the majority of studies performed evaluate the use of hepatic artery infusion chemotherapy in the treatment of metastatic colorectal carcinoma to the liver there have been several studies suggesting its usefulness in the treatment of other locally advanced primary malignancies.

In a phase II clinical trial, the efficacy and safety of hepatic artery infusion of floxuridine in combination with systemic gemcitabine and oxaliplatin was evaluated in patients with unresectable intrahepatic cholangiocarcinoma. The primary end point of this study was progression-free survival. This study found that the combination of hepatic artery infusion of floxuridine with systemic gemcitabine and oxaliplatin was well-tolerated and resulted in a median progression-free survival of 11.8 months with 84% of patients obtaining at least 6 months of progression-free survival. The median overall survival was 25 months, and the 1-year survival rate was 89% [8].

This study also evaluated the safety profile of the treatment regimen and found that the most common reason for hepatic infusion discontinuation and dose reduction were related to elevated liver function tests and abdominal pain. Systemic chemotherapy was commonly discontinued due to fatigue, thrombocytopenia and to prevent neurotoxicity. Primarily, this study showed that hepatic artery infusion with systemic chemotherapy was an effective treatment option for patients with unresectable intrahepatic cholangiocarcinoma, with a high objective response rate and favorable progression-free survival and overall survival outcomes.

Hepatocellular carcinoma is the most common primary liver malignancy. The mainstay of treatment remains surgery or locoregional therapy. The latter is generally reserved for patients with advanced disease who are not deemed to be surgical candidates. Hepatic artery infusion therapy has been shown to have a beneficial response in both patient populations with resectable and unresectable primary hepatocellular carcinoma. A meta-analysis was performed combining 26 studies and 4506 cases evaluating the usefulness of hepatic artery infusion therapy in patients with resectable and unresectable hepatocellular carcinoma. This meta-analysis found that HAI therapy was associated with a significant improvement in overall survival compared to other forms of locoregional therapy, like trans-arterial chemoembolization, or systemic therapy, like sorafenib. Analysis demonstrated a pooled hazard ratio of 0.58 and disease-free survival with a hazard ratio of 0.49. There was also an overall improvement in progression-free survival with a pooled hazard ratio of 0.52 in the hepatic artery infusion groups [9]. To summarize, this meta-analysis suggests that hepatic artery infusion may be a promising treatment option for patients with hepatocellular carcinoma as it appears to be associated with better overall survival and progression-free survival than other locoregional treatments.

In conclusion, hepatic artery infusion chemotherapy represents an important and evolving treatment approach for patients with liver metastases as well as primary liver malignancies. While the history of HAI chemotherapy dates back to the mid-twentieth century, it was not until the 1980s that significant progress was made in its development and clinical application.

Over the years, the philosophy of HAI chemotherapy has evolved to incorporate new drugs, delivery techniques, concurrent systemic chemotherapy, and patient selection criteria, leading to improved outcomes and quality of life for patients with liver metastases and primary liver cancers. Despite the potential benefits, HAI chemotherapy remains a complex and specialized treatment approach, requiring expertise and collaboration among healthcare providers across multiple disciplines.

Moving forward, ongoing research and clinical trials are expected to further refine the use of hepatic artery infusion chemotherapy, with a focus on optimizing treatment efficacy while minimizing adverse effects. Ultimately, continued progress in HAI chemotherapy holds promise for improving outcomes for patients with liver metastases and enhancing our understanding of cancer at a molecular level.

References

1. Meta-Analysis Group In Cancer, et al. Efficacy of intravenous continuous infusion of fluorouracil compared with bolus administration in advanced colorectal cancer. J Clin Oncol. 1998;16(1):301–8. https://doi.org/10.1200/JCO.1998.16.1.301.
2. Allen PJ, et al. Technical complications and durability of hepatic artery infusion pumps for unresectable colorectal liver metastases: an institutional experience of 544 consecutive cases. J Am Coll Surg. 2005;201(1):57–65. https://doi.org/10.1016/j.jamcollsurg.2005.03.019.
3. Kemeny NE, et al. Hepatic arterial infusion versus systemic therapy for hepatic metastases from colorectal cancer: a randomized trial of efficacy, quality of life, and molecular markers (CALGB 9481). J Clin Oncol. 2006;24(9):1395–403. https://doi.org/10.1200/JCO.2005.03.8166.
4. Kemeny NE, et al. Conversion to resectability using hepatic artery infusion plus systemic chemotherapy for the treatment of unresectable liver metastases from colorectal carcinoma. J Clin Oncol. 2009;27(21):3465–71. https://doi.org/10.1200/JCO.2008.20.1301.
5. D'Angelica MI, et al. Phase II trial of hepatic artery infusional and systemic chemotherapy for patients with unresectable hepatic metastases from colorectal cancer: conversion to resection and long-term outcomes. Ann Surg. 2015;261(2):353–60. https://doi.org/10.1097/SLA.0000000000000614.
6. Kemeny N, et al. Hepatic arterial infusion of chemotherapy after resection of hepatic metastases from colorectal cancer. N Engl J Med. 1999;341(27):2039–48. https://doi.org/10.1056/NEJM199912303412702.
7. Kemeny MM, et al. Combined-modality treatment for resectable metastatic colorectal carcinoma to the liver: surgical resection of hepatic metastases in combination with continuous infusion of chemotherapy—an intergroup study. J Clin Oncol. 2002;20(6):1499–505. https://doi.org/10.1200/JCO.2002.20.6.1499.
8. Cercek A, et al. Assessment of hepatic arterial infusion of Floxuridine in combination with systemic gemcitabine and Oxaliplatin in patients with Unresectable intrahepatic cholangiocarcinoma: a phase 2 clinical trial. JAMA Oncol. 2020;6(1):60–7. https://doi.org/10.1001/jamaoncol.2019.3718.
9. Li S, et al. The role of hepatic arterial infusion chemotherapy in the treatment of hepatocellular carcinoma: a systematic review and meta-analysis. Chemotherapy. 2021;66(4):124–33. https://doi.org/10.1159/000518257.

2 The History of Transarterial Therapies and Hepatic Arterial Infusion

Maranda Pahlkotter, Bradley Digney, Caio Max S. Rocha Lima, J. Eva Selfridge, and Noah A. Cohen

Introduction

The development of hepatic artery infusion (HAI) to its present state is a story that is much older and more interesting than one might think. It is a journey that unfolds over the course of a century, punctuated by rapid gains in knowledge and technological developments. In this chapter, we will take you through this journey by examining these developments in their historical setting of anatomy, surgery, and chemotherapy. We demonstrate how these fields have converged with our understanding of hepatic blood supply wherein the portal vein (PV) and hepatic artery (HA) perfuse and nourish the hepatocytes and cancer cells differently, with the latter receiving blood predominantly from the HA. We describe the trials that led to modern HA infusion and, as accurately as we can, based on the historical descriptions, the state of medicine in which these events occurred.

> Without bold, sometimes brash efforts, or without neglect of some of the moral and ethical ramifications of pioneering operations, we might never have developed operations on the heart, brain, or liver. Courage may accompany a lack of wisdom, but perhaps wisdom brings with it a diminution in courage. We should not dwell too long on that dilemma; else we might stop operating.—James H Foster, MD [1]

Background

The birth of HA infusion closely follows the development of modern anatomic and physiologic understandings of the liver. This, in turn, is largely due to the advancement and convergence of multiple fields of medicine. It begins with the development of surgery as a legitimate practice in the late 1800s. Operations only made possible by the recent development of general anesthesia and aseptic surgical techniques [2, 3]. Early operations on the liver took place in the same era as the development of gastric resection by Billroth [4] and the radical mastectomy by Halsted [5]. But

M. Pahlkotter · N. A. Cohen (✉)
Division of Surgical Oncology, Department of Surgery, Icahn School of Medicine at Mount Sinai, New York, NY, USA
e-mail: Maranda.Pahlkotter@mountsinai.org; noah.cohen@mountsinai.org

B. Digney
Steward Surgical Specialists, Jordan Valley Medical Center, West Jordan, UT, USA

C. M. S. Rocha Lima
Medical Oncology and Hematology, Atrium Health Wake Forest Baptist Comprehensive Cancer Center, Winston-Salem, NC, USA
e-mail: crochali@wakehealth.edu

J. E. Selfridge
University Hospitals Seidman Cancer Center and Case Comprehensive Cancer Center, Case Western Reserve University, Cleveland, OH, USA
e-mail: Jennifer.Selfridge@UHhospitals.org

M. D'Angelica, M. Lidsky (eds.), *Hepatic Arterial Infusion for Malignancy*,
https://doi.org/10.1007/978-3-031-74935-3_2

these surgeries were limited by poor anatomic understanding of the liver.

As knowledge of the anatomy progressed over the first half of the twentieth century, other remarkable developments were taking place. Aortography and imaging of the vascular system flourished. With the introduction of the Seldinger technique in 1953 [6], arteriography became safer and easier to accomplish. Further refinement in technique allowed for imaging of the hepatic arterial tree and paved the way for vascular interventions.

The last and most crucial development was taking place in the chemical treatment of cancer. The myelosuppressive effects of mustard gas were well known after its use in World War I. Over the course of the 1940s, experiments in the use of nitrogen mustards began [7]. This, in turn, was followed by the development of antimetabolic agents such as 5-fluorouracil (5-FU) and 5-fluoro-2′-deoxyuridine (floxuridine, FUDR) in the 1950s [8].

Over the course of this chapter we will review the historical developments that ultimately led to the modern practice of hepatic resection, liver-directed chemotherapy, and systemic chemotherapy for patients with cancer.

Early Liver Resection and Hepatic Anatomy

The first liver resection was reported by Luckenbach in 1888, the same surgeon who was also the first to perform a cholecystectomy in 1882. In 1892, WW Keen described these early experiences including his own, "Both experiments on animals and operation on man have shown that tumors of the liver, and even large portions of the liver itself, can be removed without undue disturbance of the function of the liver." [9] He also prepared a table with all the published cases of liver resection up until that time. There were 20 in all. However, throughout this early period mostly nonanatomic resections were attempted, and by the time of Keen's early American textbook *Surgery: Its Principles and Practices* [10] in 1916, no descriptions followed segmental anatomy of the liver, which would be described in later decades.

Cantlie as well as a German physician Rex are generally credited as the founders of the modern study of intrahepatic anatomy. In 1892, Cantlie described the anatomy of the liver as split by a line from the gallbladder to where the inferior vena cava grooves the back of the liver. He stated, "There can be no doubt that any surgical interference with the liver will be much more readily tolerated as it approaches that line, which I have termed the mid-line of the liver, and that the hemorrhage has less to be dreaded as the liver is incised or torn in the neighbourhood of that line." [11]

Segall reviewed the literature up until 1923 and found dramatic implications for the dual blood supply of the liver and noted opportunities for hepatic arterial intervention in the treatment of hepatic neoplasms. He reviewed the reports of hepatic arterial thrombosis due to an aneurysm in 1856 where the liver was described as unaltered as well as hepatic arterial ligations for aneurysms by Kehr in 1905 and Kaeding in 1919, both whose patients recovered. He suggested that the PV was sufficient for the survival of hepatic parenchyma. In his own postmortem examinations, he suggested, "portal blood takes no part in the nutrition of tumor metastases and that bile ducts are either entirely replaced or pushed aside by metastases of new-growth within the liver, while arterial blood alone is responsible for the nutrition of the metastases." [12] This finding was later confirmed by Breedis in 1949 using pigment injection into the PVs and HAs of rabbits and mice. The liver would be stained by PV injection and spare the tumors while HA injection of pigment would stain mainly the tumors and adjacent hepatic tissue [13, 14].

By the end of the 1950s, hepatic anatomy and anatomical resections would finally proceed to our modern understanding. The ability for the liver to survive after ligation of the HA as well as dozens of potential routes for hepatic arterial collateralization after ligation were recognized [15]. The first right hepatic lobectomies were reported at the beginning of the decade with Lortat-Jacob in France in 1952 [16] and Quattlebaum's and

Pack's right hepatic lobectomies in the United States in 1953 [17, 18]. Couinaud published his formal and extensive description of the segmental anatomy of the liver in 1957, becoming the standard by which hepatic anatomy was described [19]. However, despite these operations and anatomical discoveries of the 1950s, their application in surgical practice was limited. No clinical methods existed that could detect the existence of small liver tumors [20]. Thus, treatment of hepatic metastases was mostly palliative, driven by emerging interventional techniques and chemotherapy.

Chemotherapy and the Beginning of Arterial Infusion

The initial clinical trial of chemotherapy occurred in collaboration between Yale University and the Office of Scientific Research and Development to investigate chemical warfare agents. In 1942, the first patient with a lymphosarcoma refractory to radiation treatment was given nitrogen mustard (HN_2) over 10 days. There was a dramatic response, but it also resulted in leukopenia, thrombocytopenia, and cutaneous purpura. He relapsed in a month, was given a lower dose with a lesser response, then treated again and had no response [7]. By 1946, 160 patients with various neoplasms had been treated with HN_2 and some early conclusions reached: it was not a cure, tumor regression was temporary, and their largest effects were exerted on rapidly growing tissue. Major toxic effects included severe local inflammatory reactions, various degrees of nausea and vomiting, and damage to the blood forming organs [21].

In the following years, numerous trials began reporting on the results of HN_2, mostly with similar results. It was recognized early that leukemias and lymphomas were much more responsive to treatment than solid tumors, although Karnofsky found that anaplastic and epidermoid carcinomas of the lung had the favorable response of a temporary improvement in symptoms in ¾ of patients [22]. Up until 1950, no trials of intra-arterial administration had been performed due to the severe local inflammatory response observed with infiltration into soft tissue, which was thought to preclude regional administration. However, after accidentally administering HN_2 into the brachial artery of a patient with Hodgkin's disease, the hand and forearm of the patient became erythematous for days, then vesiculation and ulceration occurred. Eventually the reaction subsided and no irreversible changes were observed, suggesting a new method for treating regional carcinoma with an accessible arterial blood supply [23].

Using an experimental technique designed for intra-arterial administration of heparin [24], in 1950, Klopp introduced polyethylene tubing through a proximal arterial branch directly into the artery selected for injection (Fig. 2.1). Ten patients with varying pathology were treated using HN_2: seven head and neck cancers, two brain metastases, one extremity sarcoma. Three patients were excluded and died within 24 h of treatment, reportedly from complications of their disease. The patients with extremity sarcoma and head and neck cancers had variable responses. Relief of pain was the primary endpoint and was achieved in most [23].

Interestingly, the contemporaneous development of angiography led Bierman to the same conclusion regarding regional chemotherapy in

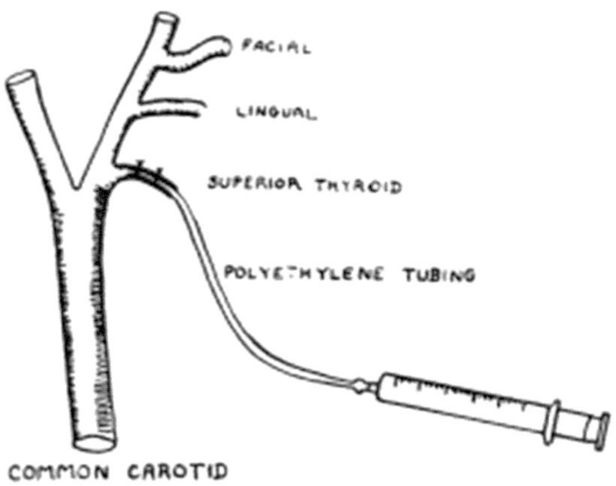

Fig. 2.1 Diagram illustrating introduction of polyethylene tube into the external carotid artery. Klopp CTR, Alford C, Bateman J, et al. Fractionated intra-arterial cancer chemotherapy with methyl bis amine hydrochloride; a preliminary report. Ann Surg 1950;132(4):811–832

1951. Angiography had its roots in cerebral angiograms, pioneered in Portugal in 1927 by Egas Moniz (the same neurologist who would win a Nobel Prize in 1949 for the development of the prefrontal lobotomy) [25]. The first aortography soon followed, and by the 1940s percutaneous techniques of aortography were becoming widely spread [26]. By 1950, increased vascularity of neoplasms had been noticed in brain, bone, renal, and other visceral neoplasms [27].

In 1951, a series of groundbreaking applications of angiography were developed at the National Cancer Institute by Bierman and colleagues. First, the group injected major arteries leading to tumor sites with fluorescein and demonstrated that some cutaneous lesions exhibited increased fluorescence compared to surrounding normal tissue. They hypothesized that arterial delivery of chemotherapy may be advantageous in delivering higher concentrations directly to neoplastic tissue [28]. Next, they gave intra-arterial HN_2 to "17 hopelessly incurable patients with far advanced neoplastic lesions involving the skin." Those neoplasms with increased vascularity, such as mycosis fungoides (cutaneous T-cell lymphoma), showed a prompt decrease in size, while the areas without increased vascularity did not respond. Importantly, they found fewer severe toxic hematologic changes than after intravenous administration [29]. The group went on to perform hepatic arteriography via a catheter introduced into the brachial artery. They confirmed that the arterial pattern in the liver with metastases was characterized by increased vascular outlines in the tumor masses, opening a new field of investigation for diagnostic and therapeutic purposes [27].

The earliest reports of treatment of abdominal neoplasms using HN_2 came from Sullivan in 1953. Using a brachial approach, a polyvinyl catheter was introduced into the upper or lower abdominal aorta depending on the site of disease. Abdominal lymphosarcoma and locally invasive cervical cancer, both refractory to radiation therapy, were treated in this method. A partial response followed by a rapid regrowth was seen in the lymphosarcoma. A dramatic response was seen in the cervical cancer, although the patient died just over a week later from urosepsis [30].

In 1956, Ariel reported the specific treatment of primary and metastatic cancer of the liver using intra-arterial chemotherapy delivered at the level of the celiac axis. The primary benefit was palliation of symptoms such as pain or anorexia. The best responses were observed in patients with ovarian carcinoma, while patients with metastases from the gastrointestinal tract had worse responses [31]. Abdominal administration was also reported in 1958 and resulted in the disappearance of jaundice in metastatic gastric cancer [32]. However, it was not until 1961 that a formal approach to isolated hepatic arterial infusion was described by Byron. Of the 39 patients treated, the catheter tip was placed just below the diaphragm in 19, in the celiac in 12, the HA in seven, and the right renal artery in one. Due to the small sample size and multiple types of tumors, treatment conclusions were difficult to reach. However, of the seven patients with HA infusion, four patients had metastases from colorectal cancer and three had an objective response to chemotherapy [33].

Antimetabolites and Prolonged Infusion

The 1960s saw the decline of nitrogen mustards and the rise of antimetabolites. By the 1950s, the antineoplastic effects of folic acid antagonists such as methotrexate were recognized [34]. In the latter part of the 1950s, the use of fluorine substitution for hydrogen on purines and pyrimidines had shown to have promising antitumor activity [35]. Early trials of intravenous 5-FU found that objective regression of neoplasms was only observed with doses that also produced systemic side effects. The authors suggested using the development of stomatitis as a guide for termination of therapy as it may have prevented the two deaths from chemotherapy in the series [8]. These early studies demonstrated that the alkylating agents, such as nitrogen mustards, had rapid antitumor effects even in a single dose, while antimetabolites require a more prolonged period of action before antitumor effects are produced. 5-FU and FUDR were found to have short serum half-lives and were effective against colorectal cancer, which often metastasizes to the liver [36]. It was also suggested that toxicity was reduced by longer infusion periods [37].

Sullivan began experiments with continuous intra-arterial antimetabolites in 1959 using one of the earliest models of an electric pump designed for infusion, a Bowman pump (Fig. 2.2), though hospitalization was required for the extent of treatment [37]. He also found that toxicity from 5-FU was dramatically decreased with continuous intravenous infusion, while toxicity from FUDR was enhanced [38]. Clarkson reported on the first results of continuous hepatic arterial infusion of antimetabolites, mostly methotrexate, 5-FU and FUDR. Catheters were placed via Bierman's method of using the brachial artery and left in place for as long as 16 weeks. Several infusion bottles were connected in tandem, one always kept full as a reserve bottle to avoid air embolism (Fig. 2.3). Patients were treated to the level of some degree of systemic toxicity (leukopenia, stomatitis, nausea, vomiting, diarrhea), thereby considered eligible for therapeutic evaluation. A total of 24 patients were successfully catheterized with 21 starting treatment. Five patients died before a complete course could be given, three from progressive liver failure, one from a perforated duodenal ulcer, one from hemorrhagic gastritis. Sixteen completed treatment and nine patients showed some beneficial response [39].

Placement of brachial artery catheters for hepatic infusion continued as the most common method of hepatic infusion throughout the 1960s. Using this method, Brennan infused 5-FU over 7 days at monthly intervals via an external Barron pump. He reported no instances of leukopenia below 2500/mm^3, enteritis or other complications of 5-FU, with two-thirds of patients having an objective response. He concluded that,

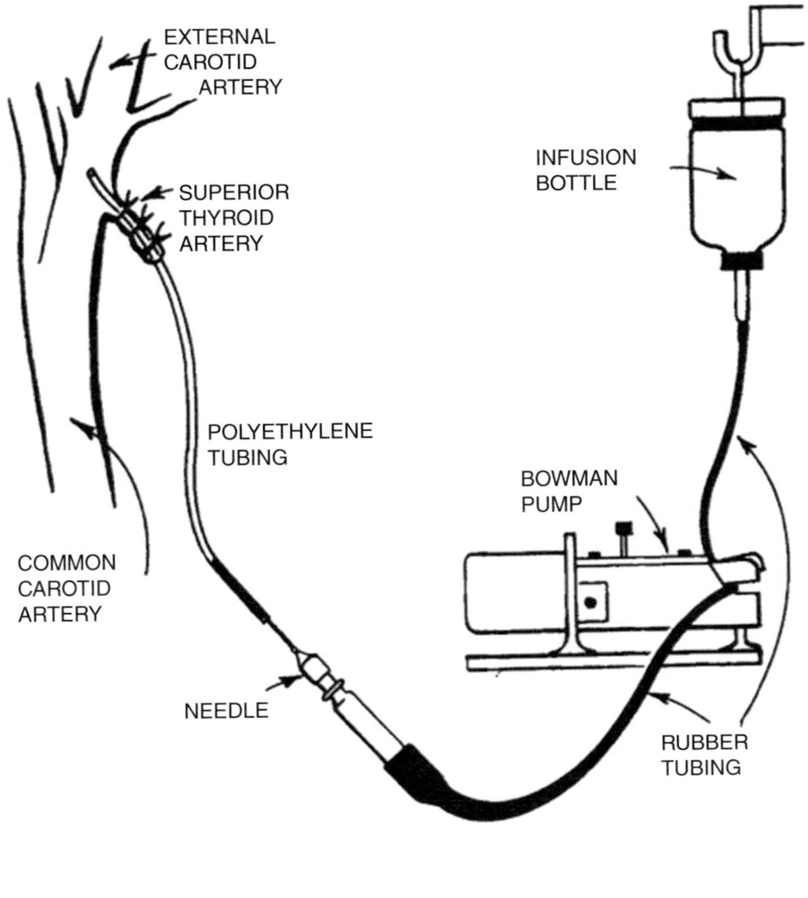

Fig. 2.2 Diagram of Bowman pump and catheter assembly. Sullivan RD, Mille E, Sikes MP. Antimetabolite-metabolite combination cancer chemotherapy; Effects of intra-arterial methotrexate-intramuscular citrovorum factor therapy in human cancer. Cancer 1959; 12:1248–1262

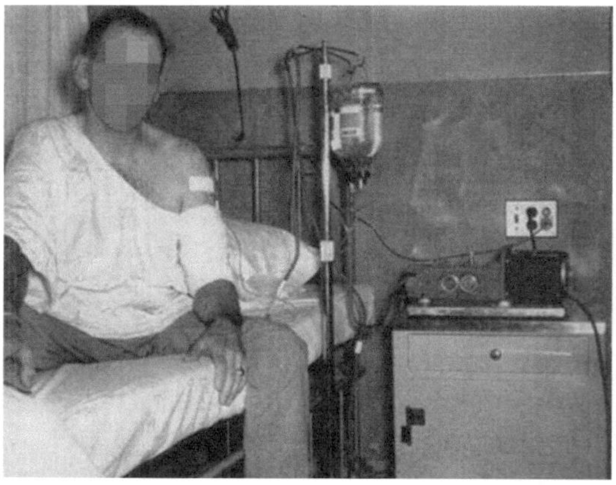

Fig. 2.3 Administration via left brachial access. Infusion bottles connected in tandem. Clarkson B, Young C, Dierick W, et al. Effects of continuous hepatic artery infusion of antimetabolites in primary and metastatic cancer of liver. Cancer 1962;15(3):472–488

"Establishment of a beachhead in the liver constitutes the critical strategic maneuver for many of these cancers. If they can be prevented from consolidating that position, a considerable proportion of them may be set back in their course for long periods of time." [40]

Refining Placement Techniques

Until 1964, the only reported method of arterial infusion into the HA was percutaneous, primarily via the brachial artery, until Sullivan and Watkins began open placement of HA infusion catheters. Their method involved surgical exposure of the HA, ligation of non-hepatic branches, and fluorescein dye infusion with ultraviolet illumination to demonstrate the distribution in the liver. Once placed, it was attached to a wearable, refillable pump that allowed continuous infusion over 21–41 day [41]. They defined objective tumor response as regression of measured tumor size and improvements in liver function tests. Clinical benefit was defined as improved performance status. This study included 21 patients but five did not receive adequate treatment (defined as satisfactory antitumor effects or local toxicity, or both): three died from hepatic coma and two had complications of the catheter interrupting treatment. Of the 16 that received adequate treatment, 13 had objective tumor regression and ten had an appreciable clinical benefit (defined as increase in functional performance status) from 2 to 12 months. They concluded, "The results of this study afford convincing evidence that the liver detoxifies FUDR when the drug is given by hepatic-artery infusion." [42]

Concurrently, a series of investigations into the consequences of the dual hepatic blood supply began to emerge. In 1962, Tygstrup clamped the HA and PV while measuring hepatic venous blood flow and oxygenation. He noted that arterial blood flow constituted 35% of hepatic venous flow and the HA supplied 50% of hepatic oxygen, but when hepatic arterial blood flow is interrupted, it is compensated for by portal venous oxygen and this is enough to maintain normal liver function [43]. These findings were in contrast to the earlier animal studies involving rabbits, all of which died with hepatic arterial division, and dogs, which sometimes lived after hepatic arterial division with administration of antibiotics [44].

With this emerging body of evidence that the HA could be sacrificed and that hepatic neoplasms were more susceptible to disruptions of arterial blood supply, a series of attempts were made to downsize hepatic tumors to allow for palliation of unresectable hepatic metastases as well as perform anatomic resections based on the advances in hepatic anatomy realized over the prior decade.

In 1966, Almersjo described a leiomyosarcoma in the liver with compression of the porta hepatis by two tumors in the right and left lobe, making radical resection impossible. The proper HA was divided, as were the falciform, lesser omentum and phrenohepatic ligaments to ensure division of major arterial collaterals. After 5 weeks the tumors were small enough to allow a left lobectomy and extirpation of the right lobe tumor [45]. This was followed by another study of four patients with hepatic arterial ligation, three with clinical improvement and one dying from hepatic failure. Ligation of either the right or left HA was performed in three patients with tumor degeneration in two patients [46].

Similarly, Murray-Lyon approached unresectable metastases by ligation of the HA and infusion of the PV with 5-FU, ten of the 11 patients had relief of their abdominal pain for up to 10 months [47].

However, despite some success in arterial ligation in downsizing tumors for resection as well as palliation of abdominal pain, an angiographic study of the collateral circulation to the liver after HA ligation showed that collateral flow, primarily from the phrenic arteries, occurred within months of ligation. This suggested that ischemia of the hepatic tumors is of short duration, and that within a short time tumor cells will develop an arterial blood supply sufficient to enable them to grow [48]. This also suggested that longer term control of tumor growth may be achieved by keeping the arterial supply of the tumor intact so that it could be used to deliver chemotherapy.

In a seminal paper on arterial infusion published in 1970, Watkins described in extensive detail the placement of hepatic arterial catheters by laparotomy. He stated that it was advantageous to ensure proper positioning, easily identify accessory arteries that may need to be ligated to prevent extrahepatic infusion and obtain information about the extent of disease (Fig. 2.4). A Polytetrafluoroethylene (PTFE) catheter was secured into the artery, usually placed in the gastroduodenal artery if feasible, with the tip lying upstream to any bifurcation of the HA. The catheter was externalized at the subxiphoid location and attached to a chronometric infusion pump. Continuous infusions of FUDR were given in 3–6 week courses. A total of 195 patients were initially enrolled in their trial. A few patients were excluded for various reasons such as misdiagnosis or too extensive disease. Five patients were excluded due to advanced hepatic decom-

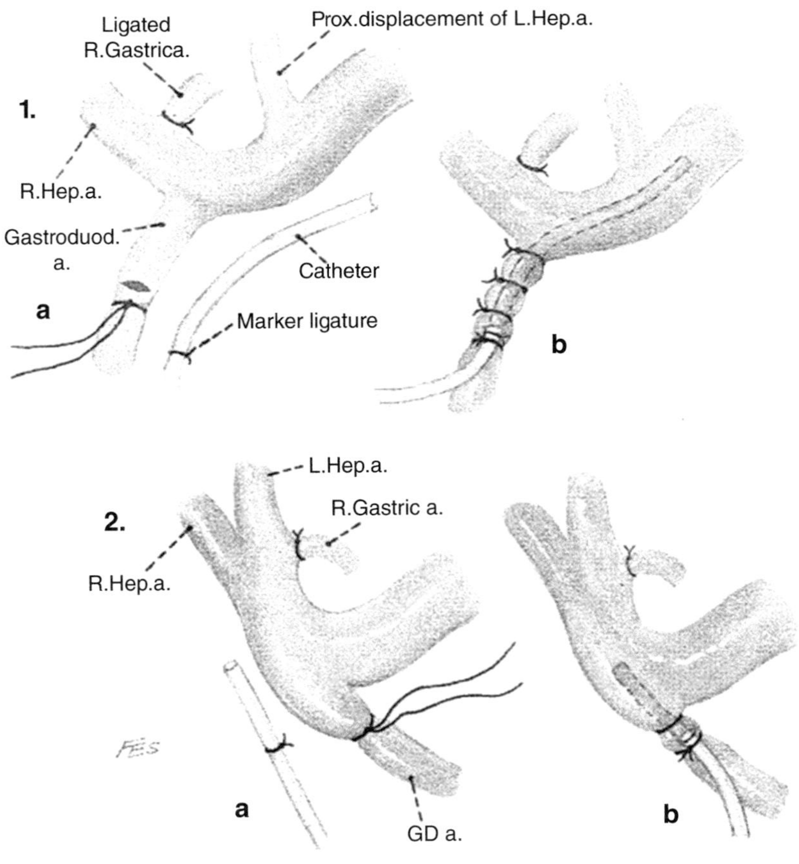

Fig. 2.4 Variations of catheter placement. Adapted from Watkins E, Khazei AM, Nahra KS. Surgical basis for arterial infusion chemotherapy of disseminated carcinoma of the liver. Surg Gyn Obs 1970;130(4):581–605

pensation, two of which had percutaneous catheter placement and further decompensation, suggesting that patients too ill to tolerate operative placement of catheters are also too ill to tolerate regional chemotherapy. Of the 184 patients with satisfactorily placed catheters, 32% had early complications preventing completion of a course of treatment. In the remaining patients, 71% had a favorable response, defined as significant decrease in liver size with relief of symptoms, improvement in liver function tests and improvement in functional capacity for more than 3 months. Median overall survival from various malignancies with hepatic metastases was reported at 14 months [49].

Subsequent studies examined the morbidity of hepatic arterial infusion delivery by percutaneously placed catheters and open catheters. Ansfield described 200 patients treated with 5-FU delivered via catheters introduced via the brachial artery. Catheters became displaced in 16.5% of patients, mycotic aneurysms and septic emboli occurred in 2.5%, entry site infections occurred in 2.5%, catheters were clotted in 2.5% and upper GI bleeds occurred in 2% [50]. Cady reported on complications from open placement and found that hepatic arterial thrombosis was more common than previously reported, but about 90% of patients had long-term catheter and arterial patency. He also found the rate of gastrointestinal hemorrhage to be 11% with two thirds of these patients dying from massive hemorrhage [51]. These studies took place years before cimetidine would be approved for use in the United States in 1977 [52].

A New Infusion Mechanism

With the growing acceptance that prolonged infusions of chemotherapeutic agents directly into the liver was an effective means of palliating advanced cancer, the delivery mechanism became improved as well. In 1970, Blackshear, a missile engineer at the University of Minnesota, reported a new design of a permanently implantable low flow infusion pump with an inexhaustible power source that could function independently of vascular pressure to provide continuous infusions [53]. This was later tested in canines using heparin and they suggested it could be used for continuous insulin administration as well as delivery of chemotherapy [54, 55]. In 1980 it was first used to deliver intra-arterial chemotherapy for primary and metastatic carcinomas of the liver (Fig. 2.5). Five patients had infusion cannulas placed in the HA via a laparotomy via methods described by Watkins [49] a decade earlier. One pump malfunctioned and was removed, but the four other patients received FUDR for

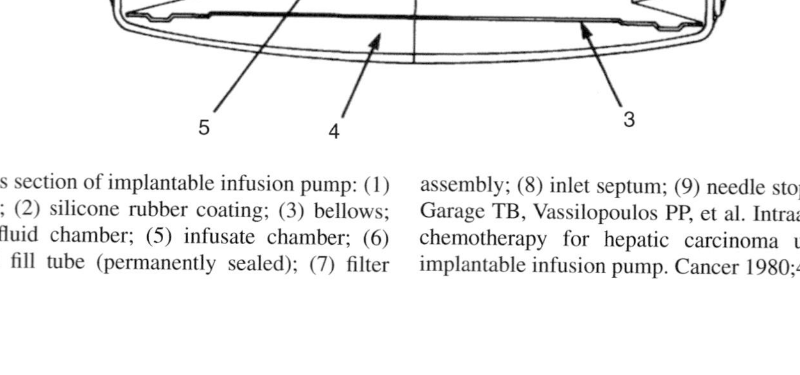

Fig. 2.5 Cross section of implantable infusion pump: (1) flow restrictor; (2) silicone rubber coating; (3) bellows; (4) charging fluid chamber; (5) infusate chamber; (6) charging fluid fill tube (permanently sealed); (7) filter assembly; (8) inlet septum; (9) needle stop. Buchwald H, Garage TB, Vassilopoulos PP, et al. Intraarterial infusion chemotherapy for hepatic carcinoma using a totally implantable infusion pump. Cancer 1980;45(5):866–869

5–33 weeks. FUDR toxicity involving pancytopenia, nausea, vomiting, anorexia, and stomatitis were reported, but the pump itself was tolerated by all patients. Tumor responses were not reported [56].

In 1978, Ensminger described the one pass phenomenon with FUDR when he compared hepatic arterial infusion of FUDR and 5-FU. Using hepatic venous sampling, he found that 94–99% of FUDR was extracted from the hepatic arterial circulation while only 19–51% of 5-FU was extracted [57]. This established FUDR as the chemotherapy of choice for hepatic arterial infusion due to high hepatic concentration and extraction compared to systemic administration, thereby providing a regional delivery advantage. He then reported the first use of an implantable pump with documented patient outcomes in 1981. Infusaid pumps, designed based on Blackshear's model, were placed in 13 patients: 11 with colorectal metastases, one carcinoid, and one hepatoma. FUDR was given for 5–17 months. Partial responses were reported in 85% of patients. Additionally, while the tumor in the liver was still controlled, four of these patients developed progressive extrahepatic disease. The median response duration and survival had not been reached at the time of publication [58].

Hepatic Arterial Chemotherapy Up to the Twenty-First Century

> No new chemotherapy agents have been developed recently that present hope for improving survival in patients with colon or rectal cancer.—Paul Sugarbaker [59]

By the early 1980s, 5-FU continued to be the only approved chemotherapy agent for metastatic colorectal cancer. Combination therapies using semustine, dacarbazine, vincristine, and hydroxyurea had shown no statistical difference in tumor response rates or survival, and were associated with higher incidences of life-threatening toxicities [60]. It would be another two decades until combining irinotecan or oxaliplatin with 5-FU would be shown to increase response rates, time to progression, and survival [61, 62]. In the absence of more active systemic chemotherapy regimens, hepatic arterial infusion emerged as a promising treatment for unresectable hepatic metastases.

In 1981, Reed published a ten-year retrospective evaluation of HA infusion. Catheters were initially placed via the brachial artery, but this approach was abandoned in favor of placement by laparotomy and infusion using Watkin's chronometric infusor. Seventy-three percent of patients with colorectal metastases obtained clinically significant remission, defined as objective and subjective improvement for at least 3 months. Seventy percent of hepatomas, 80% of gallbladder and bile duct cancers, and 50% of pancreatic cancers also achieved clinically significant responses [63]. After Ensminger's popularization of the implantable pump in the same year, the stage was set for larger studies that would explore the applications and limits of this treatment.

In 1983, a phase II trial of continuous arterial FUDR for colorectal liver metastases evaluated survival compared to a historical control group. The HAI pump patients received continuous chemotherapy on an outpatient basis and had an 88% response rate. Median and 1-year survival in the HAI pump patients was higher compared to the historical control population, 26 months versus 8 months and 82% versus 36%, respectively. However, only 41% of the control patients received systemic chemotherapy, severely limiting the applicability of this study [64].

In 1987, N. Kemeny published the first randomized trial of intravenous versus intrahepatic chemotherapy for colorectal metastases to the liver. Intrahepatic therapy produced a significantly higher response rate than intravenous therapy, 50% versus 20%, respectively. After tumor progression, 60% of the systemic therapy patients crossed over to intrahepatic therapy, 25% having a partial response and 33% a minor response or stabilization of disease [65]. However, because systemic therapy consisted of continuous FUDR via an infusion pump, their findings could not be adequately compared to standard intravenous chemotherapy regimens using 5-fluorouracil.

Another randomized trial in 1990 directly compared intra-arterial FUDR with systemic 5-fluorouracil for colorectal metastases.

Objective tumor response was observed in 48% versus 21% of patients receiving intra-arterial versus systemic therapy, respectively. Time to hepatic progression was significantly longer in the intra-arterial arm: 15.7 months versus 6 months. However, overall progression and survival were not statistically different, leading the authors to recommend against routine intra-arterial FUDR. They also found no significant difference in improvement of symptoms, ECOG performance scores, or weight gain [66].

The finding that intra-arterial FUDR did not improve survival compared to intravenous 5-fluorouracil shed considerable doubt on the wider adoption of this practice. The potential complications of HAI pump placement and side effects of the treatment were increasingly understood. In earlier studies, severe gastrointestinal toxicity was endoscopically documented in 46% of patients with ulcers, gastritis, or duodenitis. Hepatic enzyme abnormalities were seen in 71% of patients and elevated bilirubin in 22% [67]. In another study, biliary strictures resembling those in idiopathic sclerosing cholangitis were seen in 17.4% of patients, requiring treatment cessation and drainage of the biliary tree if it was dilated. Twenty-five percent of those patients died of complications [68]. Routine cholecystectomy was already advised due to the known complication of chemical cholecystitis. In 1992, concurrent hepatic arterial dexamethasone administration was shown to be associated with an increased response rate and trend toward increased survival and decreased bilirubin levels [69].

A 1996 meta-analysis of the five existing trials comparing HAI using FUDR with intravenous FUDR or 5-FUl found a significant response rate of 41% with HAI versus 14% with systemic therapy, but no survival advantage was present [70]. By the end of the 1990s, no trials had been performed that studied HAI plus systemic chemotherapy to systemic chemotherapy alone for unresectable colorectal liver metastases.

The role of HAI chemotherapy in nearly every study in the twentieth century was for palliation of unresectable disease. Adjuvant HAI chemotherapy after resection of hepatic metastases from colorectal cancer had just begun to be explored, and no trials on neoadjuvant HAI chemotherapy to convert unresectable hepatic tumors to resectable had been performed. A multi-arm trial by M. Kemeny in 1985 was the first to compare resection of colorectal liver metastases to resection plus HAI chemotherapy, but this arm of the trial enrolled five patients, and clinical benefit could not be determined [71]. However, in 1999, N. Kemeny compared HAI FUDR and systemic 5-FU to 5-FU alone after resection of colorectal liver metastasis. The complications of dual therapy were significant, with 29 patients needing hospitalization during treatment compared to 18 with monotherapy. Only 26% of the dual therapy patients received more than 50% of the planned dose of FUDR due to hepatic toxicity. Despite these issues, the median survival was 72.2 months in the dual therapy group and 59.3 months in the monotherapy group ($P = 0.03$). At 2 years, rates of survival free of hepatic recurrence was 90% with dual therapy and 60% with monotherapy ($P < 0.001$) [72]. This was the first trial that showed a conclusive survival benefit from HAI versus standard chemotherapy and marked the beginning of the modern era of hepatic arterial infusion.

Conclusion

Modern hepatic arterial infusion has emerged over the last century through the convergence of new understandings of hepatic anatomy and physiology, development of interventional techniques, and advancement of chemotherapies.

After trials using multiple chemotherapeutic regimens, FUDR had been established as the preferred agent for regional hepatic chemotherapy due to its short half-life and extensive hepatic metabolism allowing for high regional hepatic concentration, and proven efficacy in patients with colorectal metastases. Percutaneous approaches to liver-directed chemotherapy administration were all but abandoned in favor of open placement ensuring reliable hepatic perfusion and limiting extrahepatic perfusion via identification and ligation of collateral arterial branches. The methods of delivery evolved from infusion bottles hooked together in tandem and large external pumps, to wearable infusion devices allowing for easier ambulatory administration, and finally to implantable pumps. The pumps themselves have transitioned from Infusaid models for most of the 1980s and 1990s to others, such as the SynchroMed, Arrow and Codman 3000 pumps in subsequent decades, but all rely on Blackshear's original mechanism of delivery [73, 74].

At the close of the twentieth century, despite nearly 50 years of experimentation with regional therapy of hepatic metastases, the indications for HAI remained uncertain. The twenty-first century would see the rise of new chemotherapeutic regimens to treat metastatic colorectal cancer and intrahepatic cholangiocarcinoma, the adoption of laparoscopic [75] and robotic techniques [76] for minimally invasive placement of implantable pumps, and a proliferation of studies that would begin to define the role of HAI chemotherapy in the modern treatment of primary and secondary tumors of the liver.

References

1. Foster JH. History of liver surgery. Arch Surg. 1991;126:381–7.
2. Duncum B. The development of inhalation anaesthesia in the second half of the nineteenth century. Proc R Soc Med. 1946;40(2):68–74.
3. Lister J. On the antiseptic principle in the practice of surgery. Br Med J. 1867;21(2):246–8.
4. Professor billroth as an operator. Br Med J. 1894;1(1729):376–7.
5. Halsted WS. The results of operations for the cure of cancer of the breast performed at the Johns Hopkins Hospital from June, 1889, to January, 1894. Ann Surg. 1894;20(5):497–555.
6. Seldinger SI. Catheter replacement of the needle in percutaneous arteriography: a new technique. Acta Radiol. 1953;39(5):368–76.
7. Gilman A. The initial clinical trial of nitrogen mustard. Am J Surg. 1963;105:574–8.
8. Curreri AR, Ansfield FJ, McIver FA, et al. Clinical studies with 5-fluorouracil. Cancer Res. 1958;18(4):478–84.
9. Keen WW. On resection of the liver, especially for hepatic tumors. Boston Med Surg J. 1892;126:405–9.
10. Keen WW. Surgery: its principles and practices 1916.
11. Cantlie J. On a new arrangement of the right and left lobes of the liver. J Anat Physiol. 1897;32(1):iv–x.
12. Segall HW. An experimental anatomical investigation of the blood and bile channels of the liver. Surg Gynecol Obstet. 1923;37:152–78.
13. Breedis C, Young G. Blood supply of neoplasms in the liver. Am Soc Exp Path Fed Proc. 1949;8:351.
14. Breedis C, Young G. The blood supply of neoplasms in the liver. Am J Pathol. 1954;30(5):969–77.
15. Mechels NA. Collateral arterial pathways to the liver after ligation of the hepatic artery and removal of the celiac axis. Cancer. 1953;6(4):708–24.
16. Lortat-Jacob JL, Robert HG. Well defined technic for right hepatectomy. Presse Med. 1952;60(26):549–51.
17. Quattlebaum JK. Massive resection of the liver. Ann Surg. 1953;137(6):787–95.
18. Pack GT, Baker HW. Total right hepatic lobectomy. Ann Surg. 1953;138(2):253–8.
19. Couinaud C. Le foie; études anatomiques et chirurgicales. Paris: Masson; 1957.
20. HM B, Eshkenazy R, Arish A. Milestones in the evolution of hepatic surgery. RMMJ. 2011;2(1):e0021.
21. Rhoads CP. Nitrogen mustards in the treatment of neoplastic disease. JAMA. 1946;131(8):656–8.
22. Karnofsky DA, Abelmann WH, Craver LF, et al. The use of the nitrogen mustards in the palliative treatment of carcinoma with particular reference to bronchogenic carcinoma. Cancer. 1948;1(4):634–56.
23. Klopp CTR, Alford C, Bateman J, et al. Fractionated intra-arterial cancer chemotherapy with methyl bis amine hydrochloride; a preliminary report. Ann Surg. 1950;132(4):811–32.
24. Donovan TJ. The uses of plastic tubes in the reparative surgery of battle injuries to arteries with and without intra-arterial heparin administration. Ann Surg. 1949;130:1024.
25. Tondreau R. The retrospectoscope, Egas Moniz 1874-1955. Radiographics. 1985;5(6):994–7.
26. Tillander H. Selective angiography of the abdominal aorta with a guided catheter. Acta Radiol. 1956;45(1):21–6.
27. Bierman HR, Byron RL, Kelley KH, Grady A. Studies on the blood supply of tumors in mann. III. Vascular patterns of the liver by hepatic arteriography in vivo. J Natl Cancer Inst. 1951;12(1):107–31.
28. Bierman HR, Kelly KH, Dod KS, Byron RL. Studies on the blood supply of tumors in man. I. Fluorescence of cutaneous lesions. J Natl Cancer Inst. 1951;11(5):877–89.
29. Bierman HR, Kelly KJ, Byron RL, et al. Studies on the blood supply of tumors in man. II. Intra-arterial nitrogen mustard therapy of cutaneous lesions. J Natl Cancer Inst. 1951;11(5):891–905.
30. Sullivan RD, Jones R, Schnabel TG, Shorey JM. The treatment of human cancer with intra-arterial nitrogen mustard, methylbis (2-chloroethyl) amine hydrochloride, utilizing a simplified catheter technique. Cancer. 1953;6(1):121–34.

31. Ariel IM. The treatment of primary and metastatic cancer of the liver. Surgery. 1956;39(1):70–91.
32. Karnofsky DA. Summary of results obtained with nitrogen mustard in the treatment of neoplastic disease. Ann N Y Acad Sci. 1958;68:899–914.
33. Byron R, Perez F, Yonemoto R, et al. Left brachial arterial catheterization for chemotherapy in advanced intra-abdominal malignant neoplasms. Surg Gynecol Obstet. 1961;112:689–96.
34. Farber S. Some observations on the effect of folic acid antagonists on acute leukemia and other forms of incurable cancer. Blood. 1949;4(2):160–7.
35. Heidelberger C, Chaudhuri NK, Danneberg P, et al. Fluorinated pyrimidines, a new class of tumor-inhibitory compounds. Nature. 1957;179(4561):663–6.
36. Clarkson B, O'Connor A, Winston L, Hutchinson D. The physiologic disposition of 5-fluorouracil and 5-fluoro-2′-deoxyuridine in man. Clin Pharmacol Ther. 1964;5(5):581–610.
37. Sullivan RD, Mille E, Sikes MP. Antimetabolite-metabolite combination cancer chemotherapy; effects of intra-arterial methotrexate-intramuscular citrovorum factor therapy in human cancer. Cancer. 1959;12:1248–62.
38. Sullivan RD, Young CW, Miller E, et al. The clinical effects of the continuous administration of fluorinated pyrimidines (5-fluorouracil and 5-fluoro-2′-deoxyuridine). Cancer Chemother Rep. 1960;8:77–83.
39. Clarkson B, Young C, Dierick W, et al. Effects of continuous hepatic artery infusion of antimetabolites in primary and metastatic cancer of liver. Cancer. 1962;15(3):472–88.
40. Brennan MJ, Talley RW, Drake EH, et al. 5-fluorouracil treatment of liver metastases by continuous hepatic artery infusion via cournand catheter: results and suitability for intensive postsurgical adjuvant chemotherapy. Ann Surg. 1963;158(3):405–17.
41. Watkins E. Chronometric infusor - an apparatus for protracted ambulatory infusion therapy. N Engl J Med. 1963;269:850–1.
42. Sullivan RD, Norgcross JW, Watkins E. Chemotherapy of metastatic liver cancer by prolonged hepatic-artery infusion. N Engl J Med. 1964;270:321–7.
43. Tygstrup N, Winkler K, Mellemgaard K, Andreassen M. Determination of the hepatic arterial blood flow and oxygen supply in man by clamping the hepatic artery during surgery. J Clin Invest. 1962;41(3):447–54.
44. Markowitz J, Rappaport A, Scott AC. Prevention of liver necrosis following ligation of hepatic artery. Proc Soc Exp Biol Med. 1949;70(2):305–15.
45. Almersjo O, Bengmark S, Engevik L, Hafstrom LO, Nilsson LAV. Hepatic artery ligation as pretreatment for liver resection of metastatic cancer. Rev Surg. 1966;23(5):377–80.
46. Nilsson LA. Therapeutic hepatic artery ligation in patients with secondary liver tumors. Rev Surg. 1966;23(5):374–6.
47. Murray-Lyon IM, Dawson JL, Parsons VA, et al. Treatment of secondary hepatic tumors by ligation of hepatic artery and infusion of cytotoxic drugs. Lancet. 1970;2:172–5.
48. Bengmark S, Rosengren K. Angiographic study of the collateral circulation to the liver after ligation of the hepatic artery in man. Am J Surg. 1970;119(6):620–4.
49. Watkins E, Khazei AM, Nahra KS. Surgical basis for arterial infusion chemotherapy of disseminated carcinoma of the liver. Surg Gynecol Obstet. 1970;130(4):581–605.
50. Ansfield FJ, Ramirez G, Skibba JL, et al. Intrahepatic arterial infusion with 5-fluorouracil. Cancer. 1971;28(5):1147–51.
51. Cady B. Hepatic arterial patency and complications after catheterization for infusion chemotherapy. Ann Surg. 1973;178(2):156–61.
52. Clayman CB. Evaluation of cimetidine (tagamet), an antagonist of hydrochloric acid secretion. JAMA. 1977;238:1289–90.
53. Blackshear PJ, Blackshear PL, Varco RL, Buchwald H. A permanently implantable self-recycling low flow constant rate multipurpose infusion pump of simple design. Surg Forum. 1970;21:136–7.
54. Blackshear PJ. The design and initial testing of an implantable infusion pump. Surg Gynecol Obstet. 1972;123(1):51–6.
55. Rhode TD, Blackshear PJ, Varco RL, Buchwald H. Chronic heparin anticoagulant in dogs by continuous infusion with a totally implantable pump. Trans Am Soc Artif Intern Organs. 1975;21:510–5.
56. Buchwald H, Garage TB, Vassilopoulos PP, et al. Intraarterial infusion chemotherapy for hepatic carcinoma using a totally implantable infusion pump. Cancer. 1980;45(5):866–9.
57. Ensminger W, Rosowsky A, Raso V, et al. A clinical-pharmacological evaluation of hepatic arterial infusions of 5-fluoro-2′-deoxyuridine and 5-fluorouracil. Cancer Res. 1978;38:3784–92.
58. Ensminger W, Niederhuber J, Dakhil S, et al. Totally implanted drug delivery system for hepatic arterial chemotherapy. Cancer Treat Rep. 1981;65:393–400.
59. Sugarbaker PH, et al. Prospective, randomized trial of intravenous versus intraperitoneal 5-fluorouracil in patients with advanced primary colon or rectal cancer. Surgery. 1985;98(3):414–22.
60. Engstrom PF, Macintyre JM, Douglass HO, et al. Combination chemotherapy of advanced colorectal cancer utilizing 5-fluorouracil, semustine, dacarbazine, vincristine, and hydroxyurea: a phase III trial by the eastern cooperative oncology group (EST: 4275). Cancer. 1982;49:1555–60.
61. Douillard JY, Cunningham D, Roth AD, et al. Irinotecan combined with fluorouracil compared with fluorouracil alone as first-line treatment for metastatic colorectal cancer: a multicentre randomised trial. Lancet. 2000;355:1041–7.
62. De Gramant A, Figer A, Seymour M, et al. Leucovorin and fluorouracil with or without oxaliplatin as first-

line treatment in advanced colorectal cancer. J Clin Oncol. 2000;18(16):2938–47.
63. Reed ML, Vaitkevicius VK, Al-Sarraf M, et al. The practicality of chronic hepatic artery infusion therapy of primary and metastatic hepatic malignancies: ten-year results of 124 patients in a prospective trial. Cancer. 1981;47:402–9.
64. Balch CM, Urist MM, Soon SN, McGregor M. A prospective phase II clinical trial of continuous FUDR regional chemotherapy for colorectal metastases to the liver using a totally implantable drug infusion pump. Ann Surg. 1983;198(5):567–73.
65. Kemeny N, Daly J, Reichman B, et al. Intrahepatic or systemic infusion of fluorodeoxyuridine in patients with liver metastases from colorectal carcinoma: a randomized trial. Ann Intern Med. 1987;107:459–65.
66. Martin JK, O'Connel MJ, Wieand HS, et al. Intra-arterial floxuridine vs systemic fluorouracil for hepatic metastases from colorectal cancer: a randomized trial. Arch Surg. 1990;125:1022–7.
67. Kemeny N, Daly J, Oderman P, et al. Hepatic artery pump infusion toxicity and results in patients with metastatic colorectal carcinoma. J Clin Oncol. 1984;2(6):595–600.
68. Kemeny MM, Battifora H, Blayney DW, et al. Sclerosing cholangitis after continuous hepatic artery infusion of FUDR. Ann Surg. 1985;202(2):176–81.
69. Kemeny N, Seiter K, Niedzwiecki D, et al. A randomized trial of intrahepatic infusion of fluorodeoxyuridine with dexamethasone versus fluorodeoxyuridine alone in the treatment of metastatic colorectal cancer. Cancer. 1992;69(2):327–34.
70. Meta-Analysis Group in Cancer. Reappraisal of hepatic arterial infusion in the treatment of nonresectable liver metastases from colorectal cancer. J Natl Cancer Inst. 1996;88(5):252–8.
71. Kemeny MM, Goldberg DA, Browning S, et al. Experience with continuous regional chemotherapy and hepatic resection as treatment of hepatic metastases from colorectal primaries: a prospective randomized study. Cancer. 1985;55:1265–70.
72. Kemeny N, Huang Y, Cohen AM, et al. Hepatic arterial infusion of chemotherapy after resection of hepatic metastases from colorectal cancer. N Engl J Med. 1999;341(27):2039–48.
73. Kemeny M. The surgical aspects of the totally implantable hepatic artery infusion pump. Arch Surg. 2001;136:348–52.
74. Strnad BS, Ludwig DR, Gilcrease-Garcia B, et al. Contemporary imaging of the surgically placed hepatic arterial infusion chemotherapy pump. AJR Am J Roentgenol. 2021;2017(3):633–43.
75. Feliciotti F, Paganini A, Guerrieri M, et al. Laparoscopic intra-arterial catheter implantation for regional chemotherapy of liver metastasis. Surg Endosc. 1996;10(4):449–52.
76. Dhir M, Magge D, Novak S, et al. Robotic-assisted placement of an hepatic artery infusion pump and catheter for regional chemotherapy of the liver. Ann Surg Oncol. 2016;23:S755–6.

HAI Device Development: The Implantable Reservoir-Based Pump

3

Jacob Lambdin, Macie Enman, Vikas Dudeja, and Jonathan Hernandez

The first efforts toward the development of a fully implantable reservoir-based hepatic artery infusion pump (HAIP) began in earnest in the 1960s. Throughout the 1950s there was growing interest in the idea of regional chemotherapy. Calvin Klopp, a surgeon from George Washington University, published a report describing the potential role of arterial infusions as regional chemotherapy. This report was inspired by an accidental infusion of nitrogen mustard into the brachial artery and the observation that it produced only local toxicity in an arterial distribution [1]. This observation suggested the possibility of administering higher doses of drugs to an area of interest while limiting systemic toxicity. That publication prompted investigation of the potential role of arterial administration of chemotherapeutic agents for various pathologies, including primary liver tumors and isolated liver metastases. Another key advancement that paved the way for the development of a fully implantable HAIP was the refinement of the surgical techniques of hepatic artery cannulation. A publication in 1961 detailed a technique wherein a ureteral catheter could be placed into the hepatic artery via retrograde passage through the gastroepiploic artery and gastroduodenal artery [2]. The original application of this technique allowed for a stump of the gastrocolic omentum to be brought through the abdominal wound in order to allow for repeated infusions without the need for repeat laparotomy or angiography. This technique was further refined and subsequently outlined in a publication that described ligation of all non-hepatic branches of the hepatic artery in order to limit non-hepatic toxicity along with the use of a fluorescent dye to confirm isolated perfusion of the liver [3].

Around the same time researchers began to investigate the role of mechanical pumps (Fig. 3.1) to deliver continuous infusions of intra-arterial chemotherapy in order to overcome arterial pressure, and to limit the peaks and troughs associated with intermittent drug dosing [4]. The earliest described use of a mechanical pump for this purpose was in 1961 at the University of Wisconsin. In this protocol, a modified food pump was connected to either a surgically placed hepatic artery catheter, or an angiographically placed transbrachial/transfemoral catheter and

Supplementary Information The online version contains supplementary material available at https://doi.org/10.1007/978-3-031-74935-3_3.

J. Lambdin · J. Hernandez (✉)
Surgical Oncology Program, National Cancer Institute, National Institutes of Health, Bethesda, MD, USA
e-mail: jacob.lambdin@nih.gov; Jonathan.hernandez@nih.gov

M. Enman · V. Dudeja
Division of Surgical Oncology, Department of Surgery, University of Alabama at Birmingham, Birmingham, AL, USA
e-mail: vdudeja@uabmc.edu

M. D'Angelica, M. Lidsky (eds.), *Hepatic Arterial Infusion for Malignancy*,
https://doi.org/10.1007/978-3-031-74935-3_3

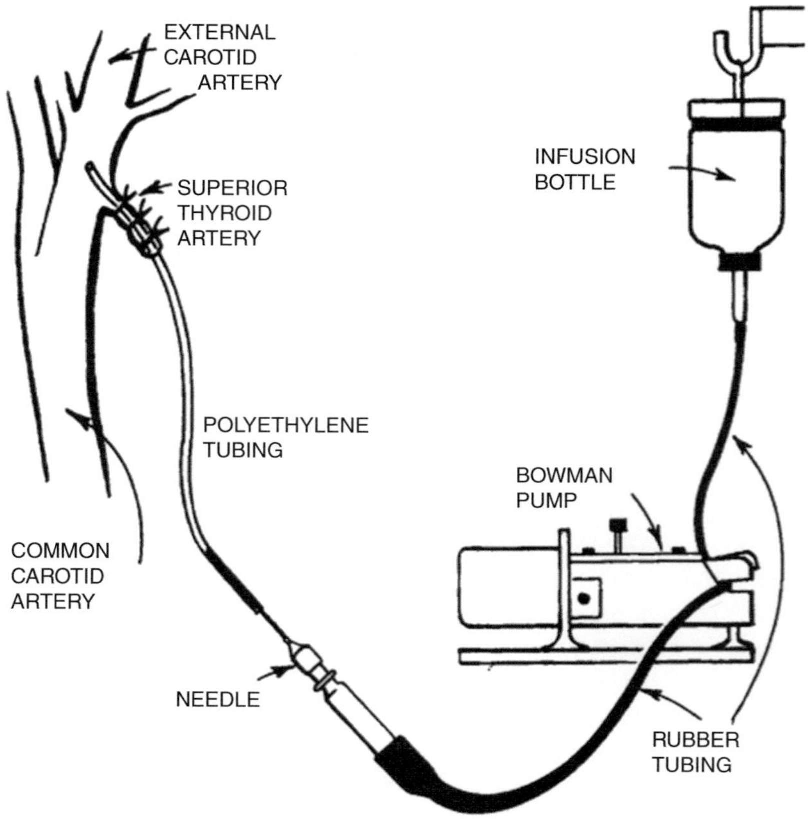

Fig. 3.1 Illustration showing how a Bowman feeding pump could be utilized to deliver intra-arterial infusion

5-fluorouracil was infused continuously [5]. This technique required near constant supervision and resulted in frequent air embolisms and was subsequently abandoned in 1963 in favor of a closed IV system with a pressure bag (Fig. 3.2). While this technique did serve to limit the complications associated with early pumps, it still required hospitalization for the duration of treatment [6]. The first description of an ambulatory arterial infusion pump appeared in 1963 when Dr. Elton Watkins of the Lahey Clinic published a report describing a new "chronometric infusor" [7]. The device housed a 25 mL reservoir and employed an internal roller pump, governed by a clock mechanism, to provide continuous infusion of drug. The device was attached to a tunneled catheter and secured to the chest wall with a harness, allowing patients to receive liver directed therapy on an ambulatory, outpatient basis. Although the initial results of liver directed therapy seemed promising, these pumps did not see wide or continued use for liver directed therapy as they required significant time and effort from physicians and patients alike in order to function properly. These pumps were a significant improvement over prolonged hospitalization, however, they still imposed considerable lifestyle restrictions on patients.

The first description of a completely implantable, drug infusion pump appeared in a brief paper published in 1970 [8]. Perry Blackshear Jr., a mechanical engineer at the University of Minnesota, described a multipurpose, permanent, implantable infusion pump capable of delivering a continuous infusion of drug at a set rate. The method of drug deliver was entirely novel in that, rather than relying on roller pumps or an external pressure bag, the driving force for drug infusion was a pressure gradient created entirely by vapor pressure. Initial in vitro testing demonstrated excellent constancy of infusion rates. Later in vivo testing demonstrated that the pump was able to provide a consistent enough infusion of heparin that, when implanted in dogs, the partial

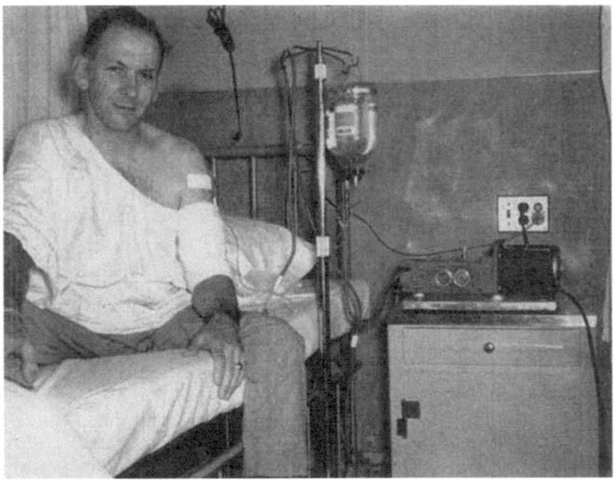

Fig. 3.2 Patient receiving liver-directed therapy by continuous infusion into a catheter inserted through the brachial artery into the common hepatic artery

thromboplastin times remained at twice the control values. The author envisioned that this technology would be useful for a variety of applications including heparin infusion, insulin infusion, vasoactive therapies, and delivery of regional chemotherapy. A subsequent publication in 1972 shed further light on the specifics of the pump design [9]. The authors set out to design a permanent implantable infusion pump with a few key principles in mind. First, the pump should be capable of maintaining constant low flow rates with the ability to alter the flow rate with the pump remaining in situ. They also recognized that the power source would need to be essentially inexhaustible and that the drug reservoir would need to be large enough to avoid the need for frequent refills. The ingenious design of the pump capitalized on the principle of vapor-liquid equilibrium, the concept wherein a vapor in equilibrium with its liquid phase exerts a constant pressure, at a given temperature, regardless of volume. The pump was designed such that the vapor pressure from an evaporating fluorocarbon would exert a force on the pump's internal bellows, propelling the drug through a capillary pressure limiter, then out into the patient's artery via a silicone catheter [10]. The rate of the infusion would then be governed by Poiseuille's Law ($Q = \frac{\pi P r^4}{8nl}$), which describes the relationship of a flow of fluid to a number of factors including viscosity of the fluid, dimensions of the tubing, and the driving pressure gradient. In the case of the implantable infusion pumps, temperature is held nearly constant at body temperature, and the force exerted by the vapor pressure is constant. Flow rates of the pumps would therefore be set by altering the length of the capillary pressure limiter as well as the viscosity of the drug [10]. The reservoir of the pump was designed such that it could be refilled via a percutaneous injection through a self-sealing silicon septum (Fig. 3.3) [11]. The re-filling of the reservoir would then compress the fluorocarbon vapor, causing it to condense back into liquid form, allowing for "recharging" of the power-source of the pump. Blackshear and his team of engineers at the University of Minnesota continued to refine this technology and in 1975 they published a paper describing a newly designed infusion pump. This new pump was tested in a canine model and demonstrated the ability to safely and reliably deliver a continuous heparin infusion for a 1 year period [12]. The study reported consistent and predictable elevations in partial thromboplastin times over the duration of the study period. Rates of infection, cannula thrombosis, and hemorrhage were all sufficiently low for the authors to conclude that it was reasonable to trial use of their pump in human patients.

In 1980, Dr. Henry Buchwald, one Blackshear's co-inventors at the University of Minnesota, published the first paper describing the use of a totally implantable arterial infusion pump to deliver chemotherapy directly to the liver [10]. He described his results using the implantable HAIP he helped create in four patients (three with isolated liver metastases and one with a primary liver cancer) using 5-fluorodeoxyuridine (FUDR). While this treatment did result in a "beneficial response" in two of the four patients, the main triumph of this work was to demonstrate the feasibility of the use of a fully implantable HAIP for delivery of liver-directed chemotherapy. In that publication, Buchwald noted that optimization of the pump was ongoing, and described plans to add a side port to the pump to allow for bolus injections via the catheter (Fig. 3.4) [11]. Soon after, the modi-

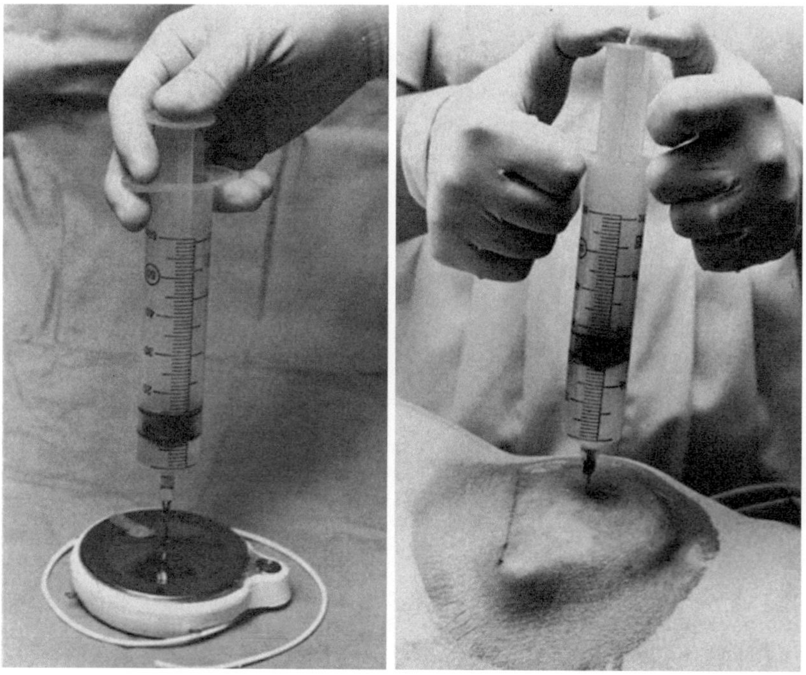

Fig. 3.3 Photographs of Blackshear's pump being filled prior to implantation and refilled after implantation by a percutaneous injection

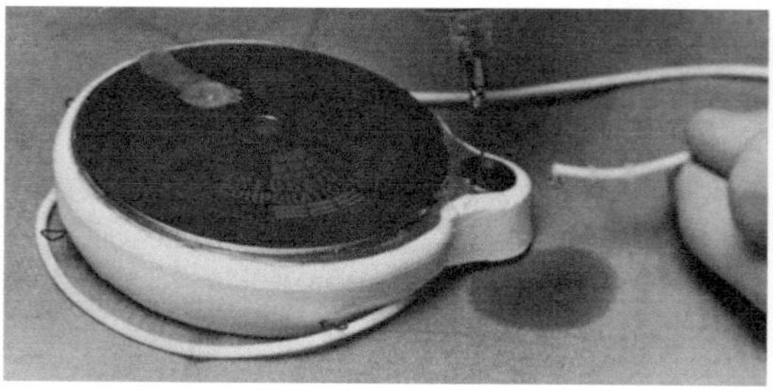

Fig. 3.4 Photograph demonstrating the ability to provide bolus injections via the catheter by injecting the side port

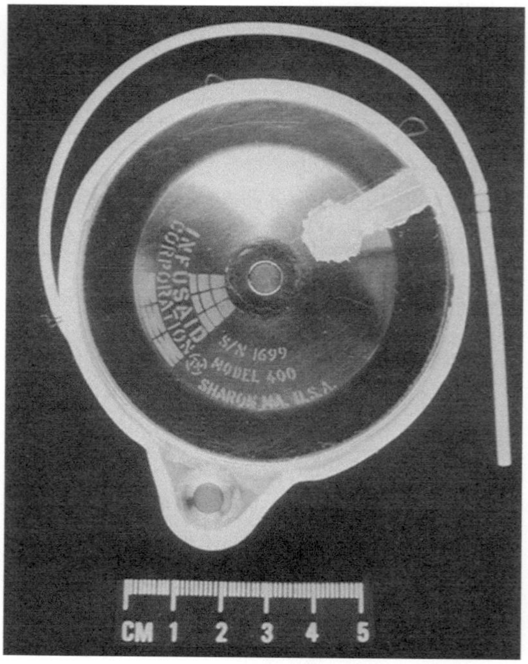

Fig. 3.5 The Infusaid Model 400 implantable infusion pump

fied implantable infusion pump gained commercial approval, marketed as the "Infusaid Model 400 pump" (Figs. 3.5 and 3.6) and the public interest in fully implantable HAIPs grew [13]. Many studies on the use of HAIPs were subsequently published in the mid- and late-1980s [11, 14–17]. Dr. Buchwald went on to describe many of the issues inherent with HAIPs and their catheters (Fig. 3.7) in efforts to improve the design [18].

Modern Pumps Modern implantable infusion pumps are of two general types. The first type is a non-programmable, constant flow pump that uses the pressure applied on the collapsible central drug-containing compartment. The second type of modern pumps are programmable electronic motor-driven pumps.

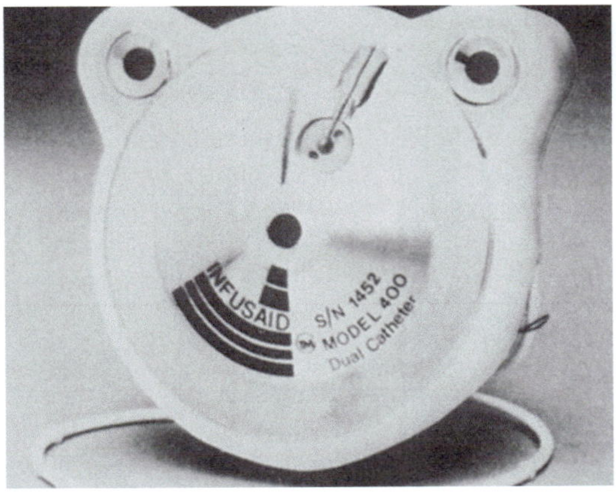

Fig. 3.6 Later version of Infusaid Model 400 featuring dual side ports

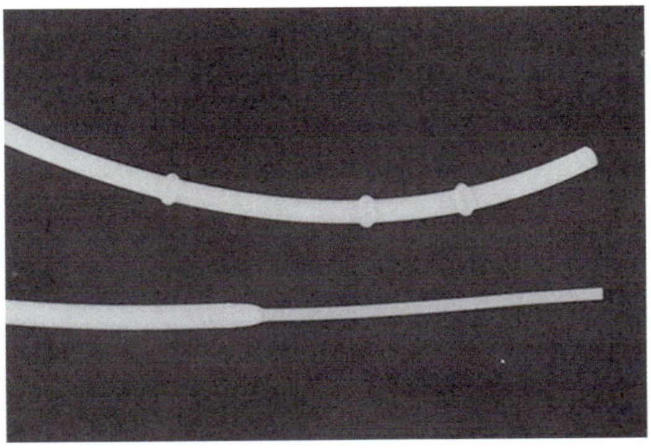

Fig. 3.7 Photograph of two different types of catheters available for use with the Infusaid Model 400

Intera 3000 Pump This pump represents an evolution of the early work outlined above, with key milestones outlined in Table 3.1. The device is structured like a circular disk or a "hockey puck". It is about 3 in. wide and about 1 inch thick (78 mm wide, 34 mm high in the center, 19.5 mm high in periphery). It is made of titanium and has a central "nipple like" protrusion on its superior surface. The center of this protrusion has an access hole, which is guarded by a silicone septum. The inner cavity of the pump is divided into inner and outer chambers, by accordion-like bellows (Fig. 3.8). The inner chamber holds the drug, while the outer propellant chamber holds the two-phase (liquid-vapor) chlorofluorocarbon propellant (Freon). Drug can be filled into the inner chamber through a non-coring needle (refill needle), which is pushed through the septum until it hits the needle stop plate. The refill needle has a hole at the end of its tip. As the pump is filled, the inner drug reservoir expands, compressing the propellant in the outer chamber. Once the drug reservoir is filled, the vapor pressure of the propellant exerts pressure on the reservoir bellows, forcing the drug from the reservoir through a bacterial retentive filter and capillary flow restrictor out of the pump, and through a catheter to the intended site within the body. The flow rate is determined and regulated by passage through the flow restrictive capillary tubing and can only be regulated by changing the viscosity of fluid. This pump can also be used to infuse drug directly into the catheter through the use of a bolus needle. Unlike the refill needle, the special bolus needle has a side hole and no hole at the tip (solid core distal to side hole). When properly placed, the side hole of the bolus needle aligns with the bolus path and the infusate goes directly into the catheter, instead of the inner chamber (Fig. 3.9).

Table 3.1 Timeline of the major events in the history of the development of hepatic artery infusion pumps

1970	Perry Blackshear Jr. publishes the first description of fully implantable constant flow pump
1975	Blackshear publishes results showing that an updated version of his pump (Infusaid M-400) is able to safely and effectively deliver heparin to dogs over a 1-year period
1980	Dr. Henry Buchwald publishes the first paper describing the use of a totally implantable arterial infusion pump to deliver chemotherapy directly to the liver
1982	Infusaid M-400 receives FDA approval for liver-directed FUDR therapy
1986	Pfizer acquires Infusaid
1988	Clinical trials begin with new pump "Model 3000"
1995	Arrow acquires rights to the Model 3000 pump
1996	Arrow Model 3000 receives FDA approval for delivery of intra-arterial chemotherapy
2001	Codman (Johnson & Johnson) acquires rights to Arrow Model 3000, renames pump the Codman 3000
2018	Production of Codman 3000 ends
2021	Intera Oncology obtains rights to resume production of the Codman 3000 under new name, the Intera 3000

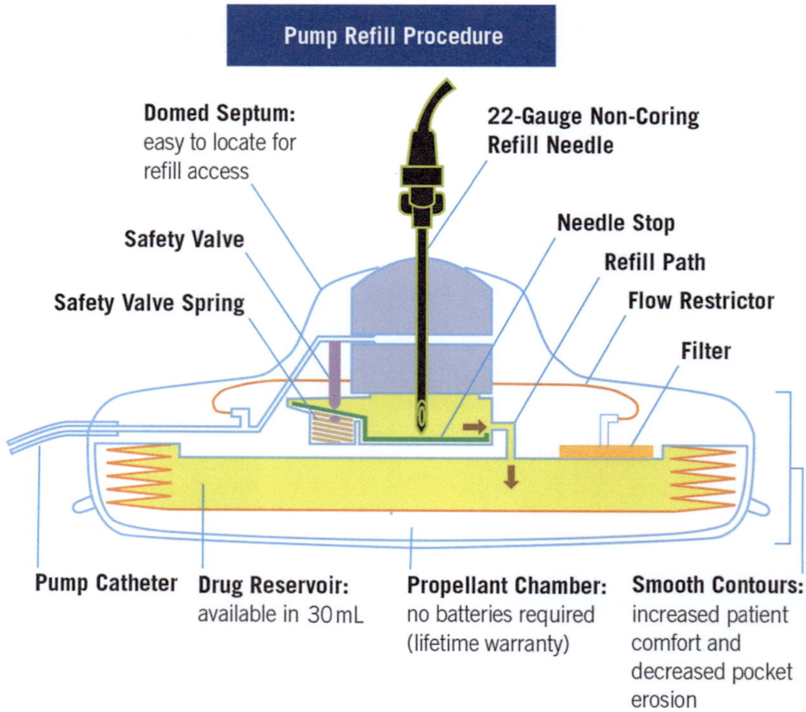

Fig. 3.8 Cross-sectional schematic of Intera 3000 showing core components and pump refill procedure. (© Intera Oncology. Used with permission)

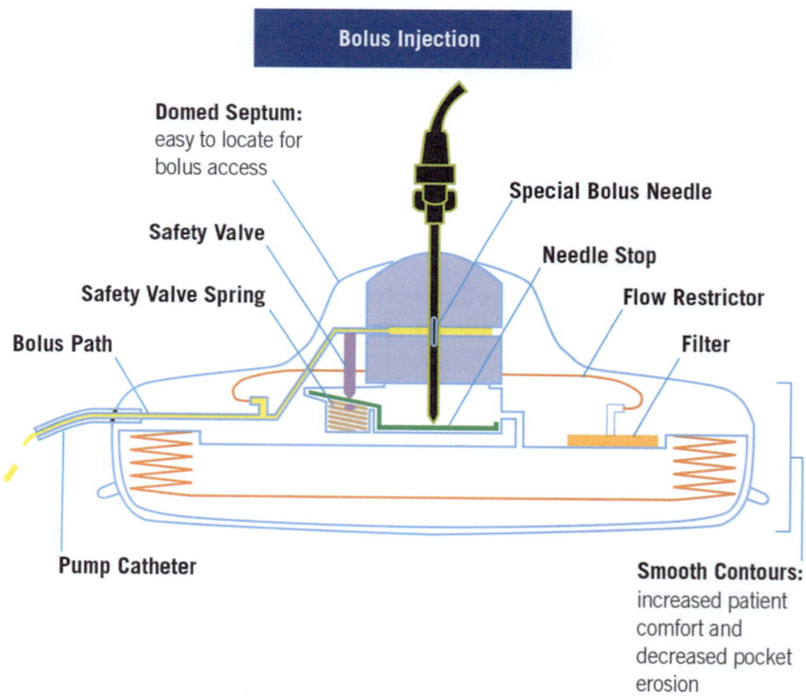

Fig. 3.9 Cross-sectional schematic of Intera 3000 showing core components with use of a special bolus needle. (© Intera Oncology. Used with permission)

As mentioned above, the non-programmable constant flow pumps do not have any mechanism to adjust the flow rate. Thus, the pump needs to be serviced (i.e., the reservoir needs to be refilled) either with drug or with heparinized saline, every 14 days, such that the reservoir does not completely empty. Drying of the pump leads to the absence of constant flow, causing the catheter to clot off, rendering the pump unusable. A workaround for this issue is to fill the pump with glycerin, which leads to an increased time interval of up to 8 weeks between pump refills due to glycerin's higher viscosity and therefore lower flow rate. The use of glycerin obviates the need for patients to be seen for pump refill every 2 weeks.

SynchroMed II Production of the Codman pump (the identical predecessor to the Intera pump) was permanently halted by J&J on April 1, 2018. Cerenovus, a subsidiary of J&J, which manufactured the pump, cited raw material shortage as the primary reason for device discontinuation [19]. Given that the Codman 3000 pump was the only FDA-approved pump for HAI, this situation led surgeons to use the Medtronic SynchroMed™ II pump in combination with Codman Tapered Silicone Rubber Catheter. The SynchroMed II pump is currently FDA-approved for intrathecal infusions only but was demonstrated to be safe when employed for HAI by a small pilot study from MSKCC. This pump differs drastically from the Intera 3000 pump in design. As mentioned above, the non-programmable constant flow pumps do not have any mechanism to adjust the flow rate, but flow can be adjusted with an electronic programmable pump (increasing or decreasing the duration over which the pump empties, and thus customizing the frequency with which pump needs to be serviced). The SynchroMed II pump pairs via Bluetooth with a touchscreen tablet that allows clinicians to set appropriate doses for their individual patients. The programming device features automated calculations of volume and flow rates to help ensure appropriate dosing. In addition to infusion rates, dosages, and volumes, the device can be programmed to provide bolus dosing if desired. The SynchroMed II pump itself is offered with either a 20 mL or a 40 mL reservoir. Unlike constant flow pumps such as the Intera 3000 pump, the flow rate of infusate delivered by the SynchroMed II pump is governed by a battery powered peristaltic pump. The peristaltic pump draws the infusate from the reservoir, through the indwelling catheter into the infusion site. Battery life is variable, ranging from 4 to 7 years, depending on the power requirement of a patient's individualized treatment plan. The SynchroMed II pump also features a catheter access port which allows for direct injections into the indwelling catheter for therapeutic or diagnostic purposes.

References

1. Klopp CT, Alford TC, Bateman J, Berry GN, Winship T. Fractionated intra-arterial cancer; chemotherapy with methyl bis amine hydrochloride; a preliminary report. Ann Surg. 1950;132(4):811–32.
2. Miller TR, Griman OR. Hepatic artery catheterization for liver perfusion. Arch Surg. 1961;82:423–5.
3. Sullivan RD, Norcross JW, Watkins E Jr. Chemotherapy of metastatic liver cancer by prolonged hepatic-artery infusion. N Engl J Med. 1964;270:321–7.
4. Sullivan RD, Miller E, Sikes MP. Antimetabolite-metabolite combination cancer chemotherapy. Effects of intraarterial methotrexate-intramuscular Citrovorum factor therapy in human cancer. Cancer. 1959;12:1248–62.
5. Wirtanen GW, Bernhardt LC, Mackman S, Ramirez G, Curreri AR, Ansfield FJ. Hepatic artery and celiac axis infusion for the treatment of upper abdominal malignant lesions. Ann Surg. 1968;168(1):137–41.
6. Clarkson B, Young C, Dierick W, Kuehn P, Kim M, Berrett A, et al. Effects of continuous hepatic artery infusion of antimetabolites on primary and metastatic cancer of the liver. Cancer. 1962;15:472–88.
7. Watkins E Jr. Chronometric infusor—an apparatus for protracted ambulatory infusion therapy. N Engl J Med. 1963;269:850–1.
8. Blackshear PJ, Dorman FD, Blackshear PL Jr, Varco RL, Buchwald H. A permanently implantable self-recycling low flow constant rate multipurpose infusion pump of simple design. Surg Forum. 1970;21:136–7.
9. Blackshear PJ, Dorman FD, Blackshear PL Jr, Varco RL, Buchwald H. The design and initial testing of an implantable infusion pump. Surg Gynecol Obstet. 1972;134(1):51–6.
10. Buchwald H, Grage TB, Vassilopoulos PP, Rohde TD, Varco RL, Blackshear PJ. Intraarterial infusion chemotherapy for hepatic carcinoma using a totally implantable infusion pump. Cancer. 1980;45(5):866–9.
11. Balch CM, Urist MM, McGregor ML. Continuous regional chemotherapy for metastatic colorectal cancer using a totally implantable infusion pump. A feasibility study in 50 patients. Am J Surg. 1983;145(2):285–90.

12. Blackshear PJ, Rohde TD, Varco RL, Buchwald H. One year of continuous heparinization in the dog using a totally implantable infusion pump. Surg Gynecol Obstet. 1975;141(2):176–86.
13. Johnston J, Reich S, Bailey A, Sluetz J. Shiley INFUSAID pump technology. Ann N Y Acad Sci. 1988;531:57–65.
14. Barone RM, Byfield JE, Goldfarb PB, Frankel S, Ginn C, Greer S. Intra-arterial chemotherapy using an implantable infusion pump and liver irradiation for the treatment of hepatic metastases. Cancer. 1982;50(5):850–62.
15. Niederhuber JE, Ensminger W, Gyves J, Thrall J, Walker S, Cozzi E. Regional chemotherapy of colorectal cancer metastatic to the liver. Cancer. 1984;53(6):1336–43.
16. Rothmund M, Brückner R, Keller E, Quint B, Knuth A, Schicketanz KH. Regional chemotherapy of liver metastases of colorectal carcinoma using implanted gas pressure pumps. Results of a prospective phase II study. Dtsch Med Wochenschr. 1986;111(17):652–8.
17. Shepard KV, Levin B, Karl RC, Faintuch J, DuBrow RA, Hagle M, et al. Therapy for metastatic colorectal cancer with hepatic artery infusion chemotherapy using a subcutaneous implanted pump. J Clin Oncol. 1985;3(2):161–9.
18. Oliver GC, Shorb PE Jr. The totally implantable infusion pump in treatment of metastatic colorectal cancer. Dis Colon Rectum. 1985;28(1):18–23.
19. Denise Grady SK. A lifesaving pump for cancer patients is being phased out. New York Times. 2018. Accessed 25 Apr 2018.

4 Optimization of Therapy: Drug Development, Pharmacokinetics, and Pharmacodynamics

Fidel David Huitzil-Meléndez,
Monica Isabel Meneses-Medina,
Emilio Conde-Flores, and Vanessa Rosas-Camargo

The conceptual advantage of regional over systemic delivery of therapeutic agents is critically dependent on pharmacologic properties and emphasizes the need for a comprehensive understanding of the principles of optimal drug selection. These concepts are important for the development of a successful hepatic artery infusion (HAI) program. If a drug does not exhibit pharmacokinetics and pharmacodynamics that provide a regional delivery advantage, the expected tumor response would be virtually identical to that of drugs administered via simple intravenous delivery. Interestingly, these principles have not always been considered, jeopardizing the results of historic and even contemporary clinical trials. For proper interpretation of HAI literature and clinical trials evaluating the merits of HAI chemotherapy, only trials that used drugs with a known advantage for regional delivery should be considered [1].

Successful liver-directed therapy relies on several assumptions that must be fulfilled to expect an advantage. In brief, the model assumes (1) higher doses of certain drugs are expected to result in higher responses, (2) higher doses result in higher toxicity, (3) regional delivery results in improved therapeutic index by achieving higher local concentrations and decreased systemic toxicity [2]. Candidate drugs for hepatic artery administration should be evaluated as follows:

1. Is the HAI drug candidate expected to achieve a greater response by increasing the dose and concentration?

   The determinant pharmacological parameter is the dose-response curve of a given agent (Fig. 4.1). Only chemotherapy agents that exhibit a steep dose-response curve, where a higher dose results in better tumor response through higher concentration of the drug are good candidates. Chemotherapy agents are therefore ideal HAI drug candidates [2]. On the contrary, therapeutic antibodies do not exhibit a steep dose-response curve. Systemic administration achieves serum levels usually above the therapeutic level, although higher doses do not increase the efficacy or toxicity. Higher doses of antibodies only result in prolonged dosing interval for convenient administration. Therefore, therapeutic antibodies are not ideal HAI drug candidates [3, 4].

2. Is the HAI drug candidate's dose associated with systemic toxicity?

   The typical characteristics of chemotherapy agents are that higher doses result both in higher tumor response and increased

F. D. Huitzil-Meléndez (✉) · M. I. Meneses-Medina
V. Rosas-Camargo
Departamento de Hematología y Oncología, Instituto Nacional de Ciencias Médicas y Nutrición Salvador Zubirán, Ciudad de México, México

E. Conde-Flores
Centro Oncológico Diana Laura Riojas de Colosio, Medica Sur, Ciudad de México, México

M. D'Angelica, M. Lidsky (eds.), *Hepatic Arterial Infusion for Malignancy*,
https://doi.org/10.1007/978-3-031-74935-3_4

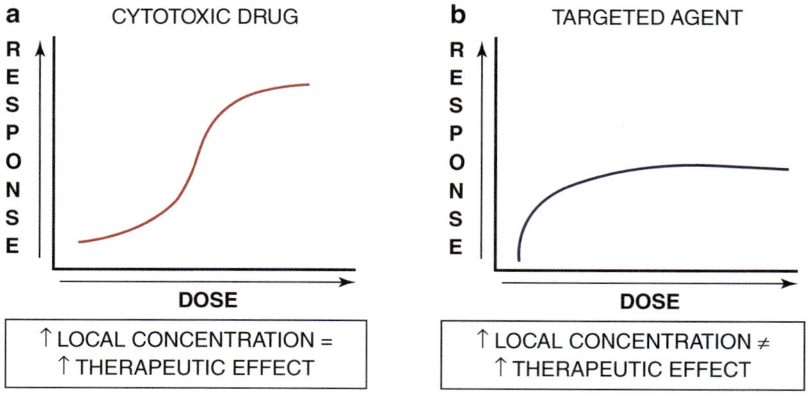

Fig. 4.1 Dose-response curves for cytotoxic and targeted therapies. (**a**) Cytotoxic drugs exhibit a steep dose-response curve. By increasing local concentrations of the drug, an advantage in therapeutic effect can be obtained by regional delivery. (**b**) Targeted drugs do not exhibit steep dose-response curve, therefore no advantages in therapeutic effect can be expected by regional delivery. (Created with BioRender)

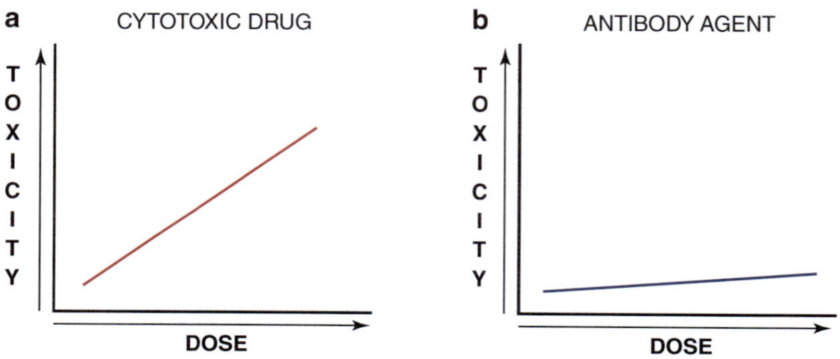

Fig. 4.2 Dose-toxicity curves for cytotoxic and targeted therapies. (**a**) Dose-toxicity curve for cytotoxic chemotherapy agents. Higher toxicity is expected from higher dose. Regional delivery represents an advantage if increased local concentration can be achieved without increased systemic concentration and toxicity. (**b**) Dose-toxicity curve for therapeutic antibodies. High concentrations do not result in increased toxicity. No advantage can be expected from regional delivery to limit systemic exposure. (Created with BioRender)

toxicity (Fig. 4.2). Regional delivery to increase local drug concentration without increased systemic toxicity may improve the therapeutic index. Therefore, chemotherapy agents are suitable HAI drug candidates with regard to this principle. Some drugs, however, do not result in increased systemic toxicity even at supratherapeutic doses, in which case there is no need to attempt increased local concentration of the drug by means of regional delivery. Specifically, therapeutic antibodies do not result in increased systemic toxicity when administered at higher doses. Phase I clinical trials usually fail to define a dose-limiting toxicity and maximal tolerated dose with intravenous antibody administration. Therefore, therapeutic antibodies are not ideal HAI drug candidates to improve the therapeutic index as systemic toxicity is not a dose-limiting factor [3].

3. Do the HAI drug candidate's pharmacokinetic parameters predict an advantage for regional drug delivery over systemic administration?

The Collins formula [2] summarizes the determinants of an advantage of regional drug delivery over systemic administration.

$$\text{Advantage} = 1 + \frac{\text{Total body clearance of the drug}}{\left(\text{HA flow rate}\left[1 - \text{fraction of drug extracted across liver}\right]\right)}$$

Within the liver model of regional drug delivery, the hepatic artery flow rate becomes a constant. Therefore, the advantage is determined by clearance and hepatic extraction of the drug. From the formula, it is deduced that higher total body clearance and higher hepatic extraction directly correlate with the regional delivery advantage. Drug clearance is defined as the volume of blood cleared of drug per unit of time (e.g., mL/min) and describes the efficiency of elimination of a drug from the body. The total body clearance of a drug is an independent pharmacokinetic parameter. It does not depend on the volume of distribution, half-life, or bioavailability and is constant for a particular drug in a specific patient. As noted, regarding total body clearance, floxuridine ranks at the top among candidate HAI drugs [5].

The second determinant of HAI advantage is the hepatic extraction rate of the drug, meaning the extent of metabolism or elimination of the drug during first-pass. Hepatic extraction is responsible for decreased systemic exposure despite increased local concentration of the drug (Fig. 4.3) [6].

$$\text{Hepatic extraction ratio} = \frac{\text{Hepatic arterial level} - \text{Hepatic venous level}}{\text{Hepatic arterial level}}$$

Interestingly, the hepatic extraction ratio has been directly measured for only a small number of agents (Table 4.1). The experimental design proposed by Ensminger in 1978 should be reproduced to systematically determine hepatic extraction after hepatic arterial infusion of drug candidates (Fig. 4.4). Floxuridine, the cornerstone of HAI therapy, has a very high hepatic extraction ratio.

4. Does the HAI drug candidate maintain advantageous pharmacokinetic parameters when administered at high doses (first-order kinetics)?

For drugs that exhibit first-order kinetics, a constant fraction of drug dose remaining in the body is eliminated per unit of time (Fig. 4.5). The rate constant for the elimination phase (KE) can be calculated for any drug. However, if a drug is given in a dose large enough to exceed the capacity of enzyme systems to eliminate a *constant proportion* of the drug, the result is that a *constant amount* per unit of time is eliminated rather than a constant fraction (zero-order kinetics).

The advantage of regional therapy remains only as long as the dose rate used does not saturate either total body clearance (CLTB) or hepatic extraction. Drugs that exhibit nonlinear pharmacokinetics will yield decreased CLTB and decreased hepatic extraction at higher doses, potentially compromising HAI advantage. FUDR exhibits first-order kinetics [7].

In summary, the pharmacological profile of the ideal drug candidate for HAI requires a steep dose-response curve, high total body clearance, high hepatic extraction ratio after hepatic artery administration and first-order kinetics (Fig. 4.6). The pharmacologically predicted advantage based on Collins formula is greatest for floxuridine. In addition to pharmacokinetic advantage, effective regional drug delivery requires other drug properties to be considered, such as stability at body temperature, high solubility to be infused in small volumes and compatibility with titanium, stainless steel, silicone rubber and polyurethane if the drug is to be administered via an implantable pump [7].

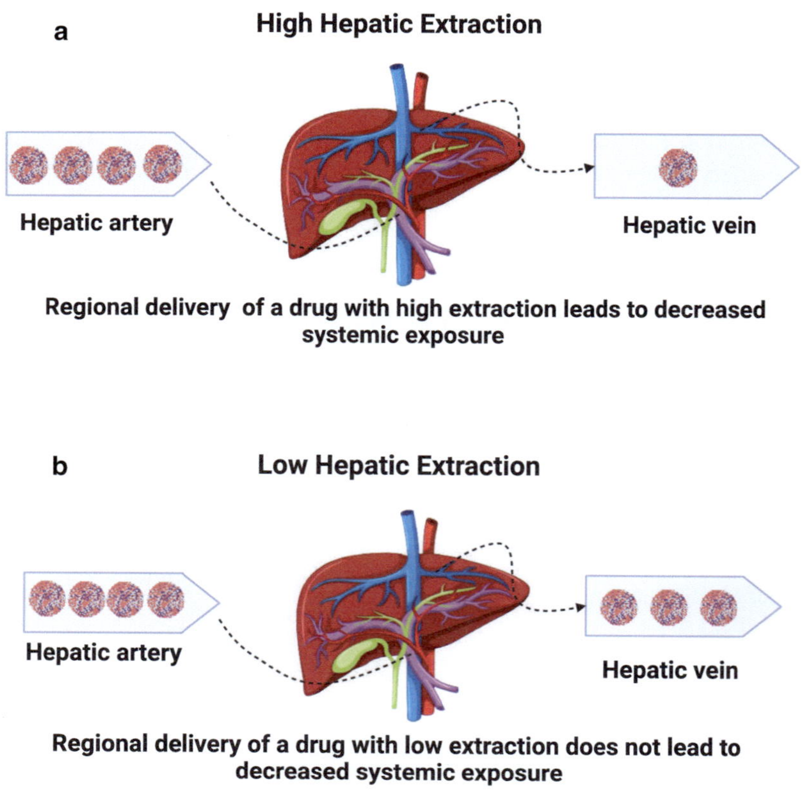

Fig. 4.3 Hepatic extraction and systemic exposure of different drugs. In the HAI model, decreased systemic exposure to an active agent depends on the hepatic extraction ratio for that particular drug. (**a**) Drugs with high hepatic extraction will result in decreased systemic exposure and potentially less systemic toxicity. If hepatic extraction exhibits linear pharmacokinetics, and the effect is dose dependent, the dose can be increased to achieve a combined benefit of increased efficacy and decreased systemic exposure. (**b**) Drugs with low hepatic extraction will not result in decreased systemic exposure. If the drug exhibits nonlinear pharmacokinetics when administered at high doses, the advantage of decreased systemic exposure may decrease as the dose is escalated. (Created with BioRender)

Table 4.1 Half-life and hepatic exposure of agents investigated for trans-arterial delivery

Drug	Half-life (min)	Estimated increased hepatic exposure with HAI[a]
5FU	<10	5- to 10-fold
FUDR[b]	<10	100- to 400-fold
Carmustine	<5	6- to 7-fold
Mitomycin-C	<10	6- to 8-fold
Cisplatin	20–30	4- to 7-fold
Doxorubicin	60	2-fold

[a]Based on hepatic extraction, total body drug clearance, and hepatic artery blood flow
[b]99% Hepatic clearance

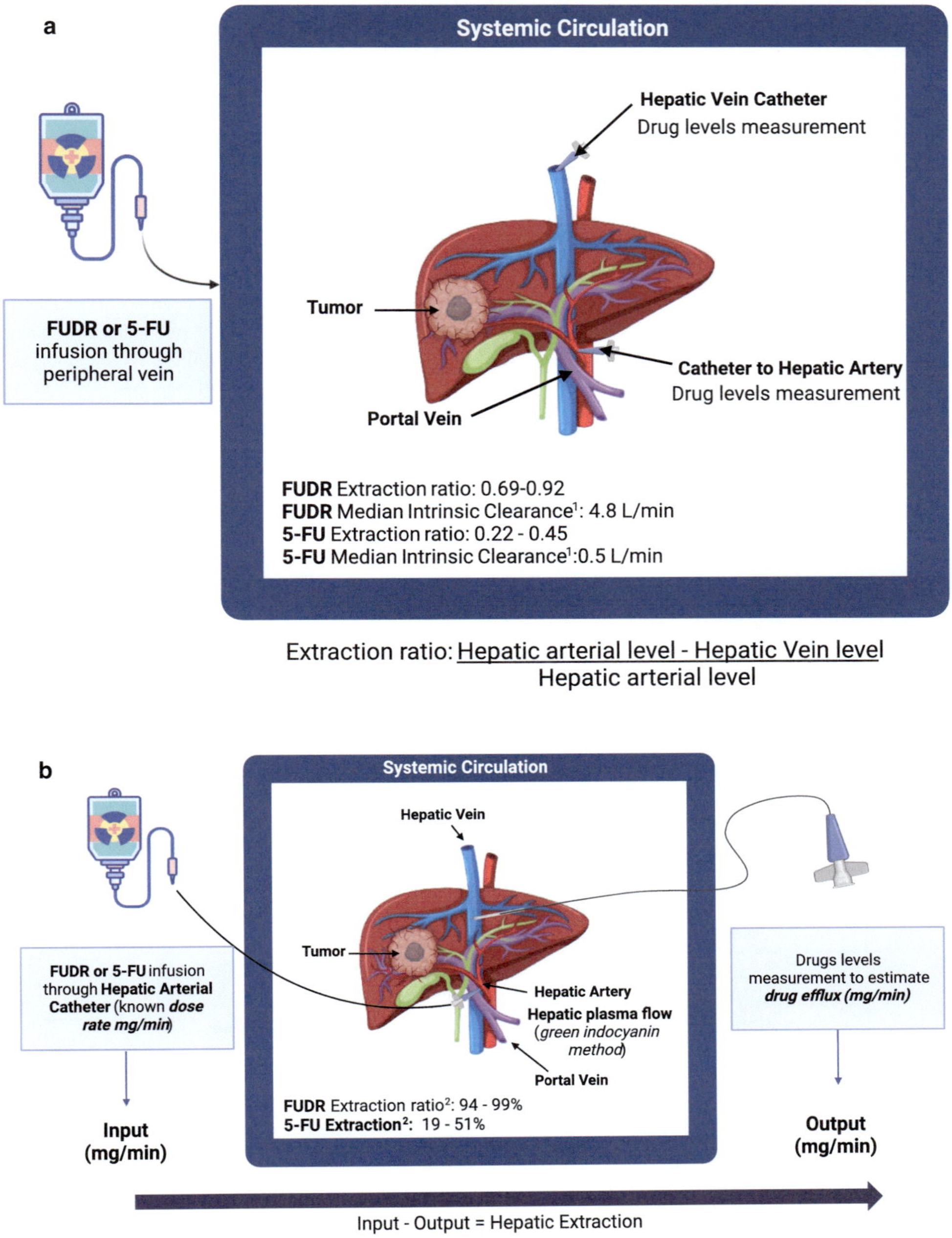

Fig. 4.4 Schematic for studying extraction ratio, intrinsic clearance, and hepatic extraction of drugs by route of administration. (**a**) Administration via peripheral vein: After FUDR or 5FU systemic infusion, drug levels were measured through catheters placed at the hepatic vein and hepatic artery to calculate the extraction ratio and intrinsic clearance. FUDR exhibits both a high extraction ratio and high intrinsic clearance, while 5FU exhibits a lower extraction ratio and lower intrinsic clearance. (**b**) Administration via hepatic artery: After FUDR or 5FU infusion through a hepatic arterial catheter, hepatic vein drug levels were measured to calculate hepatic extraction. Known dose rate (mg/min), estimated hepatic plasma flow and measured drug concentrations at hepatic vein are required to estimate hepatic drug extraction. FUDR exhibits high hepatic drug extraction, while 5FU exhibits lower hepatic drug extraction. (Created with BioRender). *Legends:* [1]Intrinsic clearance is a measurement of the maximal ability of the liver to remove drug in the absence of any flow limitations. [2]Drug efflux was determined as the product of the estimated hepatic blood flow and hepatic vein drug concentration. Hepatic drug extraction was calculated as the difference between the drug infused into the hepatic arterial catheter and the total drug effluent measured by hepatic vein sampling

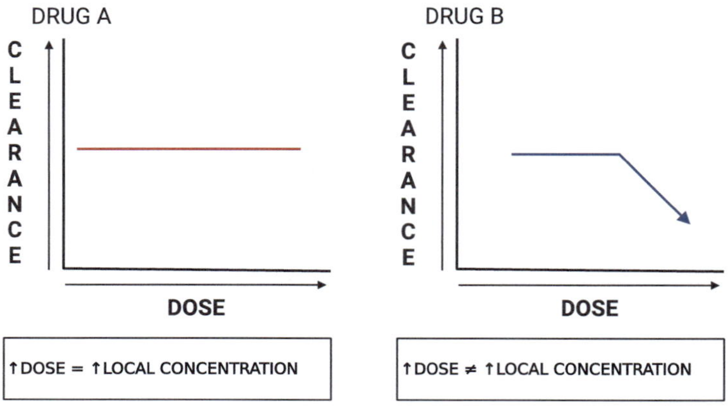

Fig. 4.5 Drug clearance is dependent on drug pharmacokinetics. Drug A shows first-order kinetics, with constant clearance despite the dose, which can result in increased local concentrations compared with systemic concentration. Drug B shows zero-order kinetics, where clearance decreases after a certain dose level, which will not result in increased local concentrations if the dose is administered at higher doses, limiting the potential advantage of increased dose with HAI delivery. (Created with BioRender)

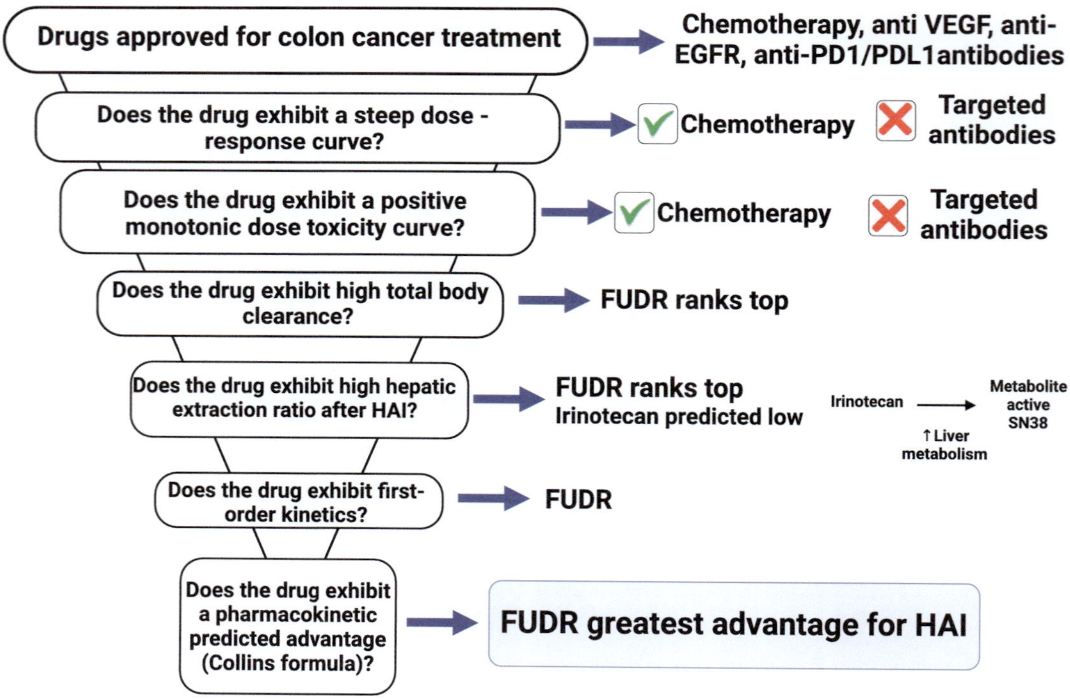

Fig. 4.6 Proposed checklist to evaluate drug candidates for HAI. (Created with BioRender)

Clinical Development of HAI

FUDR

Research led by Dr. Nancy Kemeny at Memorial Sloan-Kettering Cancer Center refined FUDR HAI therapy for colon cancer liver metastasis through the years. The pillars of the program were (1) the use of implantable pumps, (2) 14-day continuous infusion of FUDR followed by a 2–3 week period of rest [8], (3) Concurrent administration of dexamethasone to decrease the risk of biliary toxicity, and (4) combination with the ever-evolving standard of care systemic chemotherapy [9].

As an S-phase-specific cytotoxic agent, FUDR continuous infusion maximizes efficacy of the drug. Dosing of FUDR was optimized for pump infusion taking into consideration the pump flow rate. This consideration is important as commercially available implantable pumps vary in volume capacity (20–30 mL) and flow rate (provided by the manufacturer, usually around 1.2 mL/day). The flow rate may be affected by changes in altitude and/or temperature and must be confirmed for every patient. At the time of pump placement, the reservoir is filled with saline solution and heparin (1000 IU/mL). The flow rate is thereafter estimated by subtracting the residual volume from the starting volume divided by the number of days.

$$\text{Flow rate determination}: \frac{\text{pump volume day 1} - \text{pump volume on refill day}}{\text{number of days of continuous infusion}}$$

Example 1: (reservoir 30 mL for Intera Oncology implantable pump)

$$\text{Pump flow rate}: \frac{30\,\text{mL}\left(\text{initial volume}\right) - 13.2\,\text{mL}\left(\text{residual volume}\right)}{\text{After }14-\text{day infusion}}$$

$$\text{Pump flow rate} = 16.8/14 = 1.2\,\text{mL}/\text{day}.$$

Example 2: (reservoir 20 mL for an alternative implantable pump)

$$\text{Pump flow rate}: \frac{20\,\text{mL}\left(\text{initial volume}\right) - 13\,\text{mL}\left(\text{residual volume}\right)}{\text{After }7-\text{day infusion}}$$

$$\text{Pump flow rate} = 7/7 = 1\,\text{mL}/\text{day}.$$

The Medtronic® pump is programmable and the flow rate is constant. If a programmable pump is used, we recommend that the flow rate be set to 1 mL/day.

FUDR dosing regimens have evolved over time, including imputation of flow rate and the addition of dexamethasone to mitigate the risk of biliary sclerosis [8]. It is important to note that initial trials used FUDR doses that exceed those currently used, and systemic regimens that are now considered to be suboptimal (Table 4.2).

Table 4.2 Summary of clinical trials of combination systemic chemotherapy with FUDR hepatic arterial infusion: recommended dose for phase 3 trials

Reference	Study	Systemic regimen	Doses studied	Recommended dose	Comments
Unresectable liver metastases from colorectal cancer					
Kemeny, 2005 [11]	Phase I	Oxaliplatin/irinotecan	Oxaliplatin dose levels: 85, 100, 130 mg/m^2 **MTD 100 mg/m^2** Irinotecan dose levels: 150, 200 mg/m^2 **MTD 150 mg/m^2**	Oxaliplatin 100 mg/m^2 IV and irinotecan 150 mg/m^2 IV on day 1 and 15 of each cycle Concurrent HAI FUDR	Preferred regimen for first-line treatment or limited oxaliplatin exposure (<2 months) Previous chemotherapy: 81% Bilirubin elevation >3 mg/dL in 5% Response rate 90% Median survival 35.8 months
Kemeny, 2005 [11]	Phase I	5FU/folinic acid/ oxaliplatin	Oxaliplatin dose level: 100 mg/m^2 Folinic acid dose level: 400 mg/m^2 5FU dose levels: 1000, 1200, 1400, 1600 mg/m^2 48-h infusion **MTD 1400 mg/m^2**	Oxaliplatin 100 mg/m^2 IV Folinic acid 400 mg/m^2 IV 5FU 1400 mg/m^2 IV On day 1 and 15 of each 28-day cycle Concurrent HAI FUDR	DLT was diarrhea. 5FU systemic exposure is low compared to standard systemic regimens Previous chemotherapy 100% Bilirubin elevation >3 mg/dL in 7% Response rate 87% Median survival 22 months
Kemeny, 2001 [12]	Phase I	Weekly irinotecan	Irinotecan dose levels: 60, 80, 100, 125 mg/m^2 weekly × 3 **MTD 100 mg/m^2** FUDR dose levels: 0.12, 0.14, 0.16 mg/kg/d × 30 mL/flow rate **MTD 0.16 mg/kg/d × 30 mL/flow rate**	Irinotecan 100 mg/m^2 IV weekly for 3 weeks every 28 days Concurrent HAI FUDR	Early regimen, currently every 2-week regimen favored Bilirubin elevation >3 mg/dL in 4% Previous chemotherapy: 97% Response rate 74% Median survival 17 months
D'Angelica, 2015 [13]	Phase II	Oxaliplatin/Irinotecan or Irinotecan/folinic acid/5FU (for oxaliplatin pretreated patients) *Bevacizumab	Oxaliplatin 85 mg/m^2, irinotecan 125 mg/m^2 or Irinotecan 150 mg/m^2, folinic acid 400 mg/m^2, 5FU 2000 mg/m^2 48 h infusion On day 1 and 15 of a 4-week cycle Concurrent HAI FUDR	Chemotherapy-naïve: oxaliplatin 85 mg/m^2 IV or irinotecan 125 mg/m^2 IV on day 1 and 15 of each 28-day cycle Pretreated patients (>2 months of oxaliplatin): Irinotecan 150 mg/m^2 IV, Folinic acid 400 mg/m^2 IV, 5FU 2000 mg/m^2 48 h infusion IV on day 1 and 15 of each 28-day cycle Concurrent HAI FUDR Bevacizumab is not recommended	*Bevacizumab increases biliary toxicity and is not recommended Grade 3–4 bilirubin elevation: 12% (bevacizumab) vs, 4% (non-bevacizumab) Median number tumors: 14 Pretreated patients: 65% Response rate chemotherapy-naïve: 82% Response rate pretreated: 72% Resection rate: 47% 3-year survival (chemo-naïve): 75% 3-year survival (pretreated): 44%

Adjuvant treatment after resection of liver metastases from colorectal cancer					
Kemeny, 1999	Phase III	5FU/folinic acid	Folinic acid 200 mg/m^2, 5FU 325 mg/m^2 daily for 5 days On day 15: 0.25 mg of floxuridine per kilogram of body weight per day for 14 days in combination with 20 mg of dexamethasone, 50,000 U of heparin, and enough normal saline to result in a volume of 50 mL	If single agent 5FU clinically appropriate, updated infusional 5FU regimen is recommended: FUDR 0.12 mg/kg × pump volume (30 mL)/pump flow rate + dexamethasone 25 mg flat dose for a 30 mL pump volume on day 1–14 On day 15 and 29 Folinic acid 400 mg/m^2 5FU 2000 mg/m^2 48-h infusion Six 5-week adjuvant cycles	Note that pump volume was 50 mL in this trial FUDR dose was not adjusted by pump flow rate Dose was higher than currently recommended (FUDR dose 0.25 mg × kg × 14 days) Dexamethasone dose was low Systemic 5FU regimen outdated 18% of patients developed increased bilirubin >3 mg/dL 2-year survival was 86% 2-year hepatic recurrence-free survival was 90% 2-year progression-free survival was 57% 10-year survival was 41%
Kemeny N, 2003 [14]	Phase I/II	Irinotecan	Irinotecan 60, 80, 100 mg/m^2 weekly × 3, 1 week off MTD irinotecan 100 mg/m^2 On day 1 FUDR, 0.12 mg/kg; dexamethasone 1.0 mg × pump volume; 35,000 units of heparin; and normal saline in a quantity sufficient to fill the pump reservoir On day 14 residual volume removed from the pump and heparinized saline instilled. When the maximum tolerated dose of weekly irinotecan was reached, the FUDR dose was escalated to 0.14 mg/kg 4-week cycles **MTD FUDR 0.12 mg/kg** Irinotecan 150, 200, 225, 250 mg/m^2 every other week concurrent with HAI FUDR at 0.12 mg/kg MTD 200 mg/m^2	Irinotecan 200 mg/m^2 IV every other week FUDR 0.12 mg/kg × pump volume/pump flow rate Dexamethasone 1 mg × pump volume/pump flow rate and heparin plus saline for 14 days of a 28-day cycle	Lacks systemic 5FU Relies on potential value of irinotecan to decrease local and systemic recurrence although this has not been determined in adjuvant systemic trials 7% of patients developed increased bilirubin >3 mg/dL 2-year survival rate is 89% Hepatic disease-free survival at 18 months is 88% Disease-free survival at 18 months is 47%

(continued)

Table 4.2 (continued)

Reference	Study	Systemic regimen	Doses studied	Recommended dose	Comments
Kemeny N, 2009 [15]	Phase I	5FU/folinic acid/ oxaliplatin	Oxaliplatin 85, 100 mg/m^2 **MTD oxaliplatin 100 mg/m^2** Folinic acid 400 mg/m^2 5FU 1000, 1200, 1400, 1600, 1800, 2000 mg/m^2 48-h continuous infusion **MTD 5FU 1600 mg/m^2** on day 15 and 29 of a 5-week cycle On day 1, FUDR 0.12 mg/kg/d × 30 mL/ flow rate 6 cycles scheduled	Oxaliplatin 85 mg/m^2, folinic acid 400 mg/m^2, 5FU 2000 mg/m^2 on day 15 and 29 of a 5-week cycle Concurrent HAI FUDR on day 1, FUDR 0.12 mg/kg/d × 30 mL/flow rate On day 15 pump emptied and filled with heparin and saline 6 adjuvant cycles recommended	FUDR dose considered pump flow rate and adjustment for overweight patients 8.5% had bilirubin elevation 4-year survival is 88% 4-year hepatic-progression-free survival is 86% 4-year progression-free survival is 50%
Kemeny N, 2011 [16]	Randomized phase II	5FU/folinic acid/ oxaliplatin 5FU/ folinic acid/irinotecan (oxaliplatin pretreated patients) +/− bevacizumab	Oxaliplatin 85 mg/m^2, folinic acid 400 mg/m^2, fluorouracil 2000 mg/m^2 infusion for 2 days irinotecan 150 mg/m^2 was used) or Irinotecan 150 mg/m^2, folinic acid 400 mg/m^2, fluorouracil 2000 mg/m^2 infusion for 2 days +/−Bevacizumab 5 mg/kg On day 15 and 29 of a 5-week cycle concurrent with HAI FUDR On day 1, fluorodeoxyuridine 0.12 mg/ kg × pump volume (30 mL) divided by pump flow rate Dexamethasone 1.0 mg × kg × pump volume (30 mL) divided by pump flow rate with 30,000 units of unfractionated heparin and normal saline in a quantity sufficient to fill the pump reservoir to 30 mL. On days 15 and 29 of each cycle, the residual was removed from the pump and the pump was refilled with heparin and saline 30 mL	Combination with systemic bevacizumab is not recommended	FUDR dose was adjusted for overweight patients FUDR dose adjusted to pump flow rate 14% of bevacizumab treated patients developed >3 mg/dl bilirubin elevations vs. 0% of non-bevacizumab patients 1-year recurrence free survival was 83 vs, 71% ($p = 0.15$) 4-year survival is 85% vs, 81% ($p = 0.5$)—Non-bevacizumab vs. bevacizumab, respectively

Kemeny N, 2021 [17]	Randomized phase II	FOLFIRI +/− Panitumumab	Irinotecan 125–150 mg/m^2 Folinic acid 400 mg/m^2 5FU 2000 mg/m^2 48-h infusion Panitumumab 6 mg/kg On day 15 and 29 of a 5-week cycle, 6 cycles scheduled	FUDR 0.12 mg/kg × pump volume (30 mL)/pump flow rate + dexamethasone 25 mg flat dose for a 30 mL pump volume on day 1–14 on day 15 and 29 Irinotecan 125–150 mg/m^2 Folinic acid 400 mg/m^2 5FU 2000 mg/m^2 48-h infusion Panitumumab 6 mg/kg 6 adjuvant cycles recommended	Regimen suitable for RAS wild-type patients FUDR dose was adjusted for overweight patients FUDR dose (0.12 mg/kg) adjusted to pump flow rate 3-year recurrence-free survival was 57% vs. 42% 3-year overall survival was 97% vs. 91%

FUDR + Standard of Care Systemic Therapy

At the time when single agent 5FU + folinic acid represented standard of care for advanced colon cancer, CALGB 9481 study randomized colon cancer patients with unresectable liver metastasis and no extrahepatic disease to systemic 5FU or HAI FUDR without systemic. The trial did not allow crossover and was able to demonstrate improved survival and quality of life for HAI FUDR treated patients [10]. Interestingly, this trial demonstrated that: (1) FUDR lacks both systemic activity and toxicity and (2) better regional control improves survival despite suboptimal extrahepatic control associated with HAI. Nonetheless, suboptimal extrahepatic control could be addressed by concurrent administration of systemic therapy, given nonoverlapping toxicities between systemic and regional delivery of chemotherapy. Therefore, all subsequent HAI research has focused on development of combination strategies to improve outcomes, though some clinical circumstances may exist where HAI FUDR without systemic treatment may be appropriate, including elderly patients with limited tolerance to chronic systemic chemotherapy and/or heavily pretreated patients who have demonstrated hepatic only disease and/or have developed significant toxicity from systemic therapy.

Phase I and phase II clinical trials have been conducted to evaluate the safety of combining HAI FUDR with systemic 5FU, oxaliplatin, irinotecan and panitumumab, both for unresectable colon cancer liver metastases and as adjuvant treatment after liver resection (Table 4.2). Data for treatment of primary liver cancer, in particular intrahepatic cholangiocarcinoma are also available. Below, data from these trials will be reviewed, though different FUDR doses were explored in these reference trials (see Chap. 11 for full FUDR dosing details). Table 4.2 summarizes clinical trials with emphasis on maximal tolerated dose (MTD) and recommended dose of systemic agents for further development. The maximal tolerated dose (MTD) is conceptually the highest dose that most patients can tolerate, usually producing grade 3 or greater toxicity in less than 33% of patients. As phase II trials have already been conducted in some clinical scenarios, a recommended dose for phase III trials is provided.

The most active concurrent systemic chemotherapy regimen for unresectable liver metastasis combines irinotecan and oxaliplatin with HAI FUDR in the first-line setting. The primary objective of this regimen is response rate and secondary resection rate. The prospective phase 2 trial conducted at MSKCC included 49 patients with unresectable liver metastasis from CRC [13]. Chemotherapy-naïve patients received systemic oxaliplatin (85 mg/m^2) and irinotecan (125 mg/m^2) every 2 weeks with HAI FUDR for 14 days of every 28 day cycle and achieved a response rate of 82%. For oxaliplatin pretreated patients, systemic 5FU (2000 mg/m^2 48 hr. infusion), folinic acid (400 mg/m^2) and irinotecan (150 mg/m^2) every 2 weeks with HAI FUDR was administered and achieved 72% response rate. Bevacizumab was part of systemic treatment for the first 24 patients, but resulted in increased biliary toxicity and was removed. Conversion to resection was 47% and median overall survival was 38 months. After an expansion cohort was included, outcomes on 64 patients were updated: conversion to resection was 52%, median progression-free survival was 13 months and median overall survival was 38 months and 5-year overall survival was 36%. Of note, for chemotherapy-naïve patients 5-year overall survival was 51%. Grade 3–4 diarrhea occurred in 13% of patients and neutropenia in 2%. A biliary stent was required for 13% treated with bevacizumab and 2.5% patients treated without. This systemic toxicity profile compares favorably to systemic triplet regimens.

Current systemic standard of care for advanced colon cancer includes the addition of anti-VEGF or anti-EGFR antibodies to duplet or triplet chemotherapy regimens. However, more complex systemic regimens have failed to provide advantage: modified FOLFOXIRI panitumumab was not better than FOLFOX with panitumumab in the phase III TRIPLETE study [18]. The trial randomized 435 RAS and BRAF wild-type advanced colorectal cancer patients to be treated in the first-line setting. No improvement in response rate, R0 resection rate, progression-free survival or overall survival was observed. The CAIRO5 study aimed to determine the optimal induction systemic regimen for patients with unresectable colorectal cancer liver metastases [19, 20]. Primary tumor sidedness and RAS and BRAF status were considered. Patients with right-sided primary tumor site or RAS or BRAF mutated tumors were randomly assigned (1:1) to receive FOLFOX or FOLFIRI plus bevacizumab (group A) or FOLFOXIRI plus bevacizumab (group B). Patients with left-sided and *RAS* and *BRAF*V600E wild-type tumors were randomly assigned (1:1) to receive FOLFOX or FOLFIRI plus bevacizumab (group C) or FOLFOX or FOLFIRI plus panitumumab (group D), every 14 days for up to 12 cycles. Primary endpoint was progression-free survival and group C and group D were prematurely closed for futility. Median progression-free survival was 9.0 months (95% CI 7.7–10.5) in group A versus 10.6 months (9.9–12.1) in group B (stratified hazard ratio [HR] 0.76 [95% CI 0.60–0.98]; $p = 0{\cdot}032$) at the expense of increased grade 3–4 toxicity: neutropenia (19 [13%] patients in group A vs. 57 [40%] in group B; $p < 0{\cdot}0001$) and diarrhea (five [3%] vs. 28 [19%]; $p < 0{\cdot}0001$). Response rate (33% vs. 54%, $p < 0.01$), R0/R1 resection or ablation rate (37% vs. 51%, $p = 0.01$) were increased but survival was not different at median follow-up of 58 months and 79% of events (23.6 months vs. 24.1 months, $p = 0.52$). Regarding group C and group D patients, panitumumab increased response rate but not resection rate when compared to bevacizumab.

As such, most active systemic chemotherapy regimens failed to provide a survival advantage for patients with liver metastases from colorectal cancer and the need for a better regimen is recognized. These negative results highlight the importance of ongoing phase III clinical trials testing the survival benefit of HAI FUDR plus systemic combination regimens in the unresectable disease setting.

For resectable disease, adjuvant HAI FUDR has shown a survival advantage [21, 22]. On the contrary, survival benefit from any systemic regimen remains to be proven [23–27]. Nonetheless, fluoropyrimidine-based chemotherapy either perioperative or adjuvantly after liver resection is recommended in guidelines. To fully combine systemic 5FU with HAI FUDR, 5-week chemotherapy cycles were developed. In this schedule, FUDR 14-day continuous infusion is followed by a 3-week HAI rest period. On day 15 and 28, patients receive systemic treatment. One week after the second dose of systemic chemotherapy, a new cycle begins with day 1 FUDR. In this way, concurrent systemic chemotherapy and FUDR is avoided, as first dose of systemic starts when the pump is emptied and second dose occurs on day 15 of the 3-week HAI rest period.

We have clinical trial data to safely combine HAI FUDR with different systemic regimens in the adjuvant setting. As is the case for unresectable disease, dosing has evolved through time and the currently recommended adjuvant FUDR dose is lower to minimize biliary toxicity and to safely combine with systemic regimens. After resection of colon primary or liver metastases, systemic regimens have focused on the efficacy of the combination of fluoropyrimidines and oxaliplatin. In contrast, HAI FUDR adjuvant regimens more frequently rely on the combination of systemic 5FU and irinotecan and more recently, with panitumumab for RAS wild-type patients. Contemporary phase III trials in the adjuvant setting may select as experimental treatment arm safe HAI FUDR combinations defined in MSKCC adjuvant trials [14–17].

In conclusion, when 5FU was the only approved systemic drug for colon cancer treatment, phase III randomized trials showed survival benefit from HAI FUDR in both unresectable colon cancer liver metastasis and adjuvant setting. The standard of care has evolved and updated phase III clinical trials are needed. In the

United States, a randomized phase III trial is now open as an ECOG-ACRIN cancer research group trial (NCT05863195). Patients with liver-only metastatic colorectal cancer that remain technically unresectable after 3–6 months of first-line chemotherapy will be randomized 2:1 to standard of care chemotherapy with or without HAI-FUDR. Stratification factors are RAS status and primary tumor sidedness. Primary end-point is overall survival, sample size is 408 patients and no cross-over is allowed. In the Netherlands, a phase III trial will randomize 224 patients with unresectable colorectal liver metastasis in the first-line setting to systemic chemotherapy or primary tumor resection + HAI FUDR + systemic chemotherapy. Currently, primary endpoint is progression-free survival. Stratification factors will be RAS status, primary tumor sidedness, inclusion center and whether doublet or triplet systemic therapy is used. In Norway, a trial will randomize patients with CRLM and heavy tumor burden with insufficient response to first-line systemic chemotherapy to allow for resection (NCT04898504). Treatment arms will be (1) Second-line systemic chemotherapy + liver transplantation, (2) Second-line systemic chemotherapy + HAI FUDR, and (3) Second-line chemotherapy as standard of care. The primary outcome is 2-year overall survival. In the adjuvant setting, a phase III trial is recruiting in the Netherlands. Patients with resected low-risk CRLM are randomized to adjuvant HAI-FUDR without systemic treatment vs. surgery alone (EudraCT number:2019–003966-42). These contemporary trials are expected to validate HAI-FUDR in the context of evolving systemic therapy.

Oxaliplatin

Oxaliplatin is a platinum coordination complex with antitumoral activity against colorectal cancer and other gastrointestinal malignancies. Oxaliplatin is cleared equally by glomerular filtration and tissue distribution. Preclinical evidence suggests a steep dose-response curve to oxaliplatin in human colon carcinoma cells. Tumor specimens from patients with isolated liver metastases from colorectal cancer were exposed to 0.1, 1, 10, and 100 μg/mL of oxaliplatin for 2 h. All specimens showed significant concentration-response effects [28]. The PKs of platinum in ultra-filtrate are triexponential, characterized by short initial α and β distribution phases (0.28 and 16.3 h, respectively) followed by a long terminal γ phase (273 h) [29]. The α and β phases represent the clinically relevant $t_{1/2}$ values of active platinum. The platinum compounds in the terminal elimination phase are comprised almost exclusively of inactive conjugates. No accumulation has been observed in plasma ultra-filtrate after 130 mg/m^2 every 3 weeks or 85 mg/m^2 every 2 weeks. The clearance of ultra-filterable platinum decreases from 18.5 +/− 4.71 L/h at 85 mg/m^2 every 2 weeks to 9.34 +/− 2.85 to 10.1 +/− 3.07 L/h at 130 mg/m^2 every 3 weeks [29].

Kern et al. performed a Phase I study to determine the maximum tolerated dose of oxaliplatin administered by hepatic arterial infusion in escalation steps of 25 mg/m^2 starting at 25 mg/m^2. The maximum tolerated dose was reported at 150 mg/m^2 every 3 weeks in combination with intravenous folinic acid 200 mg/m^2 and 5FU 600 mg/m^2 for five consecutive days in patients with isolated hepatic metastases from colorectal cancer. This study allowed determination of the following pharmacokinetic parameters of HAI oxaliplatin administration: terminal half-life of ultra-filtrable platinum at 17.75+/− 9.29 h; renal elimination, 48.8% +/− 14.1%; renal clearance 135.55 +/− 45.32 mL/min. The mean AUC increased linearly from 3.22 +/− 0.61 μg h/mL to 18.45 +/− 8.9 μg h/mL through the first five dose levels ($p < 0.0004$) [30].

The direct hepatic extraction rate of oxaliplatin has not been determined. Instead, Guthoff et al. designed a phase II trial combining HAI oxaliplatin with 5FU/FA and mitomycin C in patients with isolated non-resectable CRLM. Hepatic extraction was estimated by comparing the area under the plasma-concentration curve (AUC) values in venous blood observed after administration of oxaliplatin 130 mg/m^2 via HAI to the AUC values obtained after intravenous administration of oxaliplatin in historical controls. Liver extraction ratio was 0.47 [31].

Compared to FUDR, the predicted pharmacological advantage of oxaliplatin is limited: low total body clearance, zero-order kinetics, and a low hepatic extraction ratio. Nonetheless patients with colorectal liver metastases have been treated with HAI oxaliplatin within phase I and phase II trials [32]. Based on available data, we can conclude the following: (1) the safe HAI oxaliplatin dose appears to be near 130 mg/m^2 every 3 weeks, which is not different from standard IV dose; (2) systemic side effects of arterial oxaliplatin delivery dominate dose-limiting toxicity suggesting limited advantage of regional administration; (3) severe abdominal pain is a characteristic side effect of HAI oxaliplatin; (4) despite authors concluding that HAI oxaliplatin may be more active and less toxic compared to IV administration, the advantage of HAI oxaliplatin if any remains to be demonstrated in randomized trials.

In contrast, clinical trials in hepatocellular carcinoma have consistently demonstrated improved efficacy of intra-arterial administration of 5FU and oxaliplatin when compared to systemic administration. The development of the so called FOLFOX-HAIC regimen is an example of successful HAI approach different from FUDR administration. A phase III trial of advanced HCC showed limited activity of systemic FOLFOX: 8% response rate, 2.9 months progression-free survival and 6.4 months overall survival [33]. However, phase III trials have shown improved overall survival from FOLFOX-HAIC when compared to standard of care in different settings including BCLC B (compared to chemoembolization) [34], BCLC C (compared to sorafenib) [35] and the adjuvant setting after resection (compared to observation) [36]. Table 4.3 summarizes relevant phase III trials of FOLFOX-HAIC in HCC patients.

It is noteworthy that FOLFOX-HAIC has clinically proven results despite suboptimal pharmacological profile. This only emphasized the need to conduct confirmatory trials. Conflicting outcomes from FOLFOX-HAIC treatment between colon cancer patients and HCC patients may be partially explained by the fact that systemic FOLFOX is very active in colon cancer patients and FOLFOX-HAIC may only be relevant in a chemo-resistant scenario such as HCC. This regimen should be further explored in western countries and other neoplasms, such as cholangiocarcinoma.

Table 4.3 Summary of clinical trials of 5FU and oxaliplatin for the treatment of hepatocellular carcinoma

Author, year, n	Study phase	Clinical stage	Intra-arterial drugs	Systemic treatment	Results
Qin, S [33], 2013, $n = 371$	III	Advanced hepatocellular carcinoma	None	Oxaliplatin 85 mg/m^2, D1 + LV 200 mg/m^2, D1–2 + 5FU 400 mg/m^2 IV bolus +600 mg/m^2 in 22 h infusion, D1–2, every 2 weeks Versus Doxorubicin 50 mg/m^2 every 3 weeks	RECIST ORR: 8.15 vs. 2.67% OS: 6.4 (95% CI 5.3–7.03) vs. 4.97 (95% CI 4.23–6.03) months
Ikeda, M [37], 2023, $n = 36$	II	Locally advanced without systemic treatment	Cisplatin 65 mg/m^2 every 4–6 weeks, max. 6 cycles	Lenvatinib ≥60 kg: 12 mg/d < 60 kg: 8 mg/d	RECIST ORR: 45.7% mRECIST ORR: 64.7% PFS: 6.3 (95% CI 5.1–7.9) months OS: 17.2 (95% CI: 10.9-NA) months
Li, QJ [34], 2021, $n = 315$	III	Unresectable hepatocelular carcinoma without systemic treatment	Oxaliplatin 130 mg/m^2 + leucovorin 400 mg/m^2 + fluorouracil bolus 400 mg/m^2 + infusion 2400 mg/m^2 every 3 weeks	None	RECIST ORR: 46% PFS: 9.6 (95% CI 7.4–11.9) months OS: 23.1 m (95% CI 18.5–27.7) months
He, M [35], 2019, $n = 247$	III	Hepatocelular carcinoma with portal vein invasion without systemic treatment	Oxaliplatin 85 mg/m^2 + leucovorin 400 mg/m^2 + fluorouracil bolus 400 mg/m^2 + infusion 2400 mg/m^2 every 3 weeks + sorafenib 400 mg BID	Sorafenib 400 mg BID	RECIST ORR: 40.8% PFS: 7.03 (95% CI 6.05–8.02) months
Li, S [36], 2022, $n = 315$	III	Resected hepatocellular carcinoma with microvascular invasion	Oxaliplatin 85 mg/m^2 + leucovorin 400 mg/m^2 + fluorouracil bolus 400 mg/m^2 + infusion 2400 mg/m^2 every 3 weeks	None	DFS: 20.3 m (95% CI 10.4–30.3) 1 yr OS: 98.3% (95% CI 89.8–98.1) 2 yr OS: 86.4 (95% CI 80–93.2) 3 yr: 80.4% (95% CI 71.9–89.9%)

Irinotecan

Irinotecan (CPT-11) is a DNA synthesis inhibitor which acts by hindering topoisomerase I activity, an enzyme overexpressed in colorectal cancer. CPT-11 is further metabolized into SN-38 by carboxyl esterase and to SN-38G, an inactive metabolite, by hepatic uridine diphosphate glucuronosyltransferases. Compared to CPT-11, SN-38 has a 100- to 1000-fold greater antitumor activity. The AUC of SN-38 is approximately 4% of that of irinotecan, which suggests that a small fraction is ultimately converted into the active form. The half-life of SN-38 is 11.5 h. The molar ratio of SN-38 AUC/CPT-11 is threefold greater when administered orally than after intravenous administration, which suggests a higher exposure to SN-38 (active metabolite) due to first-pass metabolism. This is the most concerning pharmacokinetic characteristic of irinotecan for HAI administration as first-pass metabolism predicts higher systemic exposure to the active metabolite. CPT-11 displays nonlinear pharmacokinetics. At higher doses, the molar ratio of SN-38 / CPT-11 decreases due to saturation of irinotecan conversion into SN-38. The metabolic ratio of SN-38/CPT-11 has also been shown to be significantly higher after a low-dose continuous infusion of CPT-11 than after a high-dose, short infusion of CPT-11 [38]. Investigators have tried to overcome the nonlinear pharmacokinetics pitfall by using the continuous administration of CPT-11 by HAI at low doses over 5 days. They hypothesized that increased antitumoral activity is due to increased active metabolite that is primarily active in the S-phase of the cell-cycle. However, phase I and phase II trials failed to demonstrate decreased systemic toxicity or increased efficacy with this approach [39–42]. In summary, pharmacological parameters predict no advantage for HAI irinotecan and early trials appear confirmatory.

Gemcitabine

Gemcitabine is a pyrimidine antimetabolite structurally similar to cytarabine. Cytotoxicity of gemcitabine is mediated primarily by its effects on DNA replication. Gemcitabine is cleared through metabolic elimination by cytidine deaminase and cytidylate deaminase; both are abundant in the liver. Gemcitabine exhibits linear pharmacokinetics with a half-life of 11–26 min when a short infusion schedule is used (<70 min) [43]. With longer infusion times, the half-life varies from 18.5 to 57.1 min, which has been attributable to increased tissue distribution. Systemic gemcitabine is commonly dosed at 1000 mg/m^2 weekly × 3 in a 30-min infusion. Trials have examined fixed-dose rate gemcitabine at 10 mg/m^2/min to maximize the phosphorylation of gemcitabine and the incorporation of its active metabolite, dFdCTP, into newly synthesized DNA, with the goal of improving response for patients. Fixed-dose rate resulted in increased hematologic toxicity without improved survival.

Gemcitabine, in combination with cisplatin and immunotherapy, constitutes the current standard of care for the treatment of advanced biliary tract cancer. As a single agent, gemcitabine exhibits activity against pancreas, non-small cell lung, breast, bladder, and ovarian cancers [43]. For intrahepatic cholangiocarcinoma, HAI FUDR alone or in combination with systemic gemcitabine and oxaliplatin yield encouraging outcomes in phase II trials [44, 45].

Early trials have also explored the potential advantage of HAI gemcitabine. Compared to other drugs, gemcitabine has relatively high total body clearance and given liver metabolism, hepatic extraction was predicted. A phase I trial treated patients with intrahepatic cholangiocarcinoma or liver metastases from pancreatic cancer with HAI gemcitabine. The maximum tolerated dose was 1400 mg/m^2 and 1800 mg/m^2 (with microspheres) when given on day 1 and day 8 of a 28-day cycle, by short infusion (<20 min) through a percutaneously placed catheter. No responses were observed [46]. A subsequent phase I trial conducted at Memorial Sloan-Kettering Cancer Center further explored HAI gemcitabine using a fixed-dose rate through the side-port of implantable pumps in patients with primary or metastatic hepatic malignancies. All patients had been previously treated with FUDR. During the dose escalation phase, the gemcitabine dose could be escalated from 800 mg/m^2 to 1500 mg/m^2 without reaching dose-limiting toxicity. Observed gemcitabine concentrations following HAI were generally lower than values predicted from population PK parameters of IV gemcitabine, providing preliminary evidence for hepatic extraction of the drug when given directly into the liver. An infusion duration-escalation phase was also implemented. Patients were treated with 1000 mg/m^2 over an increasing duration of infusion, every week for 3 of 4 weeks. To estimate hepatic extraction, a single intravenous dose of gemcitabine was administered during the duration-escalation phase. Intriguingly, PK data indicated that a much lower proportion of gemcitabine is extracted and is inconsistent between patients. Reasons for high variability of hepatic extraction were discussed, including arteriovenous shunting through tumor sinusoids, genetic polymorphisms of nucleoside transporters and metabolizing enzymes among patients, and possibly errors in PK sampling. Overall, despite pharmacological prediction, hepatic extraction was not confirmed in this trial [47]. Nonetheless, phase I trials have identified a safe dose for HAI gemcitabine which can be used as a platform for further development including HAI combination therapy with either FUDR or oxaliplatin. In addition, lower doses by means of prolonged infusions through the pump reservoir remain to be tested.

Mitomycin

Mitomycin acts as an alkylating agent. It inhibits DNA synthesis and cross-links DNA at the N6 position of adenine and at the O6 and N7 positions of guanine. Attempts to repair DNA lead to strand breaks. While it is not cell cycle specific, mitomycin has its maximum effect against cells in the late G and early S phases. It exhibits a half-life of 25–90 min. Clearance is mediated by hepatic metabolism or chemical conjugation with sulfhydryls. It is administered intravenously as a bolus (6–20 mg/m^2) every 6–8 weeks [43].

Mitomycin is a well-known radiosensitizer in the management of anal carcinoma and displays activity in combination with other agents in the treatment of bladder, gastric, and hepatocellular carcinoma, among others. As HAI chemotherapy, mitomycin has been used mainly for the treatment of liver-confined metastatic colorectal, hepatocellular, and gastric cancer.

Hu et al. estimated that the hepatic extraction ratio of mitomycin was 0.3 +/− 0.12, 0.16 +/− 0.01, and 0.21 +/− 0.08 when the infusion rates were 0.4, 1.2, and 4.0 mg/m^2/min, respectively. This was performed in seven patients with metastatic carcinoma in the liver. Of note, six of them had colon carcinoma and one had metastatic melanoma. It was observed that the lower the plasma tumor flow, the higher the relative advantage of an intra-arterial infusion [48]. Addressing this, a more recent study evaluated infusion of mitomycin (20 mg/m^2 at 30 mL/min) after hepatic arterial occlusion in ten patients with hepatic metastasis from colorectal cancer. Total body clearance was 35.5 l/h/m^2 (range 25.4–50.4) with an AUC ranging from 251 to 850 Ug/h/L. When compared with intravenous and intraarterial models alone, this method showed a significant increase in total body clearance and reduction in AUC [49].

Future Developments

Systemic treatment for colon cancer, cholangiocarcinoma and hepatocellular carcinoma has evolved and trials testing safety and efficacy of new regimens when combined with HAI FUDR are needed. Figure 4.7 delineates a clinical proposal for such development of HAI strategies in the future. As an example, despite a limited predicted pharmacokinetic advantage of HAI oxali-

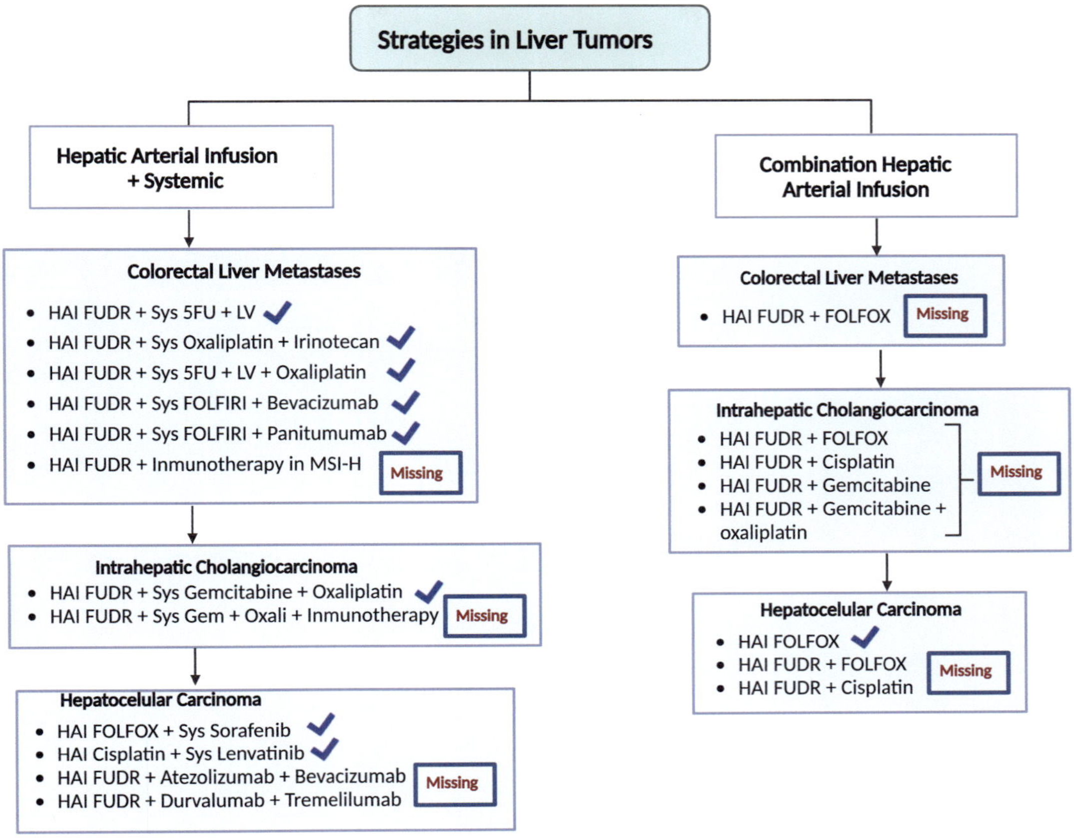

Fig. 4.7 Conceptual pathways for future HAI development. (Created with BioRender). ✓ Completed trial. Missing Trial not yet performed. *HAI* hepatic arterial infusion, *Sys* systemic treatment, *MSI-H* microsatellite instability

platin over systemic delivery, lessons learned from hepatocellular carcinoma suggest exploration of combination HAI strategies may be worthwhile. FOLFOX-HAIC in combination with HAI-FUDR appears to be a logical subsequent step. The feasibility and efficacy of this strategy are currently anecdotal, as shown in Fig. 4.8. Other drug combinations, in particular, the hepatic arterial gemcitabine and/or oxaliplatin with HAI FUDR should also be tested in patients with intrahepatic cholangiocarcinoma. Until additional data are available, given the indisputable clinical and pharmacokinetic advantage of FUDR over any other known drugs for the regional treatment of primary and secondary liver cancers, the combination of HAI FUDR with optimal systemic regimens remains the preferred clinical strategy for HAI.

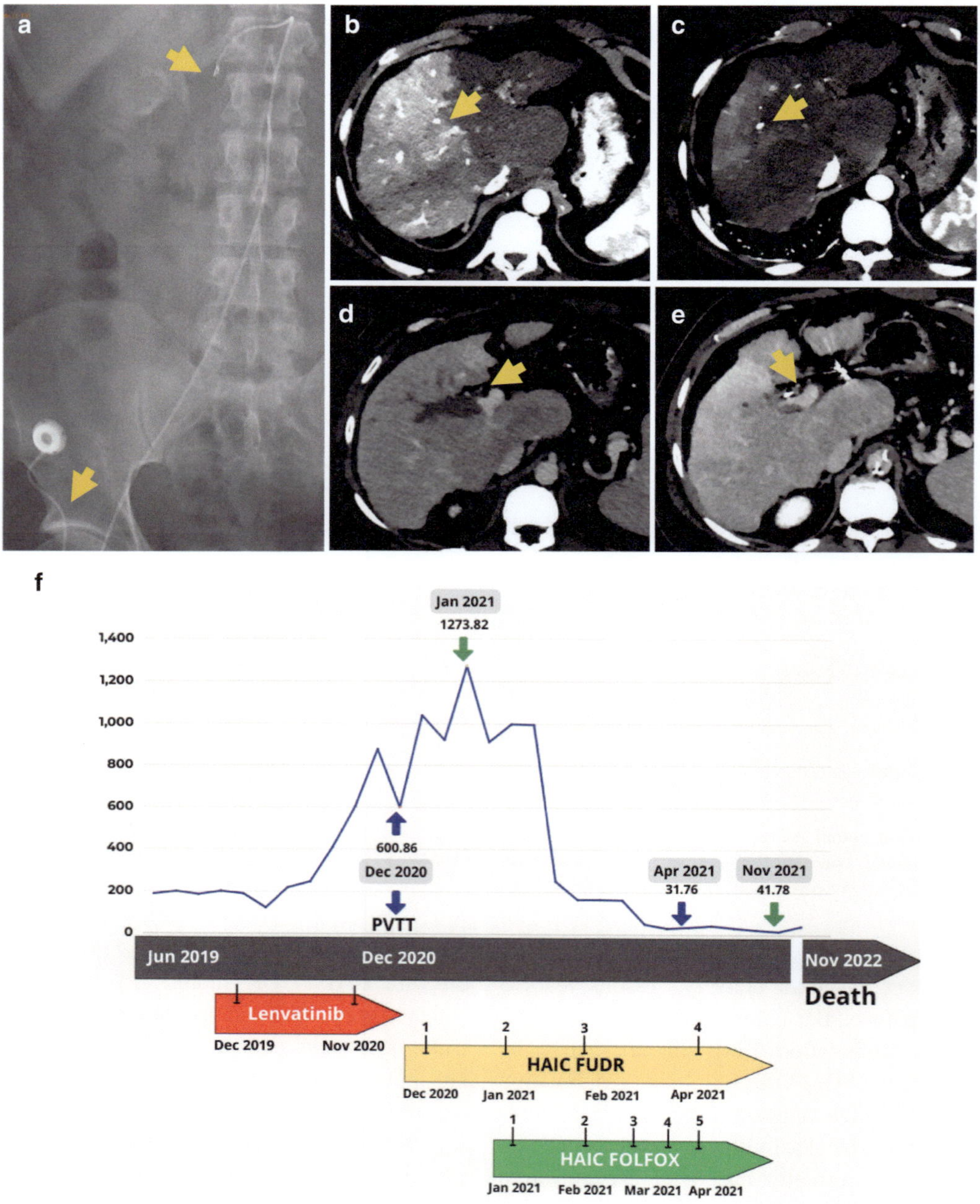

Fig. 4.8 Clinical case: feasibility of combining HAI FUDR with HAI FOLFOX. (Created with BioRender). Clinical case. A 36 y/o male, hepatitis C-related cirrhosis and unresectable hepatocellular carcinoma (HCC). After first-line lenvatinib, patient developed right portal vein tumor thrombosis and alfa-fetoprotein (AFP) levels reached 1237 ng/mL. He received 14-day FUDR hepatic arterial infusion (HAI-FUDR) combined with hepatic arterial infusional fluorouracil, leucovorin and oxaliplatin (FOLFOX-HAIC). After 5 months of therapy patient achieved clinical benefit, partial response and prolonged survival. (**a**) Placement of a permanent intra-arterial port via femoral access. (**b**) Pretreatment arterial-phase CT scan, large tumor with arterial enhancement, longest diameter was 16 cm. (**c**) The follow-up CT scan showed notorious decrement of size (6 cm) and decreased tumor arterial enhancement. (**d**) Pretreatment venous-phase CT scan showed complete obliteration of the anterior branch of the right portal vein. (**e**) Follow-up CT scan showed thrombus retraction and improvement of portal vein flow. (**f**) The overall survival of the patient from the beginning of HAIC to death was 23 months. AFP levels reflected that the AFP nadir was 31 ng/mL

References

1. Huitzil-Melendez F, Kemeny N. Pharmacologic principles of regional therapy in the treatment of liver metastases or primary liver tumors. In: Interventional oncology: principles and practice; 2008. p. 38–52.
2. Collins JM. Pharmacologic rationale for regional drug delivery. J Clin Oncol. 1984;2:498.
3. Brock K, Homer V, Soul G, Potter C, Chiuzan C, Lee S. Is more better? An analysis of toxicity and response outcomes from dose-finding clinical trials in cancer. BMC Cancer. 2021;21(1):777.
4. Iasonos A, Ostrovnaya I. Estimating the dose-toxicity curve in completed phase I studies. Stat Med. 2011;30(17):2117–29.
5. Ensminger WD, Gyves JW. Regional chemotherapy of neoplastic diseases. Pharmacol Ther. 1983;21(2):277–93. https://api.semanticscholar.org/CorpusID:15075601.
6. Ensminger WD, Rosowsky A, Raso V, Levin DC, Glode M, Come S, Steele G, Frei E 3rd. A clinical-pharmacological evaluation of hepatic arterial infusions of 5-fluoro-2'-deoxyuridine and 5-fluorouracil. Cancer Res. 1978;38(11 Pt 1):3784–92.
7. Ensminger WD. Intrahepatic arterial infusion of chemotherapy: pharmacologic principles. Semin Oncol. 2002;29(2):119–25.
8. Kemeny N, Seiter K, Conti JA, Cohen A, Bertino JR, Sigurdson ER, et al. Hepatic arterial floxuridine and leucovorin for unresectable liver metastases from colorectal carcinoma. New dose schedules and survival update. Cancer. 1994;73(4):1134–42.
9. Huitzil-Melendez FD, Kemeny N. Clinical management of patients with colorectal liver metastases using hepatic arterial infusion. In: Interventional oncology: principles and practice; 2008.
10. Kemeny NE, Niedzwiecki D, Hollis DR, Lenz HJ, Warren RS, Naughton MJ, et al. Hepatic arterial infusion versus systemic therapy for hepatic metastases from colorectal cancer: a randomized trial of efficacy, quality of life, and molecular markers (CALGB 9481). J Clin Oncol. 2006;24(9):1395–403.
11. Kemeny N, Jarnagin W, Paty P, Gönen M, Schwartz L, Morse M, et al. Phase I trial of systemic oxaliplatin combination chemotherapy with hepatic arterial infusion in patients with unresectable liver metastases from colorectal cancer. J Clin Oncol. 2005;23(22):4888–96.
12. Kemeny N, Gonen M, Sullivan D, Schwartz L, Benedetti F, Saltz L, et al. Phase I study of hepatic arterial infusion of Floxuridine and dexamethasone with systemic irinotecan for unresectable hepatic metastases from colorectal cancer. J Clin Oncol. 2001;19:2687–95.
13. D'Angelica MI, Correa-Gallego C, Paty PB, Cercek A, Gewirtz AN, Chou JF, et al. Phase ii trial of hepatic artery infusional and systemic chemotherapy for patients with unresectable hepatic metastases from colorectal cancer conversion to resection and long-term outcomes. Ann Surg. 2015;261(2):353–60.
14. Kemeny N, Jarnagin W, Gonen M, Stockman J, Blumgart L, Sperber D, et al. Phase I/II study of hepatic arterial therapy with floxuridine and dexamethasone in combination with intravenous irinotecan as adjuvant treatment after resection of hepatic metastases from colorectal cancer. J Clin Oncol. 2003;21(17):3303–9.
15. Kemeny N, Capanu M, D'Angelica M, Jarnagin W, Haviland D, Dematteo R, et al. Phase I trial of adjuvant hepatic arterial infusion (HAI) with floxuridine (FUDR) and dexamethasone plus systemic oxaliplatin, 5-fluorouracil and leucovorin in patients with resected liver metastases from colorectal cancer. Ann Oncol. 2009;20(7):1236–41.
16. Kemeny NE, Jarnagin WR, Capanu M, Fong Y, Gewirtz AN, DeMatteo RP, et al. Randomized phase II trial of adjuvant hepatic arterial infusion and systemic chemotherapy with or without bevacizumab in patients with resected hepatic metastases from colorectal cancer. J Clin Oncol. 2011;29(7):884–9.
17. Kemeny NE, Chou JF, Capanu M, Chatila WK, Shi H, Sanchez-Vega F, et al. A randomized phase II trial of adjuvant hepatic arterial infusion and systemic therapy with or without Panitumumab after hepatic resection of KRAS wild-type colorectal cancer. Ann Surg. 2021;274:248–54.
18. Rossini D, Antoniotti C, Lonardi S, Pietrantonio F, Moretto R, Antonuzzo L, et al. Upfront modified fluorouracil, Leucovorin, Oxaliplatin, and irinotecan plus Panitumumab versus fluorouracil, Leucovorin, and Oxaliplatin plus Panitumumab for patients with RAS/BRAF wild-type metastatic colorectal cancer: the phase III TRIPLETE study by GONO. J Clin Oncol. 2022;40:2878.
19. Bond MJG, Bolhuis K, Loosveld OJL, de Groot JWB, Droogendijk H, Helgason HH, et al. First-line systemic treatment strategies in patients with initially unresectable colorectal cancer liver metastases (CAIRO5): an open-label, multicentre, randomised, controlled, phase 3 study from the Dutch Colorectal Cancer Group. Lancet Oncol. 2023;24(7):757–71.
20. Punt CJA, Bond MJG, Bolhuis K, Loosveld OJL, de Groot JW, Droogendijk H, et al. LBA27 first-line systemic treatment in patients with initially unresectable colorectal cancer liver metastases (CRLM): overall survival of the phase III CAIRO5 study of the Dutch Colorectal Cancer Group. Ann Oncol. 2023;34:S1268.
21. Kemeny N, Huang Y, Cohen AM, Shi W, Conti JA, Brennan MF, et al. Hepatic arterial infusion of chemotherapy after resection of hepatic metastases from colorectal cancer. N Engl J Med. 1999;341:2039.
22. Kemeny NE, Gonen M. Hepatic arterial infusion after liver resection. N Engl J Med. 2005;352(7):734–5.
23. Portier G, Elias D, Bouche O, Rougier P, Bosset JF, Saric J, et al. Multicenter randomized trial of adjuvant fluorouracil and Folinic acid compared with surgery alone after resection of colorectal liver metastases:

FFCD ACHBTH AURC 9002 trial. J Clin Oncol. 2006;24(31):4976–82.
24. Mitry E, Fields ALA, Bleiberg H, Labianca R, Portier G, Tu D, et al. Adjuvant chemotherapy after potentially curative resection of metastases from colorectal cancer: a pooled analysis of two randomized trials. J Clin Oncol. 2008;26(30):4906–11.
25. Kanemitsu Y, Shimizu Y, Mizusawa J, Inaba Y, Hamaguchi T, Shida D, et al. Hepatectomy followed by mFOLFOX6 versus hepatectomy alone for liver-only metastatic colorectal cancer (JCOG0603): a phase II or III randomized controlled trial. J Clin Oncol. 2021;39(34):3789–99.
26. Nordlinger B, Sorbye H, Glimelius B, Poston GJ, Schlag PM, Rougier P, et al. Perioperative FOLFOX4 chemotherapy and surgery versus surgery alone for resectable liver metastases from colorectal cancer (EORTC 40983): long-term results of a randomised, controlled, phase 3 trial. Lancet Oncol. 2013;14(12):1208–15.
27. Ychou M, Hohenberger W, Thezenas S, Navarro M, Maurel J, Bokemeyer C, et al. A randomized phase III study comparing adjuvant 5-fluorouracil/folinic acid with FOLFIRI in patients following complete resection of liver metastases from colorectal cancer. Ann Oncol. 2009;20(12):1964–70.
28. Kornmann M, Fakler H, Butzer U, Beger HG, Link KH. Oxaliplatin exerts potent in vitro cytotoxicity in colorectal and pancreatic cancer cell lines and liver metastases. Anticancer Res. 2000;20(5):3259.
29. Graham MA, Lockwood GF, Greenslade D, Brienza S, Bayssas M, Gamelin E. Clinical pharmacokinetics of Oxaliplatin: a critical review. Clin Cancer Res. 2000;6(4):1205–18. http://aacrjournals.org/clincancerres/article-pdf/6/4/1205/2301806/df040001205.pdf.
30. Kern W, Beckert B, Lang N, Stemmler J, Beykirch M, Stein J, et al. Phase I and pharmacokinetic study of hepatic arterial infusion with oxaliplatin in combination with folinic acid and 5-fluorouracil in patients with hepatic metastases from colorectal cancer. Ann Oncol. 2001;12:599.
31. Guthoff I, Lotspeich E, Fester C, Wallin I, Schatz M, Ehrsson H, et al. Hepatic artery infusion using oxaliplatin in combination with 5-fluorouracil, folinic acid and mitomycin C: oxaliplatin pharmacokinetics and feasibility. Anticancer Res. 2003;23(6D):5203–8.
32. Ranieri G, Laforgia M, Nardulli P, Ferraiuolo S, Molinari P, Marech I, et al. Oxaliplatin-based intra-arterial chemotherapy in colorectal cancer liver metastases: a review from pharmacology to clinical application. Cancer. 2019;11:141.
33. Qin S, Bai Y, Lim HY, Thongprasert S, Chao Y, Fan J, et al. Randomized, multicenter, open-label study of oxaliplatin plus fluorouracil/leucovorin versus doxorubicin as palliative chemotherapy in patients with advanced hepatocellular carcinoma from Asia. J Clin Oncol. 2013;31(28):3501–8.
34. Li QJ, He MK, Chen HW, Fang WQ, Zhou YM, et al. Hepatic arterial infusion of Oxaliplatin, fluorouracil, and Leucovorin versus transarterial chemoembolization for large hepatocellular carcinoma: a randomized phase III trial. J Clin Oncol. 2021;40:150–60.
35. He M, Li Q, Zou R, Shen J, Fang W, Tan G, et al. Sorafenib plus hepatic arterial infusion of Oxaliplatin, fluorouracil, and Leucovorin vs Sorafenib alone for hepatocellular carcinoma with portal vein invasion: a randomized clinical trial. JAMA Oncol. 2019;5(7):953–60.
36. Li SH, Mei J, Cheng Y, Li Q, Wang QX, Fang CK, et al. Postoperative adjuvant hepatic arterial infusion chemotherapy with FOLFOX in hepatocellular carcinoma with microvascular invasion: a multicenter, phase III, randomized study. J Clin Oncol. 2023;41:1898.
37. Ikeda M, Yamashita T, Ogasawara S, Kudo M, Inaba Y, Morimoto M, et al. Multicenter phase II trial of Lenvatinib plus hepatic intra-arterial infusion chemotherapy with cisplatin for advanced hepatocellular carcinoma: LEOPARD. Liver Cancer. 2023;13:193–202.
38. Iyer L, Ratain MJ. Clinical pharmacology of camptothecins. Cancer Chemother Pharmacol. 1998;42(S1):S31–43.
39. Herben VMM, Schellens JHM, Swart M, Gruia G, Vernillet L, Beijnen JH, et al. Phase I and pharmacokinetic study of irinotecan administered as a low-dose, continuous intravenous infusion over 14 days in patients with malignant solid tumors. J Clin Oncol. 1999;17(6):1897.
40. Ohe Y, Sasaki Y, Shinkai T, Eguchi K, Tamura T, Kojima A, et al. Phase I study and pharmacokinetics of CPT-11 with 5-day continuous infusion. JNCI J Natl Cancer Inst. 1992;84(12):972–4.
41. van Riel JMGH, van Groeningen CJ, Kedde MA, Gall H, Leisink JMA, Gruia G, et al. Continuous administration of irinotecan by hepatic arterial infusion: a phase I and pharmacokinetic study. Clin Cancer Res. 2002;8(2):405–12.
42. van Riel JMGH, van Groeningen CJ, de Greve J, Gruia G, Pinedo HM, Giaccone G. Continuous infusion of hepatic arterial irinotecan in pretreated patients with colorectal cancer metastatic to the liver. Ann Oncol. 2004;15(1):59–63.
43. Brunton LL, Knollmann BC. Goodman and Gilman's the pharmacological basis of therapeutics. 14th ed; 2023.
44. Cercek A, Boerner T, Tan BR, Chou JF, Gönen M, Boucher TM, et al. Assessment of hepatic arterial infusion of Floxuridine in combination with systemic gemcitabine and Oxaliplatin in patients with Unresectable intrahepatic cholangiocarcinoma. JAMA Oncol. 2020;6(1):60.
45. Jarnagin WR, Schwartz LH, Gultekin DH, Gönen M, Haviland D, Shia J, et al. Regional chemotherapy for unresectable primary liver cancer: results of a phase

II clinical trial and assessment of DCE-MRI as a biomarker of survival. Ann Oncol. 2009;20(9):1589–95.

46. Vogl TJ, Schwarz W, Eichler K, Hochmuth K, Hammerstingl R, Jacob U, et al. Hepatic intraarterial chemotherapy with gemcitabine in patients with unresectable cholangiocarcinomas and liver metastases of pancreatic cancer: a clinical study on maximum tolerable dose and treatment efficacy. J Cancer Res Clin Oncol. 2006;132(11):745–55.
47. Tse AN, Wu N, Patel D, Haviland D, Kemeny N. A phase I study of gemcitabine given via intrahepatic pump for primary or metastatic hepatic malignancies. Cancer Chemother Pharmacol. 2009;64(5):935–44.
48. Hu E, Howell SB. Pharmacokinetics of intraarterial mitomycin C in humans. Cancer Res. 1983;43(9):4474–7.
49. Cerretani D, Roviello F, Pieraccini M, Civeli L, Correale P, Francini G, et al. Pharmacokinetics of intraarterial mitomycin C in hypoxic hepatic infusion with embolization in the treatment of liver metastases. Vascul Pharmacol. 2002;39(1–2):1–6.

Part II

Perioperative and Operative Considerations

Preoperative Evaluation

5

Gloria Y. Chang, Robert E. Roses, Adel Kardosh, and Adam C. Yopp

Introduction

Careful preoperative evaluation prior to hepatic artery infusion pump (HAIP) placement is essential for assessing the candidacy of the patient for both surgical placement of HAIP and administration of subsequent hepatic artery infusion chemotherapy (Table 5.1). The preoperative assessment must include a thorough history, physical examination and pertinent imaging studies to delineate the feasibility of HAIP placement and the appropriateness of infusional chemotherapy.

Table 5.1 Overview of the preoperative evaluation for HAIP therapy

1. **Confirm histological diagnosis and appropriate indication for HAIP therapy**
2. **General assessment**
   (a) History and physical
   (b) Routine labs, biochemical profile, tumor biomarkers (Table 5.2)
   (c) Electrocardiogram as warranted
   (d) Chest X-ray as warranted
3. **Rule out extrahepatic disease**
   (a) CT scan of the chest, abdomen, and pelvis
   (b) +/– colonoscopy, PET scan, and bone scan
4. **Rule out contraindications** (Table 5.3)
5. **Delineate hepatic arterial anatomy**
   (a) CT angiography to define the celiac and superior mesenteric arteries
   (b) Rule out the presence of portal vein thrombosis
   (c) Evaluate for aberrant hepatic arterial anatomy; exclude patients with anatomy that precludes complete perfusion of the liver

Initial Evaluation

Preoperative evaluation should begin with confirmation that the patient is an appropriate candidate for HAIP in the context of their underlying diagnosis. After histological diagnosis and appropriate indication for HAIP therapy is confirmed (see Chaps. 14–17) for disease-specific considerations for patient selection), a complete history and physical examination should be performed. The patient must have a sufficient performance status to allow general anesthesia and undergo an

G. Y. Chang · A. C. Yopp (✉)
Division of Surgical Oncology, Department of Surgery, University of Texas Southwestern Medical Center, Dallas, TX, USA
e-mail: gloria.chang@utsouthwestern.edu; adam.yopp@utsouthwestern.edu

R. E. Roses
Department of Surgery, Hospital of the University of Pennsylvania, Philadelphia, PA, USA
e-mail: robert.roses@pennmedicine.upenn.edu

A. Kardosh
Division of Hematology/Medical Oncology, Knight Cancer Institute, Oregon Health and Science University, Portland, OR, USA
e-mail: kardosh@ohsu.edu

M. D'Angelica, M. Lidsky (eds.), *Hepatic Arterial Infusion for Malignancy*,
https://doi.org/10.1007/978-3-031-74935-3_5

Table 5.2 Recommended preoperative laboratory values for HAIP placement

Recommended preoperative laboratory values for HAIP placement
WBC ≥ 3.0 K/uL
ANC > 1.5 K/uL
Platelets ≥100,000/uL
Creatinine <1.5 mg/dL
Hgb ≥ 9 g/dL
Total bilirubin ≤1.5 mg/dL

HAIP placement using either a minimally invasive or open surgical technique. Eastern Cooperative Oncology Group 0 or 1 or Karnofsky Performance Status ≥60% is generally required to proceed. Significant comorbidities should be carefully evaluated to allow counseling regarding perioperative risk. Patients undergo electrocardiography and chest X-ray as part of the routine preoperative assessment as clinically warranted. Extensive prior abdominal surgery, particularly hepatopancreaticobiliary surgery, ostomies (previous and current), and abdominal wall hernias may complicate pump placement and should be carefully considered.

Any serious medical conditions that may preclude the receipt of chemotherapy as well as any medical history that may exclude the patient from the surgical implantation of a foreign body should be elicited, including the presence of active infection, coagulopathy, nonhealing wounds, ulcers, or bone fractures [1]. Active viral hepatitis is typically considered a contraindication to HAIP therapy; however, HAIP may still be considered in select patients with treated chronic hepatitis and/or cirrhosis with underlying Child-Pugh Class A liver function and no stigmata of portal hypertension (see below).

Following the initial general assessment, candidates for HAIP placement should undergo routine bloodwork consisting of a complete blood count, coagulation profile, comprehensive metabolic profile, and appropriate tumor biomarkers as warranted. Table 5.2 describes the recommended laboratory values for HAIP pump placement to minimize perioperative complications and ensure future administration of hepatic artery infusion chemotherapy.

Table 5.3 Contraindications to HAIP therapy

Patient factors	Tumor and anatomic factors
Poor performance status: ECOG >1 or KPS < 60%	Extrahepatic disease
Poor hepatic function: Total bilirubin >1.5, presence of ascites, hepatic encephalopathy, or portal hypertension (splenomegaly, varices, recanalized umbilical vein, thrombocytopenia)	Portal vein thrombosis
Active hepatitis; Child-Pugh Class B or C cirrhosis	Extensive hepatic metastases (>70% replacement)
Active infection or nonhealing wounds	Aberrant HA anatomy that precludes complete perfusion of the entire liver
Coagulopathy	
Inability to tolerate general anesthesia and laparotomy	
Patient compliance to HAIP maintenance and follow-up schedule	

Evaluation of Extrahepatic Disease

The presence of extrahepatic disease, including metastatic disease to the portal nodes, is considered a relative contraindication to HAIP therapy and the associated high likelihood of extrahepatic recurrence or progression should be taken into consideration prior to HAIP placement [2]. Computed tomography (CT) scans of the chest, abdomen, and pelvis are obtained and reviewed as part of an extent of disease workup. Pending equivocal findings on CT, whole body FDG-18 PET scan may be obtained as clinically indicated. A bone scan can be considered if the patient reports bone pain, and a colonoscopy can also be considered to exclude the presence of second primary tumors or local recurrence for the appropriate HAIP placement indication [3].

Potential Contraindications to HAIP

In addition to the evaluation of extrahepatic disease, candidate patients must have an adequate hepatic reserve or functional volume. Ascites, portal hypertension, hepatic encephalopathy, and/or total bilirubin greater than 1.5 mg/dL are surrogate markers of hepatic dysfunction precluding HAIP placement and administration of future therapy. Extensive replacement of hepatic parenchyma with tumor burden (>70%) is also a relative contraindication [2]. Imaging should also be carefully reviewed for evidence of main portal venous occlusion as this precludes HAIP therapy due to the risk of hepatic ischemia [3]. A history of prior trans-arterial therapy such as Y90 or trans-arterial chemoembolization is typically considered a relative contraindication: the candidacy of these patients should be carefully evaluated in the context of the extent of prior embolotherapies (e.g., radiation lobectomy vs segmentectomy), their underlying liver dysfunction and access to a viable conduit as the gastroduodenal artery (GDA) may have been embolized in these patients.

Surgical Planning

Once the patient has been deemed an appropriate candidate for future hepatic artery infusion therapy based on disease status, clinical fitness, and the absence of contraindicating comorbidities, technical aspects of HAIP placement must be carefully considered, specifically the evaluation of hepatic arterial anatomy. Hepatic artery infusion chemotherapy is delivered via a solitary vessel conduit, preferably the GDA, to ensure bilobar hepatic perfusion without extrahepatic perfusion or obstruction of normal hepatic arterial inflow.

Preoperative imaging mapping the hepatic vasculature is critical for assessing the suitability of the patient for HAIP placement and planning the operative approach. Historically, direct catheter-based angiography was performed to evaluate the anatomic branching of the celiac and superior mesenteric arteries. However, with the development of high-quality cross-sectional imaging, noninvasive computed tomography angiography has become the preferred method for clarification of hepatic arterial anatomy, vascular patency/stenoses and the identification of replaced or accessory vessels to the liver. Magnetic resonance angiography may be appropriate in patients with contraindications to contrast agents, including allergic reactions or renal impairment [4].

As the GDA is the preferred insertion conduit of the HAIP catheter, the anatomic course and origin of the GDA, the caliber of its lumen, and the anatomy of its distal branches should be reviewed to ensure that the GDA is an appropriate target for cannulation and can safely accommodate the infusion catheter. Collateral branches distal to the GDA are noted on preoperative imaging so that corresponding vessels can be identified and ligated intraoperatively to minimize the risk of extrahepatic perfusion. Aberrant origin of the GDA from either the right hepatic artery, left hepatic artery, or as a trifurcation occurs in 6–11% of patients. None of these variants are considered a contraindication for the use of the GDA as a conduit, however, ligation of the contralateral hepatic artery is often necessary if adequate perfusion is not observed following catheter placement and intraoperative perfusion test.

If preoperative imaging reveals that the GDA is anatomically absent, occluded, or potentially too small to accommodate an infusion catheter, the patient can be evaluated for advanced operative techniques for pump placement (Fig. 5.1). The most common catheter (Intera silicone arterial beaded tip catheter, Intera Oncology Inc., Wellesley, MA) used during HAIP placement has a 0.6 mm inner diameter and 2.3 mm outer diameter, thus requiring a conduit vessel of at least 3 mm. Similarly, the beaded catheter requires a GDA length of at least 1 cm to ensure that at least one bead lies within the GDA and the tip of the catheter does not lie in the lumen of the common hepatic artery potentially preventing arterial flow to the liver (Fig. 5.2).

If the GDA is not a suitable conduit, strategies may include retrograde placement of the infusion catheter into the right or left hepatic artery, autol-

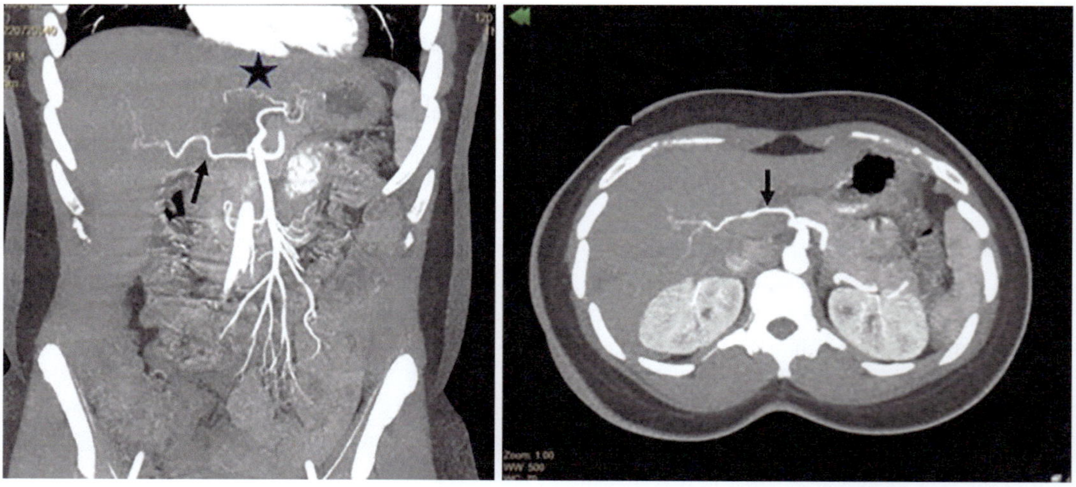

Fig. 5.1 Computed tomography angiography demonstrating absent gastroduodenal artery. Arrowhead illustrates right hepatic artery directly arising from the celiac trunk. Star illustrates replaced left hepatic artery arising from the left gastric artery

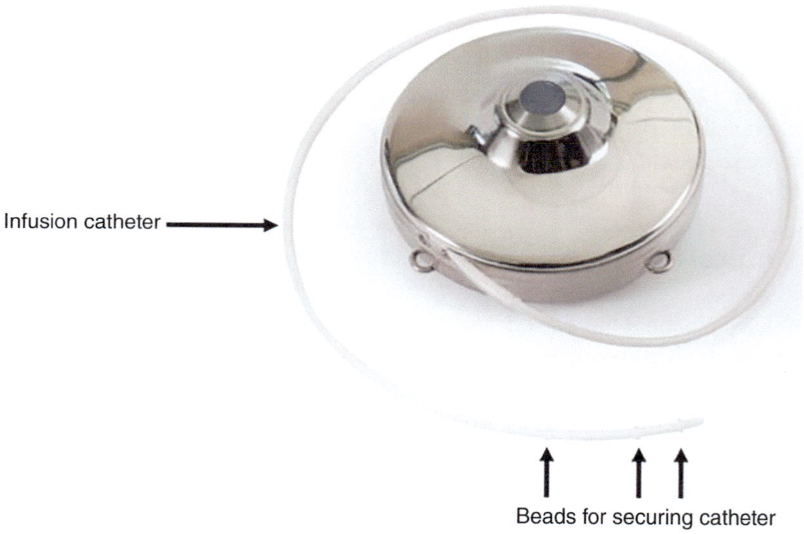

Fig. 5.2 Hepatic artery infusion pump. (Courtesy of Intera Oncology Inc., Wellesley, MA)

ogous saphenous or gonadal vein grafts, synthetic grafts, or native branches (e.g., common hepatic artery or splenic artery) used as conduits [5–7]. While the use of these techniques is described with successful perfusion for HAIP therapy, catheter placement in the GDA remains the preferred technique, as cannulation of vessels other than the GDA is associated with an increased risk of pump-related complications and failure [8].

Aside from assessment of the GDA, delineation of aberrant hepatic arterial anatomy is important as failure to adequately address accessory or replaced vessels can result in incomplete perfusion to both hepatic lobes. Variant hepatic arterial anatomy is seen in 30–50% of patients and may present as an accessory or replaced vessels with ten different categorized variants ([9, 10]). The most common variants include a replaced or accessory left hepatic artery arising from the celiac or left gastric artery (15–20%) (Fig. 5.3a) or a replaced/accessory right hepatic artery arising from the superior mesenteric artery (3–8%)

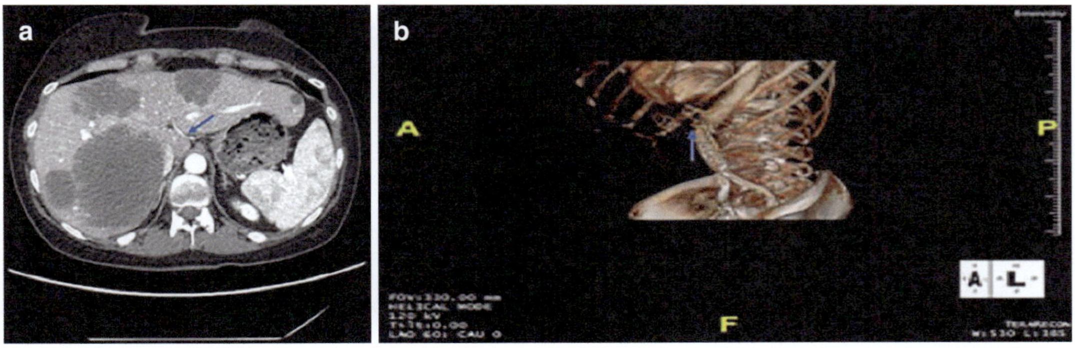

Fig. 5.3 Computed tomography angiography demonstrating variant hepatic arterial anatomy: (**a**) replaced left hepatic artery arising from the left gastric artery (arrow) and (**b**) replaced right hepatic artery arising from the superior mesenteric artery (arrow)

(Fig. 5.3b). Aberrant or accessory hepatic arterial vasculature may be intraoperatively ligated or embolized postoperatively to reduce competitive intrahepatic flow ensuring bilobar hepatic perfusion via intraparenchymal and hilar cross-perfusion between the left and right hepatic arterial systems. Ligation of accessory or replaced hepatic arterial branches is preferred and generally well tolerated especially in patients without underlying liver dysfunction. Embolization should be considered in the context of a major hepatic resection if there are concerns for impairing the future liver remnant.

Final Considerations

HAIP therapy requires careful adherence to a rigorous follow-up schedule at least every 2 weeks for regular refilling and proper maintenance of the pump, as well as appointments for clinical exams, laboratory screenings, and radiographic assessments to monitor for disease response and treatment-related complications [11–14]. The preoperative evaluation should include a candid discussion with the patient regarding the medical and logistical requirements of HAIP therapy; concern regarding treatment and schedule adherence may be an additional contraindication to successful HAIP therapy. Access to a medical oncologist with experience administering HAIP therapy as well as an institution with the infrastructure (appropriately trained surgeons, interventional radiology, nuclear medicine, gastroenterology, and diagnostic radiology) to manage the HAIP postoperatively is also paramount to successful HAIP placement and subsequent therapy administration.

References

1. Skitzki JJ, Chang AE. Hepatic artery chemotherapy for colorectal liver metastases: technical considerations and review of clinical trials. Surg Oncol. 2002;11(3):123–35. https://doi.org/10.1016/s0960-7404(02)00032-4.
2. Cohen AD, Kemeny NE. An update on hepatic arterial infusion chemotherapy for colorectal cancer. Oncologist. 2003;8(6):553–66. https://doi.org/10.1634/theoncologist.8-6-553.
3. Koea JB, Kemeny N. Hepatic artery infusion chemotherapy for metastatic colorectal carcinoma. Semin Surg Oncol. 2000;19(2):125–34. https://doi.org/10.1002/1098-2388(200009)19:2<125::Aid-ssu5>3.0.Co;2-e.
4. Saba L, Mallarini G. Multidetector row CT angiography in the evaluation of the hepatic artery and its anatomical variants. Clin Radiol. 2008;63(3):312–21. https://doi.org/10.1016/j.crad.2007.05.023.
5. Thiels CA, D'Angelica MI. Hepatic artery infusion pumps. J Surg Oncol. 2020;122(1):70–7. https://doi.org/10.1002/jso.25913.
6. Yezhelyev M, Osgood M, Egnatashvili V, Lumsden A, Staley CA, Kooby DA. Saphenous vein graft conduits for insertion of hepatic arterial infusion pumps in patients with abnormal hepatic arterial anatomy. J Surg Oncol. 2008;97(1):85–9. https://doi.org/10.1002/jso.20890.

7. Aust JC. Saphenous vein graft as a conduit for hepatic artery catheters in anomalies of the hepatic arterial system. Surgery. 1986;100(3):581–3.
8. Allen PJ, Nissan A, Picon AI, Kemeny N, Dudrick P, Ben-Porat L, et al. Technical complications and durability of hepatic artery infusion pumps for unresectable colorectal liver metastases: an institutional experience of 544 consecutive cases. J Am Coll Surg. 2005;201(1):57–65. https://doi.org/10.1016/j.jamcollsurg.2005.03.019.
9. Allen PJ, Stojadinovic A, Ben-Porat L, Gonen M, Kooby D, Blumgart L, et al. The management of variant arterial anatomy during hepatic arterial infusion pump placement. Ann Surg Oncol. 2002;9(9):875–80. https://doi.org/10.1007/bf02557524.
10. Michels NA. Newer anatomy of the liver and its variant blood supply and collateral circulation. Am J Surg. 1966;112(3):337–47.
11. Kemeny N, Seiter K, Niedzwiecki D, Chapman D, Sigurdson E, Cohen A, et al. A randomized trial of intrahepatic infusion of fluorodeoxyuridine with dexamethasone versus fluorodeoxyuridine alone in the treatment of metastatic colorectal cancer. Cancer. 1992;69(2):327–34. https://doi.org/10.1002/1097-0142(19920115)69:2<327::aid-cncr2820690209>3.0.co;2-u.
12. Hohn DC, Rayner AA, Economou JS, Ignoffo RJ, Lewis BJ, Stagg RJ. Toxicities and complications of implanted pump hepatic arterial and intravenous floxuridine infusion. Cancer. 1986;57(3):465–70. https://doi.org/10.1002/1097-0142(19860201)57:3<465::aid-cncr2820570311>3.0.co;2-s.
13. Kemeny N, Fata F. Hepatic-arterial chemotherapy. Lancet Oncol. 2001;2(7):418–28. https://doi.org/10.1016/s1470-2045(00)00419-8.
14. Lewis HL, Bloomston M. Hepatic artery Infusional chemotherapy. Surg Clin North Am. 2016;96(2):341–55. https://doi.org/10.1016/j.suc.2015.11.002.

Conduct of Open Hepatic Arterial Infusion Pump Placement

6

Ana L. Gleisner and Ronald P. DeMatteo

Placement of a hepatic artery infusion pump (HAIP) can be performed either as an isolated procedure or in combination with other procedures, such as liver resection or resection of the primary tumor in patients with colorectal liver metastasis. Hepatic arterial blood supply and its relationship with the gastroduodenal artery (GDA) should be determined preoperatively (see Chap. 5) as anatomic variants are common [1] and may require modifications in the technique. In general, the GDA is the vascular conduit of choice.

Preparation of the GDA

The operation can be performed via laparotomy, laparoscopy, or robotic approach. To mitigate the risk of pump or pocket infection, one should consider placing an Ioban drape on the abdominal wall to prevent the pump from contacting the skin or other pathogens during concurrent procedures, such as colectomy. In addition, preoperative intravenous antibiotics are always administered, and some surgeons irrigate the pump pocket with saline containing antibiotics.

Surgery starts with assessment of the entire abdomen for the presence of extrahepatic metastasis, which is typically a contraindication for HAIP placement. Next, the falciform and the round ligaments are ligated to prevent perfusion of the abdominal wall through branches from the hepatic artery. The gastrohepatic ligament is inspected for an accessory or replaced left hepatic artery, which needs to be ligated and divided to ensure bilobar perfusion. Many surgeons will empirically divide the gastrohepatic ligament to the level of the left hepatic vein to remove any competitive flow from occult aberrant arteries that may not have been detected on preoperative imaging. The gallbladder, if present, is removed to avoid chemical cholecystitis from perfusion through the cystic artery [2].

The arterial dissection begins from the patient's left. The hepatic artery lymph node is removed, exposing the common hepatic artery. Dissection then proceeds to the right. The right gastric artery is identified, ligated, and divided. The surgeon may consider ligation of the right gastric artery with ties to avoid vascular clamp malfunction at the time of arterial inflow control

Supplementary Information The online version contains supplementary material available at https://doi.org/10.1007/978-3-031-74935-3_6.

A. L. Gleisner
Division of Surgical Oncology, Department of Surgery, University of Colorado Anschutz Medical Campus, Aurora, CO, USA
e-mail: ana.gleisner@ucdenver.edu

R. P. DeMatteo (✉)
Department of Surgery, Perelman School of Medicine, University of Pennsylvania, Philadelphia, PA, USA
e-mail: Ronald.DeMatteo@pennmedicine.upenn.edu

M. D'Angelica, M. Lidsky (eds.), *Hepatic Arterial Infusion for Malignancy*,
https://doi.org/10.1007/978-3-031-74935-3_6

due to malpositioned clips. Small arterial branches are ligated and divided as the dissection continues along the common and proper hepatic arteries, as well as along the gastroduodenal artery. All soft tissue and non-hepatic branches are cleared for at least 2 cm in each direction from the origin of the GDA [3] between the hepatic artery and the GDA and the portal vein and bile duct. The tissue between the proper hepatic artery and left aspect of the common bile duct is removed by dissecting parallel to the bile duct, while balancing the risk of biliary injury with extrahepatic perfusion, with avoidance of the former as the priority. There are often small veins in this location that need to be clipped or ligated. The dissection should be carried posteriorly to identify the portal vein. Small branches of the GDA to the duodenum and pancreatic head, such as the supraduodenal artery, are carefully ligated with nonabsorbable ties, avoiding narrowing of the GDA, and then divided. In particular, the posterior superior pancreaticoduodenal artery arises from the GDA at the 7 o'clock position, about 2 cm from the GDA origin. It is ligated but does not necessarily need to be divided. A partial Kocher maneuver of the first and second portions of the duodenum allows a thorough inspection of the duodenum and pancreatic head and may further decrease the risk of extrahepatic perfusion (EHP), as the lateral portocaval nodal chain is disrupted. Although not required, we typically remove the low-lying nodes which are lateral to the bile duct and contact the pancreas in the portacaval space. These nodes can light up on postoperative perfusion studies leading to confusion and may also harbor small branches to the duodenum. The GDA is circumferentially dissected to free a length that ideally permits at two beads of the pump catheter to be positioned within the artery, although the insertion of a single bead may only be possible and that is all that is required for safe catheter placement (Fig. 6.1). The actual length of the GDA that can be cleared varies among patients. Manipulation of the GDA often induces vasospasm. Therefore, during the creation of the pump pocket, papaverine (with or without a corner of a soaked gauze pad) is placed onto the GDA to induce vasodilation.

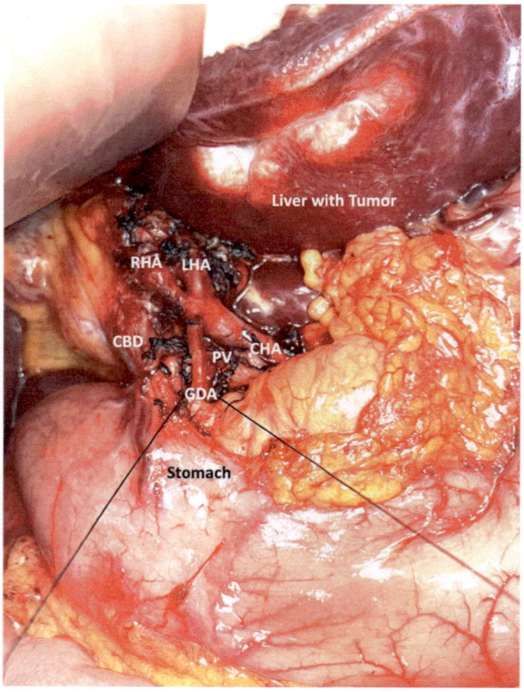

Fig. 6.1 Preparation of the GDA. In this patient with a trifurcation of the hepatic artery, the common (CHA), left (LHA), and right (RHA) hepatic arteries are dissected for at least 1–2 cm from the origin of the GDA, with removal of the lymphatic tissue and ligation and division of all small arterial branches to the duodenum and head of the pancreas. The GDA is circumferentially dissected distally 2–3 cm to the superior border of the pancreas. Care is taken to avoid injury to the common bile duct

Creation of the Pump Pocket

The subcutaneous pump pocket is typically created in the left hemiabdomen for several reasons: (1) future Kocher incisions are unobstructed; (2) negative consequences of pump artifact limiting liver imaging are minimized; and (3) the catheter can then be positioned underneath the left liver, protecting it from inadvertent disruption at the time of future exploration. However, the pump pocket location can be adjusted according to patient characteristics, such as obesity or the presence of an ostomy. In obese patients, a deep subcutaneous pocket is associated with catheter displacement and pump migration (e.g., flipping) as well as difficulties in accessing the pump reservoir. In these situations, the pump can be placed in the left anterior chest wall, although this is

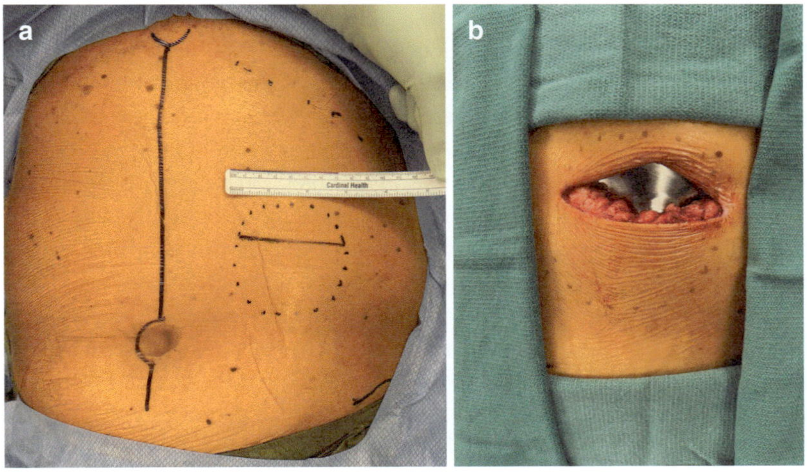

Fig. 6.2 Creation of the pump pocket. (**a**) The subcutaneous pocket is created in the left hemiabdomen, situated between the anterior superior iliac spine and costal margin. (**a**, **b**) The incision is made in the upper third of the planned pocket to avoid cannulating the pump through the pocket incision. The catheter is positioned behind the device to prevent a needle injury during percutaneous access

rarely needed. Placement of a polypropylene mesh can also be used to anchor a pump at risk of displacement, and fat debridement can be performed if the pump cannot be easily palpated [4]. The pocket should be positioned to avoid contact of the pump with the anterior superior iliac spine and the lower ribs (Fig. 6.2a). A transverse incision approximately 7 cm in length is made in the upper portion of the planned subcutaneous pocket so that the access site in the center of the pump is away from the incision. The incision is carried through the subcutaneous tissue until the anterior rectus sheath is identified. Flaps are created to fit the pump snuggly to minimize seroma formation and pump dislodgement. Care must be taken to avoid communication of the pump pocket with the laparotomy incision (if present). It is common to encounter a few small veins that exit the fascia and enter the subcutaneous fat. These vessels can be ligated and divided or cauterized. The catheter is tunneled through the abdominal wall into the abdominal cavity, minimizing the size of the passage through the abdominal wall to avoid postoperative bleeding from the muscle. The catheter should be positioned directly behind the device to prevent a needle injury when the pump is accessed percutaneously (Fig. 6.2). The pump is secured to the fascia in four quadrants with nonabsorbable sutures placed through the eyelets of the pump. Care should be taken to avoid passing the needle through the rectus muscle or in thin patients transabdominally into the abdomen. Once the pump has been secured, fat debridement can facilitate pump access, but excessive debridement increases the risk of seroma formation. Generally, all that is needed is resection of a quarter-sized portion of Scarpa's fascia over the pump access point and then the remaining fat can be morcellated to the level of the skin by pinching it. The pump is then accessed and flushed to make sure that the catheter is not kinked within the pump pocket.

Cannulation of the GDA

The pump catheter has three beads near the end. The last two beads are 1 cm apart. The catheter is cut with a straight or curved scissor to create a bevel immediately beyond the terminal bead. The GDA should be test-clamped to confirm pulsatile flow in the proper hepatic artery to rule out celiac stenosis and reversed flow through the GDA. However, reversed flow is typically suspected on preoperative imaging or intraoperatively if the GDA is unusually large in caliber. The GDA is ligated as far distally as possible with a 2-0 silk tie and the tie is subsequently used for traction while inserting the catheter. We prefer to place a clip in this location to further mitigate retrograde perfusion of chemotherapy to the pancreas or duodenum, and it also serves as a potential marker for future radiologic studies of the pump catheter. Proximal vascular control is then obtained through one of several common approaches. The authors prefer to use a blue vessel loop to lift up the GDA origin and then place a soft, plastic bulldog clamp to occlude flow. Alternatively, bulldog clamps are applied to the hepatic artery proximal and distal to the GDA origin. Metal clamps, including bulldog clamps and vascular clamps (e.g., Satinsky clamps) can also be used. Nearly any form of vascular control is reasonable to consider however rough clamps that may injure the artery (and theoretically increase the risk of dissection) should be avoided (Fig. 6.3a).

A transverse arteriotomy is created using a #11 blade as far distal in the GDA as possible, 2–3 mm cephalad to the silk ligature on the distal GDA. This may have to be altered depending on the width of the GDA at that level. About one-third but no more than one-half of the anterior artery should be incised to avoid complete disruption of the intima which would result in a dissection when inserting the catheter. The pump catheter is inserted into the GDA with the aid of a vein pick, avoiding disruption of the intima. Dilating the arteriotomy with a mosquito clamp prior to using the vein pick can be considered. The tip of the catheter is positioned at the junction of the common hepatic artery and the GDA. At least one bead needs to be located completely within the vessel. Positioning of the catheter tip into the lumen of the hepatic artery should be avoided since it may result in turbulent flow and thrombosis. On the other hand, if the catheter tip is left within the GDA, there can be pooling of the infused drug, which can result in arteritis. The catheter is then secured with a 2-0 silk suture just proximal to the terminal bead (never between the terminal bead and beveled tip). The vascular clamp(s) is removed and the catheter is gently flushed with heparinized saline (100 U/ml). Injection into the catheter is accomplished according to the pump being utilized. At least two 2-0 silk ties are serially placed around the GDA for additional security, one of which is just

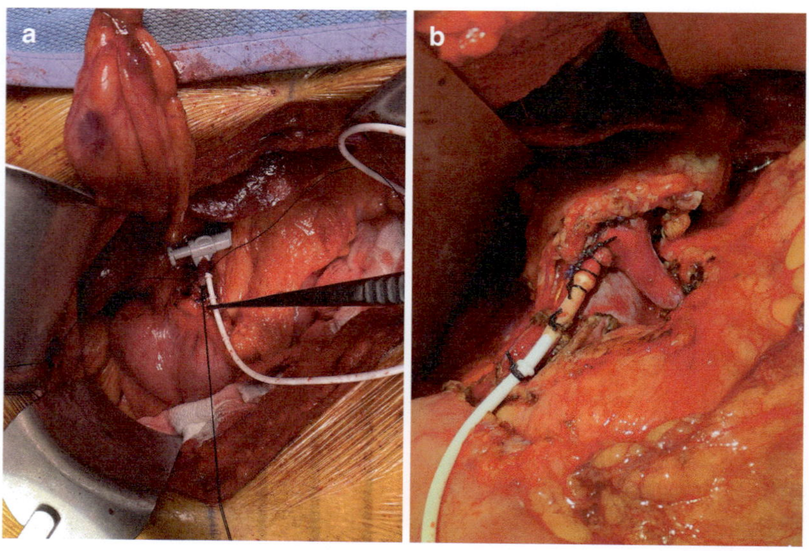

Fig. 6.3 Cannulation of the GDA. (**a**) Bulldog clamps are applied to the common and proper hepatic arteries for inflow control. The beaded silastic catheter with a beveled tip is inserted through a small distal GDA transverse arteriotomy and positioned such that the tip terminates at the junction of the common hepatic artery and the GDA. (**b**) A series of nonabsorbable ties are used to secure the catheter in place. The beads on the catheter prevent catheter dislodgement, and no ties should be placed distal to the terminal bead

distal to the second bead, with the catheter being flushed following each tie to identify inadvertent occlusion of the catheter (Fig. 6.3b). Almost never can all three catheter ridges be placed inside the GDA.

Intraoperative Perfusion Assessment

Once the catheter is positioned and secured, bilateral perfusion of the liver and absence of EHP is established by slowly injecting 2–3 mL of undiluted methylene blue into the pump (Fig. 6.4a). Rapid or forceful injection should be avoided since it may result in a false-positive study due to retrograde flow into the common hepatic artery, hemilobar perfusion, and/or arterial injury or catheter dislodgement. To mitigate these risks, the authors recommend using syringes that are no smaller than 3 mL, but ideally 5–10 mL. It may take a few minutes to appreciate the blue discoloration of the liver. Typically, the liver perfusion is not uniform, but it should at least be bilateral and extend to all segments of the liver. Otherwise, there may be a missed accessory or replaced hepatic artery, the left hepatic artery may be branching prior to the GDA takeoff, or there may be an arterial dissection. Other dyes such Indocyanine green (ICG) or fluorescein can be used instead or in addition to methylene blue. ICG uptake is established with the use of a fluorescent filter and fluorescein can be visualized with a Wood's ultraviolet lamp. EHP is most commonly seen in the distal stomach, proximal duodenum, and pancreas and results from patent small vessels or lymphatic channels. Often, the culprit structures can be identified as they are stained blue or retain fluorescein or ICG. After ligation and transection of the identified structures, a repeat injection is carried out to reassess the EHP. An alternate dye can be utilized to confirm the absence of EHP if necessary. Rarely a dissection will have occurred and if not noticed will be obvious upon dye infusion: the wall of the artery will become dark blue and will often not perfuse easily into the liver. These are difficult situations and one must consider leaving the catheter to see if the dissection repairs itself over time or replacing the catheter into an alternate conduit branch (see below). Once the perfusion is satisfactory, the catheter is flushed with low dose heparinized saline (100 units/mL) and the wounds are closed. The pump catheter should be placed

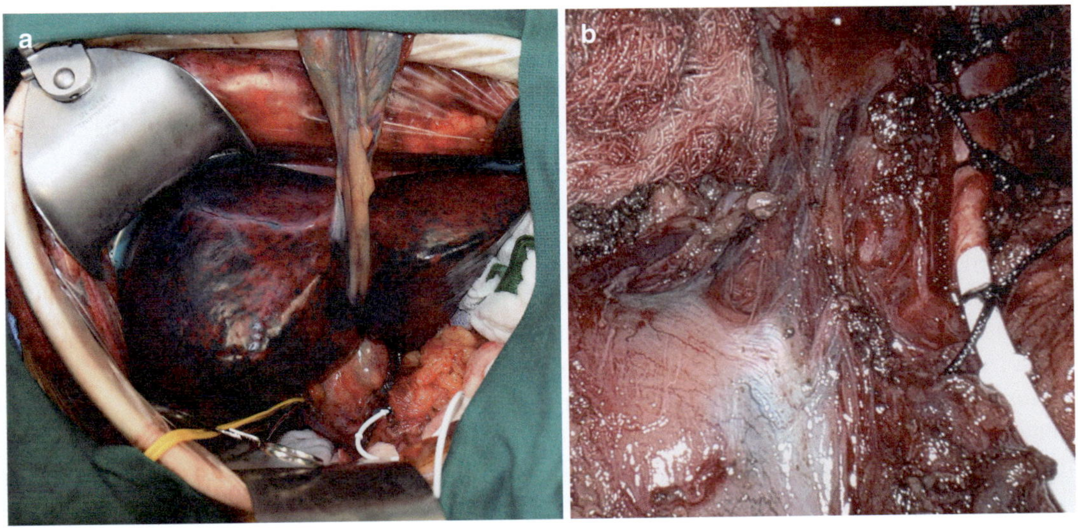

Fig. 6.4 Intraoperative perfusion assessment. The pump is injected slowly with 2–3 mL of undiluted methylene blue to confirm bilateral hepatic perfusion (**a**) and rule out extrahepatic perfusion, indicated by blue discoloration of the duodenal bulb (**b**)

along the lateral abdomen, on the side where the pump was positioned, and tucked under the ipsilateral hemiliver. The pump pocket should be closed before other wounds in three layers. Scarpa's fascia and the deep dermal layer are closed with running or interrupted absorbable suture. The skin is then closed with a running subcuticular stitch and surgical glue.

Pitfalls and Solutions

Variant Arterial Anatomy

The most common arterial variants involve a replaced or accessory right hepatic artery (6–20%) arising from the superior mesenteric artery, followed by a replaced or accessory left hepatic artery (6–10%) that originates from the celiac or left gastric arteries [1, 5, 6]. The GDA origin is typically proximal to both the left and right hepatic arteries, but the GDA can also originate from the right or left hepatic artery or exist in a trifurcation with both arteries (Fig. 6.5).

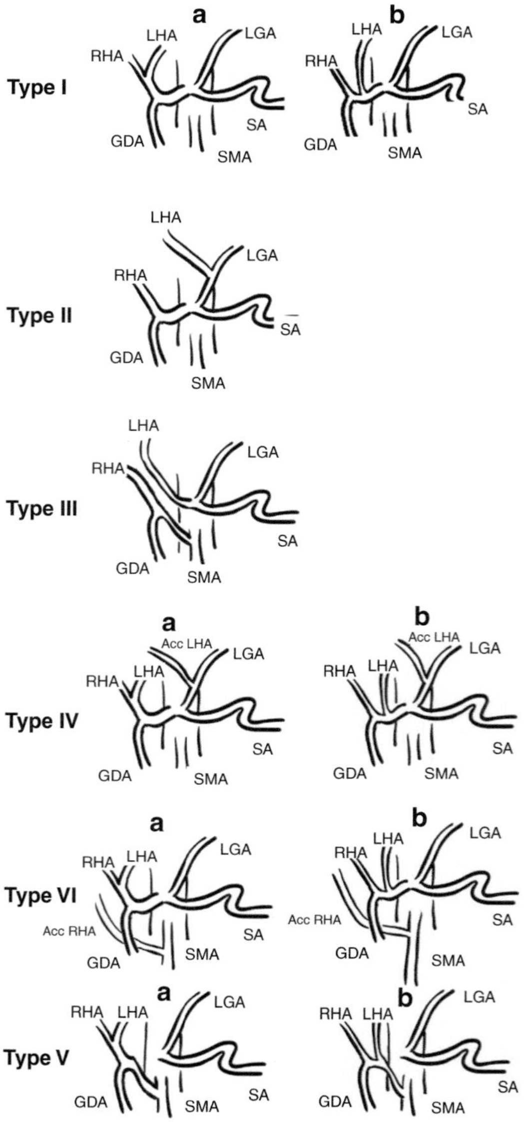

Fig. 6.5 Variations in the hepatic arterial anatomy. The many types of variations in hepatic arterial anatomy are depicted. *CA* celiac axis, *SMA* superior mesenteric artery, *LGA* left gastric artery, *SA* splenic artery, *LHA* left hepatic artery, *RHA* right hepatic artery, *GDA* gastroduodenal artery, *Acc* accessory. (From Daly et al. [1], with permission)

If GDA cannulation is feasible and has inline flow to the liver, this is the artery of choice, even in the presence of anatomic variants. Cannulation of vessels other than the GDA is associated with higher complication rates and decreased patency of the catheter [7]. Replaced or accessory vessels should be routinely ligated to remove competing flow that will result in preferential flow of chemotherapy only to the distribution of the in-line artery (chemotherapy will not perfuse the liver supplied by patent replaced or accessory hepatic arteries). In the same way, if the GDA origin is not proximal to both left and right arteries, the native vessel that is not in line with the GDA (most commonly the left hepatic artery) needs to be ligated to ensure bilateral perfusion of the liver. Prior to ligation, the aberrant or native vessel should be test clamped, and the liver observed for signs of ischemia, which is rare. Perfusion dye testing can also be performed to ensure adequate cross-perfusion. In nearly all cases, perfusion of the liver will be established through intraparenchymal and hilar cross-perfusion between the left and right hepatic arterial systems. The exception may be when there is a large central tumor that interferes with cross-perfusion. Nonetheless, lack of direct perfusion of a hemiliver needs to be taken into consideration when planning a future liver resection. Complete resection of the hemiliver that is being directly perfused is still possible, but may result in ischemia of the liver remnant. It should be stressed that even in the case of multiple accessory/replaced vessels, the GDA with ligation of these aberrant vessels remains the strategy of choice. Lastly, if a pump is being placed at the time of a major liver resection one can consider a delayed angiographic embolization of the accessory/replaced vessel if there are concerns over dividing an arterial branch to a future liver remnant.

Lack of Suitable GDA and Alternate Cannulation Strategies

Although the GDA is the conduit of choice when placing an HAIP catheter, it may not be suitable in some occasions. In these situations, an alternative vessel can be cannulated, although there is a higher risk of complications and lower patency [7, 8]. For instance, in a large single institutional experience, HAIP complications were 41% in patients whose HAIP catheter was placed in a vessel other than the GDA compared to 21% when placed in the GDA [7]. In addition, aside from surgeon experience, placement in a vessel other than the GDA was the only factor associated with HAIP failure. Therefore, before an HAIP is placed in an alternate vessel, the goals, risks, and benefits of intra-arterial treatment should be carefully considered.

Situations in which the GDA cannot be cannulated include:

1. Aberrant anatomy in which the GDA is not in line with the hepatic arterial system (Fig. 6.5).
2. A small GDA that cannot accommodate the beaded catheter, despite the use of vasodilators such as papaverine.
3. A short GDA, despite maximal distal dissection, cannot accommodate the first bead of the catheter without positioning the catheter tip into the lumen of the proper hepatic artery.
4. Arterial dissection during cannulation of the GDA, with absence of liver perfusion.
5. Presence of celiac stenosis resulting in hepatic perfusion through retrograde GDA flow.

In these circumstances, the following alternate cannulation strategies can be considered:

1. Retrograde Cannulation of the Right or Left Hepatic Arteries

   In patients with standard hepatic arterial anatomy, either artery can be utilized for retrograde cannulation. A possible future formal liver resection may dictate which artery should be preferably cannulated. Typically, extensive hilar dissection is required for the mobilization of an adequate length of the vessel. The larger the caliber of a lobar hepatic artery may make securing the catheter with ties more difficult, thereby increasing the risk of catheter dislodgement.
2. Retrograde Catheterization of the Splenic Artery

   The right gastric artery, the left gastric artery (distal to the origin of an aberrant left hepatic artery if present), and the GDA are ligated. The catheter is placed into the splenic artery, which has been ligated distally. The catheter tip is placed at origin of the splenic artery. Because of the presence of rich collateral flow, the splenic artery and the common hepatic artery must be completely dissected so that all small collateral vessels can be identified and ligated and EHP can be prevented. This approach, while feasible, is associated with a significantly higher risk of catheter-related complications.
3. Catheterization of the Common Hepatic Artery

   In patients with celiac stenosis, the first choice is to attempt correction of the stenosis, reestablishing hepatic flow through the hepatic artery. In the case of an arcuate ligament syndrome, this can be done by lysing the ligament. If this is due to atherosclerotic narrowing of the celiac, preoperative dilation/stenting can be considered. If that is not an option, the common hepatic artery can be cannulated directly after proximal ligation, such that the catheter tip is positioned at the bifurcation of the common hepatic artery into the proper hepatic artery and GDA. Both approaches can work effectively.

4. Venous Conduit to the Common Hepatic Artery

   A venous conduit (saphenous vein or the right gonadal vein can be used) is dissected for approximately 6 cm, resected, and placed in saline. The catheter is placed in the conduit with the tip flushed to the proximal end, and the conduit is tied to the catheter with two separate ties. After proximal and distal control of the proper hepatic artery, the vein graft with the catheter secured to it is anastomosed to the artery. Alternatively, the vascular anastomosis can be carried out first and then the catheter placed. This approach should only be considered when there are no other options and the therapy is considered essential.

Incomplete Perfusion or Non-Perfusion

Lack of lobar or segmental perfusion are often the result of competing flow to the liver through an unrecognized patent aberrant artery, such as a replaced or accessory hepatic artery or from a native vessel in the setting of an aberrant origin of the GDA. A high-quality preoperative CT angiogram should identify most if not all physiologically significant arterial variants. If there is incomplete perfusion of the left hemiliver, the gastrohepatic ligament should be inspected again and completely divided to the level of the left hepatic vein to avoid potential flow through an accessory or replaced left hepatic artery. For incomplete perfusion to the right hemiliver, dissection of the lateral aspect of the hepatic hilum should be performed to rule out a replaced or accessory right hepatic artery. If liver perfusion is still not bilateral, other possible causes include migration of the catheter into the left or right hepatic artery or intimal dissection of the GDA or either hepatic artery. If the issue cannot be identified or fixed, postoperative angiography should be performed for further evaluation.

If there are no signs of perfusion of the liver upon slow injection of undiluted methylene blue, another dye, such as ICG or fluorescein, should be utilized. If the dye has been injected appropriately (i.e., in the side port of the Medtronic pump or with the appropriate needle for the Intera pump), possible explanations for lack of perfusion are proximal occlusion, thrombosis or arterial dissection. If there is absence of a pulse in the hepatic artery, the catheter can be removed and the GDA can be inspected for an intimal flap. If a flap is not identified, an attempt to recannulate the GDA is recommended.

References

1. Daly JM, Kemeny N, Oderman P, Botet J. Long-term hepatic arterial infusion chemotherapy. Anatomic considerations, operative technique, and treatment morbidity. Arch Surg. 1984;119(8):936–41.
2. Kemeny MM. The surgical aspects of the totally implantable hepatic artery infusion pump. Arch Surg. 2001;136(3):348–52.
3. Perez DR, Kemeny NE, Brown KT, Gewirtz AN, Paty PB, Jarnagin WR, et al. Angiographic identification of extrahepatic perfusion after hepatic arterial pump placement: implications for surgical prevention. HPB (Oxford). 2014;16(8):744–8.
4. Sharib JM, Creasy JM, Wildman-Tobrine B, Kim C, Uronis H, Hsu SD, et al. Hepatic artery infusion pumps: a surgical toolkit for intraoperative decision-making and management of hepatic artery infusion-specific complications. Ann Surg. 2022;276(6):943–56.
5. Song SY, Chung JW, Yin YH, Jae HJ, Kim HC, Jeon UB, et al. Celiac axis and common hepatic artery variations in 5002 patients: systematic analysis with spiral CT and DSA. Radiology. 2010;255(1):278–88.
6. Noussios G, Dimitriou I, Chatzis I, Katsourakis A. The main anatomic variations of the hepatic artery and their importance in surgical practice: review of the literature. J Clin Med Res. 2017;9(4):248–52.
7. Allen PJ, Nissan A, Picon AI, Kemeny N, Dudrick P, Ben-Porat L, et al. Technical complications and durability of hepatic artery infusion pumps for unresectable colorectal liver metastases: an institutional experience of 544 consecutive cases. J Am Coll Surg. 2005;201(1):57–65.
8. Allen PJ, Stojadinovic A, Ben-Porat L, Gonen M, Kooby D, Blumgart L, et al. The management of variant arterial anatomy during hepatic arterial infusion pump placement. Ann Surg Oncol. 2002;9(9):875–80.

Robotic Approach to Hepatic Arterial Infusion Pump Placement

7

Mengyuan Liu, Mohammad Zaidi, Sabino Zani Jr, and T. Peter Kingham

Synopsis
Robotic hepatic arterial infusion pump placement has several advantages including magnified visualization and enhanced recovery while its complication rates are comparable to the open approach. This chapter describes its indications, considerations, and operative technique.

Introduction

Hepatic arterial infusion chemotherapy (HAIC) has been used as regional treatment for hepatic tumors since the 1970s [1]. In the modern era, indications for HAIC in combination with various systemic therapies continue to expand, such that the placement of hepatic arterial infusion pumps (HAIP) often occurs with simultaneous liver and colon resections [2]. As these procedures grow more complex, minimally invasive and robotic platforms have concurrently evolved to accommodate multistep operations with comparable operative times and safety profiles to open surgery. Laparoscopic HAIP placement was first described in 1995 and was shown to have similar outcomes, operative times, and pump complications as the open approach [3, 4]. Although the laparoscopic approach was a viable method for HAIP placement, early experience with laparoscopy demanded special attention to the hepatic artery vasculature, especially in the setting of variant anatomy. With the introduction of robotic platforms, difficult vascular dissections could be better navigated with articulating instruments and high-definition magnification compared with the laparoscopic method [5]. The first case report of a robotic HAIP placement was described in 2008 using the Da Vinci system [6]. The robotic platform offered three-dimensional visualization that had multiple advantages over laparoscopy, especially when making a controlled arteriotomy and placing delicate intracorporeal sutures around a small vessel.

To date, there are two case series reporting the outcomes of robotic-assisted HAIP placement. Dhir et al. reported a single institution experience of 24 patients who underwent robotic-assisted

Supplementary Information The online version contains supplementary material available at https://doi.org/10.1007/978-3-031-74935-3_7.

M. Liu · T. P. Kingham (✉)
Department of Surgery, Memorial Sloan Kettering Cancer Center, New York, NY, USA
e-mail: lium4@mskcc.org; kinghamP@mskcc.org

M. Zaidi · S. Zani Jr
Department of Surgery, Duke University, Durham, NC, USA
e-mail: mohammad.yahya.zaidi@emory.edu; sabino.zani@duke.edu

M. D'Angelica, M. Lidsky (eds.), *Hepatic Arterial Infusion for Malignancy*,
https://doi.org/10.1007/978-3-031-74935-3_7

HAIP placement for colorectal cancer metastases and intrahepatic cholangiocarcinoma between 2008 and 2015 [5]. In this series, they reported a learning curve of eight cases, after which they observed a steep decline in operative times. This observation, however, was among a limited group of operating surgeons. Qadan et al. subsequently published a single institution case series of 24 patients between 2011 and 2016, 16 of which were for colorectal cancer liver metastases [7]. This second series compared preoperative, operative, and postoperative data between open, laparoscopic and robotic approaches for HAIP patients. Data on the robotic performance from both studies are outlined in Table 7.1.

In the later series from Qadan et al., outcomes from the first half of the observational period were compared to the second half [7]. The median operative time decreased from 282 to 232 min and the median length of stay decreased from 5.5 to 3.5 days. The robotic approach was associated with shorter median lengths of stay compared to the open approach (6.4 vs. 4 days). Selective performance of concomitant hepatic or colorectal surgery and aberrant anatomy identification were shown to be feasible in both series.

Table 7.1 Two case series on robotic hepatic artery infusion pump placement

	Preoperative					Operative				Postoperative		
	Dates	*n*	Indication	Age	Aberrant arterial anatomy	Mean OR time (min)	Mean EBL (mL)	Hepatectomy	Colectomy	Median LOS (days)	Complications Grade 1–2	Complications Grade 3–5
University of Pittsburgh	2008–2016	24	17 (71%) CRCLM	61 (median)	4 (17%)	282	100	6 (25%)	8 (33%)	6	5 (21%)	3 (13%)
MSKCC	2011–2016	24	16 (66%) CRCLM	58 (average)	8 (33%)	297	170	4 (17%)	4 (17%)	4	15 (79%)	4 (21%)

OR operating room, *EBL* estimated blood loss, *LOS* length of stay, *CRLM* colorectal liver metastases

Considerations

Variant hepatic artery anatomy presents particular challenges during robotic-assisted HAIP placement and should routinely be evaluated preoperatively with CT angiography. As with the open approach, the gastroduodenal artery (GDA) is the conduit of choice, and replaced or accessory hepatic arteries are ligated [8]. Difficult vascular dissections involving aberrant hepatic arteries, especially in the setting of prior radiation and surgery can be treated with postoperative embolization if intraoperative ligation is impossible [5]. In instances where the GDA cannot be cannulated or after an intraoperatively recognized arterial dissection, the HAIP catheter can be placed retrograde in either the left or right hepatic artery as cross-perfusion occurs via interlobar collateral vessels. Although these solutions exist for difficult vascular anatomy, it has been reported that cannulation of a vessel other than the GDA and aberrant anatomy are associated with more frequent postoperative pump complications [9]. A relative contraindication to the robotic approach is the need for vascular reconstruction as most robotic surgeons are still gaining familiarity with these techniques.

Given the lower morbidity of the robotic approach, a broader patient population may be considered for HAIP placement. With less surgical trauma and faster recovery times, robotic HAIP placement may be employed in patients with existing comorbidities, although it must be recognized that conversion to open surgery is always a possibility. Furthermore, a robotic approach may be preferable in patients who would benefit from shortened time to initiation of systemic chemotherapy [10]. In addition, for patients undergoing staged procedures with anticipated future hepatectomy, robotic techniques anecdotally limit adhesion formation in the porta hepatis and may facilitate safer subsequent surgery.

When performing concomitant hepatic resection, sequencing of the steps should consider the complexity of the hepatectomy along with the ease of exposing the porta hepatis. For example in major hepatic resections, robotic hepatectomy is usually performed first to allow for resuscitation during HAIP placement as maintaining a low central venous pressure is only necessary during liver parenchymal transection. In other cases, liver retraction is needed to expose the porta hepatis and portal dissection occurs prior to liver resection. It may also be preferable to start with portal dissection as blood loss from hepatectomy may hinder visualization of the porta hepatis later.

If colectomy is planned during the same operation, this is frequently performed after HAIP placement as pump infection rates may be lower if the pump pocket is closed completely prior to bowel surgery. Additionally, robotic HAIP implantation allows for both open and minimally invasive primary colorectal tumor resections, which can limit the wound morbidity, especially for left sided and rectal resections that may require lower midline laparotomy for exposure. Stoma creation may also interfere with trocar placement if preformed prior to HAIP. If the HAIP is placed first, special attention should be paid during the colorectal portion to not dislodge the catheter or inadvertently transect it. Regardless of sequence, during simultaneous colorectal surgery, special care should be taken to protect the pump and the catheter from contamination at all times.

Technique

Positioning and Setup

The patient is placed supine on the operating table on a nonslip pad with both arms tucked and feet secured to a footboard to minimize movement during 20° reverse Trendelenburg. Range of motion of the robotic bed is tested to ensure safety prior to the start of the operation.

Before incision, the ideal pump pocket site is marked to prevent inadvertent placement of a port through the pocket. Typically, the pump is placed in the left hemiabdomen between the costal margin and anterior superior iliac spine along the midclavicular line. A 7 × 7 cm pump pocket is marked with the superior border approximately 2–3 fingerbreadths below the costal margin. The pump is inserted through a transverse incision within this pocket such that two-thirds of the pump lies below the incision. In thin patients, care is taken to mark the pocket with enough space above the anterior superior iliac spine and lateral to the midline. For obese patients, the pocket may be moved superiorly onto the chest wall where the subcutaneous fat layer is thinner to mitigate pump migration or flipping [8].

After safely entering the abdomen, a diagnostic laparoscopy is performed to rule out any extrahepatic disease, which would preclude pump placement. Four robotic ports are placed with one accessory port, sometimes with modifications if a concomitant hepatic or colorectal resection is necessary (Fig. 7.1). The patient is then placed in 20° of reverse Trendelenburg, and the robot is docked from the patient's right for liver cases or from the left for combined colorectal cases, when room setup allows. The liver can be retracted with either a Nathanson or by suspending it from the falciform ligament. Alternatively, the fourth robotic arm can be used to expose the porta hepatis by retracting the gallbladder. Typical robotic instruments used for dissection are the ProGrasp forceps, the hook cautery, and bipolar cautery. Additional robotic instruments include the vessel sealer, metal clip applier, hemolock clip applier, and large suture cut.

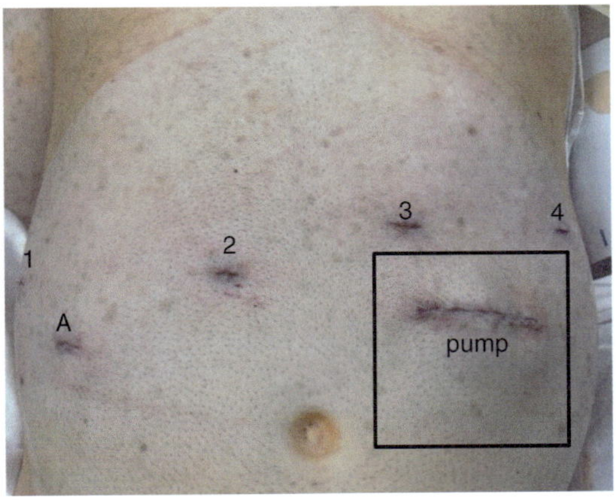

Fig. 7.1 Port placement for robotic hepatic artery infusion pump placement with four ports (1–4), an accessory AirSeal port (A) and the pump pocket highlighted

Procedure

Dissection of the porta hepatis starts with entry into the lesser sac through the pars flaccida and division of the gastrohepatic ligament up to the level of the left hepatic vein. This maneuver will control unrecognized accessor or replaced left hepatic arteries that if missed could result in incomplete hepatic perfusion. Commonly, the right gastric artery is isolated and ligated and the hepatic artery lymph node is removed, providing exposure to the common hepatic artery. The common hepatic artery is dissected and traced to the origin of the GDA. All vessels in the vicinity of the GDA are ligated with silk sutures close to their origin so as not to interfere with the cannulation. The GDA is skeletonized for at least 2 cm distally to maximize length for arteriotomy and four silk ties. Dissection is then carried distally from the proper hepatic artery to its bifurcation until the common bile duct is encountered on the right side. The common hepatic artery, proper hepatic artery, and GDA are freed from collateral branches, including the supraduodenal and superior posterior pancreaticoduodenal arteries and dissected circumferentially to provide adequate space around the vessels to allow for a bulldog clamp. Failure to identify and ligate collateral branches can result in extrahepatic perfusion and need for subsequent angiography and embolization. Accessory or replaced hepatic arteries are also identified but not divided until after cannulation and pump placement.

A cholecystectomy is performed while the pump is prepared, but not fully resected if it is used for retraction purposes (cystic duct and artery can be ligated but gallbladder is otherwise left attached to the cystic plate for retraction). Indocyanine green (ICG) dye may be given intravenously at the start of the case to facilitate identification of biliary structures, though this may negate use of ICG to assess for extrahepatic perfusion. The pump is assembled and primed in the standard fashion. The pump pocket is created with the abdomen desufflated. The pump is anchored to the anterior abdominal fascia with four silk or prolene sutures and the catheter is introduced into the abdomen either bluntly or by using the Seldinger technique with a 10F peel away sheath (Fig. 7.2). Some authors prefer to leave the abdomen insufflated during pocket creation to not undock the robot, but careful attention must be paid to not over dissect the pocket, and the anchoring sutures are not tied down until the end of the case when pneumoperitoneum is evacuated. Prior to cannulation, the bedside assistant ensures all necessary equipment are easily accessible, including silk ties cut to 12 or 15 cm (for multiple uses), bulldog clamps attached to a silk tie, the vein pick attached to a silk tie and the #11-blade attached to a silk tie.

The sequence of cannulation starts with ligating the distal GDA near the pancreatic head with a silk tie reinforced with a small metal clip. Bulldog clamps are placed on the common and proper hepatic arteries as well as on any aberrant hepatic artery. Alternatively, a single curved bulldog clamp can be placed such that it tangentially traverses the hepatic artery and occludes inflow to the GDA. A silk tie is then passed behind the proximal GDA and left untied. An arteriotomy is made in the distal GDA with the #11-blade just proximal to where the vessel is ligated (Fig. 7.3). Other devices such as robotic scissors have been used for the arteriotomy but may have a higher risk of GDA dissection compared to a fresh blade. The blade should either have a long silk tie attached to it so that it remains retrievable even if it goes out of field, or the blade should be removed from the abdomen immediately after its use. A vein pick dilates the arteriotomy and guides the catheter insertion just beyond the second bead. The assistant stabilizes the catheter while the aforementioned silk tie is tied behind the terminal bead. The bulldogs are removed and additional silk sutures are placed just distal to the second bead and between the first and second beads (Fig. 7.2). The pump is flushed after each suture to ensure patency of the catheter.

If not already performed, the pars flacida and falciform ligament are completely transected to reduce collateral flow. Afterwards, methylene blue is slowly instilled through the pump to confirm bilobar liver perfusion and assess extrahepatic perfusion. If the latter is present, the porta hepatis is dissected further to identify persistent

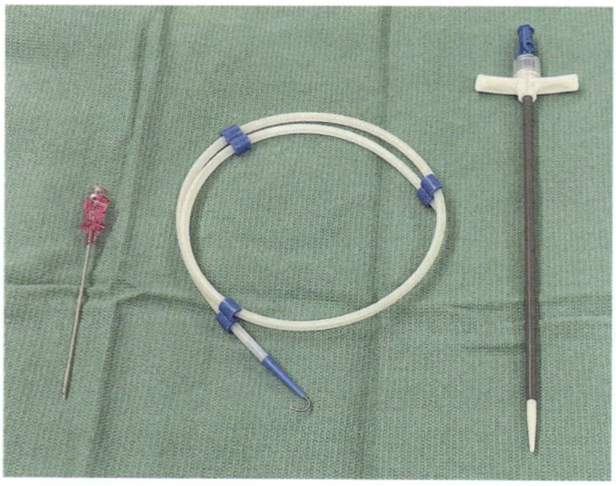

Fig. 7.2 A 10 F peel away sheath used to introduce the hepatic artery infusion pump catheter via the Seldinger technique with introducer needle, guidewire, and peel away sheath (shown from left to right)

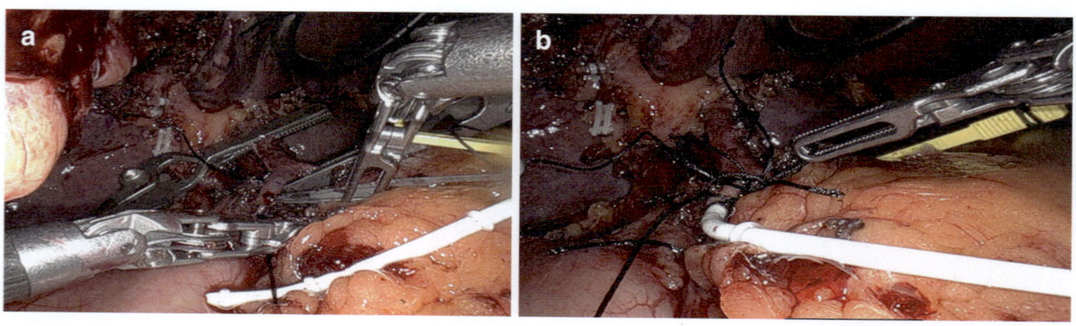

Fig. 7.3 Sequence of cannulation during robotic hepatic artery infusion pump placement. (**a**) After distal GDA ligation and proximal vascular control with bulldog clamps, an 11-blade is used to create a small anterior arteriotomy in the GDA. (**b**) The vein pick is used to facilitate insertion of the beaded tip catheter into the GDA which is subsequently secured with nonabsorbable ties

collaterals. ICG can be used if there are perfusion issues with methylene blue as it is more sensitive. At this time, if the procedure was successful, replaced or accessory hepatic arteries are ligated. The catheter is checked again for adequate redundant length prior to desufflation and port closure. Specimens are removed at the end of the case with an Endocatch bag or can be removed at the completion of concomitant colorectal surgery. If not already done, the four-quadrant anchoring stitches are tied down to secure the pump in the pocket. The pump is then flushed once more with low-dose heparin (100 units/mL) for patency before closing the pocket.

Conversion from robotic to open is uncommon, with reported at rates of 4–17% [3, 5]. It is difficult to distinguish between those conversions that occur due to concomitant surgery and those from HAIP pump placement. Pump complications also occur at similar rates as the open approach and include hematomas, arterial thrombosis, arterial dissection, and biliary sclerosis.

Postoperative Care

Patients can undergo a nuclear medicine scan to assess for extrahepatic perfusion as early as the first postoperative day. Recovery largely depends on the concomitant surgery and most patients can be safely discharged once their pain is well controlled, usually as early as postoperative day two although some patients may reach all milestones on postoperative day one. Recent data shows a trend towards decreased length of stay from 5.5 to 3.5 days [7].

Conclusion

Robotic HAIP placement can be safely performed, even in the setting of aberrant anatomy and concomitant liver or colorectal surgery. Advantages to this minimally invasive approach include faster recovery and decreased length of stay.

References

1. Daly JM, et al. Long-term hepatic arterial infusion chemotherapy. Anatomic considerations, operative technique, and treatment morbidity. Arch Surg. 1984;119(8):936–41.
2. Creasy JM, et al. Implementation of a hepatic artery infusion program: initial patient selection and perioperative outcomes of concurrent hepatic artery infusion and systemic chemotherapy for colorectal liver metastases. Ann Surg Oncol. 2020;27(13):5086–95.
3. Franklin MNR Jr, Stubbs R. Laparoscopic approach for regional hepatic chemotherapy in the treatment of primary or metastatic malignancy. In: Minimal access surgical oncology; 1995. p. 153–7.
4. Franklin ME Jr, Gonzalez JJ Jr. Laparoscopic placement of hepatic artery catheter for regional chemotherapy infusion: technique, benefits, and complications. Surg Laparosc Endosc Percutan Tech. 2002;12(6):398–407.
5. Dhir M, et al. Robotic assisted placement of hepatic artery infusion pump is a safe and feasible approach. J Surg Oncol. 2016;114(3):342–7.
6. Hellan M, Pigazzi A. Robotic-assisted placement of a hepatic artery infusion catheter for regional chemotherapy. Surg Endosc. 2008;22(2):548–51.
7. Qadan M, et al. Robotic hepatic arterial infusion pump placement. HPB (Oxford). 2017;19(5):429–35.
8. Shin PJ, Kingham TP. Minimally invasive approaches to hepatic arterial infusion pump placement in metastatic colorectal cancer. Laparosc Surg. 2019;4:5.
9. Allen PJ, et al. Technical complications and durability of hepatic artery infusion pumps for unresectable colorectal liver metastases: an institutional experience of 544 consecutive cases. J Am Coll Surg. 2005;201(1):57–65.
10. Cercek A, et al. Assessment of hepatic arterial infusion of Floxuridine in combination with systemic gemcitabine and Oxaliplatin in patients with unresectable intrahepatic cholangiocarcinoma: a phase 2 clinical trial. JAMA Oncol. 2020;6(1):60–7.

8 Concurrent Procedures and Perioperative/Postoperative Care

Angela L. Hill, Patrick Grierson, Kian-Huat Lim, Gregory Wilson, Georgios Karagkounis, and Ryan C. Fields

Introduction

Since the 1970s, implantable hepatic artery infusion pumps (HAIPs) have been used for the treatment of intrahepatic malignancy. Since these tumors predominantly derive blood flow from the hepatic artery, whereas liver parenchyma is primarily perfused by the portal vein, hepatic arterial infusion (HAI) can selectively target tumors with increased drug concentrations while limiting systemic exposure and side effects due to high first pass metabolism [1, 2]. Although HAI was initially associated with a high complication rate, the accumulation of technical experience led by Memorial Sloan Kettering Cancer Center (MSKCC) and others has resulted in improved morbidity risk, and this modality has become increasingly popular amongst many high-volume tertiary cancer centers [2–6].

Despite the growing popularity of HAI, details regarding patient selection, optimal timing of HAI and postoperative care have yet to be defined. As such, this chapter reviews the rationale for HAIP use, patient eligibility criteria, surgical timing inclusive of concurrent procedures, and postoperative considerations unique to the HAI patient population.

Oncologic Indications

The indications for HAIP therapy have been primarily focused on colorectal liver metastases (CRLM) in the adjuvant and unresectable settings. Over the last two decades HAIP for intrahepatic cholangiocarcinoma (iCCA) has also been developed in the palliative setting.

Thirty to 60% of patients with colorectal adenocarcinoma will develop liver-only or liver-predominant metastatic disease, and of these, only 10–20% present with resectable tumors [7]. HAIP

A. L. Hill
Division of General Surgery, Department of Surgery, Washington University School of Medicine, St. Louis, MO, USA
e-mail: Angela1@wustl.edu

P. Grierson · K.-H. Lim
Division of Oncology, Department of Medicine, Washington University School of Medicine, St. Louis, MO, USA
e-mail: grierson@wustl.edu; Kian-huat.lim@wustl.edu

G. Wilson
Division of Surgical Oncology, Department of Surgery, University of Cincinnati Medical Center, Cincinnati, OH, USA
e-mail: Wilsong3@ucmail.uc.edu

G. Karagkounis
Department of Surgery, Hepatopancreatobiliary Service, Memorial Sloan Kettering Cancer Center, New York, NY, USA
e-mail: KaragkoG@mskcc.org

R. C. Fields (✉)
Section of Surgical Oncology, Division of General Surgery, Department of Surgery, Washington University School of Medicine, St. Louis, MO, USA
e-mail: rcfields@wustl.edu

M. D'Angelica, M. Lidsky (eds.), *Hepatic Arterial Infusion for Malignancy*,
https://doi.org/10.1007/978-3-031-74935-3_8

therapy has been shown to be effective in this patient population, as adjuvant therapy following definitive resection, as a bridge to resection, or to palliate or control incurable disease. Previously, when coadministered with systemic chemotherapy in the adjuvant setting after resection of CRLM, HAIP was associated with an increased median overall survival (OS) by approximately 2 years compared to systemic chemotherapy alone [3, 8, 9]. In patients with unresectable CRLM, the most recent randomized trial comparing HAIP with floxuridine (FUDR) alone versus systemic systemic 5-FU and leucovorin alone demonstrated improved median OS, despite shorter time to extrahepatic progression [10]. This trial suggested the importance of controlling hepatic disease burden to improve survival. Contemporary studies, albeit nonrandomized, have since used concurrent systemic chemotherapy with HAI/FUDR, and have yielded encouraging survival outcomes. In part, the improved overall survival may be due to the high rate of conversion to resection: when combined with systemic chemotherapy, patients with unresectable CRLM treated with HAI achieved 52% conversion to resection in a single contemporary phase 2 study which yielded survival rates similar historical controls with resectable disease at diagnosis [11, 12]. HAIP has also been shown to be effective in chemo-refractory patients, with a 33% response rate amongst highly selected patients with liver-only or liver-predominant metastases who have failed at least three lines of systemic therapy [13].

HAIP has also demonstrated promising results in locally advanced, unresectable intrahepatic cholangiocarcinoma (IHC). HAIP combined with systemic chemotherapy has yielded disease control at 6 months in 84% of patients and was associated with a median OS of 25 months in a single arm phase 2 study [14]. In patients with multifocal IHC, HAIP has also been associated with comparable overall survival compared to resection, suggesting that the poor prognostic feature of multifocality (e.g., intrahepatic metastases) may be appropriately managed with aggressive liver-directed therapy using HAIP chemotherapy, rather than resection of what is considered by most to be biologically unresectable [15]. In several case series, HAI was shown to elicit a high response rate when compared to other locoregional therapies, such as transarterial chemoembolization (TACE) and transarterial radioembolization (TARE) [16]. Although these findings have been documented by several retrospective studies and single arm prospective trials, randomized controlled trials are lacking [17].

Preoperative Considerations

Patients with CRLM or IHC should be assessed for HAI eligibility. In general, patients best suited for HAIP placement are those with normal liver function and no evidence of extrahepatic metastases. HAI can be also considered in highly selected patients with liver dominant disease and minimal extrahepatic disease. Preoperative workup requires basic laboratory tests including complete blood count (CBC) and liver function tests (LFTs). Furthermore, all patients should have dedicated multiphasic cross-sectional imaging of the liver (to include CT angiography of the hepatic arteries) inclusive of the chest and pelvis prior to HAIP placement, which provides critical information about hepatic arterial anatomy and assesses for distant disease [8].

Given that HAIP chemotherapy is administered via the hepatic artery, which in turn perfuses both tumor implants and the biliary system, patients with elevated liver function tests (LFTs) run an increased risk of therapeutic toxicity, resulting in early cessation of treatment. Additionally, toxicity to the liver and biliary tree may have downstream implications for systemic chemotherapy and subsequent liver-directed interventions (e.g., ablation, embolization, hepatectomy, etc.).

Intraoperative Considerations

Concurrent Procedures and Associated Perioperative Care

This section reviews intraoperative considerations a surgeon may face and how concurrent operations may alter operative planning and postoperative care.

Generally, it is recommended that patients undergo any concurrent liver-related operations, such as anatomic or nonanatomic resection and ablations, prior to pump catheter placement. Arterial anatomy should be dissected prior to opening and preparing the pump to ensure proper anatomy and patent vessels, and prior to performing hepatic resections when possible to avoid contaminating dissection planes with blood. The pump should be placed in a pocket in the left hemiabdomen to avoid proximity to future liver-related incisions and to avoid interference with subsequent liver imaging due to artifact. Typically, the pocket is placed subcutaneously such that it avoids contact with the costal margin and anterior superior iliac spine. Occasionally patients present with an abdominal wall that precludes pump placement in the conventional location (e.g., due to prior ostomy placement); in this case, the pump can be placed in the right hemiadomen or on the lower left chest wall.

Pump placement is often performed with concurrent colorectal resection and/or ostomy creation or reversal. In such cases, colorectal resection should be performed after pump placement and pump pocket closure to decrease the risk of pump contamination by enteric fluora. Some surgeons also place skin glue with or without non-adherent air-tight dressings over the glue to provide additional protection from enteric contamination.

Should the patient require an ostomy, it should ideally be placed in the right abdomen to avoid the pump and to again minimize the risk of pump contamination. Alternatively, should the patient require ostomy reversal and concurrent pump placement, pump implantation should be completed first in a site distant from the existing ostomy (contralateral hemiabdomen vs chest wall). In preparing for such a combined case, the ostomy may be oversewn, the surgical site prepped, followed by ostomy draping, reprepping, and finally ioban placement. Despite these measures, concurrent ostomy reversal may theoretically be associated with additional infectious morbidity, though data are lacking.

Incision placement and length will depend on these concurrent operations. For surgeons utilizing an open approach for HAIP implantation, upper midline, right subcostal and right hockey stick incisions all facilitate pump placement. A right hockey stick incision may be best suited for simultaneous liver resection and can also be used for a right colon resection. An upper midline incision can also be used for a simultaneous right-sided colonic resection. For patients requiring concurrent left colon or rectal resection, a larger midline incision is usually necessary. Similarly, surgeons performing pump implantation robotically can often use the same port placement for pump, liver and primary resections; however, undocking and redocking and sometimes additional port placement may be required for concurrent left-sided colorectal resections.

When Should I Perform Primary Tumor Resection?

Asymptomatic primary tumors are often resected at the time of pump placement. Theoretically, this allows for consolidation of remaining disease to the liver as a single site, yet balances the risk and benefit of primary tumor resection at the time of HAIP placement. Furthermore, upfront colorectal resection may decrease the risk of complications attributable to an intact primary tumor, such as bleeding, obstruction and fistulization [18]. Symptomatic primary tumors are routinely resected, or diverted, at the time of HAIP implantation.

Although staging primary and liver resections was originally thought to decrease perioperative risk compared to that of a concurrent colorectal and liver resection, the latter has been found to be safe provided surgeons exercise good judgement. Studies comparing colonic/hepatic resections with simultaneous HAIP placement versus colorectal and/or hepatic resections alone did not find increased postoperative risk. One retrospective matched cohort study using a national dataset comparing patients who underwent liver and/or colon resection with or without HAIP placement found no significant differences in mortality or serious morbidity rates (22.7% versus 26.0%, respectively), as well as no differences in wound complications (13.7% versus 10.6%) and infectious complications (15.0% versus 14.6%), suggesting the liver and colorectal components of these operations drive morbidity and mortality, not pump placement [19]. Similarly, institutional level data comparing patients who had HAIP placement alone versus combined pump placement and primary colorectal resection suggest rates of general postoperative and pump-specific complications to be similar between groups, including infectious complications, and importantly concurrent colorectal resection does not delay time to initiate HAI or systemic chemotherapy postoperatively [18, 20].

Despite an acceptable safety profile with pump implantation and concurrent colorectal resection, primary tumor resection may not be necessary in all patients. Unresectable, asymptomatic rectal tumors can be closely monitored, especially in the era of organ preservation with multimodal therapy (chemotherapy and radiation), which is often preferable—when feasible—to major operations such as low anterior resection (LAR) and abdominal perineal resection (APR). It should also be noted that in patients with unresectable CRLM broadly, primary tumor resection does not improve overall survival. However, it is unclear if such data extend to patients with unresectable CRLM treated with HAI [18]. Although it is common practice to resect the primary tumor in patients receiving HAI, the decision to resect the primary tumor remains nuanced, highlighting the need for optimizing patient selection based on symptoms attributed to the primary tumor, the magnitude and risk of resection that may derail initiation of HAI, and input and expertise from a multidisciplinary team.

When Should I Resect Liver Disease and What Can I Expect?

HAI can facilitate resection both in patients who are initially deemed unresectable or potentially resectable (Fig. 8.1). Specific to patients with potentially resectable CRLM, surgeons may opt for a two-stage hepatectomy (TSH) approach, which typically entails two partial hepatectomies separated in time, often by interval chemotherapy, which may include HAI chemotherapy, and portal vein embolization-induced liver remnant hypertrophy. Patients who are not considered resectable upfront, even with TSH, may become resectable after HAIP chemotherapy. In patients requiring a TSH, the future liver remnant is usually the lobe with lesser disease burden, which is cleared during the first operation, leaving the metastases in the more diseased lobe to be cleared at the time of the second and definitive resection [21]. TSH can be performed with a number of nuanced strategies, including the sequential timing of the first and second hepatectomy (short versus long interval between stages) and whether chemotherapy is utilized in between these stages [22]. HAI chemotherapy can be used in such patients; when HAI is used in this fashion, the pump is implanted at the time of the first stage hepatectomy, and the primary tumor, if present, should also be resected during the first operation, unless the primary is a rectal cancer that is either asymptomatic or well controlled with chemoradiation. In general, primary resection avoids the added risk and complexity at the time of the second stage resection which oftentimes requires major hepatectomy. HAI as a bridge to TSH provides three theoretical benefits: (1) decreases the likelihood of hepatic progression, especially in the remnant; (2) may downstage remaining disease to facilitate a parenchymal preserving operation at the second stage; and (3) provides a 2–3+ month window to ensure there is no extrahepatic progression. This extended duration between staged liver resections contrasts what is often a relatively shorter time (often within 4–6 weeks) when TSH requires only portal vein embolization. Depending on the extent of prior HAI, either in the purely unresectable setting or during TSH, additional HAI and/or systemic therapy may be considered after definitive resection, however, the risk of cumulative biliary toxicity must be weighed.

Of note, patients undergoing partial hepatectomy after HAI (e.g., second stage of TSH or after conversion in the initially unresectable patient) may theoretically be at an increased risk for complications. Due to biliary toxicity from intra-arterial FUDR, patients may be at increased

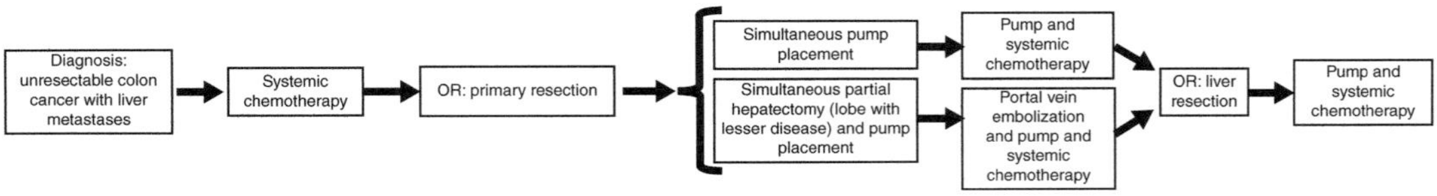

Fig. 8.1 Potential treatment pathway for colorectal cancer with liver metastases

risk for bile leak, especially if preoperative liver function tests are abnormal (e.g., elevated alkaline phosphatase) and/or imaging shows some degree of biliary dilatation. Additionally, while the normal hepatic parenchyma tolerates HAI relatively well, subclinical hepatic toxicity can occur, especially when compounded by extensive durations of systemic cytotoxic chemotherapy (e.g., irinotecan), resulting in an increased risk of postoperative hepatic insufficiency and hepatic failure.

When Should Ablation Be Performed in HAI Patients?

In the modern era of liver surgery, thermal ablation has become commonplace to facilitate parenchymal preserving operations [23]. Specific to HAI patients, ablation after pump chemotherapy does have a higher risk of biliary complications and biloma [15, 24]. Therefore, the ideal time to ablate is prior to HAI initiation, including at the time of pump implantation. Although a major consideration, HAI is not an absolute contraindication to future ablation; should post-HAI ablation be performed, clinicians should consider smaller ablation zones more peripherally rather than larger ablation zones centrally and avoidance of proximity to any dilated bile ducts.

Perioperative Care: Days Following Pump Implantation Through Discharge

Following HAIP implantation, patients can typically follow an institutionally guided minor liver procedure or colonic resection Enhanced Recovery After Surgery (ERAS) protocol, depending on concurrent operations. Patients should receive daily chemical deep venous thrombosis (DVT) prophylaxis while inpatient, multimodal pain regimens, and gradual diet advancement. As with other abdominal operations, patients are at risk of ileus and PO tolerance should be monitored. While admitted, the pump pocket incision should be monitored closely by the surgical team for any evidence of infection (e.g., increasing erythema, induration and warmth, drainage) or hematoma (e.g., excessive bruising overlying the pump or tracking toward the flank, rapid expansion of the pocket) [25]. Any suspicion of infection is managed with early initiation of antibiotics, but in the event of gross contamination, operative management may be required including washout of the pocket, pump re-siting, or perhaps pump removal [26]. The management of pocket hematomas depends on the severity: small/minor hematomas can be treated conservatively with compression while large/major hematomas require re-exploration to achieve hemostasis and evacuate blood products, thereby alleviating pressure on the skin flaps and reducing any nidus for subsequent infection.

Either prior to discharge or in the outpatient setting, patients should also undergo a nuclear medicine perfusion scan to assess the distribution of pump perfusion. Should there be any evidence of extrahepatic perfusion, this can often be treated with catheter-directed embolization by interventional radiology [27]. Ongoing extrahepatic perfusion can lead to direct toxicity of surrounding organs, resulting in gastrointestinal ulcers, gastroduodenitis, or pancreatitis [28, 29]. Therefore it is critical that such findings are adequately corrected prior to initiation of HAI chemotherapy.

At the time of discharge, the decision for extended duration chemical DVT prophylaxis is an individualized one, contingent on concurrent operations and patient factors increasing the risk for a venous thromboembolic event [26]. Specifically, patients who underwent a combined left-sided resection and were positioned in lithotomy for several hours or those whose operations were long in duration should be considered for extended duration postoperative DVT prophylaxis, contingent on clinician judgment regarding the relative risks of complications, such as pocket hematomas, versus benefits.

Upon discharge, patients should be cautioned to avoid any conditions that may alter the temperature or pressure of the pump, given that such activity may affect the pump flow rate. Activities to avoid include flying in unpressurized planes, scuba diving, applying heating pads to the abdominal wall, and submersing in water hotter than body temperature. Since it is critical that the pump be filled every 2 weeks to ensure patency, appointments for pump filling should be ensured at the time of discharge.

Conclusion

HAI chemotherapy is an effective liver-directed therapy in patients with CRLM and intrahepatic cholangiocarcinoma. Patient selection is critical to optimize the likelihood of benefit from this therapy, which is best achieved in a multidisciplinary setting. Whether HAI is used between staged hepatectomies, as an adjuvant therapy, or purely for palliation, the indication and timing for primary tumor resection and subsequent hepatectomy or ablation hinges on therapeutic response. In select patients, HAI may result in downstaging to definitive resectability with possibility for cure, though surgeons should be prepared for a theoretically increased risk of postoperative morbidity.

References

1. Chaudhry S, Fields RC, Grierson PM, Lim K-H. Combined systemic and hepatic artery infusion pump chemo-therapy as a liver-directed therapy for colorectal liver metastasis-review of literature and case discussion. Cancer. 2021;13(6):1283.
2. Muaddi H, D'Angelica M, Wiseman JT, et al. Safety and feasibility of initiating a hepatic artery infusion pump chemotherapy program for unresectable colorectal liver metastases: a multicenter, retrospective cohort study. J Surg Oncol. 2021;123(1):252–60.
3. Karanicolas PJ, Metrakos P, Chan K, et al. Hepatic arterial infusion pump chemotherapy in the management of colorectal liver metastases: expert consensus statement. Curr Oncol. 2014;21(1):e129.
4. Creasy JM, Napier KJ, Reed SA, et al. Implementation of a hepatic artery infusion program: initial patient selection and perioperative outcomes of concurrent hepatic artery infusion and systemic chemotherapy for colorectal liver metastases. Ann Surg Oncol. 2020;27(13):5086–95.
5. Dhir M, Jones HL, Shuai Y, et al. Hepatic arterial infusion in combination with modern systemic chemotherapy is associated with improved survival compared with modern systemic chemotherapy alone in patients with isolated unresectable colorectal liver metastases: a case–control study. Ann Surg Oncol. 2017;24:150–8.
6. Walker BS, Sutton TL, Eil RL, et al. Conventional hepatic arterial anatomy? Novel findings and insights of a multi-disciplinary hepatic arterial infusion pump program. Am J Surg. 2021;221(6):1188–94.
7. Chapelle N, Matysiak-Budnik T, Douane F, et al. Hepatic arterial infusion in the management of colorectal cancer liver metastasis: current and future perspectives. Dig Liver Dis. 2018;50(3):220–5.
8. Napier KJ, Lidsky ME, James OG, Wildman-Tobriner B. Hepatic arterial infusion pumps: what the radiologist needs to know. Radiographics. 2021;41(3):895–908.
9. Groot Koerkamp B, Sadot E, Kemeny NE, et al. Perioperative hepatic arterial infusion pump chemotherapy is associated with longer survival after resection of colorectal liver metastases: a propensity score analysis. J Clin Oncol. 2017;35:1938.
10. Kemeny NE, Niedzwiecki D, Hollis DR, et al. Hepatic arterial infusion versus systemic therapy for hepatic metastases from colorectal cancer: a randomized trial of efficacy, quality of life, and molecular markers (CALGB 9481). J Clin Oncol. 2006;24(9):1395–403.
11. D'Angelica MI, Correa-Gallego C, Paty PB, et al. Phase II trial of hepatic artery infusional and systemic chemotherapy for patients with unresectable hepatic metastases from colorectal cancer: conversion to resection and long-term outcomes. Ann Surg. 2015;261(2):353.
12. Pak LM, Kemeny NE, Capanu M, et al. Prospective phase II trial of combination hepatic artery infusion and systemic chemotherapy for unresectable colorectal liver metastases: long term results and curative potential. J Surg Oncol. 2018;117(4):634–43.
13. Cercek A, Boucher TM, Gluskin JS, et al. Response rates of hepatic arterial infusion pump therapy in patients with metastatic colorectal cancer liver metastases refractory to all standard chemotherapies. J Surg Oncol. 2016;114(6):655–63.

14. Cercek A, Boerner T, Tan BR, et al. Assessment of hepatic arterial infusion of floxuridine in combination with systemic gemcitabine and oxaliplatin in patients with unresectable intrahepatic cholangiocarcinoma: a phase 2 clinical trial. JAMA Oncol. 2020;6(1):60–7.
15. Franssen S, Soares KC, Jolissaint JS, et al. Comparison of hepatic arterial infusion pump chemotherapy vs resection for patients with multifocal intrahepatic cholangiocarcinoma. JAMA Surg. 2022;157:590.
16. Karanicolas PJ, Ko Y-J. Transarterial therapy for primary liver carcinomas: a crack in the armor? Ann Surg Oncol. 2015;22(13):4111–2.
17. Holster JJ, El Hassnaoui M, Franssen S, et al. Ann Surg Oncol. 2022;29:5528.
18. Turley MC, Moore C, Creasy JM, et al. Combined primary resection with hepatic artery infusion pump implantation is safe for Unresectable colorectal liver metastases. J Gastrointest Surg. 2022;26(4):764–71.
19. Brajcich BC, Bentrem DJ, Yang AD, et al. Short-term risk of performing concurrent procedures with hepatic artery infusion pump placement. Ann Surg Oncol. 2020;27(13):5098–106.
20. Verheij FS, Soares KC, Beets GL, et al. Timing of primary tumor resection in synchronous metastatic colon cancer patients undergoing hepatic arterial infusion pump placement. Ann Surg Oncol. 2022;29(3):2044–51.
21. Chavez MI, Gholami S, Kim BJ, et al. Two-stage hepatectomy for bilateral colorectal liver metastases: a multi-institutional analysis. Ann Surg Oncol. 2021;28(3):1457–65.
22. Cardona K, Donataccio D, Peter Kingham T, et al. Treatment of extensive metastatic colorectal cancer to the liver with systemic and hepatic arterial infusion chemotherapy and two-stage hepatic resection: the role of salvage therapy for recurrent disease. Ann Surg Oncol. 2014;21(3):815–21.
23. Kingham TP, Correa-Gallego C, D'Angelica MI, et al. Hepatic parenchymal preservation surgery: decreasing morbidity and mortality rates in 4,152 resections for malignancy. J Am Coll Surg. 2015;220(4):471–9.
24. Kurilova I, Bendet A, Petre EN, et al. Factors associated with local tumor control and complications after thermal ablation of colorectal cancer liver metastases: a 15-year retrospective cohort study. Clin Colorectal Cancer. 2021;20(2):e82–95.
25. Sharib JM, Creasy JM, Wildman-Tobriner B, et al. Hepatic artery infusion pumps: a surgical toolkit for intraoperative decision-making and management of hepatic artery infusion-specific complications. Ann Surg. 2022;276(6):943–56.
26. Thiels CA, D'Angelica MI. Hepatic artery infusion pumps. J Surg Oncol. 2020;122(1):70–7.
27. Allen PJ, Nissan A, Picon AI, et al. Technical complications and durability of hepatic artery infusion pumps for unresectable colorectal liver metastases: an institutional experience of 544 consecutive cases. J Am Coll Surg. 2005;201(1):57–65.
28. Shi L, Zhao J, Lu Q, et al. Initial hepatic artery infusion and systemic chemotherapy for asymptomatic colorectal cancer with un-resectable liver metastasis. Int J Clin Exp Med. 2015;8(1):1000.
29. Wells JJ, Nostrant TT, Wilson JAP, Gyves JW. Gastroduodenal ulcerations in patients receiving selective hepatic artery infusion chemotherapy. Am J Gastroenterol. 1985;80:425.

9 Hepatic Arterial Infusion Pumps for Malignancy From a Molecular Imaging and Therapy Perspective

Humberto G. Mendoza, Patrick Silveira, Terence Z. Wong, and Heiko Schöder

Introduction

Hepatic arterial infusion pumps (HAIPs) are used for the administration of targeted liver-directed chemotherapy in patients with hepatic metastases from colorectal cancer and intrahepatic cholangiocarcinoma (ICC). Chemotherapy is delivered directly to the liver, thus achieving higher drug concentrations in liver parenchyma. In contrast to selective therapies, such as surgical segmentectomy or interventional radiology-based ablations of liver lesions, chemotherapy administered via HAIPs treats the entire liver parenchyma. While randomized data for ICC are not available, patients with colorectal liver metastases who receive HAIP therapy have been shown to have superior outcomes [1].

In contrast to normal liver parenchyma, for which most of the blood supply is delivered by portal venous circulation, malignant hepatic tumors are preferentially perfused by branches of the hepatic artery. Administration of chemotherapy via HAIP takes advantage of this differential circulation. HAIPs are surgically implanted devices consisting of a subcutaneously placed pump containing a reservoir, which is attached to a catheter that runs through the peritoneal cavity, with the tip implanted into the hepatic arterial system—typically via the gastroduodenal artery. Any agent administered through the HAIP therefore reaches the hepatic arterial circulation (Fig. 9.1).

The HAIP reservoir serves as the entry point for chemotherapy infusion, which then progresses via the catheter and is ultimately delivered to the liver via the proper hepatic artery. Some HAIPs have an additional access port, allowing for bolus injection and delivery of contrast material as well as heparinized saline into the hepatic artery via the implanted catheter. After HAIP placement, but prior to initiation of liver-directed chemotherapy, it needs to be ensured that agents injected into the pump reach the liver parenchyma, and only the liver parenchyma. HAIP chemotherapy is given in high concentration, and distribution to other organs should be avoided. Distribution of chemotherapy can be simulated by the administration of a radiopharmaceutical that is also injected into the HAIP and then gets trapped in the liver. This is performed by the administration of ^{99m}Tc-macroaggregated albumin (^{99m}Tc-MAA) into the HAIP. The particles of this radiopharmaceutical are larger in diameter than capillaries (range, 10–90 μm; mean, 30–50 μm) and cannot permeate the intrahepatic capillary beds. Therefore, these particles

H. G. Mendoza · P. Silveira · H. Schöder (✉)
Molecular Imaging and Therapy Service, Memorial Sloan Kettering Cancer Center, New York, NY, USA
e-mail: schoderh@mskcc.org

T. Z. Wong
Division of Nuclear Medicine and Radiotheranostics, Department of Radiology, Duke University, Durham, NC, USA
e-mail: terence.wong@duke.edu

M. D'Angelica, M. Lidsky (eds.), *Hepatic Arterial Infusion for Malignancy*,
https://doi.org/10.1007/978-3-031-74935-3_9

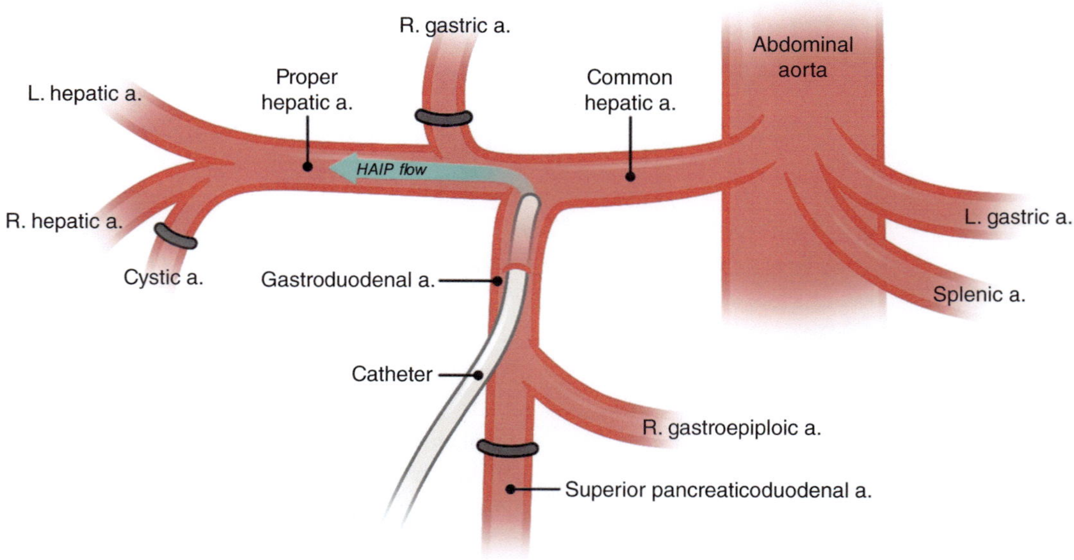

Fig. 9.1 The most common placement of the catheter into the gastroduodenal artery (GDA) in the setting of normal anatomy allows for perfusion of the entire liver without obstructing hepatic artery flow. As part of the surgical procedure, patients undergo cholecystectomy, and the cystic artery as well as any accessory and aberrant hepatic arteries (whose presence is known from pre-surgical contrast enhanced CT imaging) are ligated to prevent extrahepatic perfusion and ensure perfusion to the entire liver

become trapped (for some time, before their breakdown into smaller particles), providing sufficient time for imaging. ^{99m}Tc-MAA therefore serves as a surrogate marker for chemotherapy delivery, to ensure adequate functioning and integrity of the hepatic pump and arterial catheter; to demonstrate that therapy is delivered to the entire liver, and to exclude that chemotherapy reaches other organs. Ideally, the radiopharmaceutical should be distributed homogeneously throughout the entire liver. Of note, the HAIP treatment targets the entire liver, regardless of the sites of metastatic disease. In contrast to other liver-directed therapies, such as ^{90}Y microspheres, radiotracer (and by implication, chemotherapy) should distribute throughout the entire liver parenchyma, not sparing any segments. If certain liver segments are supplied by accessory hepatic vessels, these vessels require intraoperative ligation at the time of pump placement or perioperative embolization prior to HAIP treatment, which will lead to formation of intrahepatic arterial collaterals from the orthotopic hepatic artery circulation.

Today, images of the ^{99m}Tc-MAA distribution are acquired with single photon emission computed tomography/computed tomography (SPECT/CT) cameras. As the name indicates, this method hybridizes two tomographic techniques, for which the camera heads of the SPECT as well as the X-ray tube of the CT rotate around the patient. This initially yields two sets of images—nuclear medicine images showing the distribution of the radiopharmaceutical, and X-ray CT images showing structural anatomic detail. The two datasets are then fused into one, whereby the nuclear medicine images are overlaid on the X-ray CT images (see case examples). As stated before, the radiopharmaceutical should only accumulate in the liver. On fused SPECT/CT images, it is easy to identify sites of undesired extrahepatic perfusion from HAIP-based agent administration, along with their exact location. Prior to widespread availability of SPECT/CT other nuclear medicine techniques were employed; these will be explained in brief below for historical reasons. If extrahepatic perfusion is identified, the vessel(s) through which the radiopharmaceuticals reach those extrahepatic sites will require embolization by an interventional radiology procedure (see cases below) prior to the initiation of HAIP chemotherapy.

MAA

MAA is radiolabeled with the ^{99m}Tc isotope, which has a photon energy of 140 KeV and a physical half-life of 6 h. While the ^{99m}Tc-MAA reported biological half-life varies widely in the literature, a range of 3–6 h has been reported most. The effective dose of ^{99m}Tc-MAA is 2.04 mSv/185 MBq or 0.204 rem/ 5 mCi (calculating for 0% lung shunt in an average 70 kg person). If administered *intravenously*, more than 90% of MAA particles will be trapped in lung capillaries during first pass metabolism, while particles that are less than 10 μg are phagocytosed by the liver and spleen; therefore, this agent is used for the diagnostic nuclear medicine imaging of pulmonary embolism. Although a small portion of systemic capillaries are temporarily occluded by MAA, these radioisotope particles break down over time, then enter systemic circulation and are taken up by the reticuloendothelial system (RES) [2].

In *HAIP studies*, MAA particles are administered into the hepatic artery via the catheter coming from the HAIP. As such, and because MAA particles have a predilection for the RES, these particles first accumulate in the liver, oftentimes with preferential accumulation at sites of metastatic disease. In another liver-directed therapy, the intra-arterial administration of ^{90}Yttrium microspheres, MAA intrahepatic distribution prior to treatment can predict the distribution of such microspheres and help in estimating the radiation dose to hepatic metastases and healthy liver from this therapy [3–5]. Few studies on metastatic colorectal cancer and cholangiocarcinoma and multiple studies on hepatocellular carcinoma have demonstrated a strong relationship between MAA tumor absorbed dose and selective internal radiation therapy efficacy [6–8]. For liver pump therapy, Daly et al. demonstrated MAA activity to be a predictor of metastatic colorectal tumor response to arterially administered chemotherapy in 1985 [9].

Imaging Protocol for HAIP Assessment

Hepatic infusion pump structural and functional perfusion assessments can be performed either on an inpatient basis during the patient's hospitalization for pump placement, or as an outpatient procedure following discharge. The study can usually be completed in 45 min. The subsequent paragraph narrates our protocol for HAIP assessment studies using MAA. Radiotracer is injected into the pump. Since the pump is implanted superficially in the abdominal wall, it can generally be palpated. In some instances, there can be overlying postsurgical edema, which may make it difficult to access the HAIP by palpation. In these more difficult cases, fluoroscopic guidance can be helpful for accessing the pump with the injection needle.

MAA protocol: With the patient on the imaging table, the dome of the access port is localized via palpation. Following aseptic technique, a dedicated bolus needle is utilized to access the pump, which has direct access to the catheter pathway. For patients with larger body habitus or for patients with edema at the surgical site, a longer bolus needle (2″) may need to be utilized for access. Once the bolus needle is inserted, 5 mCi of ^{99m}Tc MAA is injected followed immediately by a 10 cc saline flush. Simultaneously, the dynamic images of the upper abdomen, covering a field of view of about 40 cm are acquired, followed by static images of the injection site at the pump, as well as of the liver. In some cases, e.g., difficult port accesses or if radiologic assistance (fluoroscopy) is utilized to access the port, a test injection of either radiographic contrast or 0.5 mCi ^{99m}Tc pertechnetate is performed via the bolus needle to confirm placement. If successful, with orthograde progression of the radiotracer from the HAIP reservoir to the liver via the catheter system, the full dose of 5 mCi of ^{99m}Tc-MAA is injected to assess the structure and function of the HAIP. On the gamma camera, dynamic images are acquired for 1 min (1 s per frame; low energy/high resolution (LEHR) collimator; energy window of 140 keV ± 15%; matrix 64 × 64 × 16). Dynamic images are then compressed (2:1) and displayed in a 12-zone dynamic format. Subsequently, static images of the liver can be obtained for approximately 5 min (512 × 512 × 16 matrix) in the anterior, posterior, and right lateral projections, with a ^{57}Cobalt point marker placed over the umbilicus and a circular lead marker on the xiphoid process, for anatomic correlation. However, recent technological developments now allow this step to be eliminated. Rather, immediately after the initial dynamic imaging sequence, SPECT/CT images of the upper abdomen may be obtained (low dose CT at about 80 kV, 40 mA, 0.5 s/rot), covering an ~40 cm axial field of view. The effective radiation dose to the patient from the low-dose CT is about 6 mSv.

Image Display, Radiological Analysis, and Reporting

Images are reviewed at a standard nuclear medicine workstation using one of the various commercial software programs. The initial dynamic images are reviewed in a cine loop and should demonstrate rapid progression of injected activity from the pump reservoir, via the pump catheter, into the liver. CT, SPECT, and fused SPECT/CT (color overlay of the radioactivity distribution over the gray level CT images) images are then displayed in the transaxial, coronal, and sagittal projections. Ideally, all the injected radioactivity should only accumulate within the liver. Any extrahepatic activity indicates suboptimal placement of the pump catheter tip and/or the presence of hepatic arterial branches perfusing extrahepatic organs, as shown in the case examples below. Undesired extrahepatic activity can be accurately localized on CT images, allowing for the identification of accessory vessels to be embolized via interventional radiology procedures.

The report generated by a nuclear medicine physician should address the transport of activity from the HAIP to the liver, the possibility of a leak, pattern of intrahepatic tracer distribution (homogeneous versus heterogeneous, as well as possible preferential accumulation in any subsection of the liver), the exact location of any undesired extrahepatic activity (e.g., in the head of pancreas), as well as any incidental CT findings.

Celiac Axis and HAIP Study Patterns of Perfusion

Variations in the Anatomy of the Celiac Trunk

The liver has a dual blood supply. Approximately 75% of physiologic blood flow to the liver parenchyma comes from the portal vein while the other 25% originates from the hepatic artery. Unlike normal hepatic parenchyma, liver malignancies are preferentially perfused by branches of the hepatic artery due to their pathologic sprouting neovasculature, providing the rationale for HAIP therapy [10–12]. In conventional hepatic anatomy, the celiac axis trifurcates from the abdominal aorta at the level of T12, branching into the common hepatic artery, left gastric artery and splenic artery. Variations from conventional celiac axis anatomy can lead to abnormal findings on HAIP studies. Wide ranges in the prevalence of hepatic artery anatomic variations have been reported. Some studies note that variations in celiac axis can be greater than 33% [13–16]. A recent retrospective study evaluating more than 5000 patients who underwent TACE demonstrated an aberrant right and/or left hepatic artery in 36% of patients, while 4.5% of patients had both [17].

Normal and Normal Variant Patterns

Normal perfusion and normal variant perfusion patterns of HAIP perfusion are summarized in Fig. 9.2. Case 1 shows a normal, homogeneous perfusion pattern. However, even in normal liver parenchyma, radiotracer distribution is often somewhat heterogeneous (Cases 2). Moreover, preferential tracer accumulation may be seen at known sites of hepatic metastases (Case 3). Although such lesions may not be discernable on the non-contrast enhanced, low-dose companion CT of the acquired SPECT/CT, their location is usually known from previously obtained contrast enhanced CT or MRI scans. Common findings that do not require any intervention include mild pooling of tracer activity at the catheter tip (Case 4); *low level* tracer activity at the proximal common bile duct (Case 5); tracer uptake within a periportal node (Case 6, medically inconsequential).

Since this imaging study is performed shortly after surgical HAIP placement, postoperative CT findings are expected. These may include pneumoperitoneum proportional to postoperative time interval; subcutaneous emphysema; trace pneumobilia; fluid and/or air in hepatic resection bed(s); small volume ascites (typically perihepatic and in the vicinity of viscera involved during the surgery); hemidiaphragm elevation ipsilateral to surgically manipulated viscera; small pleural effusions with adjacent atelectasis; and occasional postsurgical ileus.

Abnormal Patterns

Abnormal HAIP study findings can be categorized into vascular and nonvascular-related abnormalities (Fig. 9.3). Vascular abnormalities can be further characterized into abnormal intrahepatic or extrahepatic perfusion. Nonvascular-related abnormalities occur due to failure of the catheter and/or pump system.

Abnormal Intrahepatic Perfusion

Metastatic liver disease affects the right lobe more than the left lobe, and most commonly involves segment VI [18, 19]. Multiple studies have reported that the right lobe receives more blood flow from the portal vein, given its larger size and volume, thus providing a possible explanation for the higher incidence of metastatic disease in the right lobe [18, 20, 21]. This may also, in part, be the reason for heterogeneous intrahepatic distribution of tracer administered via HAIP.

While some heterogeneity in intrahepatic radiotracer distribution is a common finding, lack of perfusion to an entire segment should not occur. Such can be the case when liver segments are perfused by accessory vessels not originating from the common hepatic artery. Examples of those vessels include other branches of the celiac trunk, diaphragmatic artery, and superior mesenteric artery (Case 7). These remaining accessory vessels identified on SPECT/CT require embolization prior to HAIP therapy, in order for chemo-

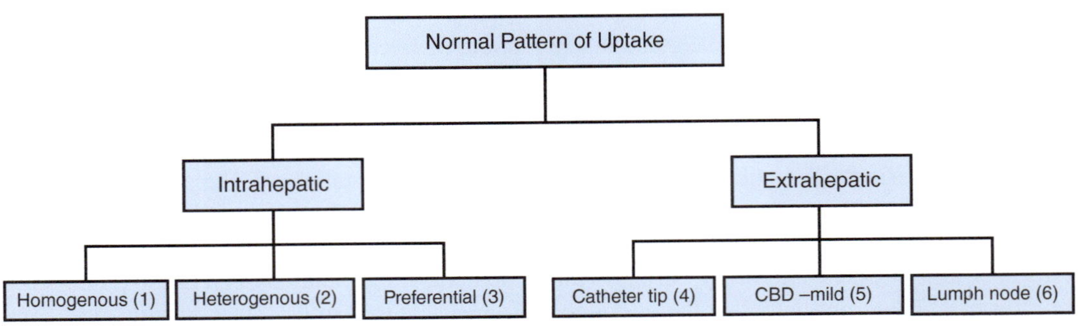

Fig. 9.2 Summary of normal patterns of radiotracer uptake in HAIP studies. Numbers in parenthesis indicate case examples

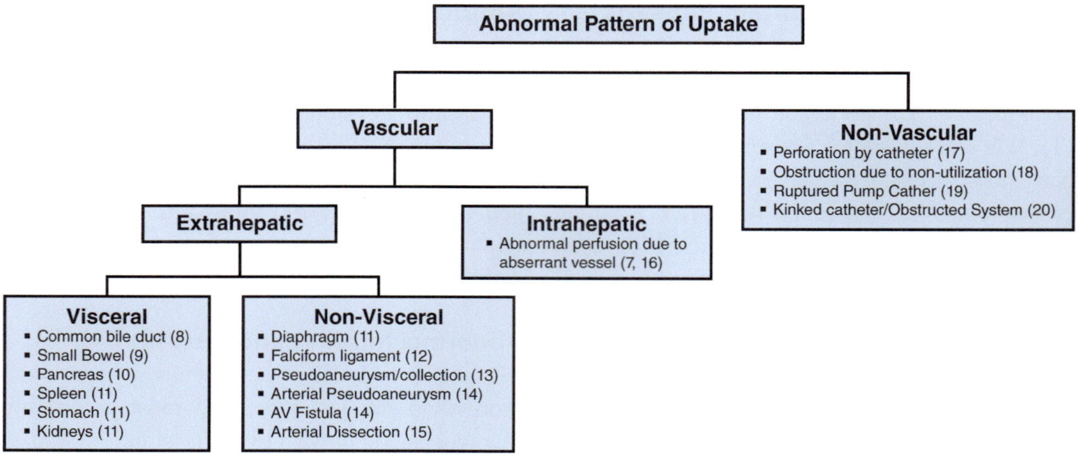

Fig. 9.3 Summary of abnormal patterns of radiotracer uptake in HAIP studies. Numbers in parenthesis indicate case examples

therapy to reach the entire liver parenchyma [2]. Additionally, if accessory or replaced arteries are ligated at the time of HAIP placement there can be related preferential perfusion which usually improves over time.

Extrahepatic Perfusion: Visceral and Non-Visceral

Any extrahepatic perfusion from the HAIP system is abnormal. The most common sites of extrahepatic *visceral* perfusion include *intense* uptake along the common bile duct (Case 8), as well as any uptake in duodenum (Case 9), pancreas (Case 10), stomach (Case 11), spleen (Case 11), and kidneys (Case 11). Such extrahepatic perfusion has been reported to occur in 2–9% of cases [22].

Additionally, extrahepatic *non-visceral* perfusion can be noted. Rarely, skeletal muscle (including diaphragm) perfusion can be seen, usually requiring surgical revision of the catheter tip's placement. Extrahepatic perfusion can also occur via the hepatic falciform artery (Case 12), a vascular variant most commonly arising from the middle hepatic artery. The falciform artery courses anteriorly through the falciform ligament and supplies the supraumbilical region of the abdominal wall. Although some angiographic studies have reported an incidence of 40–50%, this is far less commonly observed in nuclear medicine HAIP imaging studies yet is the justification for empirically dividing the ligamentum teres and falciform ligament during HAIP placement [23, 24]. Occasionally, extrahepatic activity may also be seen adjacent to surgical clips, for instance, from formation of arterial dissection or pseudoaneurysm (Cases 13–15). These may occur in the first few months following HAIP placement and may result in incomplete or nonperfusion of the liver and formation of fluid filled cavities outside the artery.

Patients with extrahepatic perfusion are more likely to develop adverse effects from HAIP chemotherapy at sites where abnormal radiotracer activity is noted [25]. Depending on the site of extrahepatic perfusion, these side effects may include gastritis, enteritis, gastrointestinal ulceration, pancreatitis, and periumbilical soft tissue inflammation associated with pain, skin changes and possibly ulceration.

Patients with extrahepatic perfusion will require embolization of the culprit accessory vessel(s) responsible for extrahepatic radiotracer accumulation, prior to the initiation of HAIP chemotherapy. In a study by Perez et al., the branch responsible for extrahepatic perfusion most commonly arose from the proper hepatic artery, while most other branches originated from the right hepatic artery [26].

Aberrant arteries (not coming from the proper hepatic artery but, for instance, from other branches of the celiac trunk) may perfuse portions of the liver. These aberrant arteries need to be ligated or embolized prior to initiation of HAIP therapy (Case 16), whereupon intrahepatic collaterals will ensure that drugs given through the HAIP will in fact reach the entire liver parenchyma.

HAIP System and CT Imaging Abnormalities

Nonvascular HAIP System Abnormalities

Pump catheters can be occluded, dislodged, or erode the vessels in which they are placed. These complications can commonly present as the lack of fluid return or greater than expected residual volume upon accessing the reservoir, inability to flush the catheter/resistance to flushing, or with pain upon flushing the catheter. Initial decreases in infusion rate are treated with fibrinolytic agents via the catheter. If infusion rate fails to improve, further evaluation and intervention follows, sometimes requiring embolization, stenting, or surgical intervention to salvage the HAIP.

Faulty integrity and mechanical malfunction of the HAIP system includes the following: severed/disconnected/abandoned catheter; flipped external reservoir/pouch of the hepatic arterial pump system within the abdominal wall; perforation of the stomach by the HAIP catheter system (Case 17); and nonfunctioning pump system due to catheter thrombosis after long non-utilization (Case 18). Finally, a discontinuity within the catheter system may lead to extravasation of tracer activity into the peritoneal cavity (Case 19). This requires surgical revision of the entire catheter or removal of the pump. In the case of a kinked or obstructed catheter system, transient or permanent stagnation of tracer activity will be noted on dynamic images (Case 20).

Pump reservoir-related complications such as infection, hematoma, wound dehiscence, and device malpositioning are often discovered on physical exam during outpatient follow-up visits or when the patient presents to have their pump accessed in the nuclear medicine suite. Addressing these complications may only require minor intervention such as antibiotics for infection, incision and drainage for hematomas, wound care for dehiscence, or manual manipulation for a malpositioned (flipped) pump reservoir. However, these complications can become more severe and require more extensive intervention, such as surgical relocation of the pump or even pump removal. When the pump reservoir is removed, the catheter is clipped. The abandoned catheter, without further intraluminal flow, will eventually clot. On subsequent imaging, the location of the abandoned catheter can be in the region of the removed reservoir or anywhere in the peritoneal cavity.

CT Imaging Abnormalities

In addition to molecular imaging findings on SPECT/CT, some CT findings are unexpected and abnormal in the postsurgical period. These abnormal findings include the following: pneumomediastinum, pneumothorax; pneumatosis coli; pneumobilia; bowel herniation, such as through the diaphragm or rectus abdominis musculature; bowel obstruction; and perforated viscus.

Historical Utilization of Sulfur Colloid in HAIP Studies

Historically, before the advent and utilization of SPECT/CT machines, HAIP imaging required a two-part study using ^{99m}Tc sulfur colloid (SC) and ^{99m}Tc-macroaggregated albumin (MAA) and were less accurate. In those days, 1 mCi of ^{99m}Tc SC was administered intravenously to outline relevant anatomic structures: this radiotracer only accumulates within the reticuloendothelial system of the liver and spleen, and in the bone marrow. Planar images of the upper abdomen were acquired in the anterior, posterior and both lateral projections, with a ^{57}Cobalt point marker used to indicate the position of the umbilicus and a circular lead marker on the xiphoid process. ^{99m}Tc-MAA was then injected into the HAIP reservoir and dynamic images were obtained as described above. This was followed by an additional set of planar images. For analysis, four sets of images were reviewed: (a) ^{99m}Tc SC images; (b) ^{99m}Tc-MAA dynamic images; (c) ^{99m}Tc-MAA planar images; (d) overlay of the two static (SC and MAA) image sets. Extrahepatic activity would be recognized by any difference between the MAA and the overlay images. The widespread clinical introduction of SPECT/CT machines has shortened the overall imaging time and has allowed for a more accurate description of extrahepatic activity.

Summary

HAIPs are surgically placed to deliver chemotherapeutic agents directly to liver in the setting of metastatic colorectal cancer and unresectable intrahepatic cholangiocarcinoma, thus maximizing intrahepatic drug concentration while limiting systemic toxicity. After surgical placement and prior to initiation of HAIP-based chemotherapy, imaging studies are performed to confirm distribution of activity throughout the entire liver and a lack of extrahepatic perfusion. Both the SPECT and CT components provide vital information prior to the chemotherapeutic infusion. Nuclear medicine physicians interpreting these imaging studies need to be aware of potential pitfalls and complications of HAIP, including reasons for malfunction and the various sites of undesired extrahepatic perfusion that require embolization of aberrant vessels prior to initiation of chemotherapy.

Cases

Case 1

Normal, relatively homogeneous uptake. A 59-year-old male with metastatic colorectal cancer, status post distant low anterior resection, two-stage liver resection, HAIP placement, and progression of disease refractory to multiple lines of chemotherapy. HAIP study was performed prior to reinitiating pump therapy. Non-contrast axial CT demonstrates (A) postsurgical changes from prior liver resections and the partially visual HAIP catheter passing within the left of midline anterior abdomen. Fused SPECT/CT (B) and anterior planar images (C) demonstrate normal homogenous activity throughout the liver without evidence of extrahepatic perfusion.

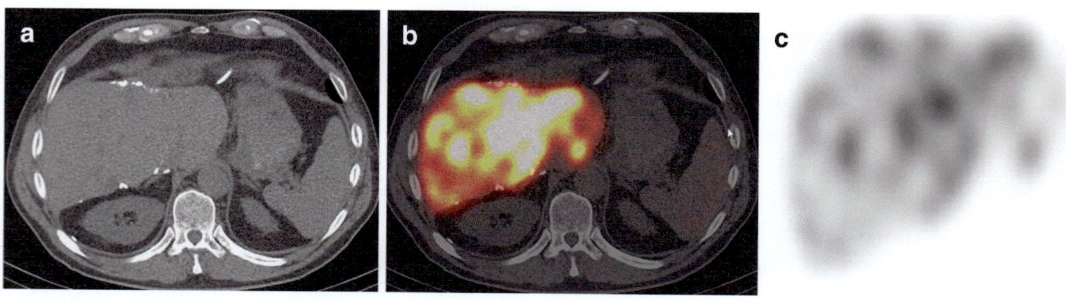

Case 2

Normal, heterogenous tracer distribution with preferential accumulation in the right lobe. A 51-year-old female with metastatic colorectal cancer status post systemic chemotherapy, recent resection of cecal primary, and HAIP placement for unresectable hepatic metastases. Hypodense areas on the non-contrast axial CT image (A) correspond to hepatic metastases. Fused axial SPECT/CT (B) and anterior planar images (C) are also shown. There is no extrahepatic perfusion.

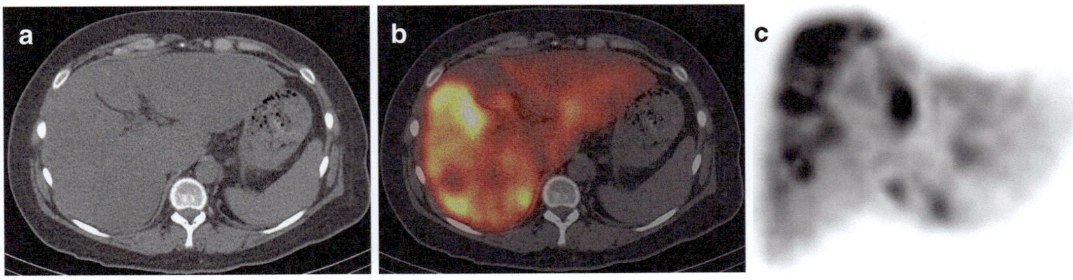

Case 3

Normal, heterogeneous uptake with preferential localization around sites of metastatic disease. A 67-year-old female with metastatic colorectal cancer as seen on non-contrast axial CT (A), status post resection of primary and systemic chemotherapy with progression of disease. HAIP was placed due to unresectable liver metastases. Fused axial SPECT/CT (B) and coronal SPECT images (C) are shown.

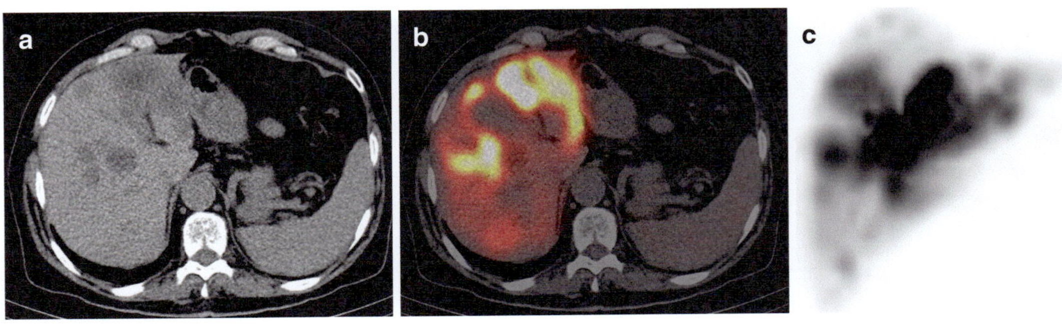

Case 4

Pooling of radiotracer activity at the HAIP catheter tip, a frequent normal radiographic finding. A 37-year-old female with metastatic colorectal cancer with unresectable bilobar hepatic metastases, status post cholecystectomy, systemic chemotherapy, and robotic HAIP placement. Non-contrast axial CT (A) demonstrates the partially visualized HAIP catheter tip (arrow) in the region of porta hepatis, and postsurgical subcutaneous emphysema in the right abdominal wall. Fused axial SPECT/CT images (B) and anterior planar image (C) demonstrate focal activity in the porta hepatis region (arrow). There is relatively homogenous distribution of activity throughout the liver.

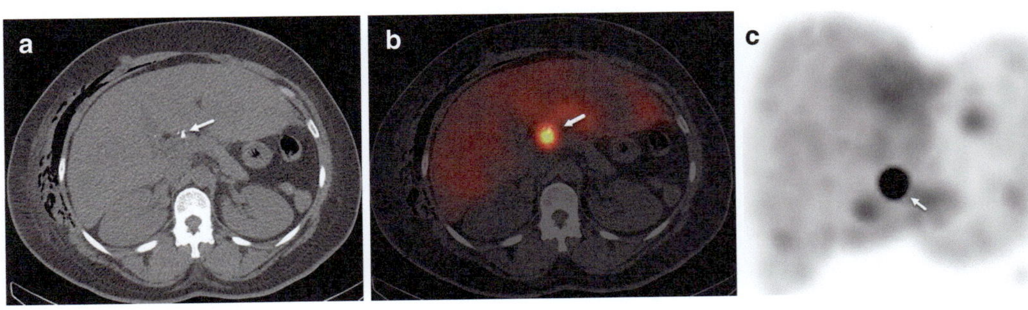

Case 5

Mild activity in the region of the proximal common bile duct (arrow), which can be seen as a normal radiographic finding. A 50-year-old male with metastatic colorectal cancer, status post right hemicolectomy, partial hepatectomy, cholecystectomy, systemic chemotherapy, and recent HAIP placement for unresectable hepatic metastatic disease. Non-contrast axial (A) and coronal (C) CT images demonstrate a partially visualized HAIP catheter terminating in the porta hepatis region. Fused axial (B) and coronal (D) SPECT/CT images, as well as the anterior planar image (E), demonstrate heterogenous activity in the liver in addition to mild activity in the region of the common bile duct (arrow).

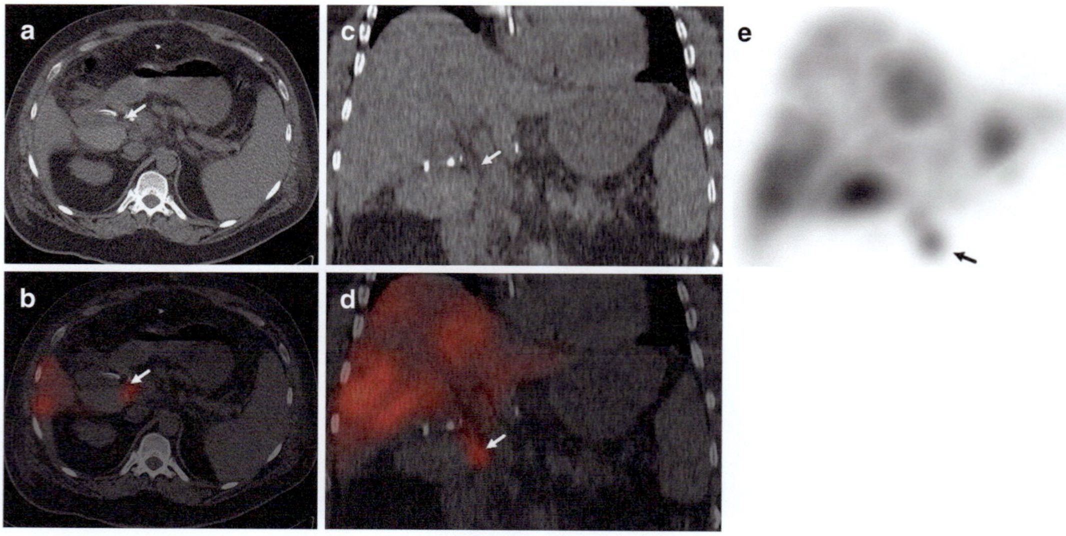

Case 6

Mild tracer uptake in periportal nodes. A 37-year-old female with metastatic colorectal cancer, status post systemic therapy, left hemicolectomy, partial hepatectomy, cholecystectomy, and HAIP placement for unresectable bilobar hepatic metastases. (A) Non-contrast axial CT. (B) Fused SPECT/CT. There is heterogenous activity throughout the liver with focal activity in porta hepatis corresponding to a small lymph node (arrow). This finding is clinically inconsequential and does not require embolization of aberrant vessels prior to initiation of chemotherapy.

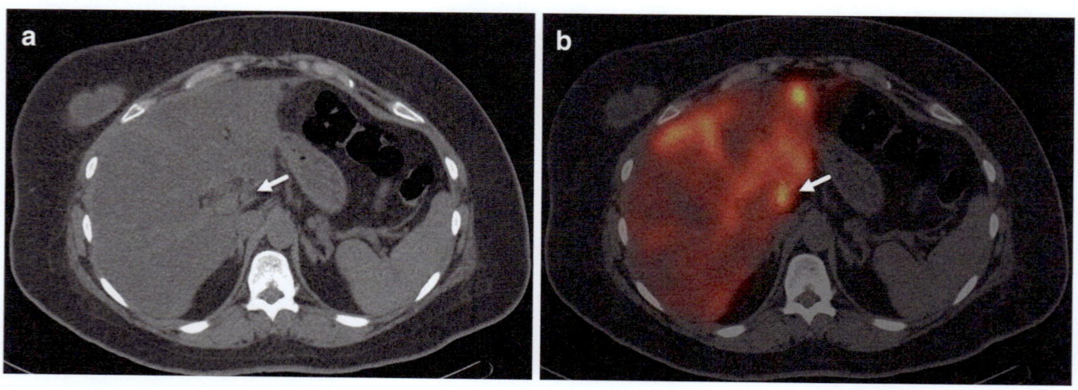

Case 7

Aberrant left hepatic artery resulting in incomplete hepatic perfusion. An 83-year-old female with metastatic colorectal cancer status post partial colectomy, cholecystectomy, multiple liver resections and systemic therapy, with course complicated by treatment-related toxicity. Non-contrast axial CT (A) and fused axial SPECT/CT images (B) depict heterogenous activity in the right lobe with no activity in the left lobe, consistent with an abnormal origin of the left hepatic artery. CT angiography (C) showed an aberrant left hepatic artery arising from the left gastric artery. This vessel needs to be embolized in order to ensure perfusion of chemotherapy to the entire liver parenchyma.

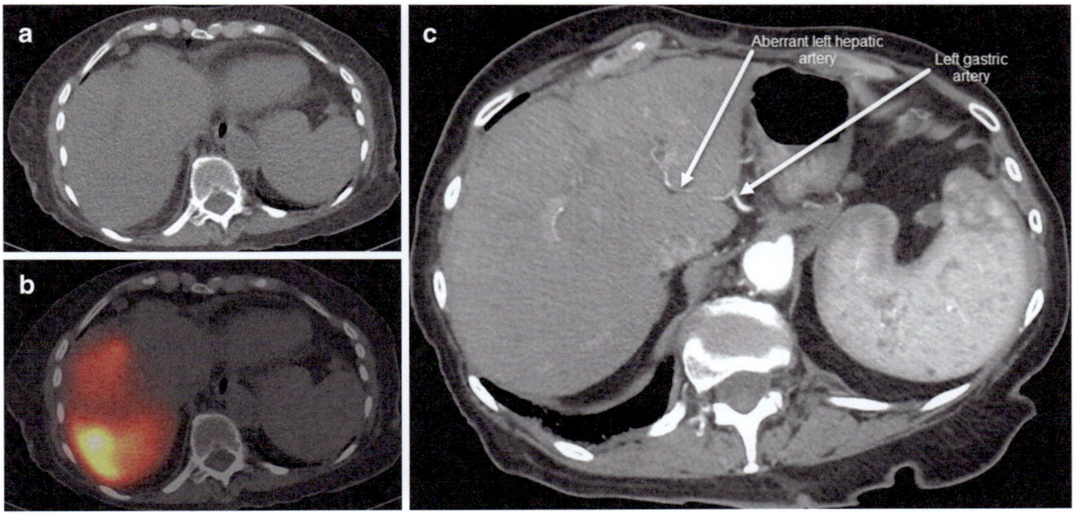

Case 8

Intense abnormal focal activity, with an intensity greater than liver, involving the proximal common bile duct. A 75-year-old male with metastatic colorectal cancer status post systemic chemotherapy, cholecystectomy, and HAIP placement for treatment of unresectable bilobar hepatic metastases. Non-contrast axial (A) and coronal (C) CT images demonstrate a partially visualized HAIP catheter in the right anterior abdomen, as well as small postsurgical pneumoperitoneum. Fused axial (B) and coronal (D) SPECT/CT, in addition to an anterior planar image (E), illustrate homogenous activity in the liver with intense abnormal focal activity, much greater than the liver, involving the common bile duct (arrow).

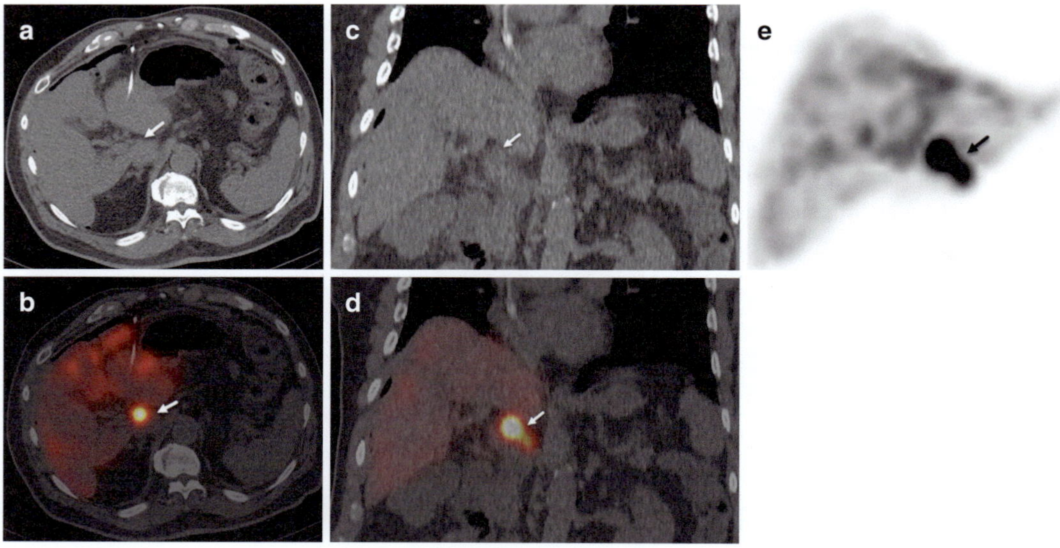

Case 9

Abnormal extrahepatic perfusion to the duodenum. A 41-year-old female with metastatic colorectal cancer status systemic chemotherapy, low anterior resection, partial hepatectomy, and HAIP placement for refractory metastatic disease in the liver. Non-contrast axial CT (A) demonstrates postsurgical pneumoperitoneum, subcutaneous air locules and evidence for anasarca. Axial SPECT/CT (B) shows extrahepatic radiotracer localization to the second and third portions of the duodenum (arrow and star).

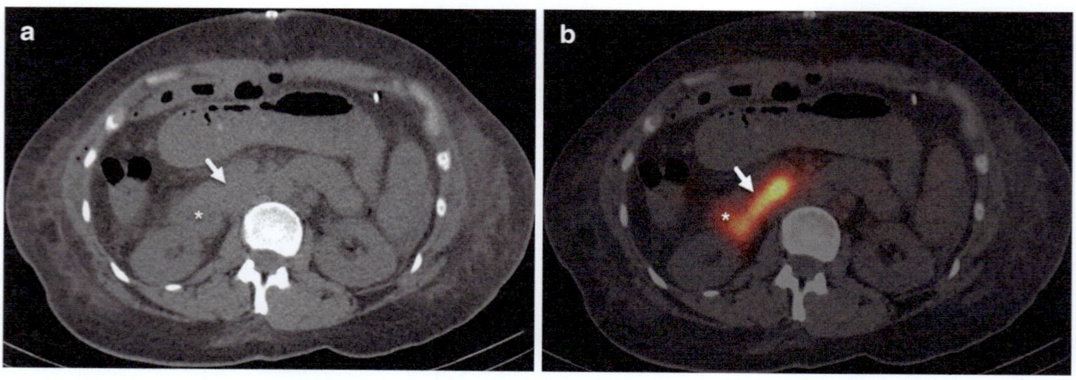

Case 10

Extrahepatic perfusion to pancreas. A 61-year-old woman with metastatic colorectal cancer who initially received neoadjuvant chemotherapy, LAR, left partial hepatectomy, and HAIP placement. HAIP study following her initial surgery was normal and she went on to complete neoadjuvant concurrent HAIP and systemic chemotherapy. For approximately two years she was disease free but then developed recurrent disease involving the rectum and vagina and underwent partial sigmoidectomy and partial vaginectomy. Shortly after surgery she underwent HAIP pump study. Given no evidence of liver disease, no intervention was undertaken to fix the pump and she was started on systemic chemotherapy. Non-contrast axial (A) CT images demonstrate surgical clips from prior partial left hepatectomy near pancreatic head (arrow). Fused axial (B) and coronal (C) SPECT/CT), illustrate intense abnormal activity within the pancreatic head and no activity within the liver (*).

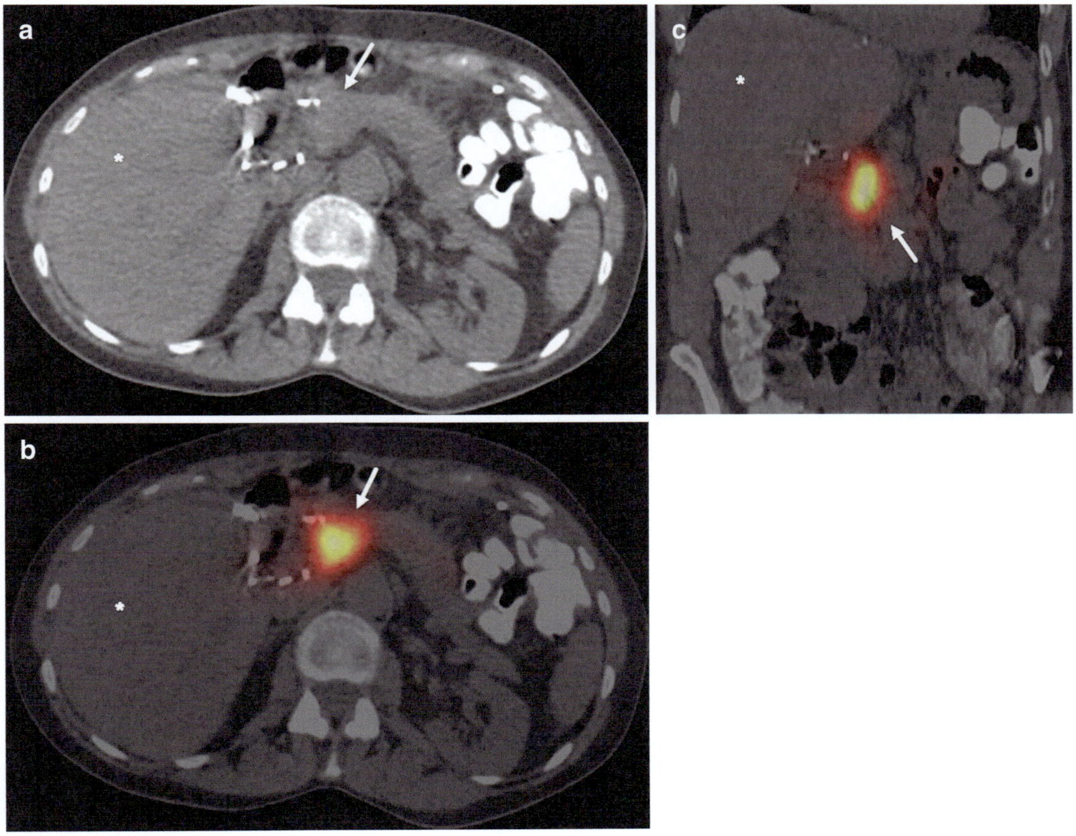

Case 11

Abundant extrahepatic perfusion to various organs. A 68-year-old female with intrahepatic cholangiocarcinoma status post systemic therapy, cholecystectomy, and HAIP placement for unresectable intrahepatic metastases. Initial HAIP study demonstrated perfusion to the spleen, pancreas, and stomach so the patient underwent angiography which demonstrated preferential flow to a large splenic artery and its branch vessels. Splenic artery embolization with coils was performed and angiography following embolization was remarkable for flow from the celiac artery that demonstrated preferential flow to the common hepatic with near complete stasis of contrast to the splenic artery. Repeat HAIP study (shown below) demonstrated even more sites of extrahepatic perfusion. Non-contrast coronal (A, C) and axial (E, G) CT images demonstrate a HAIP catheter tip in the porta hepatitis region (arrow), large low attenuation hepatic tumor conglomerate (long arrow), coil within the splenic artery (arrowhead), and leiomyomatous uterus. Fused SPECT/CT images in the coronal (B, D) and axial (F, H) planes show multifocal extrahepatic activity as a result of injected activity reaching the systemic circulation, with perfusion to spleen, bilateral (right greater than left) kidneys (B), diffuse small bowel perfusion (D) with some focal uptake at the catheter tip (arrow, D), stomach and right diaphragmatic crus (crus: arrow; F), and right gluteal musculature (*, H). Liver activity is abnormally low due to the systemic distribution of radiotracer. She underwent angiography once again and the HAIP was deemed unsalvageable and the reservoir was later removed.

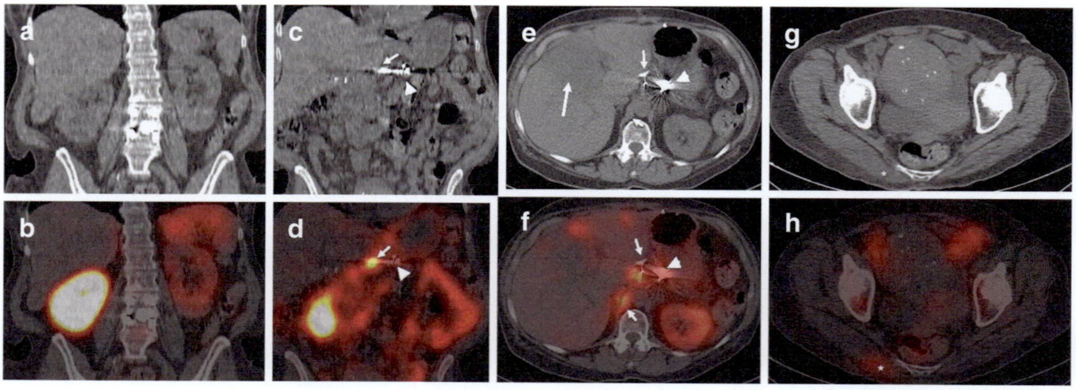

Case 12

Abnormal perfusion through falciform artery. A 35-year-old male with metastatic colorectal cancer status post low anterior resection with new hepatic metastases status post partial hepatectomy, cholecystectomy, and HAIP placement for targeted liver-directed therapy. Non-contrast axial (A) and sagittal (C) CT images are provided. Axial (B) and sagittal (D) SPECT/CT images demonstrate heterogenous activity with the liver and linear uptake (arrow) extending to the right anterior abdominal wall, probably within the hepatic falciform ligament artery.

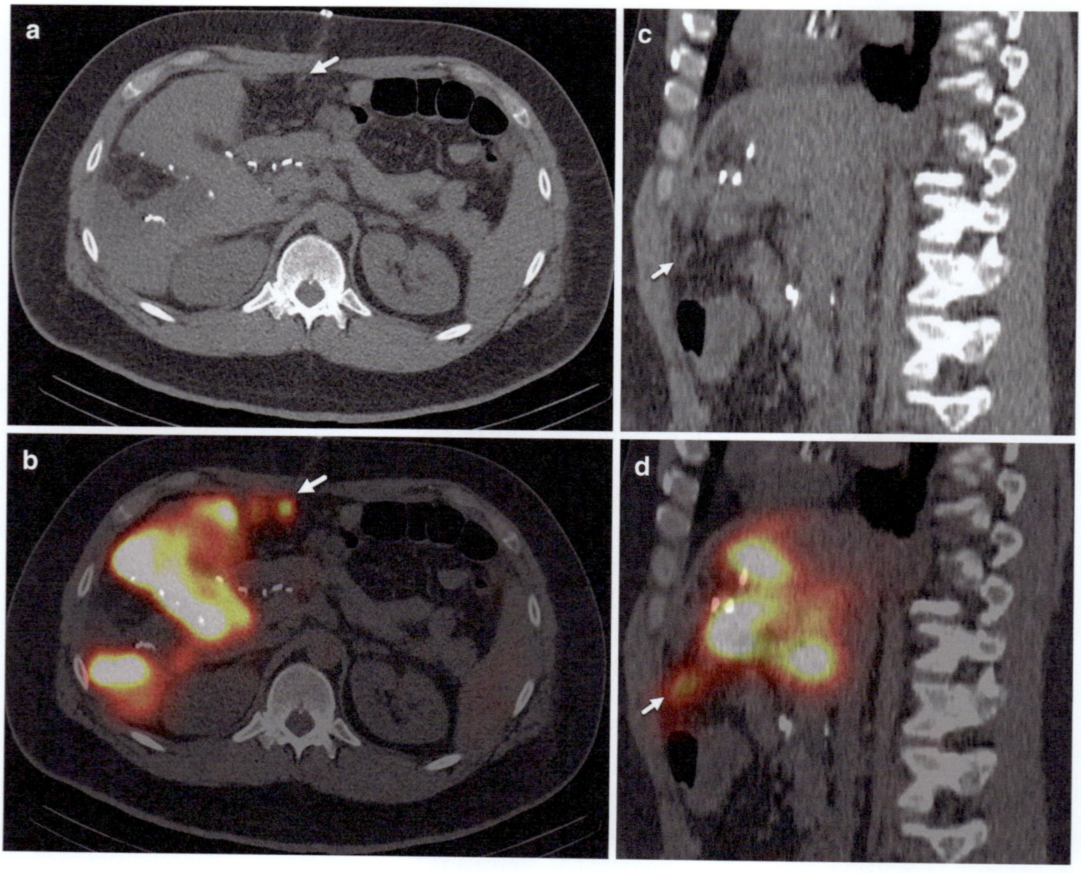

Case 13

Pseudoaneurysm with loculated extrahepatic activity accumulation. A 48-year-old male with colorectal cancer status post resection, cholecystectomy, and systemic therapy. Patient underwent HAIP placement for new unresectable bilobar hepatic metastases and presented one month later for HAIP assessment. Axial (A) and coronal (C) CT images are provided. Fused axial (B) and coronal (D) SPECT/CT images (D) demonstrate tracer accumulation within the porta hepatis, corresponding to a low-density collection (*) in the surgical bed. No tracer activity is seen in the liver. Follow-up contrast enhanced axial CT (E) shows a hypodense collection (*) adjacent to the catheter tip, consistent with localized leak into pseudoaneurysm, probably secondary to migration of the catheter tip out of the GDA.

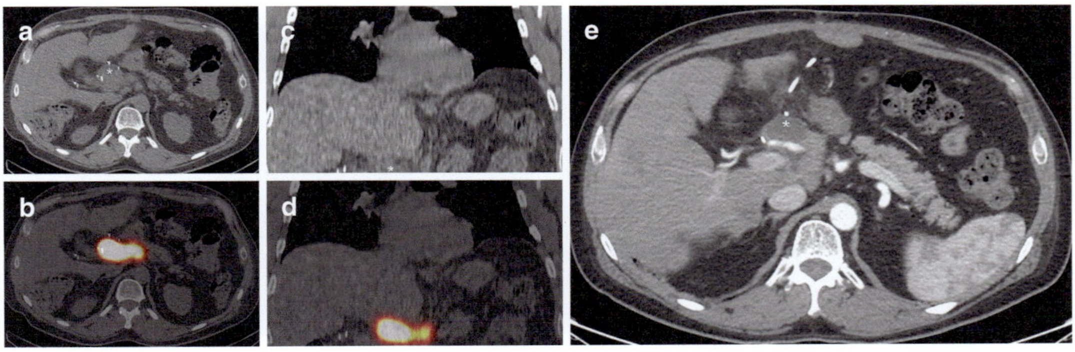

Case 14

Arterial pseudoaneurysm and arterio-venous fistula. A 53-year-old female with colorectal cancer treated with low anterior resection and chemoradiation, with subsequent recurrent hepatic metastatic disease status post left hepatectomy, multiple ablations, and HAIP placement. Initial HAIP study had shown mild activity to the pancreatic head and a stent was placed in the right hepatic artery excluding perfusion to the tiny branch supplying the pancreas. The patient went on to complete her HAIP chemotherapy, and a follow-up surveillance scan demonstrated no active disease. Eighteen months following completion of HAIP-directed chemotherapy, the patient presented for follow-up surveillance CT imaging, which showed no evidence of disease but incidentally demonstrated an intra-/perihepatic fluid collection. The contrast enhanced axial CT (A) demonstrates an intra-/perihepatic fluid collection (*). Subsequently, an HAIP study was performed to evaluate for possible extravasation. Non-contrast axial CT (B) demonstrates a partially visualized HAIP catheter in the anterior abdomen. Axial (C) and coronal (D) SPECT/CT images demonstrate tracer activity within the fluid collection (*), consistent with vascular leak into a pseudoaneurysm. In addition, there is intense activity accumulation throughout the lungs, consistent with arterio-venous fistula (MAA particles reaching the venous circulation will get trapped in the lungs because they are larger than the pulmonary capillary diameter). No hepatic tracer activity is noted. The patient then underwent angiography and stent placement. Angiography of CHA (E) demonstrates complete occlusion of right hepatic artery stent (*), collateralization of flow within right liver via the LHA (arrow), without active extravasation, and the HAIP catheter terminating in the region of the non-visualized GDA with multiple surgical clips in the region (arrowhead). A covered stent was then placed from the proper hepatic artery to the origin of the left hepatic artery to exclude the expected origin of the gastroduodenal artery (E, arrow). The aforementioned conditions precluded the use of the HAIP, and the pump reservoir was removed. Follow-up CT scans demonstrated resolution of the fluid collection. CHA: common hepatic artery, GDA: gastroduodenal artery, LGA: left gastric artery, PHA: proper hepatic artery, SA: splenic artery.

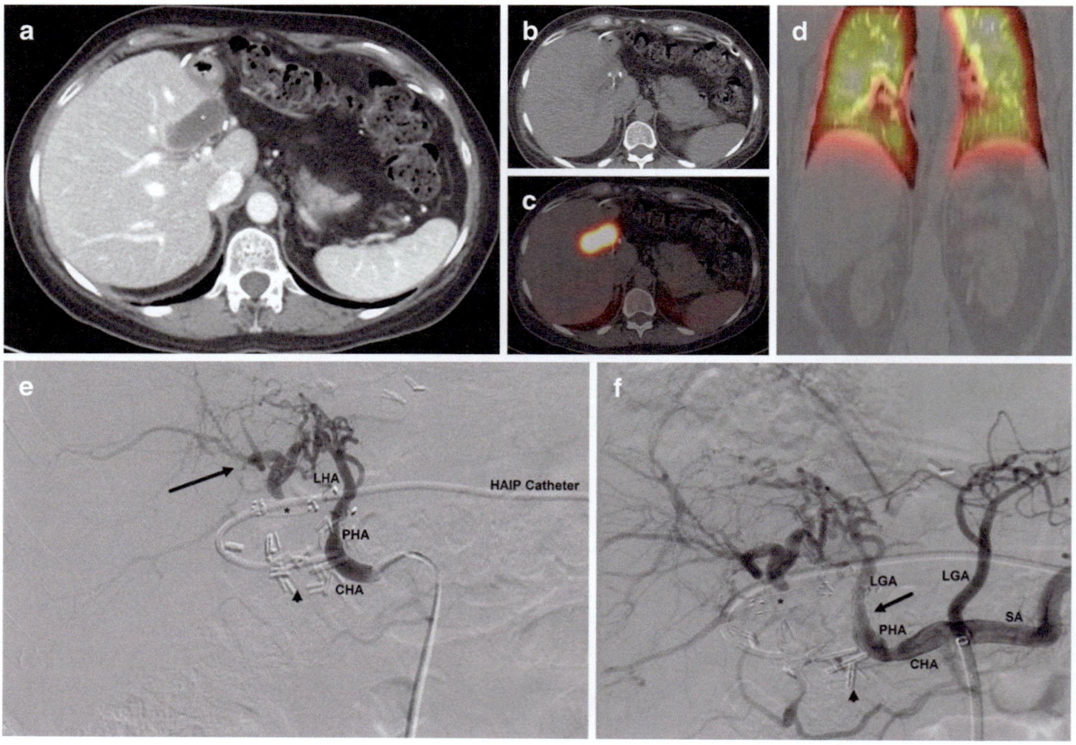

Case 15

Arterial dissection with extrahepatic stasis and near exclusive perfusion of left hepatic lobe. A 62-year-old male with metastatic colorectal cancer status post chemotherapy, sigmoidectomy, irreversible electroporation of segments II and IV, microwave ablation of the caudate lobe, cholecystectomy, and HAIP placement for adjuvant chemotherapy. Non-contrast axial CT (A, C) demonstrates a partially visualized HAIP catheter, and difficult to characterize treated hepatic metastases. Fused SPECT/CT images (B, D) depict accumulation of activity in the left lobe, minimal activity within segment 4 and the right hepatic lobe, abnormal activity involving the pancreatic tail (D, arrow) and spleen, as well as intense stasis of tracer activity in the periportal region (arrowhead) consistent with partial obstruction. Planar image (E) predominant accumulation in the left lobe (arrow) and intense activity without the periportal region (arrowhead). A subsequent pump angiogram demonstrated contrast material predominantly flowing retrograde towards the celiac axis with a small amount of contrast flowing antegrade through the liver, both likely in a false lumen of a dissected vessel, opacified vessel surrounding the catheter tip severely narrowed, and no antegrade flow towards the intrahepatic arteries, consistent with dissection of the proper hepatic artery. Follow-up CT (F) demonstrated narrowing of the proper hepatic artery (arrow) consistent with known dissection. The HAIP was removed.

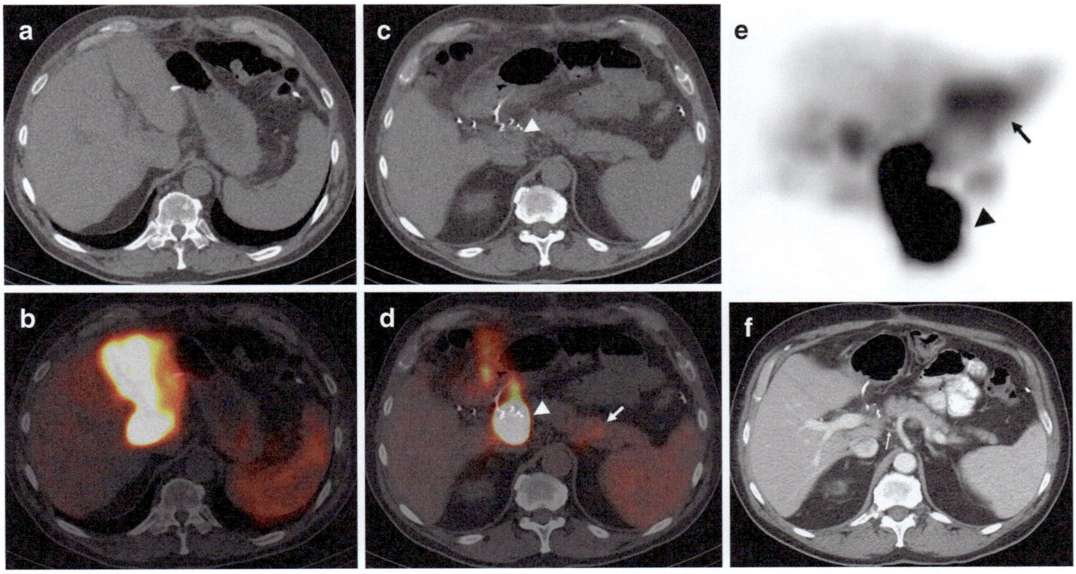

Case 16

Accessory left hepatic artery (ALH) with initial lack of perfusion to left lobe of liver by the HAIP system, with perfusion of entire liver after embolization of the aberrant artery. A 43-year-old male with metastatic colorectal cancer to the liver status post left hemicolectomy, systemic chemotherapy, segmentectomy (VI/VII, II), and wedge resections (segments V and VIII). HAIP was placed for adjuvant liver-directed chemotherapy.

Non-contrasted axial CT (A) demonstrates postsurgical changes in the liver. Pre-embolization fused axial SPECT/CT (B) demonstrates activity in the right posterior liver and caudate lobe, with no perfusion to segments II–IV.

The patient then underwent angiography and embolization (C–G).

- Catheterization of celiac artery (E): Patent CHA, splenic artery (SA), ligated GDA posthepatic pump placement, ALH arising from the LGA.
- Catheterization of ALH (F): Perfusion of left hepatic lobe and a proximal branch of the ALH communicating with LHA arising from the proper hepatic artery (PHA).
- Embolization of ALH (H).
- Catheterization of LGA following embolization (G): Occlusion of ALH with preserved flow to gastric branches.

Post-embolization non-contrasted axial CT (H) demonstrates postsurgical changes in the liver, and the fused axial SPECT/CT (I) demonstrates heterogenous activity throughout the entire liver. ALH: accessory left hepatic artery CHA: common hepatic artery GDA: gastroduodenal artery LGA: left gastric artery PHA: proper hepatic artery SA: splenic artery.

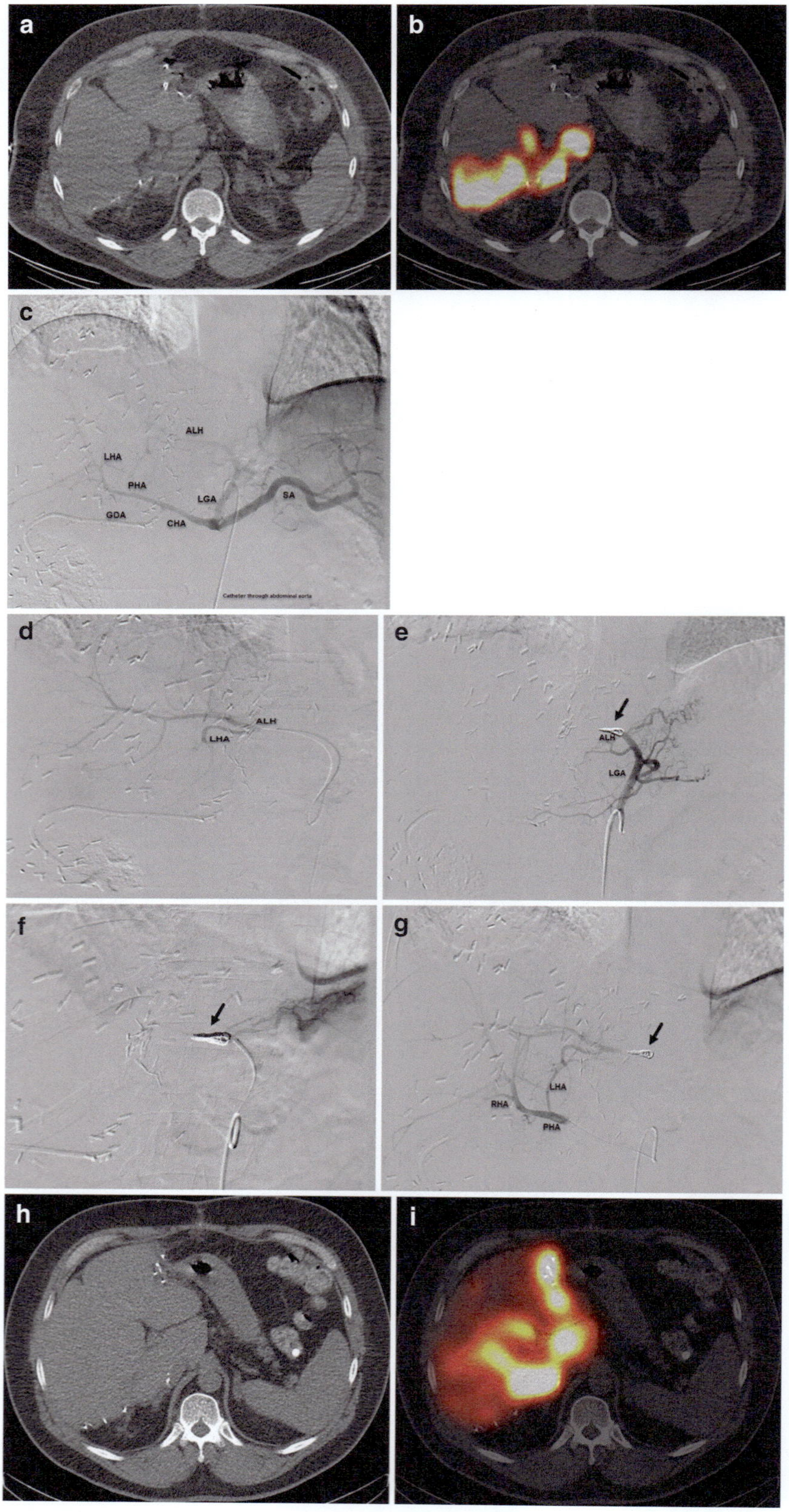
a
b
c
ALH
LHA
PHA
LGA
SA
GDA
CHA
Catheter through abdominal aorta
d
ALH
LHA
e
ALH
LGA
f
g
LHA
RHA
PHA
h
i

Case 17

Gastric perforation by the HAIP catheter. A 66-year-old male with metastatic colorectal cancer treated with primary resection and right hepatectomy, with development of unresectable metastatic liver disease status post segment III wedge resection and HAIP placement. Shortly after presenting with weakness and fatigue, labs revealed anemia, and imaging demonstrated GDA stump hemorrhage, for which the patient underwent interventional radiology embolization. HAIP evaluation was done to determine whether the catheter was salvageable. Snapshots of dynamic images were acquired at 5-s intervals for a total of 60 s (A), demonstrating the immediate presence of tracer activity in the stomach (black arrow), followed by activity in the duodenum at 40–45 s (red arrow). Findings are consistent with gastric perforation by the HAIP catheter. Non-contrast enhanced axial (B) and coronal images (D) demonstrate post-procedural changes, embolization clips in the antrum of the stomach (arrow), and the catheter traversing through the stomach. Fused axial (B) and coronal SPECT/CT images (E) show intense activity in the gastric antrum (arrow) and throughout small bowel without any activity in the liver.

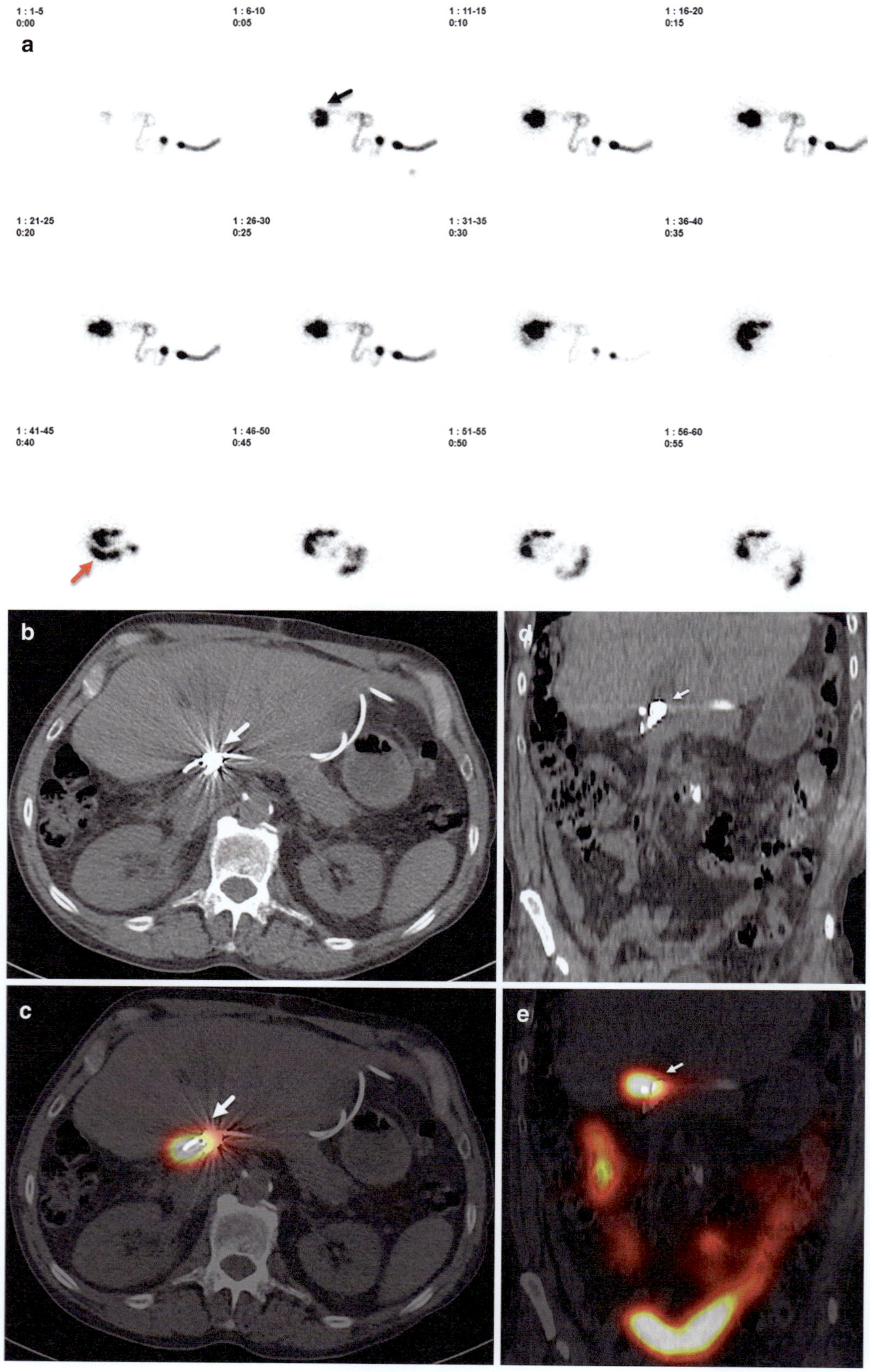
1 : 1-5
0:00
a
1 : 6-10
0:05
1 : 11-15
0:10
1 : 16-20
0:15
1 : 21-25
0:20
1 : 26-30
0:25
1 : 31-35
0:30
1 : 36-40
0:35
1 : 41-45
0:40
1 : 46-50
0:45
1 : 51-55
0:50
1 : 56-60
0:55
b
c
d
e

Case 18

Obstruction of hepatic pump system. A 47-year-old male with metastatic colorectal cancer to liver and lung who was initially treated with systemic chemotherapy, primary tumor resection, partial hepatectomy, and lung metastasectomy. A few years later, he developed recurrent metastatic disease to the liver and underwent wedge resection and HAIP placement for adjuvant intrahepatic pump therapy. Following completion of adjuvant therapy, the patient continued to demonstrate no evidence of disease; the HAIP system was flushed monthly to maintain its patency. Approximately 2.5 years following the last treatment, flushing of the pump system was found to be difficult. An HAIP study was performed. Dynamic images acquired at 5-s intervals for a total of 60 s (A) show activity within line accessing the pump reservoir (black triangle) and in the HAIP reservoir (arrow) but no further transport into the liver. Subsequent fused axial (B) and coronal (C) SPECT/CT confirms tracer activity solely within the pump reservoir, consistent with catheter obstruction. The HAIP reservoir was removed.

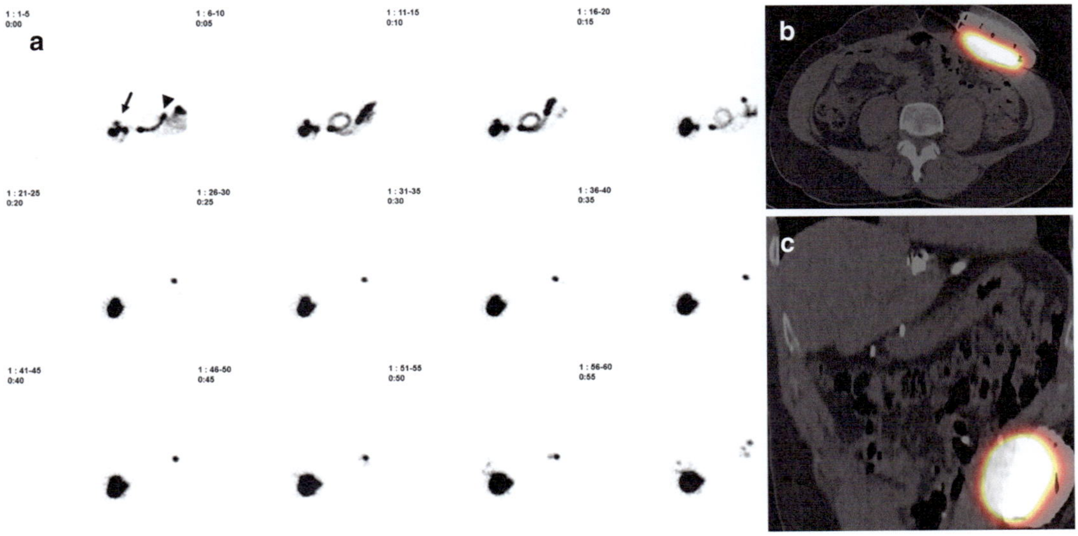

Case 19

Ruptured pump catheter. A 68-year-old male with metastatic colorectal cancer treated with systemic chemotherapy, primary tumor resection, partial left hepatectomy, and HAIP-based chemotherapy for unresectable liver metastases. Patient presented with bleeding from the HAIP access site and an HAIP study was done to evaluate for possible obstruction. Non-contrast axial CT (A) demonstrates the HAIP reservoir within the subcutaneous tissues of the left lower quadrant abdominal wall. Fused axial (B) and coronal (C) SPECT/CT depicts extravasation of radiotracer into the peritoneal cavity (red arrow) and no activity within the liver (*).

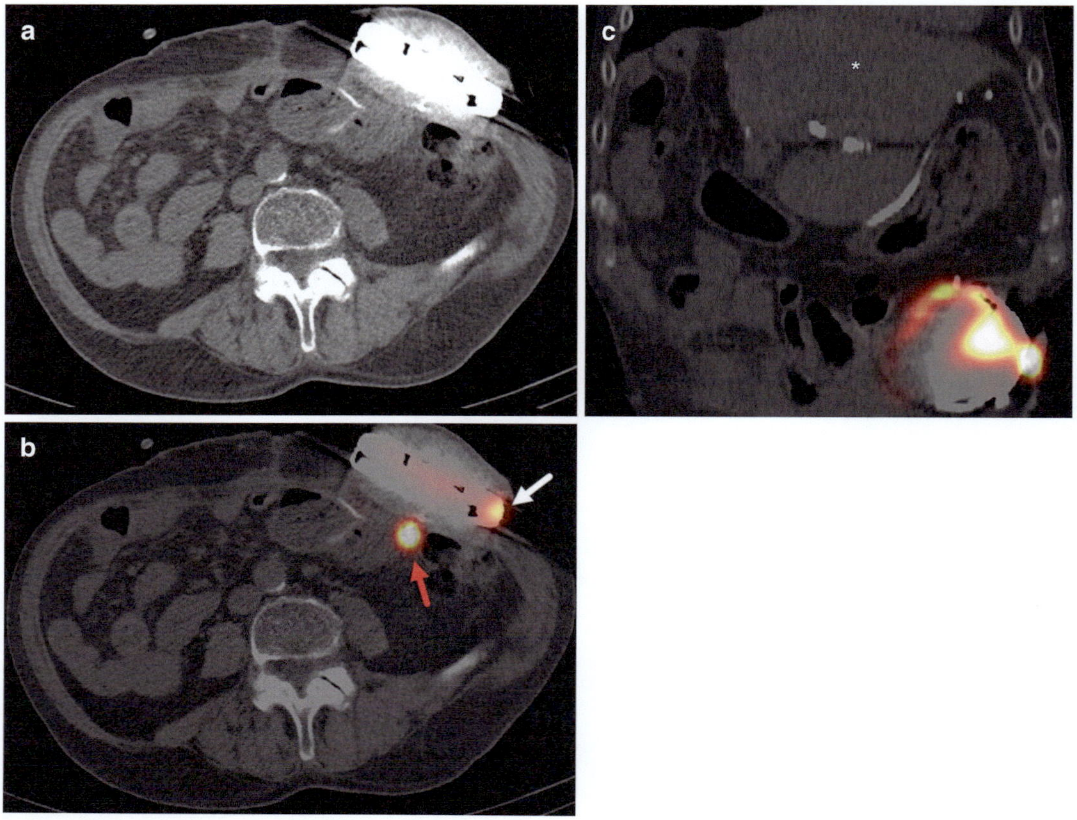

Case 20

Kinked HAIP catheter causing obstruction. A 48-year-old female with metastatic colorectal cancer treated with hemicolectomy, partial hepatic resection, systemic therapy, with new liver metastases status post segment 2 resection and HAIP placement. Initial HAIP study following surgery was normal and the patient received a few cycles of hepatic pump chemotherapy. Subsequently the patient developed increasing pump mobility and flipping, requiring manual reorientation. She presented for a pump check and the pump was difficult to access, requiring multiple attempts. Upon successful pump access, high residual was present, and patient developed tenderness at her pump site prompting a HAIP study. Non-contrast axial (A) and sagittal CT images (C) demonstrate the proximal pump catheter (arrow) at the level of reservoir (A) circumscribing about the pump pouch (C) prior to traversing the abdominal wall and entering the intraabdominal cavity. Fused axial SPECT/CT (B) and sagittal images (D) demonstrate activity surrounding the pump reservoir without distal progression of the radiotracer and no activity within the liver (*). The patient then underwent fluoroscopy (E) which demonstrated the catheter flipped multiple times upon itself (arrow) probably causing obstruction and extravasation into the subcutaneous tissues of the abdominal wall (arrowhead) from the catheter possibly due to needle puncture during multiple access attempts. Shortly after, the patient underwent catheter repair. On follow-up visit, the pump was easily accessible, and the patient went on to receive additional cycles of chemotherapy via the HAIP.

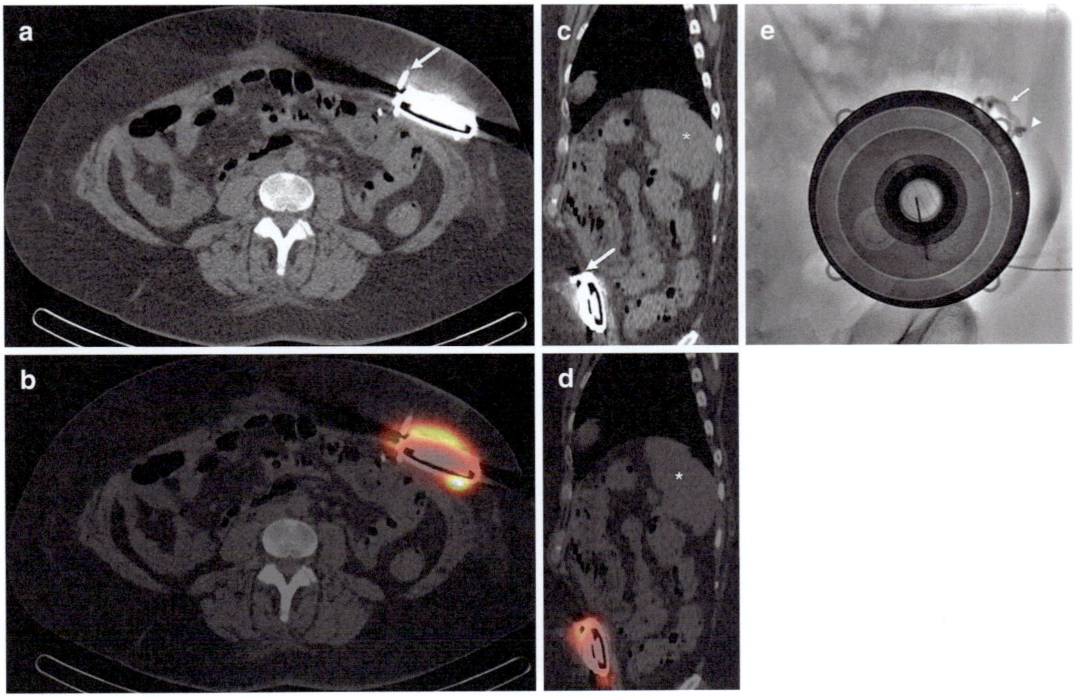

References

1. Qadan M, D'Angelica MI, Kemeny NE, Cercek A, Kingham TP. Robotic hepatic arterial infusion pump placement. HPB. 2017;19:429–35. https://doi.org/10.1016/j.hpb.2016.12.015.
2. Lee AJ, Gomes AS, Liu DM, Kee ST, Loh CT, McWilliams JP. The road less traveled: importance of the lesser branches of the celiac Axis in liver Embolotherapy. Radiographics. 2012;32:1121–32. https://doi.org/10.1148/rg.324115114.
3. Gates VL, Singh N, Lewandowski RJ, Spies S, Salem R. Intraarterial hepatic SPECT/CT imaging using ^{99m} Tc-macroaggregated albumin in preparation for Radioembolization. J Nucl Med. 2015;56:1157–62. https://doi.org/10.2967/jnumed.114.153346.
4. Sancho L, Rodriguez-Fraile M, Bilbao JI, Beorlegui Arteta C, Iñarrairaegui M, Moran V, et al. Is a technetium-99m macroaggregated albumin scan essential in the workup for selective internal radiation therapy with Yttrium-90? An analysis of 532 patients. J Vasc Interv Radiol. 2017;28:1536–42. https://doi.org/10.1016/j.jvir.2017.07.019.
5. Kao YH, Hock Tan AE, Burgmans MC, Irani FG, Khoo LS, Gong Lo RH, et al. Image-guided personalized predictive dosimetry by artery-specific SPECT/CT partition modeling for safe and effective ^{90} Y Radioembolization. J Nucl Med. 2012;53:559–66. https://doi.org/10.2967/jnumed.111.097469.
6. Piasecki P, Narloch J, Brzozowski K, Zięcina P, Mazurek A, Budzyńska A, et al. The predictive value of SPECT/CT imaging in colorectal liver metastases response after 90Y-radioembolization. PLoS One. 2018;13:e0200488. https://doi.org/10.1371/journal.pone.0200488.
7. Bourien H, Palard X, Rolland Y, Le Du F, Beuzit L, Uguen T, et al. Yttrium-90 glass microspheres radioembolization (RE) for biliary tract cancer: a large single-center experience. Eur J Nucl Med Mol Imaging. 2019;46:669–76. https://doi.org/10.1007/s00259-018-4199-5.
8. d'Abadie P, Walrand S, Lhommel R, Hesse M, Jamar F. A Theranostic approach in SIRT: value of pretherapy imaging in treatment planning. J Clin Med. 2022;11:7245. https://doi.org/10.3390/jcm11237245.
9. Daly JM, Butler J, Kemeny N, Yeh SDJ, Ridge JA, Botet J, et al. Predicting tumor response in patients with colorectal hepatic metastases. Ann Surg. 1985;202:384. https://doi.org/10.1097/00000658-198509000-00017.
10. Buisman FE, Homs MYV, Grünhagen DJ, Filipe WF, Bennink RJ, Besselink MGH, et al. Adjuvant hepatic arterial infusion pump chemotherapy and resection versus resection alone in patients with low-risk resectable colorectal liver metastases—the multicenter randomized controlled PUMP trial. BMC Cancer. 2019;19:327. https://doi.org/10.1186/s12885-019-5515-6.

11. Thiels CA, D'Angelica MI. Hepatic artery infusion pumps. J Surg Oncol. 2020;122:70–7. https://doi.org/10.1002/jso.25913.
12. Taylor I, Bennett R, Sherriff S. The blood supply of colorectal liver metastases. Br J Cancer. 1978;38:749–56. https://doi.org/10.1038/bjc.1978.283.
13. Löschner C, Nagel S, Kausche S, Teichgräber U. Hepatic arterial supply in 1297 CT-angiographies. Rofo. 2015;187:276–82. https://doi.org/10.1055/s-0034-1385816.
14. Koops A, Wojciechowski B, Broering DC, Adam G, Krupski-Berdien G. Anatomic variations of the hepatic arteries in 604 selective celiac and superior mesenteric angiographies. Surg Radiol Anat. 2004;26:239–44. https://doi.org/10.1007/s00276-004-0229-z.
15. Abdullah SS, Mabrut J-Y, Garbit V, De La Roche E, Olagne E, Rode A, et al. Anatomical variations of the hepatic artery: study of 932 cases in liver transplantation. Surg Radiol Anat. 2006;28:468–73. https://doi.org/10.1007/s00276-006-0121-0.
16. Gümüs H, Bükte Y, Özdemir E, Sentürk S, Tekbas G, Önder H, et al. Variations of the celiac trunk and hepatic arteries: a study with 64-detector computed tomographic angiography. Eur Rev Med Pharmacol Sci. 2013;17:1636–41.
17. Choi TW, Chung JW, Kim H-C, Lee M, Choi JW, Jae HJ, et al. Anatomic variations of the hepatic artery in 5625 patients. Radiol Cardiothorac Imaging. 2021;3:e210007. https://doi.org/10.1148/ryct.2021210007.
18. Wigmore SJ, Madhavan K, Redhead DN, Currie EJ, Garden OJ. Distribution of colorectal liver metastases in patients referred for hepatic resection. Cancer. 2000;89:285–7.
19. Kadiyoran C, Cizmecioglu H, Cure E, Yildirim M, Yilmaz P. Liver metastasis in colorectal cancer: evaluation of segmental distribution. Gastroenterol Rev. 2019;14:188–92. https://doi.org/10.5114/pg.2019.88168.
20. Rhu J, Heo JS, Choi SH, Choi DW, Kim JM, Joh J-W, et al. Streamline flow of the portal vein affects the lobar distribution of colorectal liver metastases and has a clinical impact on survival. Ann Surg Treat Res. 2017;92:348. https://doi.org/10.4174/astr.2017.92.5.348.
21. Holbrook RF, Rodriguez-Bigas MA, Ramakrishnan K, Blumenson L, Petrelli NJ. Patterns of colorectal liver metastases according to Couinaud's segments. Dis Colon Rectum. 1995;38:245–8. https://doi.org/10.1007/BF02055595.
22. Doussot A, Kemeny NE, D'Angelica MI. Hepatic arterial infusional chemotherapy in the management of colorectal cancer liver metastases. Hepat Oncol. 2015;2:275–90. https://doi.org/10.2217/hep.15.9.
23. Ozaki K, Kobayashi S, Matsui O, Minami T, Koda W, Gabata T. Extrahepatic arteries originating from hepatic arteries: analysis using CT during hepatic arteriography and visualization on digital subtraction angiography. Cardiovasc Intervent Radiol. 2017;40:822–30. https://doi.org/10.1007/s00270-017-1568-6.
24. Song S-Y, Chung JW, Lim HG, Park JH. Nonhepatic arteries originating from the hepatic arteries: angiographic analysis in 250 patients. J Vasc Interv Radiol. 2006;17:461–9. https://doi.org/10.1097/01.RVI.0000202718.16416.18.
25. Ziessman H, Wahl R, Juni J, Gyves J, Ensminger W, Thrall J, et al. The utility of SPECT for 99mTc-MAA hepatic arterial perfusion scintigraphy. Am J Roentgenol. 1985;145:747–51. https://doi.org/10.2214/ajr.145.4.747.
26. Perez DR, Kemeny NE, Brown KT, Gewirtz AN, Paty PB, Jarnagin WR, et al. Angiographic identification of extrahepatic perfusion after hepatic arterial pump placement: implications for surgical prevention. HPB (Oxford). 2014;16:744–8. https://doi.org/10.1111/hpb.12208.

10 HAI-Specific Complications and Management

Isabella Guajardo, Peter Allen, James Pingpank, and Jason K. Sicklick

Introduction

Hepatic artery infusion therapy has had complication rates as high as 35–80%, but these improved after the introduction of the subcutaneous implantable pump [1, 2]. The complication rate was further reduced with increased experience and placement of hepatic artery infusion pumps (HAIPs) by high-volume surgeons. These devices can now be placed with acceptable morbidity (22%) and low mortality (<1%) [3] that are most often associated with the simultaneous procedures (e.g., partial hepatectomy and partial colon resections) rather than the pump placement itself [3, 4].

Complication rates have continued to remain low, as high-volume centers gain experience with HAIP placement and application. For example, two recent series reported pump-related complications in 22–28% of patients, and a salvage rate of up to 45% if intervention occurs promptly [4–6]. Despite these advances, one series still reported pump failure of 9% at 1 year and 16% at 2 years [6], while another reported a complication rate of 35.1%, although only 4.6% of those were Clavien-Dindo grade ≥3b to 4 [7]. Such HAIP-related complications can especially occur in the early postoperative period or after initiating infusional therapy. Awareness of pitfalls that can occur with placement and management of these pumps is vital to prevent delays in treatment, while recognition of delayed complications most often associated with liver directed therapy is crucial for successful long-term utilization of this approach.

Supplementary Information The online version contains supplementary material available at https://doi.org/10.1007/978-3-031-74935-3_10.

I. Guajardo
Department of Surgery, University of California San Diego, San Diego, CA, USA
e-mail: iguajardo@health.ucsd.edu

P. Allen
Department of Surgery, Duke University, Durham, NC, USA
e-mail: peter.allen@duke.edu

J. Pingpank
Department of Surgery, University of Pittsburgh Medical Center, Pittsburgh, PA, USA
e-mail: pingpankjf@upmc.edu

J. K. Sicklick (✉)
Department of Surgery, University of California San Diego, San Diego, CA, USA

Division of Surgical Oncology, University of California San Diego, San Diego, CA, USA

Moores Cancer Center, University of California San Diego, La Jolla, CA, USA

Department of Pharmacology, University of California San Diego, San Diego, CA, USA
e-mail: jsicklick@health.ucsd.edu

M. D'Angelica, M. Lidsky (eds.), *Hepatic Artery Infusion for Malignancy*,
https://doi.org/10.1007/978-3-031-74935-3_10

The aims of this chapter are to review complications encountered when caring for patients with HAIPs, as well as to discuss troubleshooting and management of each of these issues. We will review the following six topics outlined below (Table 10.1):

1. Pump- and pocket-related positional complications.
2. Pump pocket fluid collections.
3. Catheter complications.
4. Vascular complications.
5. Biliary complications.
6. Infusion rate-related considerations.

Brief Overview of Hepatic Artery Infusion Pump Construction and Function

The pump most commonly utilized in the United States and only device with FDA approval for intra-arterial therapy is manufactured by Intera Oncology (Wellesley, MA, USA; Fig. 10.1). The Intera 3000 is a circular device made of titanium that measures about 3 inches in diameter and includes two chambers. One chamber is the drug reservoir with a capacity of 30 mL, and is accessible via a resealable septum for drug loading, with an outlet to the catheter for drug delivery. The other chamber is adjacent to the drug reservoir and is permanently sealed with a charging fluid. This fluid contains a fluorocarbon liquid (freon) that converts to a gas phase when heated by the body's temperature and exerts pressure on the drug chamber, akin to a bellows, forcing the drug to flow into the catheter at a slow continuous rate [8, 9].

Table 10.1 Differential diagnosis of HAIP-associated complications

Pump- and pocket-related positional complications
Difficult access
Pump flipping
Pump migration
Pump pocket fluid collections
Seroma
Infection (cellulitis, abscess)
Hematoma
Catheter-related complications
Kinking
Thrombosis (early)
Thrombosis (late)
Migration
Dislodgement from pump
Breakage
Erosion into bowel
Vascular complications
Arterial dissection
Arterial pseudoaneurysms
Incomplete perfusion
Extrahepatic perfusion
Biliary complications
Transaminitis
Hyperbilirubinemia
Elevated alkaline phosphatase
Biliary sclerosis with unifocal or multifocal bile duct stenosis and intrahepatic biliary ductal dilation
Cholangitis
Hepatic failure
Infusion rate-related complications
Diminished flow rate
Increased flow rate
Pump dry out
Pump failure/loss

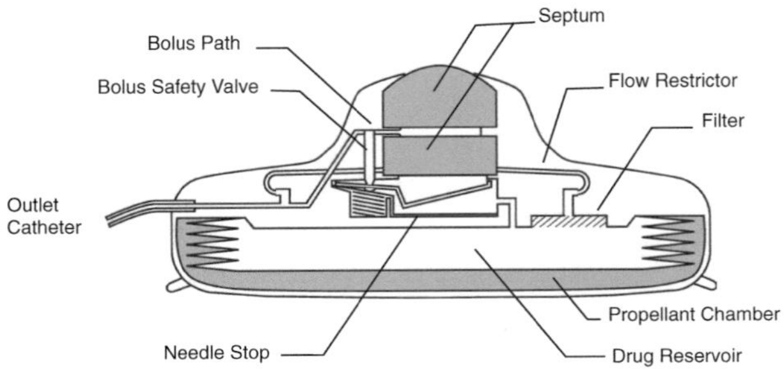

Fig. 10.1 Components and construction of the hepatic artery infusion pump (Intera 3000)

Complications: Diagnosis, Workup, and Management

This chapter is organized in the manner that one might expect when approaching any pump malfunction, starting with the accessible portion (i.e., the pump in the subcutaneous space). We then systematically follow the course of the medication infusion into the pump, along the course of the catheter, and through the hepatic arterial blood supply. After systematically reviewing various pump elements and their common pitfalls, the chapter will conclude with a discussion of issues previously encountered with the mechanics of the pump itself, including how inadequate understanding of HAIP function can lead to issues with medication delivery and ultimate pump loss. The overall management of complications is summarized in Table 10.2.

Pump- and Pocket-Related Positional Complications

Difficult Access

When placing the pump, it is important to ensure that the tissue overlying the pump permits palpation of the pump itself and the reservoir ports for ongoing use. Patient characteristics that may preclude or complicate pump placement and subsequent use include obesity, prior surgical incisions or mesh, and ostomy presence or concurrent ostomy creation at the time of pump placement. In cases where the pump pocket is deep due to copious subcutaneous tissue, defatting the tissue between the access port and the dermis should be performed to allow for easier palpation and device cannulation [4, 10, 11]. In situations where there is significant abdominal wall fat and the pump may be too deep to access, one should consider placement on the lower chest wall. This is a particularly feasible option in male patients without significant breast tissue.

Pump Flipping/Migration

The device is positioned superficial to the fascia and secured flat against the fascia with four sturdy nonabsorbable sutures (e.g., silk or Prolene). When accessing the device, if the raised access septum itself cannot be palpated, then the pump may have flipped or rotated within the pocket. This is typically identified when a distinct metal sound is made when the needle tip hits metal while trying to access the chamber. Pump flipping or swirling (i.e., rotating along its axis more than once) can occur if: (1) any of the sutures have loosened or pulled through the fascia; (2) sutures have broken; or (3) the pump is

Table 10.2 Diagnosis and management of complications

Category	Complication	Timing	Diagnosis and management		Considerations
			Medical	Surgical	
Pump- and pocket-related positional complications	Difficult access	Early	Evaluate location of port with ultrasound or obtain cross-sectional imaging	Consider pocket re-creation for easier accessibility or re-location to chest wall for firmer floor	
	Pump flipping	Late	Manual repositioning can be done under image guidance	Device re-securement to fascia or chest wall	
	Pump migration, swirling or twisting	Late		Device untwisting and re-securement to fascia or chest wall; thorough evaluation of catheter	
Pump pocket fluid collections	Seroma	Early	Antibiotics if concern for development of secondary infection	Aspiration of fluid collection	Drain placement should not be performed
	Cellulitis	Early/late	Antibiotics and close monitoring		
	Abscess	Early/late		Pump site debridement and culture; replacement of old pump within pocket after soaking with betadine (considered temporary measure) vs new pump spliced to old catheter and re-sited at remote pocket (contralateral abdominal wall or chest wall)	If recurrent infection, removal of original device and replacement at new location
	Bleeding/hematoma		Compression therapy	Washout and hemostasis	Temporary cessation of anticoagulation
Catheter	Kinking	Early/late		Splicing of catheter and re-connection to pump if kinking at pump end	
	Thrombosis	Early	Systemic anticoagulation and pump heparinization	Pump injection under fluoroscopy; heparinized saline flushes to dislodge fresh clot	
	Thrombosis	Late	Systemic anticoagulation and pump heparinization	Catheter tPA under imaging guidance	Salvage rate approx. 30%
	Migration		Discontinuation of therapy	Consider catheter removal to avoid further complications	Consider alternative catheter insertion sites for HAIP continuation
	Dislodgement from pump or breakage		Temporary cessation versus discontinuation of treatment	Assessment of catheter patency under fluoroscopic guidance; attempts at dislodging clot can be made but unsalvageable complication if catheter is occluded	
	Erosion into bowel		Discontinuation of therapy	Endoscopic evaluation of erosion into viscera; surgery for catheter removal, bowel repair or resection	

Vascular	Arterial dissection	Early	Watchful waiting; anticoagulation	Consider fenestration of dissection flap	
	Arterial pseudoaneurysm	Early/late	Discontinuation of therapy; Management of liver injury/ischemia	Occlusive stent or angioembolization versus direct surgical intervention	
	Incomplete perfusion	Early	Evaluation for systemic therapy in addition to HAIP	IR consultation for possible transarterial embolization options	
	Extrahepatic perfusion	Early	Temporary postponement of treatment initiation	Angioembolization of collateral branches	
	Extrahepatic perfusion	Late	Temporary cessation of treatment, supportive care of possible side effects (gastritis, duodenitis, pancreatitis, etc.)	Angioembolization of collateral branches	
Biliary complications	Transaminitis	Early	Supportive care; FUDR dose adjustment, dexamethasone in pump		
	Hyperbilirubinemia and elevated phosphatase		Supportive care; FUDR adjustment, dexamethasone in pump		
	Unifocal biliary stricture		Temporary cessation of treatment, supportive care, dexamethasone in pump	GI consult for decompressive ERCP (alternatively IR consult for percutaneous intervention)	
	Multifocal biliary sclerosis		Complete cessation of treatment, dexamethasone in pump	GI consult for decompressive ERCP (alternatively IR consult for percutaneous intervention)	
	Cholangitis	Late	Temporary cessation of treatment; antibiotics, supportive care	GI consult for decompressive ERCP (alternatively IR consult for percutaneous intervention)	
	Liver failure		Complete cessation of treatment; supportive care		

(continued)

Table 10.2 (continued)

Category	Complication	Timing	Diagnosis and management: Medical	Diagnosis and management: Surgical	Considerations
Infusion rate-related complications	Diminished flow rate	Early/late	Early pump heparinization or re-filling; avoidance of ice packs on or near pump site	Consider IR consult for pump angiography (+/− tPA infusion)	Replace pump if related to device malfunction
	Increased flow rate	Early/late	Avoid circumstances that would increase temperature around pump	Consider pump replacement if device determined to be malfunctioning	Close monitoring of febrile patient and possible toxicity due to increased infusion rate
	Pump dry-out	Early/late	Unsalvageable—Prevent with glycerin solution	Consider pump removal	
	Pump failure/loss	Early/late	Unsalvageable—Prevent with glycerin solution	Consider pump removal	

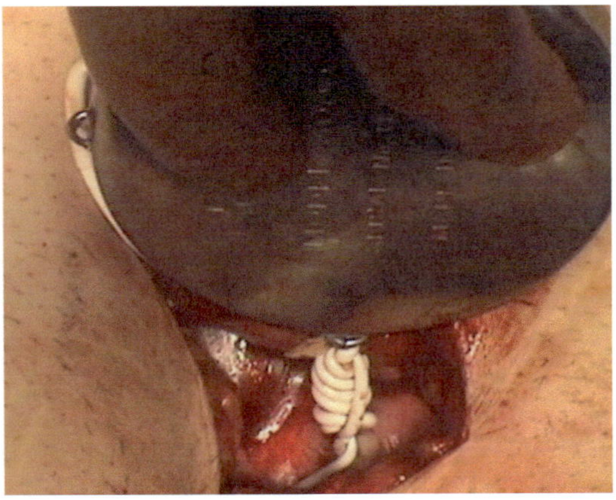

Fig. 10.2 Catheter twisting after the pump swirled/flipped on its axis several times resulting in catheter occlusion

loose-fitting within the pocket (Fig. 10.2). The latter can occur if the surgeon is overly aggressive with defatting the pocket or creates an initial pocket that is much larger than the pump. This is a challenge in obese patients in whom there is often a thicker abdominal wall requiring deeper dissection at the time of pump placement. Over time, this increases the risk of suture loosening, and with prolonged pump use, this can lead to migration within the pocket itself. Physical exam findings of a migrated or flipped pump can include device displacement, an inability to palpate or access the pump, an inability to cannulate the ports, blistering or erosion of the skin, or even skin ulceration.

Plain films or fluoroscopy can be helpful in confirming whether a pump has flipped or migrated. A flipped pump may be manually re-positioned at the bedside by an experienced clinician. This should only be considered a temporary solution, as repeated bedside re-positioning risks kinking the catheter or dislodging it altogether [8, 11]. More definitive solutions to a flipped pump include reoperation to re-secure the pump more tightly to the fascia within the same pocket, relocating it to a newly created and snugger pocket if the original was loose-fitting, or using mesh to keep the device in place and well-positioned against the fascia. As obese patients require the creation of a deeper pocket to secure the device to the fascia, the pump can be placed on the chest wall over the ribs. This ensures that the pump is within a more superficial pocket and secured over a more fixed "floor," making it more easily accessible and less likely to flip. This can also be considered in patients at high risk for complications associated with pump relocation, such as multiple prior abdominal surgeries or the presence of an ostomy or wounds that may risk pump infection if placed nearby.

Finally, if the device is exposed, one should consider the pump infected, hence it should be removed and a new pump relocated using sterile procedures. If there is ulceration or blistering but the device is not exposed, it is still at high risk for infectious complications, and should also be removed and relocated. In the next section, we will further discuss fluid collections and infectious complications.

Pump Pocket Fluid Collections

Recent series have found that the rate of pocket complications due to seroma, hematoma, wound infection, or abscess occur in between 8% and 18% of patients [5, 6, 12–14]. Complications can occur in the early or late postoperative periods, are typically diagnosed on physical exam, and include findings of erythema, tenderness, fullness, fluctuance, or drainage from the pump pocket incision. If exam findings are inconclusive, imaging studies such as ultrasound (US) or computed tomography (CT) can be used to aid in diagnosis.

Seroma

A seroma is a common postoperative complication in which a fluid collection forms within the pump pocket. The size of the seroma can vary, but it can make the pump difficult to palpate and access without drainage of the seroma. If small, it is unlikely to affect pump function or the ability to palpate the pump. These will often resolve over time. A seroma of significant size can become a nidus for infection and may cause pressure or encroachment on the pump. In turn, this may affect pump position and subsequent access, and can also lead to catheter position changes or catheter kinking. If the seroma is large enough that the pump is not palpable and therefore not safely accessible, the fluid should be aspirated under sterile conditions with US guidance to avoid damaging the catheter, which is generally positioned posterior to the pump. The aspirate is often straw colored or serosanguinous in appearance and can be sent for culture to rule out infection. Seromas often re-accumulate and may require repeat drainage procedures. Repeat aspirations can be done if the pump remains functional, and the fluid continues to be sterile. With time, healing will often slowly occur, and with that, absorbance of the fluid. To facilitate resorption, the patient can wear an abdominal binder or be prescribed diuretics to aid in seroma resolution [8, 11]. Some also advocate for empiric antibiotics to mitigate the risk of infection with serial aspirations and may even facilitate drying of the collection. Percutaneous drain placement should not be performed as this immediately converts a sterile seroma to an infected seroma, thereby contaminating the pump.

Infection

The rate of pump infection is low (2–3%), even in the case of concurrent colorectal resection [6, 15, 16]. However, the pump pocket should be closely monitored during the early postoperative period for signs and symptoms of infection. If there is any concern for infection, early antibiotic intervention should be pursued to prevent infection of the device, and broad-spectrum antibiotics should be used that cover skin flora as well as Gram-positive and -negative organisms [11]. In cases of minor cellulitis, the patient can be treated with oral antibiotics. If no improvement is observed and there is concern for deeper infection, then they should be treated with a longer course of IV antibiotics. If the pump is grossly infected, temporary salvage can be achieved with pocket exploration and washout with an antimicrobial solution (e.g., betadine and/or antibiotic solution) with concurrent administration of IV antibiotics. However, the success of this approach is usually short-lived, and only allows for an average of 1–2 months of rescue HAI treatment [8, 10, 11]. A long-term solution to pump infection is pump removal and relocation to a new site, with a new sterile device. The infected pump is disconnected from the catheter and removed, and a new pump is placed at a new site [10]. The catheter end which was within the previously infected pocket is clipped and removed. The newly trimmed catheter is then redirected to the new site and connected to the pump via splicing with a catheter repair or extension kit. The catheter can be identified intra-abdominally and brought to the new pump location either via a traditional mini-laparotomy, or laparoscopically. Alternatively, if the abdomen is hostile, the catheter can be relocated completely extraperitoneally by tunneling to the new pump site, but this approach risks ongoing infection [11].

Pocket Bleeding/Hematoma

Postoperative bleeding, either intra-abdominally or into the pump pocket, occurs in less than 1% of patients, however, it can result in loss of the pump if not promptly treated. This happens through eventual wound breakdown and subsequent infection [9, 10]. Flank hematomas more commonly develop in cases of obesity and thicker abdominal walls, as these patients may require more extensive dissection to reach the fascia to properly secure the pump. Minor bleeding or a small pocket hematoma can be managed conservatively with compression therapy and an abdominal binder. However, if a significant hematoma develops leading to rapid expansion and subsequent pressure or tension of the overlying skin, the patient must return to the operating room immediately to obtain adequate hemostasis and evacuate the hematoma which can otherwise become a nidus for infection or create local skin breakdown. Of note, re-exploration of the pocket increases the risk of subsequent pump infection, however, the benefits of achieving hemostasis and evacuating the hematoma outweigh such risks.

Catheter Complications

Catheter-related complications are more challenging in nature. These can lead to a catheter that is unusable, thus eliminating HAI-pump therapy as a treatment option. Although catheter-related complications have decreased since the introduction of implantable devices, the placement of a foreign body within a small artery is technically challenging. Even so, catheter-related complications occur in 10–26% of patients, and can be due to either catheter occlusion (i.e., thrombosis or kinking) or migration [6]. These complications can be suspected if there is difficulty in flushing the device at the time of postoperative nuclear imaging, or if there is an unexpectedly high residual volume in the pump at the time of refilling because the drug is unable to exit the occluded catheter.

Catheter Occlusion Including Thrombosis

If there is concern for either arterial or catheter thrombosis, one can obtain a CT angiography together with pump angiogram to differentiate between them. Catheter occlusion can be ruled out with pump injection under fluoroscopy using a bolus needle. This method helps confirm proper pump position on the abdominal wall and allows for visualization of contrast flow through the catheter and into the hepatic arteries. If the catheter is indeed thrombosed, treatment depends largely on timing. If the diagnosis is made early, then a gentle heparin flush can clear the tube of freshly formed clot. However, late catheter thrombosis can also occur, which is defined as that occurring more than 30 days after insertion [6].

Late catheter thrombosis is often preceded by a decrease in the infusion rate as the fibrin sheath forms. This can manifest by gradually increasing residual volumes in the pump at the time of refilling. A late diagnosis of catheter thrombosis is unfortunately associated with high rates of pump failure, as there may already be an extensive fibrin sheath formed within the catheter lumen. If catheter thrombosis is suspected, one can consider instilling 1 mg of tissue plasminogen activator (tPA) [6, 10, 17, 18]. This should be performed with a bolus needle under controlled circumstances in the interventional radiology suite to allow proper visualization of the occlusion site. If the occlusion is found to extend into the hepatic artery, then the tPA infusion should be aborted because it can lead to pseudoaneurysm formation and bleeding. The patient should instead be treated with systemic anticoagulation and pump heparinization until the clot resolves. The use of thrombolytics and/or anticoagulants results in salvage rates of approximately 30% [9].

Catheter Migration

The catheter can also migrate or become dislodged at either its distal (i.e., the gastroduodenal artery, or GDA) or proximal (i.e., exiting the pump) ends, or erode through the GDA and into the neighboring viscera. The severity of this type of complication varies depending on the timing and the location where the migration occurs, with rates reported of 5–18% [6, 19]. Although rare, catheter-associated complications such as displacement (3.3% of the time) and vessel erosion (0.7% of the time) can often present as vague abdominal pain and require embolization, covered stent placement, and even surgical intervention [6].

Most commonly, the catheter can gradually migrate out of its insertion site in the GDA and can lead to pseudoaneurysm formation. When migration is gradual, significant bleeding is uncommon because the GDA will slowly thrombose, and a well-formed tract will develop that gradually fills with thrombus or becomes thrombosed. Patients are often asymptomatic and catheter migration is typically found incidentally on surveillance imaging, which will likely show separation of the catheter tip from the GDA. This may occur with or without pseudoaneurysm formation or perivascular fluid collection near the catheter tip due to extraluminal infusion or bleeding. These findings can require immediate discontinuation of pump treatment altogether, and consideration of interventional placement of a stent graft across the origin of the GDA. If stenting is not feasible, embolization of the hepatic artery is required. Most patients are asymptomatic, and removal may present more risk than leaving the device and catheter in place. However, the presence of a large (>2 cm) pseudoaneurysm is a finding that should prompt intervention, because rupture is one of the few complications that can result in mortality following this operation.

Catheter Dislodgement and Breakage

Some pumps require manual connection and/or splicing of the catheter to the device at the time of implantation. The catheter may become dislodged at the pump connection site and either stay within the pocket or become free floating within the abdominal cavity. This complication is often found on surveillance imaging and seems to be more common in patients that have required modular pump implantation or catheter repair or pump replacement, such as in the case of those who had Medtronic devices implanted that required splicing of two catheters together for the initial pump placement [11]. Dislodgement at the pump insertion site rarely leads to bleeding since the catheter will thrombose due to its small caliber. This is typically an unsalvageable complication which requires pump removal (Fig. 10.3), as the entire conduit for drug delivery is no longer functional. The incidence of this type of complication can be reduced by using permanent sutures to secure the catheter at both the fascia exit site and at the pump connection site, as well as by maintaining a longer loop of catheter within the pocket. The latter is especially helpful in cases where catheter splicing is needed to avoid friction or shearing of the spliced segment as the catheter traverses the abdominal wall.

Catheter Erosion into Bowel

Complications associated with the intra-abdominal portion of the catheter can also occur, but are less common. Rarely does the catheter erode into abdominal viscera, most commonly the duodenum near the insertion site, or at other more distant locations. This may be incidentally found in asymptomatic patients, or they may present with abdominal pain, gastrointestinal bleeding, infection, or even frank perforation. In these patients, chemotherapy should be stopped immediately, IV antibiotics should be started, and if full thickness erosion is confirmed on endoscopy, surgery should be considered for catheter removal and bowel repair or resection as needed.

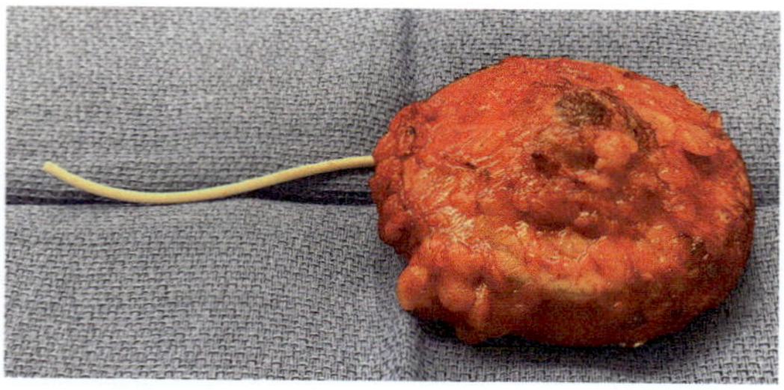

Fig. 10.3 Removed pump after ligation and division of the catheter

Vascular Complications

Vascular complications occur in less than 10% of patients, but include arterial dissection, thrombosis, pseudoaneurysm, and extrahepatic perfusion [6]. If these are not identified at the time of the index operation, they can cause liver injury or ischemia and the patient may present with right upper quadrant pain, transaminitis, hyperbilirubinemia, or alkaline phosphatemia. The first step in diagnosis is CT angiography, but if this initial CT is not diagnostic, it should be followed by hepatic arteriography in the IR suite.

Arterial Dissection

Arterial dissection can occur at the time of artery cannulation, and may be seen afterwards on surveillance imaging. Dissection will impede flow of the infusion. Attempts can be made to fenestrate the dissection flap to allow for communication between the true and false lumens. However, this is rarely successful and risks complete occlusion of the hepatic artery. Instead, it is often prudent to just leave the catheter in place and wait for further, more definitive assessment using postoperative imaging, which often will show that flow has normalized. However, it may also result in a nonfunctional pump [10]. A more detailed discussion of complications associated with artery cannulation and catheter insertion are covered in Chap. 8.

Arterial Pseudoaneurysm

As mentioned previously, pseudoaneurysms can result when the catheter tip either erodes through the GDA or is dislodged, leading to pooling of the drug and degradation of the arterial wall. Thankfully, this type of complication is rare, occurring in less than 5% of patients [11]. Although it is often asymptomatic and incidentally found at the GDA origin on surveillance imaging, patients may also present with acute abdominal pain, bleeding, hypotension, and even shock in rare circumstances. Since an unidentified pseudoaneurysm can lead to serious morbidity if left untreated, suspicion for this type of complication should be maintained until ruled out.

A CT angiogram can be obtained for workup if the patient is stable. Imaging may show the pseudoaneurysm, a fluid collection around the catheter tip and the GDA, with layering of blood products, or even active extravasation of contrast. If the patient is hemodynamically unstable, an urgent consult to interventional radiology should be obtained, and this should include diagnostic and therapeutic arteriography. Intervention will typically involve stenting the common hepatic artery across the GDA orifice to occlude the artery and prevent ongoing bleeding. If stenting is not feasible, then embolization may be necessary. In either situation, the pump must be sacrificed [11, 17].

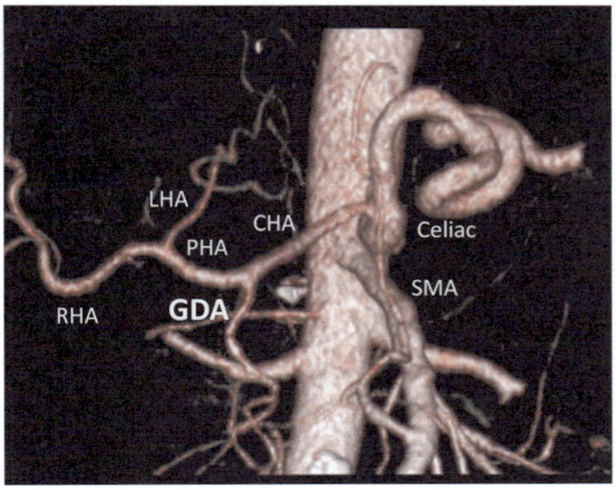

Fig. 10.4 Computed tomographic angiogram (CTA) of patient for preoperative anatomical assessment of the arterial anatomy prior to placement of HAIP. *Celiac* celiac axis, *CHA* common hepatic artery, *GDA* gastroduodenal artery, *LHA* left hepatic artery, *PHA* proper hepatic artery, *RHA* right hepatic artery, *SMA* superior mesenteric artery

Incomplete Perfusion and Extrahepatic Perfusion

HAIP placement should always include preoperative assessment of each individual patient's anatomy using CT angiography (Fig. 10.4), particularly since normal hepatic anatomy is only present in about 65% of patients [20, 21]. This is required to ensure optimal drug delivery, and to avoid incomplete perfusion or extrahepatic perfusion (EHP), often called "misperfusion." A more detailed discussion of aberrant arterial anatomy is discussed in Chapters 7 and 8.

Intraoperatively, several steps should be performed for successful pump placement and avoidance of EHP. These include dividing the ligamentum teres to avoid perfusion of the abdominal wall, and cholecystectomy to avoid chemical cholecystitis. The common hepatic artery (CHA) should be isolated circumferentially, and any small branches ligated from approximately 2 cm proximal to the origin of the GDA, and as far distally as possible, up to the branch point of the left and right hepatic arteries. This includes isolating small supra-duodenal branches from the hepatoduodenal ligament. The GDA should then be circumferentially isolated and branches proximal to the pump insertion site also divided, including the right gastric artery. If an accessory or replaced hepatic artery is present, it should also be ligated. Finally, any additional vessels arising from the celiac axis that supply the superior border of the distal stomach and proximal duodenum should also be divided [18, 22]. The division of all these branches is central to preventing any extrahepatic flow of FUDR (2′-deoxy-5-fluorouridine), which could lead to duodenitis, pancreatitis, gastritis, or gastric ulcers [23].

One must assess for EHP after placement of the catheter. This can be done by bolusing methylene blue (Fig. 10.5a), fluorescein dye (requires holding a Woods lamp over the operative field; Fig. 10.5b), or indocyanine green (ICG, requires Spy or Firefly capabilities) through the pump. If any EHP is observed, re-exploration must be carried out to ligate any remaining collateral branches, followed by re-testing of the perfusion pattern until satisfactory hepatic perfusion is achieved. The catheter should then be flushed with heparinized saline (100 units per mL) prior to closure.

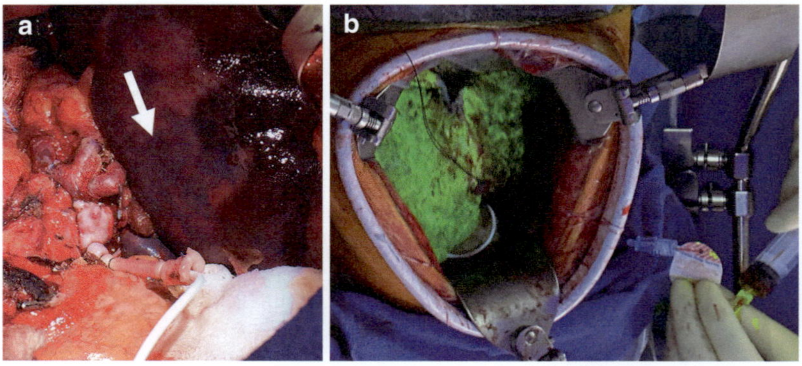

Fig. 10.5 Intraoperative perfusion assessment for appropriate intrahepatic hepatic perfusion and lack of extrahepatic perfusion using methylene blue (**a**; arrow denotes blue dye) or fluorescein dye (**b**; visualized with Woods lamp) injected using a bolus needle as shown

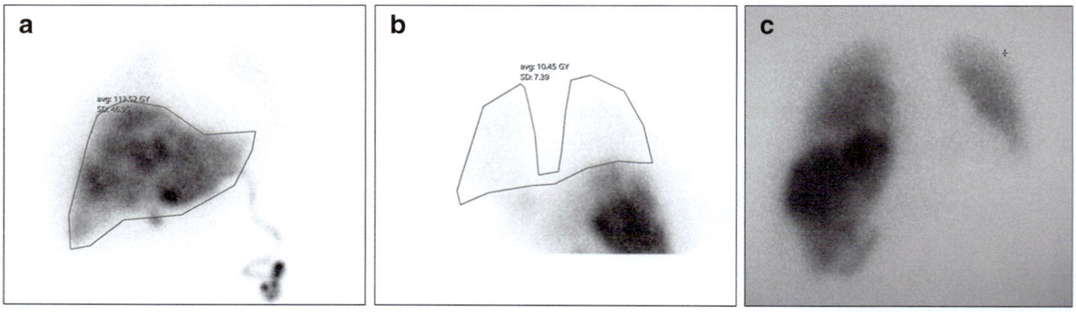

Fig. 10.6 Postoperative technetium-99 m-macroaggregated albumin pump flow scan to: (**a**) confirm bi-lobar hepatic perfusion and (**b**) absence of extrahepatic perfusion including shunt to the lungs (6.3% fraction; normal <20%). (**c**) Example of tracer shunted to the lungs (37% fraction) requiring embolization to avoid extrahepatic FUDR perfusion

Postoperatively, the patient should undergo a baseline technetium-99m macroaggregated albumin (^{99m}Tc-MAA) pump flow scan to confirm bilobar hepatic perfusion and absence of EHP (Fig. 10.6a, b). The time interval between injection of the radiolabeled marker and the acquisition of the images should be minimized. This will help avoid breakdown of the tracer and allow for accumulation of free pertechnetate, which can easily be mistaken for EHP because it will distribute to various tissues, including the kidneys, stomach, and spleen. Radiologists can also calculate the fraction of the tracer shunted to the lungs (normal is <10%) in order to calculate for appropriate dose reductions and reduce pulmonary side effects (Fig. 10.6c) [17]. SPECT/CT imaging using ^{99m}Tc-MAA can also be obtained to evaluate for extrahepatic distribution of the tracer, as these imaging studies will allow for more precise localization over just SPECT alone [25]. If EHP is confirmed, angioembolization of the culprit vessel causing extrahepatic flow can be performed. Most often, this is a branch arising from the proper, right or left hepatic arteries (Fig. 10.7) [22, 24]. Absence of extrahepatic flow must always be confirmed prior to infusing chemotherapy via the pump.

Finally, incomplete hepatic perfusion is often the result of overlooked accessory/replaced vessels or a very short/nonexistent proper hepatic artery that were not appropriately addressed in the operating room. Occasionally, incomplete perfusion may also be secondary to arterial anatomy and the positioning on the catheter in the GDA. Regardless of cause, improvement is often achieved through interventional embolization of vessels feeding the non-perfused segment.

Biliary Complications

As mentioned previously, the HAIP is used to deliver Floxuridine (2′-deoxy-5-fluorouridine; FUDR), a prodrug of 5-fluorouracil. This medi-

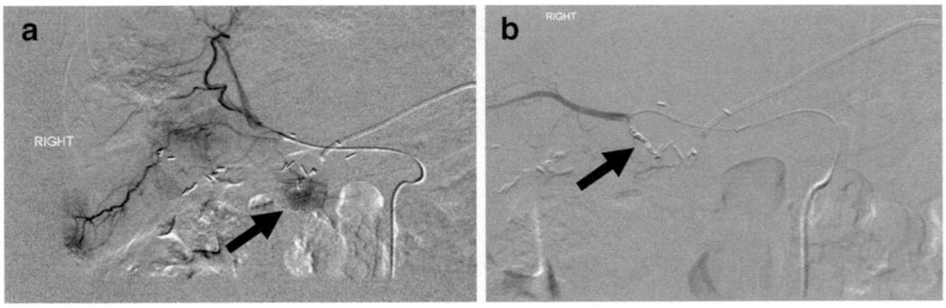

Fig. 10.7 Subtraction angiography to (**a**) identify and (**b**) coil embolize an arterial branch causing extrahepatic perfusion. The patient presented with abdominal pain shortly after filling his pump with FUDR. A supraduodenal or accessory right gastric artery originating off an accessory segment 6 artery was identified. This provided blood supply to the peripancreatic lymph node, as well as duodenum, pancreas and possibly stomach. Because this vessel was likely being perfused with chemotherapy exposure when the pump was filled, it was coil embolized

cation has a high first-pass hepatic metabolism and a short half-life, making it an ideal drug for liver directed therapy. This approach takes advantage of inherent liver physiology: while healthy liver parenchyma derives its blood supply from both the arterial and portal venous circulations, liver metastases derive their blood supply disproportionately from the hepatic arteries. By infusing chemotherapy directly into the hepatic arterial circulation, the HAIP can deliver high concentrations of the prodrug directly to the tumors while somewhat sparing normal liver parenchyma and reducing systemic toxicity [26]. However, the biliary tree is also disproportionately supplied by the hepatic arteries. Although the qualities of the prodrug make it ideal for directed therapy, delivery of this chemotherapeutic into the hepatic arterial system still places the biliary tree at risk for toxicity and subsequent irreversible biliary sclerosis. Toxicity to the biliary tree occurs in approximately 26% of patients and is often identified on routine blood work that patients undergo with each infusion cycle [6, 27]. When asymptomatic, patients will often present with elevated transaminases, bilirubin, and/or alkaline phosphatase. Some patients will present with worsening jaundice or cholangitis symptomatology.

If the patient is asymptomatic but liver enzymes are elevated, further risk can be minimized by maintaining close follow up of liver panels to guide FUDR dose reduction, concurrent dexamethasone administration with FUDR (see Chap. 11 for discussion of dosing and duration), and to allow for timely adjustment of treatment duration. However, one should suspect biliary sclerosis in patients with persistently elevated liver enzymes and bilirubin despite these measures.

HAI treatment must be terminated if ongoing biliary sclerosis is diagnosed. In these patients, MRCP (magnetic resonance cholangiopancreatography; Fig. 10.8a, b) will likely show evidence of biliary sclerosis manifesting as a common hepatic duct stenosis and/or more diffuse biliary strictures throughout the liver [28]. This complication rarely compromises survival if addressed in a timely fashion. To diminish the risk of cholangitis and hepatic failure, the biliary tree should be decompressed via stenting or dilation, which can be accomplished endoscopically (Fig. 10.8c, d) or percutaneously and must be carefully individualized to the anatomy of the stricture(s).

Despite adjustments to dosing, concurrent steroid administration, and other measures, progression of toxicity to biliary sclerosis requiring a stent still occurs in about 2–8% of patients and is highest among those receiving adjuvant HAI after hepatic resection [7, 28, 29]. Additional factors associated with biliary sclerosis include postoperative infectious complications, abnormal postoperative flow scans, and higher doses or cycles of FUDR [28]. On very rare occasions, biliary toxicity can advance to hepatic failure.

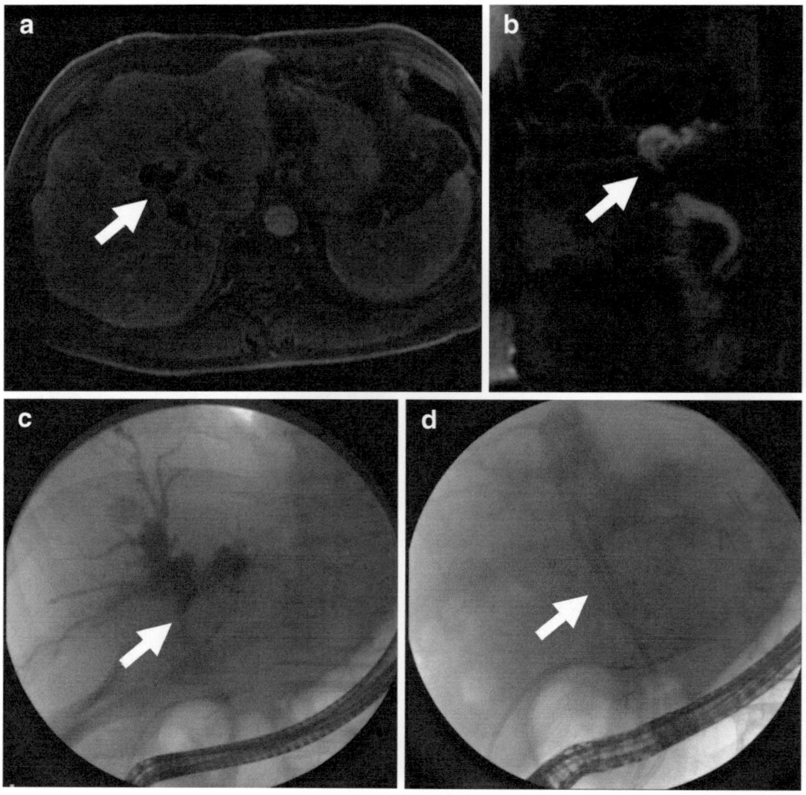

Fig. 10.8 Biliary strictures presenting with worsening jaundice. (**a**, **b**) Magnetic resonance cholangiopancreatography (MRCP) demonstrating hilar and intrahepatic biliary ductal dilatation (arrows) resulting from distal biliary stricture. (**c**) Endoscopic retrograde cholangiopancreatography (ERCP) demonstrating a tight stricture of common hepatic duct with intrahepatic ductal dilatation. (**d**) Two 7 Fr biliary stents were placed across the stricture in the right and left biliary ducts

Infusion Rate-Related Complications

The flow rate from the pump and into the catheter is dependent upon body temperature, atmospheric pressure, and the viscosity of the fluid in the drug reservoir. Together, these factors determine the interval of pump emptying and refilling. Precise drug dosing can thus be achieved by calculating an estimated flow rate. A particular dose of FUDR is instilled in the pump with heparin (100 units per mL) and normal saline to prevent catheter clotting. Treatment is then delivered over a 14-day cycle. Drug dosage is calculated based on the patient's weight, liver panel trends, and flow rate calculations (see Chap. 11).

Due to the device mechanism and design, variations in atmospheric pressure and body temperature can change the medication flow rate. Higher body temperatures and atmospheric pressures affect the behavior of the propellant and lead to increased flow rates. This can lead to faster delivery of medication and increased drug-related toxicity, as well as pump dry-out due to early emptying of the drug chamber, and this in turn can lead to unrecoverable catheter thrombosis and ultimate pump failure.

Unfortunately, there are no mechanisms in place to alert the patient that the fluid is reaching low levels. This should be kept in mind when counseling patients about their infusion pump. Drug dosage and pump refilling schedules can also be affected by traveling to or living at high altitudes. Scuba diving should be avoided, and air travel is permitted only in pressurized cabins.

Similarly, hyperbaric therapy should also be avoided. Patients should also be educated on the importance of maintaining normal body temperature and should therefore avoid hot tubs, saunas, or electric blankets, and heating pads or cold packs to the pump site. These restrictions can be frustrating for patients, who may need additional support in understanding the rationale behind these limitations. It is also important to counsel them on how the device works, as those who miss their appointments may be putting the pump at risk of running dry and, ultimately, untimely termination of HAI pump treatment [8, 30].

Finally, catheter occlusion due to prolonged nonuse can be prevented with proper refilling of the pump. For example, in cases where treatments are intentionally held for an extended period, the pump can be maintained in a functional status by instilling glycerin into the drug chamber. Glycerin, because of its high viscosity, will infuse at a slower rate and maintain catheter patency. Depending on the concentration of the glycerin used, the pump refills can last anywhere from 37 to 133 days, extending the interval between infusions. Thus, pump and catheter function can be preserved when the patient is not actively receiving chemotherapy for prolonged periods by refilling the pump with glycerin every few weeks to months [8, 11, 18, 30].

Conclusions

HAIP-based regional chemotherapy opens new avenues for treatment of colorectal liver metastases and unresectable intrahepatic cholangiocarcinoma for patients who may otherwise have dwindling options. But placement and maintenance of this device is not without its risks. Care must be taken in planning device insertion and in ensuring appropriate device placement and function. Imaging studies must be judiciously used to accomplish both of these tasks. Nevertheless, as reviewed in this chapter, there are multiple HAIP-related complications that can not only compromise device function but can limit future therapeutic options and be life-threatening. Over the years, multiple medical centers have safely and successfully delivered HAIP-based treatment to patients. These centers have gained experience and built well-prepared multidisciplinary teams trained in device management and identification of its complications. Such teams should be equipped with the resources enabling them to closely monitor patients and address issues in a timely fashion to prevent the loss of pump function.

References

1. Oberfield RA, McCaffrey JA, Polio J, Clouse ME, Lpn TH. Prolonged and continuous percutaneous intra-arterial hepatic infusion chemotherapy in advanced metastatic liver adenocarcinoma from colorectal primary. Cancer. 1979;44(2):414–23. https://doi.org/10.1002/1097-0142(197908)44:2<414::AID-CNCR2820440207>3.0.CO;2-3.
2. Reed ML, Vaitkevicius VK, Al-Sarraf M, et al. The practicality of chronic hepatic artery infusion therapy of primary and metastatic hepatic malignancies: ten-year results of 124 patients in a prospective protocol. Cancer. 1981;47(2):402–9. https://doi.org/10.1002/1097-0142(19810115)47:2<402::aid-cncr2820470231>3.0.co;2-b.
3. Brajcich BC, Bentrem DJ, Yang AD, et al. Short-term risk of performing concurrent procedures with hepatic artery infusion pump placement. Ann Surg Oncol. 2020;27(13):5098–106. https://doi.org/10.1245/s10434-020-08938-0.
4. Curley SA, Chase JL, Roh MS, Hohn DC. Technical considerations and complications associated with the placement of 180 implantable hepatic arterial infusion devices. Surgery. 1993;114(5):928–35.
5. Creasy JM, Napier KJ, Reed SA, et al. Implementation of a hepatic artery infusion program: initial patient selection and perioperative outcomes of concurrent hepatic artery infusion and systemic chemotherapy for colorectal liver metastases. Ann Surg Oncol. 2020;27(13):5086–95. https://doi.org/10.1245/s10434-020-08972-y.
6. Allen PJ, Nissan A, Picon AI, et al. Technical complications and durability of hepatic artery infusion pumps for unresectable colorectal liver metastases: an institutional experience of 544 consecutive cases. J Am Coll Surg. 2005;201(1):57–65. https://doi.org/10.1016/j.jamcollsurg.2005.03.019.
7. Muaddi H, D'Angelica M, Wiseman JT, et al. Safety and feasibility of initiating a hepatic artery infusion pump chemotherapy program for unresectable colorectal liver metastases: a multicenter, retrospective cohort study. J Surg Oncol. 2021;123(1):252–60. https://doi.org/10.1002/jso.26270.

8. Italiano D. Hepatic arterial infusion pump: complications and nursing management regarding use in patients with colorectal cancer. Clin J Oncol Nurs. 2018;22(3):340–6. https://doi.org/10.1188/18.CJON.340-346.
9. Doussot A, Kemeny NE, D'Angelica MI. Hepatic arterial infusional chemotherapy in the management of colorectal cancer liver metastases. Hepatic Oncol. 2015;2(3):275–90. https://doi.org/10.2217/hep.15.9.
10. Thiels CA, D'Angelica MI. Hepatic artery infusion pumps. J Surg Oncol. 2020;122(1):70–7. https://doi.org/10.1002/jso.25913.
11. Sharib JM, Creasy JM, Wildman-Tobriner B, et al. Hepatic artery infusion pumps: a surgical toolkit for intraoperative decision-making and management of hepatic artery infusion-specific complications. Ann Surg. 2022;276(6):943–56. https://doi.org/10.1097/SLA.0000000000005434.
12. Dhir M, Jones HL, Shuai Y, et al. Hepatic arterial infusion in combination with modern systemic chemotherapy is associated with improved survival compared with modern systemic chemotherapy alone in patients with isolated unresectable colorectal liver metastases: a case-control study. Ann Surg Oncol. 2017;24(1):150–8. https://doi.org/10.1245/s10434-016-5418-6.
13. Buisman FE, Grünhagen DJ, Homs MYV, et al. Adjuvant hepatic arterial infusion pump chemotherapy after resection of colorectal liver metastases: results of a safety and feasibility study in The Netherlands. Ann Surg Oncol. 2019;26(13):4599–607. https://doi.org/10.1245/s10434-019-07973-w.
14. Chakedis J, Beal EW, Sun S, et al. Implementation and early outcomes for a surgeon-directed hepatic arterial infusion pump program for colorectal liver metastases. J Surg Oncol. 2018;118(7):1065–73. https://doi.org/10.1002/jso.25249.
15. Roybal JJ, Feliberti EC, Rouse L, Wagman LD. Pump removal in infected patients with hepatic chemotherapy pumps: when is it necessary? Am Surg. 2006;72(10):880–4.
16. Turley MC, Moore C, Creasy JM, et al. Combined primary resection with hepatic artery infusion pump implantation is safe for unresectable colorectal liver metastases. J Gastrointest Surg. 2022;26(4):764–71. https://doi.org/10.1007/s11605-021-05195-8.
17. Napier KJ, Lidsky ME, James OG, Wildman-Tobriner B. Hepatic arterial infusion pumps: what the radiologist needs to know. Radiographics. 2021;41(3):895–908. https://doi.org/10.1148/rg.2021200130.
18. Lewis HL, Bloomston M. Hepatic artery Infusional chemotherapy. Surg Clin North Am. 2016;96(2):341–55. https://doi.org/10.1016/j.suc.2015.11.002.
19. Kemeny N, Huang Y, Cohen AM, et al. Hepatic arterial infusion of chemotherapy after resection of hepatic metastases from colorectal cancer. N Engl J Med. 1999;341(27):2039–48. https://doi.org/10.1056/NEJM199912303412702.
20. Skitzki JJ, Chang AE. Hepatic artery chemotherapy for colorectal liver metastases: technical considerations and review of clinical trials. Surg Oncol. 2002;11(3):123–35. https://doi.org/10.1016/s0960-7404(02)00032-4.
21. Michels NA. Newer anatomy of the liver and its variant blood supply and collateral circulation. Am J Surg. 1966;112(3):337–47. https://doi.org/10.1016/0002-9610(66)90201-7.
22. Perez DR, Kemeny NE, Brown KT, et al. Angiographic identification of extrahepatic perfusion after hepatic arterial pump placement: implications for surgical prevention. HPB. 2014;16(8):744–8. https://doi.org/10.1111/hpb.12208.
23. Hohn DC, Stagg RJ, Price DC, Lewis BJ. Avoidance of gastroduodenal toxicity in patients receiving hepatic arterial 5-fluoro-2′-deoxyuridine. J Clin Oncol. 1985;3(9):1257–60. https://doi.org/10.1200/JCO.1985.3.9.1257.
24. Sofocleous CT, Schubert J, Kemeny N, et al. Arterial embolization for salvage of hepatic artery infusion pumps. J Vasc Interv Radiol JVIR. 2006;17(5):801–6. https://doi.org/10.1097/01.RVI.0000217937.81939.18.
25. Bailey J, Dewaraja Y, Hubers D, Srinivasa R, Frey K. Biodistribution of 99mTc-MAA on SPECT/CT performed for 90Y radioembolization therapy planning: a pictorial review. Clin Transl Imaging. 2017;5(5):473–85. https://doi.org/10.1007/s40336-017-0245-8.
26. Gyves J, Ensminger W, Niederhuber J, et al. Totally implanted system for intravenous chemotherapy in patients with cancer. Am J Med. 1982;73(6):841–5. https://doi.org/10.1016/0002-9343(82)90774-4.
27. Power DG, Kemeny NE. The role of floxuridine in metastatic liver disease. Mol Cancer Ther. 2009;8(5):1015–25. https://doi.org/10.1158/1535-7163.MCT-08-0709.
28. Ito K, Ito H, Kemeny NE, et al. Biliary sclerosis after hepatic arterial infusion pump chemotherapy for patients with colorectal cancer liver metastasis: incidence, clinical features, and risk factors. Ann Surg Oncol. 2012;19(5):1609–17. https://doi.org/10.1245/s10434-011-2102-8.
29. D'Angelica MI, Correa-Gallego C, Paty PB, et al. Phase II trial of hepatic artery infusional and systemic chemotherapy for patients with unresectable hepatic metastases from colorectal cancer: conversion to resection and long-term outcomes. Ann Surg. 2015;261(2):353–60. https://doi.org/10.1097/SLA.0000000000000614.
30. Parks L, Routt M. Hepatic artery infusion pump in the treatment of liver metastases. Clin J Oncol Nurs. 2015;19(3):316–20. https://doi.org/10.1188/15.CJON.316-320.

Part III

Hepatic Arterial Infusion Delivery

Hepatic Arterial Infusion Drugs and Dosing

11

Louise Connell, Mary Mulcahy, and Marjolein Homs

Rationale for Hepatic Arterial Infusion of Floxuridine

The unique aspects of primary and metastatic liver cancer physiology justify the interest in liver-directed therapy. The hepatic artery is the main blood supply for liver tumors >3 mm in diameter, while the portal vein in combination with the hepatic artery supplies normal liver parenchyma [1]. This anatomical difference together with pharmacologic factors provides the rationale for liver-directed HAI therapy in the management of liver malignancies, most commonly colorectal liver metastases, as well as primary liver cancer, most commonly intrahepatic cholangiocarcinoma. The liver predominantly metabolizes certain drugs during the first pass through the hepatic arterial circulation, which results in high local concentrations of the drug within the liver and low systemic concentrations with minimal systemic toxicity.

L. Connell (✉)
Memorial Sloan Kettering Cancer Center, New York, NY, USA
e-mail: connelll@mskcc.org

M. Mulcahy
Northwestern University, Evanston, IL, USA
e-mail: mary.mulcahy@nm.org

M. Homs
Erasmus Medical Center, Rotterdam, Netherlands
e-mail: m.homs@erasmusmc.nl

Drugs with high total body clearance and a short plasma half-life are the most suitable for HAI. They facilitate the delivery of high concentrations of chemotherapy directly to liver tumors while minimizing toxicity to the remaining liver and body [2, 3]. Increased local concentration depends on the ratio of total body clearance to regional exchange [4]. The best drugs for HAI are agents that have high hepatic extraction with conversion to inactive metabolites, high total body clearance, and a short plasma half-life. If the drug is not rapidly cleared by the liver, the regional advantage is lost because of systemic recirculation.

Fluoropyrimidines have been the cornerstone of chemotherapy for colorectal cancer for more than 50 years. Much work has focused on hepatic extraction of this drug class. 5-Fluorouracil (5FU) and FUDR, the deoxyribonucleoside derivative of 5FU, are both pyrimidine antimetabolites, and both work through inhibition of thymidylate synthase. The principal mechanism of action of FUDR is through 5-fluoro-2′-deoxyuridine-5′monophate (FdUMP). However, there are significant differences in the pharmacokinetic profile between these two drugs.

5FU has saturable, nonlinear pharmacokinetics, whereas FUDR displays linear kinetics. Therefore, total body clearance and hepatic extraction of 5FU decreases at high doses [5]. Although oxaliplatin does not have superior pharmacokinetic characteristics for HAI (e.g., a

M. D'Angelica, M. Lidsky (eds.), *Hepatic Arterial Infusion for Malignancy*,
https://doi.org/10.1007/978-3-031-74935-3_11

long half-life of 15–19 h), differences were seen in tumor versus healthy hepatic tissue by a ratio of 4.3, suggesting that oxaliplatin could be administered effectively and with minimal toxicity via the intra-arterial route [6, 7].

Irinotecan is not well suited for HAI as it is converted to an active metabolite, SN-38, in the liver after first-pass extraction, and systemic effects are seen. Total body clearance of irinotecan was higher with HAI as compared to systemic administration but the levels of SN-38 were also higher [8]. Other agents, including 5-fluorouracil, mitomycin-C, cisplatin, and doxorubicin have been investigated with some advantages administered via HAI, but all have significantly less extraction compared with FUDR [9].

FUDR, a prodrug of fluorouracil (5FU), is an ideal agent for administration via HAI, and has therefore been the primary focus of research on drug therapy administered directly into the hepatic artery to treat liver tumors. Ensminger estimated that up to 99% of FUDR is extracted by the liver during the first pass which results in a hepatic/systemic ratio of 100–400, compared to a hepatic extraction rate of 19–55% for 5FU resulting in a hepatic/systemic ratio around 10 [2]. FUDR is stable at body temperature, is soluble in low volumes, and is compatible with the implantable pump materials such a titanium, silicone, rubber, and polyurethane. Systemic chemotherapy is almost always given concurrently with HAI FUDR.

The rationale behind regional HAI chemotherapy to the liver is further explained by studies using labeled FUDR showing tumoral levels of FUDR 15 times higher with HAI versus portal vein infusion [10]. In a randomized study comparing HAI versus portal vein infusion in patients with previously treated colorectal liver metastases, there were no responses in the portal vein infusion group whereas there was a 33% response in the HAI group [11]. If patients whose tumor progressed on portal infusion of FUDR were switched over to HAI of FUDR, responses occurred, demonstrating that the same drug can produce different responses just by changing the route of administration.

Prolonged, controlled infusions of drug into the hepatic artery with long-term catheter and artery patency were made possible by the development of implantable infusion pumps in the 1970s (Fig. 11.1) [12]. Prior to the development of an internal pump, catheters with external pumps were used. Responses were good, but catheter thrombosis and bleeding complications were frequent [13]. Studies have shown that implantable pumps can deliver chemotherapy for longer periods compared with surgical and percutaneous catheter placement (115 versus 31 versus 25 days, respectively) [14].

Modern implantable hepatic arterial infusion pumps are placed surgically in the subcutaneous space of the abdominal wall with the catheter inserted into the hepatic arterial system via the gastroduodenal artery (Fig. 11.1) [12] and can remain in place for years (with low complication rates). FUDR is delivered continuously over a 2-week period followed by 2 weeks of heparinized saline as part of a 4-week cycle. The pump infuses drug at a constant rate owing to the expansion of an internal bellows exerting a constant pressure on an inner chamber that is filled with drug. The reservoir of the pump is filled percutaneously by accessing a subcutaneous septum using simple palpation and a refill kit. Reservoir

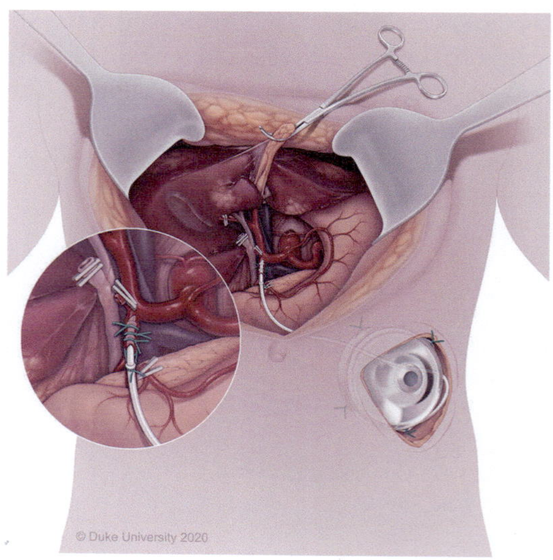

Fig. 11.1 An implantable HAI pump with a catheter in the gastroduodenal artery. Published with permission from Annals of Surgery [12]

volumes are 16–50 mL depending on the device used.

To be suitable for pump placement, patients must have no or minimal extrahepatic disease and have acceptable hepatic arterial anatomy to the liver as seen on computerized tomographic (CT) angiography. In some patients, accessory or replaced arteries supplying the liver must be ligated, thereby relying on efficient interlobar collateral flow to maintain complete hepatic perfusion. Importantly, the portal vein must be patent.

HAI FUDR Initiation

FUDR with dexamethasone is administered every 28 days (if serum liver enzymes are normal). The pump continuously infuses drug, and after 2 weeks the reservoir is emptied and then refilled with heparinized saline, which then infuses over the subsequent 2 weeks.

After implantation of an HAI pump, a single photon emission computed tomography (SPECT) CT perfusion flow scan is performed in the immediate postoperative setting. A normal flow scan shows complete liver perfusion and no evidence of extrahepatic perfusion and/or obstruction, and once confirmed, the pump can be filled with chemotherapy (see Chap. 9 for additional details regarding flow scans). If there is extrahepatic perfusion, an embolization procedure is needed to block the abberant flow, prior to commencing floxuridine.

For the first cycle, the dose of FUDR will be calculated based on the predetermined flow rate provided by the pump manufacturer. Thereafter, doses will be adjusted (lowered, if necessary, but never increased) based on the actual observed flow rate and liver function test fluctuations. The pump will be filled with FUDR, dexamethasone, heparin, and saline.

For patients with colorectal liver metastases, HAIP chemotherapy is initiated 2–12 weeks after surgery depending on patient's medical condition and liver function. In patients who do not undergo hepatic resection or ablation (unresectable CRLM), treatment can begin approximately 2 weeks postoperatively. When HAI is used as adjuvant therapy for resected CRLM, FUDR should not begin earlier than 4 weeks postoperatively. For irresectable intrahepatic cholangiocarcinoma, treatment is started 2 weeks after placement of the pump. Concurrent systemic chemotherapy, reviewed in Chap. 12, typically begins 2 weeks after initiation of FUDR, provided the patient's condition is appropriate (e.g., no concerns for poor wound healing or infection).

Concurrent systemic therapy options include 5-Fluorouracil (5FU), Oxaliplatin, Irinotecan, and EGFR inhibitors for colorectal liver metastases, depending on clinical scenario. In intrahepatic cholangiocarcinoma, gemcitabine and oxaliplatin are commonly used as the systemic option, with use of 5FU and irinotecan also possible. Bevacizumab can be considered sequentially, but should not be used concurrently with HAI FUDR, due to a high degree of biliary complications being noted in a prior study, without improvement in response or conversion rates [15].

FUDR Dosing

Systemic chemotherapy is typically dosed based on BSA (m^2). To calculate the dose of HAI FUDR, it is based on a patient's weight (kg) and the flow rate of the pump (provided by manufacturer and does not fluctuate, usually 1.2–1.4 mL/day). In patients, who have a BMI <25 kg/m^2, their actual body weight can be entered into the below formula to calculate the dose of floxuridine to be administered (formula below is for Intera 3000 pumps; modification for Medtronic Synchromed II pump includes multiplier of 0.9 in the numerator and modification of the volume to either 20 mL or 40 mL depending on which device is used; devices other than either of these may require additional modification to the dosing formula).

$$\text{Floxuridine dose formula} = \frac{(0.12\,\text{mg}/\text{kg}/\text{day}) \times (\text{weight in kg}) \times (30\,\text{mL.})}{(\text{pump flow rate mL}/\text{day})}$$

On Day 1 of active treatment, FUDR is given in combination with dexamethasone (dose calculation below), heparin and saline, to a total volume of 30 mL (provided a 30 mL reservoir is used). The inclusion of dexamethasone with each dose is based on a randomized study in patients with metastatic colorectal liver metastases which highlighted that hyperbilirubinemia occurs in about one third of patients treated with FUDR therapy alone. The addition of dexamethasone reduced the incidence of hyperbilirubinemia from 30% to 9%, while also improving response rate [16], and it is now standard of care to combine these agents during the 14 days of FUDR delivery.

$$^{*}\text{Dexamethasone dose formula} = \frac{(1\,\text{mq}/\text{day}) \times (30\,\text{mL.})}{(\text{pump flow rate mL}/\text{day})}$$

Heparin—30,000 Units.

NS—as needed to titrate volume to 30 mL.

*Some centers use a flat dose of 25 mg dexamethasone.

On Day 15 of the cycle, the pump is emptied and refilled with heparin and saline. Depending upon clinical presentation and laboratory parameters, additional dexamethasone may be considered, as discussed later in this chapter.

In patients who are overweight (defined as 25% above ideal weight), their ideal average body weight can be entered into the below formula to calculate the dose of floxuridine to be administered.

$$\text{Floxuridine dose formula} = \frac{(0.12\,\text{mg}/\text{kg}/\text{day}) \times (\text{ideal average weight in kg}) \times (30\,\text{mL})}{(\text{pump flow rate mL}/\text{day})}$$

FUDR Dose calculation for Overweight Patients.

The dose used for overweight patients is based on an Ideal Average Weight (= Actual weight + Ideal Weight/2). See formulas below for males and females.

The calculation for Ideal Weight (kg) is as follows:

Males: 50 kg + (2.3 × height in inches above 5 ft).

(i.e., for a patient who is 5′10″, use 10)

Females: 45.5 kg + (2.3 × height in inches above 5 ft).

Example: Male who is 100 kg and 5′10″.

Ideal Body Weight is 50 kg + (2.3 × 10) = 73 kg

Therefore, Ideal Average Weight = 100 kg + 73 kg = 173 kg ÷ 2 = 86.5 kg.

The Ideal Average Weight can then be used to calculate the FUDR dose, as demonstrated below. Failure to adjust for weight can result in significant dosing errors, which can inadvertently result in biliary toxicity.

Case-Based Example 1:

Pump rate—1.2 mL/day

$$\text{Real weight} - 104.6\,\text{kg}$$

$$\text{Height} - 71\,\text{in}\,(5.91\,\text{ft})$$

$$\text{Gender} = \text{Male}$$

$$\text{IBW} = 50 + (2.3 \times 11)$$
$$= 75.3\,\text{kg}$$

$$\text{Ideal Average Weight} = \frac{104.6 + 75.3}{2} = 90\,\text{kg}$$

$$\text{Floxuridine} = \frac{0.12 \times 90 \times 30}{1.2} = 270\,\text{mg}$$

If the patient's real weight was erroneously used, the dose calculated would be 314 mg, which would be 15% higher than recommended.

In addition to weight-based adjustments, a lower starting dose of FUDR may be considered per clinician judgement in the appropriate clinical context. For example, if the liver appears unhealthy in the operating room at the time of pump placement, with suggestion of chemotherapy-associated steatohepatitis (CASH) or even cirrhotic changes, starting with 0.06–0.09 mg/kg can be considered to ensure tolerance, with the potential increase to full dose in subsequent cycles provided the patient does not have lab derangements that would require further reduction. Similarly, if the lung shunt fraction is calculated to be 10–20%, it would be prudent to initiate FUDR at 0.09 mg/kg (25% reduction from full dose) and ensure the patient does not develop lung or systemic toxicity, after which subsequent cycles may allow for an increase in the dose to 100% (0.12 mg/kg). FUDR should not be administered if the lung shunt fraction >20%. On the other hand, if liver function tests (LFTs) are abnormal because of extensive liver metastases, and the hepatic metastases respond to treatment, or the liver recovers/lung shunt fraction improves, doses can often be increased after the initial courses of HAI FUDR.

HAI-Specific Complications and Toxicity of HAI FUDR

The toxicity profile for HAI chemotherapy is distinctive, and unlike what is typically seen with systemic chemotherapy agents. The toxicities of HAI can be mechanical, chemical, or a combination of both. Surgically implantable pumps have low complication rates. A retrospective study from Memorial Sloan Kettering Cancer Center, New York (MSKCC) reported on HAI pump complications in 544 patients throughout the course of treatment. Complications within the first 30 days of placement were more likely to be catheter occlusions or arterial thromboses and more likely to be salvaged [17]. The overall pump complication rate was 22%, and the majority of these complications were salvaged with 80% remaining functional for at least 2 years. For a detailed review of HAI-specific complications, see Chap. 10.

Close monitoring of liver function and routine use of proton pump inhibition is imperative. In contrast to systemic chemotherapy, myelosuppression, nausea, and vomiting do not occur with HAI FUDR. A pharmacokinetic study in the Netherlands measured very low FUDR concentrations in peripheral venous blood after HAIP chemotherapy. FUDR could only be measured 7 and 15 days after start of treatment, at earlier time points the level was below boundary of detection [18]. This confirms and explains the low systemic toxicity observed.

Hepatotoxicity from HAI depends on the drugs being used and the duration of treatment. The hepatic artery supplies the bile ducts, and therefore toxicity of HAI FUDR can be biliary in origin. Biliary toxicity (biliary sclerosis, see Chap. 18) manifests clinically as elevations of aspartate transaminase, alkaline phosphatase, and bilirubin. In the setting of jaundice, obstruction due to malignant or surgical stricture must be ruled out prior to concluding that liver dysfunction is due to HAI therapy. If a stricture is suspected, cross-sectional imaging with liver-specific computed tomography and/or magnetic resonance cholangiopancreatography are used to delineate the anatomy and extent of the biliary stricture(s). Direct cholangiography (endoscopic or percutaneous) may demonstrate sclerosis secondary to HAI therapy which, if focal, may be alleviated with interventional biliary stent insertion and/or dilation.

In the adjuvant pump studies from MSKCC, a larger than twofold increase in alkaline phosphatase was seen in 27–43% of cases. Transaminases increased by 37–59% [19, 20]. An increase in bilirubin greater than 3.0 mg/dL was seen in

Table 11.1 FUDR dose modification schema

	Reference value (RV) defined as the value obtained on D1 of previous cycle (CX-1)	% FUDR dose Relative to the dose administered in the most recent FUDR cycle
AST	2 to <3 × RV	80%
	3 to ≤4 × RV	50%
	> 4 × RV	**Hold**
ALK PHOS	1.2 to ≤1.5 × RV	50%
	> 1.5 × RV	**Hold**
[a]TOT BILI	1.2 to ≤1.5 × RV	50%
	> 1.5 × RV	**Hold**
If treatment is held for any of the above situations, treatment will not be reinstituted until values come down to 3X RV (for SGOT) or 1.2X RV (for Alk Phos, Tot Bili), at which time treatment will resume at 25% of the last dose received		

"Reference value (RV)" is defined as the value obtained on the first day of the most recent FUDR dose (CX-1D1)
To determine the dose of FUDR to be given on CXD1, the labs on CXD1 and CX-1D15 (day pump was last emptied) must be compared to labs on CX-1D1 (RV). FUDR dose modification is required if the labs on CXD1 or CX-1D15 are elevated beyond the above thresholds compared to CX-1D1 (RV). The reference value (RV) is always D1 of the last cycle (CX-1) that the FUDR was administered
[a] **If the bilirubin is increasing but within normal limits and the alkaline phosphatase is stable, dosing can continue without adjustment (FUDR dose does not need adjustment for isolated rise in bilirubin that remains within normal range). Likewise, patients with Gilbert's syndrome can be treated**
If patient develops a total bilirubin > 3.0 mg/dL, the pump should be emptied and Dexamethasone 25 mg plus 30 mL heparinized saline (30,000 units) should be placed in the pump every 14 days. Once there is no longer evidence of toxicity, the dexamethasone dose should be tapered in increments of 5 mg every 14 days. Tapering will continue unless enzymes increase. FUDR should be permanently discontinued

6–19% of cases, with biliary stents required in 3–8% of cases.

In an updated study by Kemeny and colleagues, HAI FUDR/dexamethasone was combined with oxaliplatin and irinotecan over a 5-week cycle [21]. Toxicities during the first two cycles were: grade 3 diarrhea (33%), grade 3/4 alkaline phosphatase (15% and 11%, respectively), grade 3/4 AST (19%), grade 3 bilirubin (4%), and grade 3/4 neutropenia (19% and 4%, respectively). Late toxicity (after the first two cycles) included grade 3 diarrhea (7%), grade 3 or 4 alkaline phosphatase (22% and 11%, respectively), grade 3/4 AST (7%), grade 3/4 neutropenia (15% and 11%, respectively), and neurotoxicity (19%). Thus, an algorithm for dose reductions based on liver blood tests was devised, and FUDR can be dose adjusted accordingly (Table 11.1). As mentioned above, the addition of dexamethasone to FUDR reduces biliary toxicity [16, 22].

Dose Adjustments for Liver Toxicity

Each time the HAI pump is refilled with FUDR, liver function tests should be obtained and compared with the "reference value," which is the value obtained on the first day of the most recent floxuridine dose. To determine if a dose adjustment is needed, compare the reference value to higher value between (a) the day that FUDR was emptied (CX-1D15) or (b) the day of planned FUDR refill (CXD1). The labs of importance are AST/SGOT, alkaline phosphatase (ALK PHOS), and total bilirubin (TOT BILI). The ALT/SGOT levels may also vary over time, but it is not used in making decisions on dose adjustments. In order to better understand this, a case-based example is presented below and a dose-adjustment algorithm is also visually depicted in Fig. 11.2 [23].

Case-Based Example 2: A 37-year-old male patient with descending colon cancer, metastatic

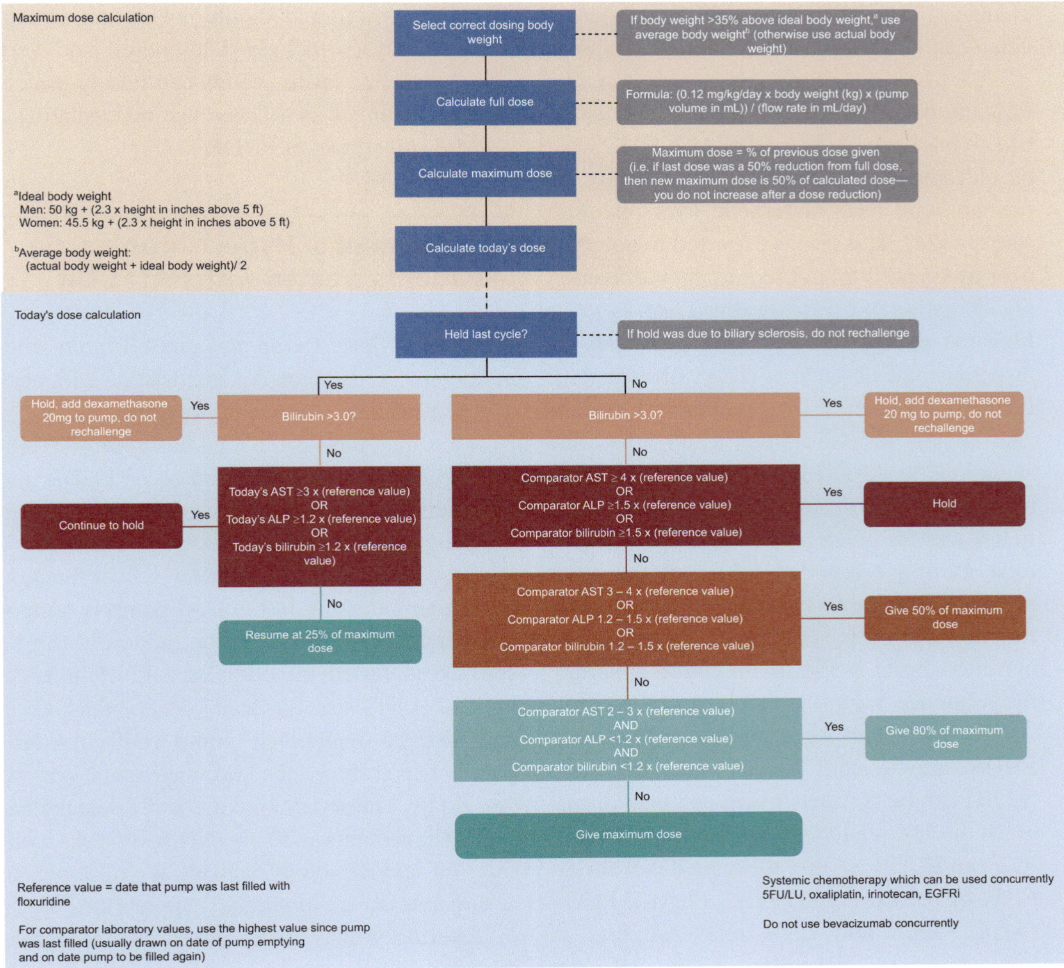

Fig. 11.2 FUDR dosing algorithm. Published with permission from JCO Clinical Practice [23]

to the liver was treated with FOLFOX x 6 cycles, with imaging evidence of response. He then underwent partial liver resection, resection of the primary tumor and HAI pump placement. FUDR was initiated in the pump on Day 14 after placement (C1D1). The trend in liver enzymes is depicted in the table below. Between C1 and C2, there was a 1.3-fold rise in ALK PHOS (120/95) and hence 50% of the original dose was administered on C2D1. Between C2 and C3, there was no significant elevation in liver function tests (LFTs) and hence C3 was administered at the same dose of floxuridine as cycle 2 (i.e., 50% of original dose). Of note, ALT levels do not direct dose adjustments.

Dose Adjustments Based on LFTs

Floxuridine dose administered compared to C1 Dose			50% ↓		50% ↓	
	C1D1	C1D15	C2D1	C2D15	C3D1	C3D15
Aspartate aminotransferase (AST), plasma	20	33	40	45	52	59
Alanine aminotransferase (ALT), plasma	22	44	68	85	104	159
Alkaline phosphatase (ALK PHOS), plasma	95	83	120	104	125	119
Bilirubin, total plasma	0.3	0.3	0.4	0.3	0.3	0.4

There are certain clinical scenarios where a clinician can refrain from FUDR dose reduction:

- Postsurgical elevation of alkaline phosphatase: It has been observed that ALK PHOS can be elevated for up to 28 days or longer, in patients who have undergone liver resection surgery [24]. This rise is expected to decrease over time and does not require a modification in calculation of C1 floxuridine dose.
- Elevated alkaline phosphatase secondary to disease (in the absence of biliary obstruction): It is not uncommon for patients with significant hepatic disease burden to have baseline elevations in ALK PHOS. If this is encountered on the day of intended FUDR initiation, FUDR can be given as planned, provided the total bilirubin is less than 1.5 mg/dL and other metrics of hepatic synthetic and metabolic function are within acceptable ranges. Such an elevation in ALK PHOS on C1D1 is simply the reference value for the subsequent cycle. As patients with such elevations in ALK PHOS are treated, lactate dehydrogenase (LDH) can be checked which can help distinguish disease-related aberrations versus toxicity from FUDR: in disease-related elevations, LDH will trend concordantly with ALK PHOS (ALK PHOS and LDH rise), whereas in toxicity-related elevations, LDH will not increase with a rising ALK PHOS (Table 11.2).
- Isolated hyperbilirubinemia can occur due to Gilbert's syndrome and this finding should be further evaluated with a direct bilirubin. Imaging can be considered to rule out evidence of biliary sclerosis, but this is typically associated with changes in AST and ALK PHOS as well and should not impact dosing. Other causes include dehydration and very low baseline levels, which can falsely project small changes as a difference necessitating a dose adjustment of FUDR.

Table 11.2 Recommencing treatment after a hold

Reason for treatment delay	Floxuridine resumed when value has returned to <=	Floxuridine dose to be administered
AST elevation	3× reference value	25% of last dose
Alk Phos elevation	1.2× reference value	25% of last dose
Total bilirubin elevation	1.2× reference value	25% of last dose

Management of Hyperbilirubinemia in Patients Treated with HAI FUDR

If a patient develops an elevated bilirubin, chemotherapy is held, and dexamethasone with heparinized saline is placed in the pump.

If a patient develops a total bilirubin ≥3.0 mg/dL, the pump should be emptied of FUDR and dexamethasone added with heparin and saline in the pump every 14 days.

If there is persistent elevation of liver function tests, chemotherapy in the HAI pump is temporarily held, and administration of steroid can be considered based on clinician's discretion. As long as LFTs are elevated, dexamethasone is administered with each pump refill. As labs improve over time, the dexamethasone can be tapered by 5 mg every 14 days. If the dexamethasone dose remains at 20 mg over 6–8 weeks, consider an endocrinology consult as you taper, to ensure assessment of adrenal suppression.

Tapering will continue unless liver enzymes increase. FUDR should be permanently discontinued unless there is evidence of disease progression (increasing CEA, worsening CT scan, worsening clinical status) and bilirubin has returned to ≤1.5 mg/dL. In this case, FUDR can be restarted as follows: Use 25% of the last FUDR dose given with dexamethasone, heparin and saline in the pump. The pump should be emptied after 7 days, and patients given a 3-week rest period. This treatment and treatment schedule should continue as long as bilirubin remains ≤1.5 mg/dL and liver enzyme values do not increase.

If the bilirubin still does not normalize, then cross-sectional imaging (typically with an MRCP) can be done to evaluate for focal strictures that may respond to dilatation.

FUDR should be held for 4 weeks prior to a surgical intervention, especially if liver surgery is planned. In these cases, when recommencing treatment, dose reduction is not routinely required.

MRI Compatibility

The Intera 3000 HAI Pump is MR-Conditional and the device can safely be used under routine MR conditions. A continuous scan longer than 15 min can result in pump temperature increasing by 6.5 °C, thereby increasing flow rate by 90%. This limit applies to continuous scan time and not to "table time" which includes the wait time between sequences.

Management of Abdominal Pain in Patients Treated with HAI FUDR

If a patient presents with abdominal pain, HAI FUDR should be withheld and, if the pump is already filled with FUDR, the FUDR should be emptied immediately.

Epigastric pain unresponsive to oral proton pump inhibitor (PPI) use is suggestive of gastroduodenal irritation or ulcer. Severe pain should prompt workup with an upper gastrointestinal endoscopy. Serum lipase/amylase should be checked along with the routine blood work (CBC, liver function tests, and creatinine) in patients with abdominal pain. If an ulcer or gastroduodenitis is documented, therapy should be held for 1 month to allow healing. If abdominal pain is severe, the pump should be emptied of FUDR until results of the workup are available. It is also prudent to repeat the nuclear medicine flow scan to rule out unrecognized extrahepatic perfusion, particularly if there is also marked diarrhea reported, which raises concern for shunting of drug to the bowels.

Maintenance of the HAI Pump

When the pump is not in use, or the planned duration of chemotherapy is completed, the pump maybe filled with glycerin (40–60%), a viscous solution which slows the rate of pump infusion and can maintain catheter patency for extended periods. Once in the maintenance/surveillance phase, the use of glycerin facilitates increasing the interval between pump refills from 2 weeks to 6–8 weeks [25]. If the pump is no longer required, it can be surgically removed by a small incision and the catheter in the hepatic artery is cut off from the pump and left in place.

Other Chemotherapeutic Agents for HAI

As mentioned previously, several other chemotherapies including 5FU, mitomycin, oxaliplatin, and irinotecan or combination of these drugs have been explored via HAI for the treatment of colorectal liver metastases to identify other safe and effective agents for use in this setting (Table 11.3).

HAI with oxaliplatin in combination with systemic 5FU has been shown to be effective for the management of CRLM with objective

Table 11.3 Chemotherapeutic agents used in hepatic arterial chemotherapy

Agent	MOA	AE	HE ratio	Comments
5-FU	Thymidylate synthase inhibitor	Leukopenia, diarrhea	0.22–0.45	19–55% extracted by liver on first pass (18)
Floxuridine	Prodrug of 5-FU. Thymidylate synthase inhibitor	Biliary toxicity	0.69–0.92	94–99% extracted by liver on first pass (18)
Oxaliplatin	Diaminocyclohexane platinum agent	Neuropathy, abdominal pain	0.47 (19)	Used in Europe where floxuridine is not approved
Irinotecan	Camptothecin analogue; topoisomerase 1 inhibitor (20)	Diarrhea, neutropenia	Lower hepatic converted to active metabolite SN-38 (20) extraction	

MOA mechanism of action, *AE* adverse effects, *HE* hepatic extraction response rates greater than 60% and conversion rates of 26% in patients with initially unresectable disease [6, 26]. A retrospective study evaluated the efficacy and toxicity of HAI or intravenous oxaliplatin amongst patients with initially unresectable CRLM that were converted to liver resection. In this study, HAI with oxaliplatin compared with intravenous oxaliplatin was associated with significantly higher rates of pathologic complete response and overall survival, but at the cost of increased risk of severe oxaliplatin-related toxicity such as grade 2 or 3 sinusoidal obstructive syndrome and/or regenerative nodular hyperplasia within non-tumorous liver. The rate of severe oxaliplatin-related injury in the HAI arm compared to intravenous arm was 66% and 20%, respectively ($p < 0.001$). Of note, almost two-thirds of the patients in each arm received concurrent cetuximab/bevacizumab therapy. While the clinical significance of the development of severe oxaliplatin-related toxicity was not reported in this study, severe postoperative complications were observed more frequently in patients who experienced severe oxaliplatin-related toxicity; however, this difference was not statistically significant (27% vs. 17%; $p = 0.26$). Notably, the presence of oxaliplatin-related liver injury did not appear to affect 3-or 5-year survival outcomes [27].

Irinotecan has also been used in HAI. Partial response rates with HAI irinotecan ranged from 14% to 40%, and stable disease was seen in ≤33% [28–30]. Pharmacokinetic data of irinotecan given via HAI showed that there was no difference in the systemic levels of the active metabolite, SN-38, when the irinotecan was given by HAI or intravenous administration [29], suggesting there was no advantage for HAI administration of this agent [8, 31].

The use of combination HAI FUDR/dexamethasone with high dose mitomycin-C via HAI was evaluated in 63 patients with unresectable colorectal liver metastases [32]. High dose mitomycin-C at 15 mg/m^2 was added via the pump sideport to HAI FUDR/dex for 14 days of a 28-day cycle. Mitomycin-C was given on Days 1 and 29. This led to a high response rate, 70%, and the median survival was 21 months, even though half of the patients were previously treated. Due to biliary toxicity issues, in practice, mitomycin-C, when now given via HAI, is administered at 10 mg/m^2. In patients with thrombocytopenia, mitomycin-C via HAI at 8 mg/m^2 is used.

HAI for Non-CRC Liver Metastases

Liver metastases are much less common in non-colorectal cancer. Some case series have evaluated the use of HAI in breast cancer patients with liver metastases after progression on systemic therapy. Drugs used via HAI include cisplatin/vinblastine, etoposide/cyclophosphamide, FU/doxorubicin/mitomycin, and FUDR.

A study of 15 patients using HAI FUDR + mitomycin-C in patients with metastatic breast cancer with chemotherapy refractory disease showed a partial response rate of 53% and overall survival of 18 months from the time of HAI initiation [33].

In hepatocellular carcinoma (HCC), HAI FUDR has been used alone, in combination with leucovorin (LV) + doxorubicin + cisplatin [34], and in combination with mitomycin-C/interferon [31]. Response rates of 41–54% were seen, and median overall survival of 15 months ($n = 29$) was reported in the HAI FUDR/LV/doxorubicin/cisplatin study by Patt and colleagues [34].

In HCC, cisplatin and 5-fluorouracil (5FU) have been used in HAI protocols because their half-lives are 20 and 10 min, respectively. The estimated increased exposure for these drugs with HAI is higher compared with systemic administration and has been estimated between 4-and seven-fold for cisplatin and 5-and ten-fold for 5FU.

At MSKCC, 34 patients with unresectable HCC ($n = 8$) and intrahepatic cholangiocarcinoma (ICC) ($n = 26$) were treated with HAI FUDR alone. Partial responses were seen in 47.1% of patients and median survival was 29.5 months. One patient with ICC went on to resection and had a complete pathological response. Median duration of response was 11.9 months (4.1–14.7 months). Median time to progression for all patients was 7.4 months. With a median follow-up of 35 months, 1-and 2-year survival is at 88% and 67%, respectively. Treatment was well tolerated with no patients requiring biliary stenting, and no significant diarrhea or neutropenia was seen [35].

Similar outcomes were obtained in a subsequent study, in which 22 patients (18 ICC; 4 HCC) were treated with HAI FUDR plus the antiangiogenic monoclonal antibody bevacizumab. In this trial, median PFS and OS were 8.5 months and 31.1 months, respectively. Despite these encouraging results, this study was prematurely terminated owing to increased biliary toxicity associated with bevacizumab [36]. In a retrospective review of 78 ICC patients who underwent treatment with combined HAI FUDR and systemic chemotherapy, HAI was associated with improved OS compared with patients who received systemic treatment alone (30.8 vs. 18.4 Months, respectively; $P < 0.001$) [37]. PFS Was Also Improved for the Combination Group although this was not statistically significant (12 months vs. 7 months). Recently, the results of a multicenter phase 2 trial assessing the efficacy and safety of HAI FUDR combined with systemic gemcitabine and oxaliplatin (GemOx) in unresectable ICC were presented. In 39 evaluable patients, the objective response rate was 46%.

PFS and 2-year OS were 11.5 months and 53%, respectively, with a median OS of 25 months. Four patients (10%) had grade 4 toxicities requiring removal from the study, including portal hypertension, gastroduodenal artery (GDA) aneurysm, GDA extravasation related to HAI catheter, and hyperbilirubinemia [38]. Further discussion on FUDR-based regimens in cholangiocarcinoma is discussed in another chapter (see Chap. 16).

Other chemotherapy drugs besides FUDR have been included in HAI protocols for ICC. Tanaka and colleagues [39] reported their initial experience of 11 ICC patients treated with three different 5FU-based combination regimens (epirubicin, mitomycin, and cisplatin). In this study, seven patients (64%) showed some degree of response in the liver, and 3-year survival was 20%. Two phase 2 trials, including altogether 50 patients, confirmed the activity of HAI with the combination of cisplatin and epirubicin in ICC. In these trials, concurrent systemic 5FU or capecitabine was administered, and response rate ranged between 32% and 40% [40, 41]. No safety concerns were described. More recently, the combination of intra-arterial 5FU and oxaliplatin also showed some activity in a phase 2 trial in which 37 patients with locally advanced biliary tract malignancies (32 ICC; 1 EHC; 4 gallbladder cancer) were included. In this trial, the response rate, PFS, and OS were 16%, 6.5 months, and 13.5 months, respectively [42].

Conclusions

Fluoropyrimidines have been the cornerstone of CRC treatment for more than 50 years. HAI is an effective way to deliver these drugs, especially FUDR, to a patient with liver metastases from CRC. This is an attractive option because high first-pass extraction of this drug given by regional perfusion in the liver limits systemic side effects. The combination of HAI FUDR with modern systemic chemotherapy may be an effective way to treat highly selected patients with liver metastases. Using well-established dosing algorithms, included herein, FUDR can be delivered safely by experienced providers. Expanding roles for HAI FUDR are emerging in other cancer types such as intrahepatic cholangiocarcinoma and HCC. Resources to educate clinicians and pharmacists on best practice in terms of management including guidelines to address the intricacies of dosing of HAI therapy are crucial for safely administering this medication in order to maximize therapeutic benefit and minimize toxicity.

References

1. Breedis C, Young G. The blood supply of neoplasms in the liver. Am J Pathol. 1954;30:969–77.
2. Ensminger WD, Rosowsky A, Raso V, et al. A clinical-pharmacological evaluation of hepatic arterial infusions of 5-fluoro-2′-deoxyuridine and 5-fluorouracil. Cancer Res. 1978;38:3784–92.

3. Ensminger WD, Gyves JW. Clinical pharmacology of hepatic arterial chemotherapy. Semin Oncol. 1983;10:176–82.
4. Collins JM. Pharmacologic rationale for regional drug delivery. J Clin Oncol. 1984;2:498–504.
5. Wagner JG, Gyves JW, Stetson PL, et al. Steady-state nonlinear pharmacokinetics of 5-fluorouracil during hepatic arterial and intravenous infusions in cancer patients. Cancer Res. 1986;46:1499–506.
6. Ducreux M, Ychou M, Laplanche A, et al. Hepatic arterial oxaliplatin infusion plus intravenous chemotherapy in colorectal cancer with inoperable hepatic metastases: a trial of the gastrointestinal group of the federation Nationale des Centres de Lutte Contre le cancer. J Clin Oncol. 2005;23:4881–7, PubMed. https://doi.org/10.1200/JCO.2005.05.120.
7. Dzodic R, Gomez-Abuin G, Rougier P, et al. Pharmacokinetic advantage of intra-arterial hepatic oxaliplatin administration: comparative results with cisplatin using a rabbit VX2 tumor model. Anti-Cancer Drugs. 2004;15:647–50, PubMed. https://doi.org/10.1097/01.cad.0000131684.06390.fe.
8. Van Riel JM, van Groeningen CJ, de Greve J, Gruia G, Pinedo HM, Giaccone G. Continuous infusion of hepatic arterial irinotecan in pretreated patients with colorectal cancer metastatic to the liver. Ann Oncol. 2004;15:59–63. https://doi.org/10.1093/annonc/mdh022.
9. Ensminger WD. Intrahepatic arterial infusion of chemotherapy: pharmacologic principles. Semin Oncol. 2002;29:119–25.
10. Sigurdson ER, Ridge JA, Kemeny N, Daly JM. Tumor and liver drug uptake following hepatic artery and portal vein infusion. J Clin Oncol. 1987;5:1836–40.
11. Daly JM, Kemeny N, Sigurdson E, Oderman P, Thom A. Regional infusion for colorectal hepatic metastases. A randomized trial comparing the hepatic artery with the portal vein. Arch Surg. 1987;122:1273–7. PubMed
12. Sharib JM, Creasy JM, Wildman-Tobrine B, et al. A surgical toolkit for intraoperative decision-making and management of hepatic artery infusion-specific complications. Ann Surg. 2022;276(6):943–56. PMID 36346892.
13. Tandon RN, Bunnell IL, Cooper RG. The treatment of metastatic carcinoma of the liver by the percutaneous selective hepatic artery infusion of 5-fluorouracil. Surgery. 1973;73:118–21.
14. Yasuda S, Noto T, Ikeda M, et al. Hepatic arterial infusion chemotherapy using implantable reservoir in colorectal liver metastasis. Gan To Kagaku Ryoho. 1990;17:1815–9.
15. Kemeny NE, et al. Randomized phase II trial of adjuvant hepatic arterial infusion and systemic chemotherapy with or without bevacizumab in patients with resected hepatic metastases from colorectal cancer. J Clin Oncol. 2011;29(7):884–9.
16. Kemeny N, Seiter K, Niedzwiecki D, et al. A randomized trial of intrahepatic infusion of fluorodeoxyuridine with dexamethasone versus fluorodeoxyuridine alone in the treatment of metastatic colorectal cancer. Cancer. 1992;69(2):327–34.
17. Allen PJ, Nissan A, Picon AI, et al. Technical complications and durability of hepatic artery infusion pumps for unresectable colorectal liver metastases: an institutional experience of 544 consecutive cases. J Am Coll Surg. 2005;201:57–65. https://doi.org/10.1016/j.jamcollsurg.2005.03.019.
18. Ijzerman NS, Filipe WF, Bruijn P, et al. Systemic exposure of floxuridine after hepatic arterial infusion pump chemotherapy with floxuridine in patients with resected colorectal liver metastases. Biomed Pharmacother. 2023;162:114625. https://doi.org/10.1016/j.biopha.2023.114625. Epub 2023 Apr 12.
19. Kemeny N, Huang Y, Cohen AM, et al. Hepatic arterial infusion of chemotherapy after resection of hepatic metastases from colorectal cancer. N Engl J Med. 1999;341:2039–48. https://doi.org/10.1056/NEJM199912303412702.
20. Kemeny N, Jarnagin W, Gonen M, et al. Phase I/II study of hepatic arterial therapy with floxuridine and dexamethasone in combination with intravenous irinotecan as adjuvant treatment after resection of hepatic metastases from colorectal cancer. J Clin Oncol. 2003;21:3303–9, PubMed. https://doi.org/10.1200/JCO.2003.03.142.
21. Kemeny N, Jarnagin W, Paty P, et al. Phase I trial of systemic oxaliplatin combination chemotherapy with hepatic arterial infusion in patients with unresectable liver metastases from colorectal cancer. J Clin Oncol. 2005;23:4888–96. https://doi.org/10.1200/JCO.2005.07.100.
22. Kemeny N, Conti JA, Cohen A, et al. Phase II study of hepatic arterial floxuridine, leucovorin, and dexamethasone for unresectable liver metastases from colorectal carcinoma. J Clin Oncol. 1994;12:2288–95.
23. Rao D, Ellis CS, Kemeny N, et al. Case-based clinical guidance on dosing and Management of the Hepatic Artery Infusion Chemotherapy Pump. JCO Oncol Pract. 2024;20(2):187–94. https://doi.org/10.1200/OP.23.00374. Epub 2023 Oct 26.
24. Nagino M, et al. Serum alkaline phosphatase after extensive liver resection: a study in patients with biliary tract carcinoma. Hepato-Gastroenterology. 1999;46(26):766–70.
25. Italiano D. Hepatic arterial infusion pump: complications and nursing management regarding use in patients with colorectal cancer. Clin J Oncol Nurs. 2018;22(3):340–6.
26. Goere D, Deshaies I, de Baere T, et al. Prolonged survival of initially unresectable hepatic colorectal cancer patients treated with hepatic arterial infusion of oxaliplatin followed by radical surgery of metastases. Ann Surg. 2010;251:686–91.
27. Allard MA, Sebagh M, Baillie G, et al. Comparison of complete pathologic response and hepatic injuries between hepatic arterial infusion and systemic administration of oxaliplatin in patients with colorectal liver metastases. Ann Surg Oncol. 2015;22:1925–32.

28. Fiorentini G, Rossi S, Dentico P, et al. Irinotecan hepatic arterial infusion chemotherapy for hepatic metastases from colorectal cancer: a phase II clinical study. Tumori. 2003;89:382–4.
29. van Riel JM, van Groeningen CJ, Kedde MA, et al. Continuous administration of irinotecan by hepatic arterial infusion: a phase I and pharmacokinetic study. Clin Cancer Res. 2002;8:405–12.
30. Vogl TJ, Eichier K, Mack MG, et al. A phase I study of hepatic arterial infusion (HAI) of irinotecan in patients with inoperable liver metastases of colorectal cancer. J Clin Oncol. 2004;22(14 suppl):298 (Abstract 3714).
31. De Jong FA, Mathijssen RH, Verweij J. Limited potential of hepatic arterial infusion of irinotecan. J Chemother. 2004;16(suppl 5):48–50.
32. Kemeny N, Eid A, Stockman J, et al. Hepatic arterial infusion of floxuridine and dexamethasone plus high-dose Mitomycin C for patients with unresectable hepatic metastases from colorectal carcinoma. J Surg Oncol. 2005;91(2):97–101. https://doi.org/10.1002/jso.20286. PMID: 16028279.
33. Maal J, Curet P, Baumer R, et al. Intra-arterial chemotherapy for hepatic metastases. Experience of the Pitie-Salpetriere hospital group. Ann Gastroenterol Hepatol (Paris). 1985;21:99–101.
34. Patt YZ, Charnsangavej C, Yoffe B, et al. Hepatic arterial infusion of floxuridine, leucovorin, doxorubicin, and cisplatin for hepatocellular carcinoma: effects of hepatitis B and C viral infection on drug toxicity and patient survival. J Clin Oncol. 1994;12:1204–11.
35. Jarnagin WR, Schwartz LH, Gultekin DH, et al. Regional chemotherapy for unresectable primary liver cancer: results of a phase II clinical trial and assessment of DCE-MRI as a biomarker of survival. Ann Oncol. 2009;20(9):1589–95.
36. Kemeny NE, Schwartz L, Gonen M, et al. Treating primary liver cancer with hepatic arterial infusion of floxuridine and dexamethasone: does the addition of systemic bevacizumab improve results? Oncology. 2011;80(3–4):153–9.
37. Konstantinidis IT, Groot Koerkamp B, Do RK, et al. Unresectable intrahepatic cholangiocarcinoma: systemic plus hepatic arterial infusion chemotherapy is associated with longer survival in comparison with systemic chemotherapy alone. Cancer. 2016;122(5):758–65.
38. Cercek A, Kemeny NE, Boerner T, et al. A bi-institutional phase II study of hepatic arterial infusion (HAI) with floxuridine (FUDR) and dexamethasone (Dex) combined with systemic gemcitabine and oxaliplatin (GemOx) for unresectable intrahepatic cholangiocarcinoma (ICC). J Clin Oncol. 2018;36(15_suppl):4092.
39. Tanaka N, Yamakado K, Nakatsuka A, et al. Arterial chemoinfusion therapy through an implanted port system for patients with unresectable intrahepatic cholangiocarcinoma–initial experience. Eur J Radiol. 2002;41(1):42–8.
40. Cantore M, Mambrini A, Fiorentini G, et al. Phase II study of hepatic intraarterial epirubicin and cisplatin, with systemic 5-fluorouracil in patients with unresectable biliary tract tumors. Cancer. 2005;103(7):1402–7.
41. Mambrini A, Guglielmi A, Pacetti P, et al. Capecitabine plus hepatic intra-arterial epirubicin and cisplatin in unresectable biliary cancer: a phase II study. Anticancer Res. 2007;27(4C):3009–13.
42. Sinn M, Nicolaou A, Gebauer B, et al. Hepatic arterial infusion with oxaliplatin and,5-FU/folinic acid for advanced biliary tract cancer: a phase II study. Dig Dis Sci. 2013;58(8):2399–405.

12 Hepatic Arterial Infusion Therapy: Considerations for Concurrent Systemic Therapy

Michael J. Raphael, Emily C. Harrold, Andrea Cercek, and John C. Krauss

Introduction

Hepatic arterial infusion (HAI) chemotherapy has been used to treat unresectable colorectal cancer liver metastases (CRLM) for over four decades [1]. The initial studies examining HAI therapy compared HAI chemotherapy alone against fluoropyrimidine single-agent systemic therapy. These studies consistently showed that HAI chemotherapy improved response rates within the liver, but this did not always translate into an improvement in overall survival (OS) [2]. Moreover, HAI therapy alone was associated with a shorter time to extrahepatic progression [3]. Therefore, all modern HAI programs now use HAI chemotherapy combined with multi-agent systemic therapy to maximize intra-and extrahepatic responses [4, 5]. More recently, based on the success in CRLM, HAI chemotherapy has also demonstrated significant response rates in the treatment of locally advanced and unresectable intrahepatic cholangiocarcinoma (IHCC) [6].

In this chapter, the seminal studies informing the modern-day treatment paradigms for HAI chemotherapy in combination with systemic therapy for treatment of CRLM and IHCC will be reviewed. Additionally, we will present a suggested approach to the integration of HAI chemotherapy in combination with systemic therapy into the management of patients with CRLM and unresectable IHCC.

M. J. Raphael (✉)
Odette Cancer Center, University of Toronto, Toronto, ON, Canada
e-mail: michaelj.raphael@sunnybrook.ca

E. C. Harrold · A. Cercek
Memorial Sloan Kettering Cancer Center, New York, NY, USA
e-mail: harrolde@mskcc.org; cerceka@mskcc.org

J. C. Krauss
University of Michigan, Ann Arbor, MI, USA
e-mail: jkrauss@med.umich.edu

HAI Chemotherapy Alone Without Concurrent Systemic Therapy for CRLM

The liver is the most common site of colorectal cancer metastases. Population-based studies estimate that 25–30% of patients with colorectal cancer will develop liver metastases during their illness [7–13]. Autopsy studies report the prevalence of colorectal liver metastases (CRLM) as high as 60% [14]. Thus, HAI chemotherapy has been studied as a treatment for patients with CRLM as way to enhance the delivery of treatment directly to where it is most needed, while sparing the body systemic side-effects. Multiple studies have been conducted to refine and optimize HAI treatments in order to maximize benefit and minimize toxicity.

M. D'Angelica, M. Lidsky (eds.), *Hepatic Arterial Infusion for Malignancy*,
https://doi.org/10.1007/978-3-031-74935-3_12

The backbone of first-and second-line chemotherapy regimens for advanced colorectal cancer for decades has been 5-Fluorouracil (5-FU). Early HAI studies aimed to determine if HAI delivery of 5-FU would result in more efficacy and less toxicity than systemic delivery. In one of the earliest and largest randomized controlled trials (RCTs) evaluating HAI therapy, the Medical Research Council (MRC) and European Organization for Research and Treatment of Cancer (EORTC) Groups randomized 290 patients with unresectable CRLM to HAI 5-FU and leucovorin (LV) or systemic 5-FU/LV [15]. HAI treatments were performed through a port on the chest wall that was attached to an external infusion pump. The LV was infused over 2 h, followed by 5-FU infusion over 46 h for both cohorts. Consistent with the limited first-pass extraction of 5-FU by the liver, the systemic levels of 5-FU were the same in the hepatic artery infused patients as the systemically infused patients. The median overall survival (OS) was the same in both groups at 15 months. In the HAI group, median progression-free survival (PFS) was 7.7 months, and it was 6.7 months in the systemic treatment group. The tumor response rates were the same for hepatic artery infusion at 22% and systemic infusion at 19%. The median duration of response was 7.6 months for the hepatic artery infusion and 7.5 months for the intravenous infusion. Over one third of patients in the hepatic artery infusion group never received hepatic artery infusion for a variety of reasons demonstrating the technical complexity of establishing and maintaining access to the hepatic artery.

Floxuridine (FUDR) has emerged as the treatment of choice in North America for HAI therapy of CRLM. FUDR is a prodrug of 5-FU which has a 95–99% first-pass hepatic extraction, allowing very high doses of treatment to be delivered, with very little systemic exposure of chemotherapy to cause systemic side-effects [16–18]. Studies have showed that FUDR delivered into the hepatic artery is more active than FUDR delivered via the portal vein, at least in part due to the blood supply of metastatic tumors coming predominantly from the hepatic artery [19]. A randomized study comparing arterial FUDR infusion to portal vein FUDR infusion was performed in patients with unresectable CRLM who had previously received systemic chemotherapy with 5-FU [20]. There was a 50% (4/8 patients) response rate in the arterial FUDR infusion group, and no responses in the portal vein FUDR infused patients. The study included a crossover from portal vein infusion to arterial infusion and there was a 33% response rate in the patients who were crossed over. The hepatic artery infusion was more toxic, with 4/8 patients developing a bilirubin greater than 34 μmol/L (2 mg/dL).

The dose of FUDR that can be administered via the hepatic artery is limited by biliary toxicity. Bile duct inflammation can be seen on blood work with transaminitis, scans, and cholestasis is suggested by hyperbilirubinemia observed from lab findings. Toxicity is first manifested with an elevation of the transaminases and alkaline phosphatase, followed by hyperbilirubinemia and in the most severe cases can progress to bile duct sclerosis and strictures. Liver biopsies from patients treated with FUDR suggests the mechanism of FUDR toxicity is ischemia of the bile ducts from inflammation of the portal triad [21, 22]. The ischemia can result in strictures which require bile duct stenting to achieve a normal bilirubin. In early studies, 70% of patients required a dose reduction of FUDR within 3 months, and 8% developed bile duct strictures [23]. To mitigate the bile duct toxicity of FUDR, all current protocols infuse FUDR admixed with dexamethasone. A randomized trial of arterial FUDR alone compared to arterial FUDR admixed with dexamethasone demonstrated that the patients receiving dexamethasone and FUDR were able to receive more FUDR with equivalent biliary toxicity. This translated to a higher complete and partial response rate of 71% in the FUDR and dexamethasone group as compared to 40% in the FUDR alone group. There was a trend towards improved OS of 23 months in the FUDR and dexamethasone group versus 14 months in the FUDR only group, but this did not reach statistical significance ($p = 0.06$) [24].

Further studies have confirmed that intra-arterial FUDR is associated with better response rates than systemically delivered FUDR. The National Cancer Institute (NCI) group reported on a randomized study of 64 patients comparing intra-arterial FUDR to systemic FUDR for patients with unresectable CRLM [25]. The response rate of the intra-arterial FUDR group was 62% compared to the 17% response rate with the IV FUDR group ($P < 0.003$). Two-year OS was not significantly different at 22% for the intra-arterial group and 15% for the systemic treatment group ($P = 0.27$). When only the patients who actually had HAI pumps placed were included in the analysis, the 2-year OS was 34% for the intra-arterial group and 17% for the systemic group ($P = 0.06$). Control of the cancer in the liver was better in the intra-arterial FUDR treated arm, with 14% of the responders relapsing in the liver only, while 80% of the patients in the systemic arm relapsed in the liver only.

Similarly, a study conducted at Memorial Sloan Kettering Cancer Center (MSKCC) randomized 99 patients with unresectable CRLM to hepatic artery FUDR or systemic FUDR [26]. The dose of FUDR was 0.15 mg/kg/day in the systemic therapy group, and 0.3 mg/kg/day in the hepatic artery infusion group. At progression, the systemic FUDR group was allowed to switch to hepatic artery delivered FUDR. Both groups were treated on a 14-day on and a 14-day off cycle, with the maximum tolerated dose of FUDR. The hepatic artery administered FUDR had a 50% response rate as compared with 19.6% for the systemically administered FUDR respectively ($p = 0.001$). Of the 60% of patients who crossed over from systemic treatment to intra-arterial treatment due to progression on systemic therapy, 25% had a partial response; 33% had a minor response or stable disease. Extrahepatic disease developed in 27 of 48 (56%) patients receiving hepatic artery therapy, compared with 19 of 51 (37%) in the systemic group ($p = 0.092$). The median OS for the intrahepatic group was 17 months compared with 12 months for the systemic group ($p = 0.424$). The apparent lack of difference in survival may have been spurious, resulting from the inclusion of the 31 patients who crossed over from systemic to intrahepatic therapy in the survival analysis of the systemic group. If the patients in the systemic arm who did not crossover were evaluated separately, their median OS was 8 months, compared with 18 months for those who crossed over.

The benefits of delivering HAI FUDR compared to systemic 5-FU were shown in the multicenter, Cancer and Leukemia Group B (CALGB) 9841 RCT [3]. In this study, 135 untreated patients with unresectable CRLM were randomized to either HAI FUDR or systemic treatment with 5 days of bolus 5-FU/LV every 28 days. Overall survival was 24.4 months in the HAI group and 20 months in the systemic therapy group ($p = 0.034$). There was a 47% objective response rate in the HAI group compared to 24% in the systemic therapy group ($p = 0.012$). The toxicity differed between the two arms, with 45% of the patient's developing neutropenia in the systemic arm as compared to 0% in the hepatic artery arm ($p < 0.0001$). A bilirubin of 51 μmol/L (3 mg/dL) developed in 38% of the HAI arm and 15% of the systemic therapy arm ($p = 0.05$). The hepatic artery FUDR was worse at controlling extrahepatic disease, with a time to extrahepatic progression of 15 months in the systemic arm vs 8 months in the hepatic artery infusion arm ($p = 0.029$). A limitation of this study is that the systemic arm has subsequently been demonstrated to be inferior to combination with infusional 5-FU and therefore bolus 5-FU/LV alone is no longer used. Further, FUDR is now given with concurrent systemic chemotherapy. Given the outdated HAI and systemic therapy regimens used in the CALGB trial, the recently activated ECOG-ACRIN clinical trial (EA2222, NCT05863195) is comparing the addition of HAI to current standard combination systemic therapies.

HAI Therapy in Combination with Concurrent Systemic Therapy for CRLM

The observation that patients treated with HAI chemotherapy alone had higher rates of extrahepatic progression prompted all modern HAI trials and treatment programs to combine HAI therapy with best available systemic therapy. It is hypothesized that the addition of systemic therapy will help improve control of the extrahepatic disease and provide synergistic effects to the intrahepatic FUDR to enhance the hepatic response.

HAI Therapy in Combination with Systemic Chemotherapy for Unresectable Colorectal Cancer Liver Metastases

HAI therapy has been safely and effectively combined with modern systemic chemotherapy agents in multiple studies. In 2009, the group at Memorial Sloan Kettering Cancer Centre (MSKCC) reported the pooled results for patients with unresectable CRLM who were treated with HAI FUDR in combination with systemic oxaliplatin and irinotecan on one of two phase 1 protocols [27]. One protocol dosed FUDR every 4 weeks and the other every 5 weeks. In both protocols, patients received a continuous infusion of FUDR dosed at 0.12 mg/kg during Day 1–14 along with systemic oxaliplatin (85–100 mg/m^2) and irinotecan (100–200 mg/m^2) every 2 weeks. Patients were treated until the extent of disease was reduced to the point where surgery was possible or until hepatic/extrahepatic progression or excessive toxicity. Among 49 enrolled patients, 92% of patients achieved a complete (8%) or partial (84%) response. Forty-seven percent of patients were able to undergo liver resection. Among chemotherapy naïve patients the response rate was 100% (23/23 patients) and the resection rate was 57%. Among previously treated patients, the response rate was 85% (22/26 patients) and resection rate was 38%. Grade 3–4 toxicities in the first two cycles included: Diarrhea (14–33%), neutropenia (18–23%) and bilirubin more than 3 mg/mL (4–5%). Grade 3–4 toxicities beyond the first two cycles included neurotoxicity (19–23%). Three patients (6%) required biliary stenting.

In 2015, the group at MSKCC reported on a phase 2 study which aimed to prospectively evaluate the rate of conversion to resection among patients with unresectable CRLM treated with HAI, systemic chemotherapy and bevacizumab [28]. Patients who had received less than 2 cycles of oxaliplatin and had no persistent neuropathy received systemic oxaliplatin (85 mg/m^2), irinotecan (125 mg/m^2) and bevacizumab (5 mg/kg) every 2 weeks. Those patients who had received more than 2 cycles of oxaliplatin or had persistent neuropathy received systemic irinotecan (150 mg/m^2), 5-fluoururacil (2000 mg/m^2 over 48 h), leucovorin (400 mg/m^2), and bevacizumab (5 mg/kg). HAI FUDR was delivered at 0.12 mg/kg/day. The first 24 patients enrolled were treated with bevacizumab, however, the investigators noted a very high rate of biliary toxicity with three patients requiring biliary stenting. Therefore, bevacizumab was removed from the treatment protocol. In updated analyses with long-term follow-up, among 64 enrolled patients, the overall response rate was 73% with 46 partial and one complete response [29]. Among chemotherapy naïve patients, the response rate was 86% (14/17) with a median volumetric response of 83%. Among previously treated patients, the response rate was 67% (23/32). Patients who did and did not receive bevacizumab had a similar response rate (73% vs 75%). In total, 52% (33 patients) were able to undergo surgical resection. The median overall survival was 76.6 months among chemotherapy-naïve patients and 29.7 months among previously treated patients ($p = 0.022$). The 5-year OS for those patients able to undergo resection was 63% compared to 12.5% for those who did not under surgery.

A major criticism against HAI therapy has been that most of the evidence comes from the MSKCC experience. Concerns have been raised that the data may not be generalizable to other centers. Recently, however, several new programs have reported on the safety and efficacy of HAI programs. In 2020, Muaddi et al. reported on a multicenter retrospective cohort study of patients with unresectable CRLM treated at six North American centers [30]. All patients in the study had previously been treated with systemic therapy (median 10 cycles; IQR 6–12). Among 154 patients enrolled, 148 patients (96%) received at least one cycle of FUDR chemotherapy. Patients received a median of 5 cycles of treatment. Fifty-three percent of patients received concurrent systemic therapy (23% FOLFIRI, 12% FOLFOX, 3% 5-FU alone, 15% other combinations). The overall response rate was 57% (18% CR, 38% PR). A total of 7.8% of patients received a liver resection with curative intent. Long-term HAIP-related complications were reported in 11% of patients, with the most common complication being biliary sclerosis (8%).

HAI Therapy in Combination with Biologic Systemic Therapies

Standard of care first-line systemic therapy for metastatic colorectal cancer includes a chemotherapy backbone in combination with a biological therapy [31]. For patients with left-sided, extended RAS wild-type cancer, an epidermal growth factor receptor (EGFR) inhibitor (cetuximab or panitumumab) is combined with chemotherapy. For patients with right-sided or RAS-mutated colorectal cancer, a vascular endothelial growth factors (VEGF) inhibitor (bevaciuzmab) is added to chemotherapy.

Bevacizumab should not be used when patients are receiving FUDR therapy because of irreversible biliary toxicity. In 2014, Cercek et al. reported on 203 patients from three prospective studies who were treated with HAI FUDR and systemic therapy including bevacizumab [32]. One study enrolled patients with resected CRLM; one study enrolled patients with unresectable CRLM; the final study enrolled patients with unresectable cholangiocarcinoma or hepatocellular carcinoma. In all three studies, the incidence of hyperbilirubinemia and biliary stent placement was higher in patients treated with concurrent bevacizumab (Table 12.1). In addition to the increased toxicity, bevacizumab was not associated with improved survival or oncological outcomes.

EGFR inhibitors (cetuximab or panitumumab) may be safely given concurrently with HAI FUDR. In 2021, Kemeny et al. reported the results of a phase 2 trial of adjuvant HAI FUDR with or without panitumumab among patients with resected oligometastatic KRAS wild-type CRC [33]. Patients were treated HAI FUDR 0.12 mg/kg infused over 14 days every 5 weeks for six doses. Patients were also treated with concurrent systemic FOLFIRI with or without panitumumab 6 mg/kg every 2 weeks for 12 doses. Three-year OS was 97% in patients treated with HAI FUDR and systemic FOLFIRI with panitumumab and 91% in patients treated with HAI FUDR and systemic FOLFIRI without panitumumab. There was no difference in grade 3 alkaline phosphatase or bilirubin elevations between those who did and did not receive panitumumab. One patient in each treatment arm required placement of a biliary stent. There was no difference in the dose intensity of FUDR or systemic chemotherapy between arms. Of note, there is no specific rationale for 5-week dosing cycles of HAI FUDR in this trial; therefore, the recommended regimen is a cycle length of 4 weeks even in combination with anti-EGFR therapy and cytotoxic chemotherapy.

HAI Therapy in Combination with Systemic Therapies for Resected CRLM

Adjuvant oxaliplatin-based chemotherapy following surgical resection of Stage 3 colorectal

Table 12.1 Biliary toxicity when systemic bevacizumab was used concurrently with intrahepatic FUDR

Patient population	Toxicity	Bevacizumab (%)	No bevacizumab (%)	*P*-value
Resectable CRLM	Bilirubin ≥2 mg/dL	14	0	0.20
	Biliary stent	11	0	0.05
Unresectable CRLM	Bilirubin ≥2 mg/dL	25	4	0.01
	Biliary stent	13	0	0.06
Unresectable CCA or HCC	Bilirubin ≥2 mg/dL	24	6	0.09
	Biliary stent	14	0	0.15

CRLM Colorectal cancer liver metastases, *CCA* Cholangiocarcinoma, *HCC* Hepatocellular carcinoma cancer is a standard of care treatment with a proven survival benefit [34, 35]. To date, there is no corresponding evidence that systemic chemotherapy given after resection of oligometastatic CRLM is associated with an improvement in survival [36, 37]. In this context, and given that over 70% of recurrences occur within the liver after initial resection of CLRM [38], intensification of liver-directed therapy with HAI therapy represents an important therapeutic option [4].

In 1999, Kemeny et al. reported the results of a single-center, randomized controlled trial which evaluated the benefit of adjuvant HAI therapy following resection of CRLM [39]. One hundred and fifty-six patients with completely resected oligometastatic CRLM were randomized to receive 6 cycles of systemic 5-FU chemotherapy with or without 6 cycles of HAI FUDR. The 2-year OS was significantly higher in the HAI arm (86% vs 72%; $P = 0.03$) and the risk ratio for death was 2.34 among patients who received systemic therapy alone (95% CI, 1.10–4.98). At 2 years, the hepatic recurrence free survival rate was 90% in the HAI arm compared to 60% in the monotherapy group ($P < 0.001$). Five percent (4/74) of patients in the HAI therapy arm required biliary stenting compared with 2% (2/82) in the systemic therapy only treatment arm. At 10 years, there remained a non-statistically significant increase in 10-year OS in the HAI therapy arm (41% vs 27%, $p = 0.10$) [40].

In 2002, a multicenter randomized controlled trial was conducted to confirm the benefits of adjuvant HAI therapy [41]. In this study, 75 patients with 1–3 CRLM were randomized to surgery with or without adjuvant HAI FUDR and systemic 5-flouoruracil. FUDR was infused over 14 days at a dose of 0.1 mg/kg/day (0.05 mg/kg/day if a lobectomy was completed) with potential for dose escalation to maximum dose of 0.2 mg/kg/day if the first cycle was well tolerated. Systemic 5-FU was administered at a dose of 200 mg/m^2/day over 14 days every 2 weeks for 4 cycles followed by 300 mg/m^2/day over 14 days for 4 further cycles. The 4-year recurrence-free rate (46% vs 25%; $p = 0.04$) and 4-year liver recurrence-free rate (67% vs 43%; $p = 0.03$) were significantly improved in the HAI arm. The median OS was not statistically different, but was numerically longer in the HAI arm (Median OS, 63.7 months vs 49 months, $p = 0.60$). In the HAI arm, nine patients developed grade 3 increases in bilirubin and two patients required biliary stenting.

In 2010, the North Central Cancer Treatment Group (NCCTG)/National Surgical Adjuvant Breast and Bowel Project (NSABP) reported the results of a phase 2 trial of adjuvant HAI FUDR and systemic CAPOX chemotherapy [42]. Fifty-five patients were treated with alternating cycles of HAI FUDR dosed at 0.2 mg/kg/day (four doses total) and CAPOX chemotherapy (six doses total). Originally, capecitabine was dosed at 1000 mg/m^2 twice a day, however, an interim review identified that 47% of patients developed grade 3 diarrhea prompting dose reduction to 850 mg/m^2 twice daily thereafter. At 2 years, OS was 89% (95% CI, 81–98%) and hepatic disease-free survival was 76% (95% CI, 65–88%). Grade 3 elevations in bilirubin were reported in 1% (3/54) of patients. There was no report of biliary stenting required. The NSABP C-09 phase 3 trial was designed to try to define the benefit of HAI FUDR by randomizing patients with resected colorectal liver metastases to adjuvant CAPOX with or without HAI FUDR [43]. However, the trial was unfortunately closed after 2 years after only accruing 22 of 400 planned patients [43].

A major criticism of the older studies of adjuvant HAI FUDR has been the inadequate systemic therapy comparator. In order to analyze the potential benefit of adjuvant HAI FUDR in the context of modern systemic therapies, in 2017, the group from MSKCC reported a retrospective study which included 2368 consecutive patients who underwent complete resection or CRLM at their institution between 1992 and 2012 [44]. In total, 785 patients received perioperative HAI therapy. Among patients receiving HAI therapy, 87% also received at least one cycle of modern perioperative systemic therapy (defined as a regimen containing oxaliplatin or irinotecan). Median OS and 10-year OS were significantly longer among patients treated with HAI (67 months vs 44 months, $P < 0.001$; 38% vs 24%, $P < 0.001$, respectively). In propensity score analyses, the hazard ratio for OS was significantly better in those patients treated with HAI therapy (0.67; 95% CI, 0.59–0.76).

Ultimately, multicenter RCTs are needed to inform whether adjuvant HAI therapy should be considered a standard of care treatment following complete resection of CRLM. Two such trials are ongoing: the PUMP [45] and PACHA-1 [46] trials. The PUMP trial is planned to enroll 230 patients with resectable CRLM. Only patients with a low clinical risk score (CRS) of 0–2 will be included. This designation of "low risk" means that patients are allowed to have no more than two out of five poor prognostic factors (disease-free interval less than 12 months, node-positive colorectal cancer, more than one CRLM, largest CRLM more than 5 cm in diameter, serum carcinoembryonic antigen (CEA) above 200 μg/L) [47]. Patients will be randomized to no further treatment after resection of CRLM or to receive 6 cycles of FUDR alone, without systemic chemotherapy. The PACHA trial is planned to enroll 220 patients who undergo resection and/or thermal ablation of at least four CRLM. Patients will be randomized to receive systemic FOLFOX or HAI oxaliplatin + systemic 5-FU and LV.

How to Integrate HAI Therapies Into the Management of CRLM

In this section, we will provide some practical advice regarding how we integrate HAI therapy into the management of patients with CRLM.

Patient Selection for HAI Therapy

All patients being considered for insertion of a HAI pump should be reviewed at a multidisciplinary consensus conference involving radiologists, hepatobiliary surgeons, and medical oncologists with experience in the management of HAI pumps [48]. Preoperative cross-sectional imaging with CT or MRI angiography is needed to define the hepatic arterial anatomy to ensure it is amenable to insertion of a HAI pump [49]. Prior to insertion of a HAI pump, it is critical to counsel patients on the importance of compliance with the treatment protocol. Failure to adhere to the strict protocol necessary to care for the HAI pump significantly increases the chance of complications and or pump clotting/failure. Prior to the administration of HAI FUDR, adequate liver remnant perfusion and lack of extrahepatic infusion should be confirmed with technectium-99-labelled nuclear medicine scanning [50].

Patient Selection for Adjuvant HAI Therapy Following Complete Resection of CRLM

Among those with suitable arterial anatomy for HAI pump placement, there are few considerations with regard to suitability for adjuvant HAI FUDR therapy. There are very limited data amongst patients who have previously experienced 5-FU coronary vasospasm. Similarly, the presence of known genetic variations in dihydropyrimidine dehydrogenase (DPYD) that predispose to severe 5-FU toxicity (the end-product of FUDR catabolism) had previously been considered a relative contraindication to HAI FUDR. A recent case report demonstrating safety in this setting provides encouraging data contradicting this assumption and provides biological rationale as to why administration of FUDR via HAI is safe. When FUDR is given via HAI, metabolism switches from deoxyuridine or thymidylate phosphorylase [51] to the thymidylate kinase 1 (TK1)/thymidylate synthase (TYMS) pathway [52]. Because of rapid exposure of FUDR to thymidine kinase in the liver, it can be converted to fluorodeoxyuridine monophosphate and inhibit TYMS which can inhibit tumor growth with minimal conversion to fluorouracil. On this biological basis and taken in conjunction with anecdotal data from large volume centers administering HAI and considering the biological mechanism of FUDR metabolism intrahepatically rather than systemically [52], this should no longer be considered a contraindication.

The presence of a RAS/RAF mutation is not a contraindication to insertion of an HAI pump for adjuvant therapy. Studies examining patients treated with HAIP FUDR following hepatectomy have shown that those with RAS/RAF mutations are at higher risk of recurrence, particularly extrahepatic recurrence [53]. However, adjuvant HAI FUDR has also been shown to be independently associated with improved OS, regardless of KRAS status. In a study from MSKCC, patients with KRAS mutations treated with HAI FUDR following hepatectomy had better 5-year OS (59% vs 40%, HR 0.53; 95% CI, 0.39–0.77) [54]. Although not a contraindication, BRAF V600E mutated colorectal cancer is associated with increased likelihood of extrahepatic disease [55], poor response to chemotherapy [56, 57], and rapid recurrence post metastatectomy [58, 59].

Administration of Adjuvant HAI FUDR Following Complete Resection of CRLM

In the adjuvant setting, HAI FUDR is started no sooner than 4 weeks after liver surgery and should not be started if the aspartate aminotransferase (AST) or alanine aminotransferase (ALT) are >5× the upper limit of normal or if the total bilirubin is >1.5 mg/dL (26 μmol) [33, 39, 60]. It is recommend that adjuvant HAI FUDR be initiated within 12 weeks, based on evidence extrapolated from the Stage 3 colorectal cancer where longer time to adjuvant chemotherapy initiation is associated worse survival outcomes [61]. In the adjuvant clinical trials, HAI FUDR was most commonly delivered over six 35-day (5 week) treatment cycles (Table 12.2) [33]. However, in current academic treatment programs, HAI FUDR is delivered on a 28-day (4 weeks) treatment cycle which greatly improves scheduling logistics. Although six adjuvant treatments of FUDR are the intended course, many patients will not be able to finish the entire course due to toxicity. In Kemeny's seminal 1999 RCT, only 26% of patients received more than 50% of the planned dose of FUDR because of dose reductions necessitated by elevations in the serum liver profile [39]. In an unplanned analysis, there was no difference in OS noted between patients who received >3 cycles of FUDR and those who received 3 cycles or fewer. Given that biliary toxicity appears to be more common with adjuvant FUDR administration compared to when it is used in the setting of unresectable CRLM, and in the absence of clinical trials directly comparing 6 to <6 cycles of FUDR, it is reasonable to consider 3–4 cycles of adjuvant FUDR an adequate treatment course, especially if there is an upward trend in the AST/ALT/Bilirubin during these early cycles of therapy compared to baseline values.

Patient Selection for HAI FUDR for Unresectable CRLM

As in the adjuvant setting, HAI FUDR should not be used for patients with metastatic disease who

Table 12.2 Treatment schedule for adjuvant FUDR following complete resection of colorectal liver metastases. Note, the 35-day cycle is mostly of historical interest, as 28-day cycles are now standard

35-Day (5-week) adjuvant cycle			
Day 1	Day 15	Day 29	Day 36 (day 1, next cycle
HAI FUDR + dexamethasone	Systemic chemotherapy + Pump emptied and filled with heparinized saline	Systemic chemotherapy	HAI FUDR + dexamethasone
28-day (4-week) adjuvant cycle			
Day 1	Day 15	Day 29 (day 1, next cycle)	
HAI FUDR + dexamethasone + systemic chemotherapy	Pump emptied and filled with heparinized saline + Systemic chemotherapy	HAI FUDR + dexamethasone + systemic chemotherapy	

FUDR Floxuridine, *HAI* Hepatic arterial infusion

have experienced coronary vasospasm attributed to 5FU. The currently available data [52] in conjunction with increasing anecdotal evidence from large volume HAI centres now suggests HAI FUDR is safe to administer in patients with DYPD (Dihydropyrimidine Dehydrogenase Deficiency, rationale provided above). A clinical trial of HAI FUDR in DYPD patients is planned to definitively address safety and efficacy

Unlike in the adjuvant setting, there is no strict cutoff for AST or ALT that is used to determine eligibility for initiation of HAI FUDR in the setting of unresectable CRLM because these lab values may be elevated due to the presence of the metastases (and may improve with therapy). However, a bilirubin <1.5 mg/dL (26 μmol) is still a standard criterion required before initiation of HAI FUDR.

There is evidence to support the use of HAI FUDR for unresectable CRLM in the first-line, second-line, and salvage settings [62]. The response rates to HAI therapy are clearly better in earlier lines of treatment, so we encourage consideration of HAI pump implantation as soon as possible after the diagnosis of unresectable CRLM [4]. The median time to best response to systemic therapy is estimated to be 12–16 weeks [63, 64], therefore, it is our practice to recommended consideration of HAI pump insertion at that time if the response to systemic therapy has been insufficient to allow surgical resection and or ablation of all visible CRLM.

As a surgical procedure, insertion of a HAI pump requires 4–8 weeks off systemic therapy including time before and after surgery. Moreover, if there are any complications from the surgery, the time off systemic therapy may be even longer. Even in experienced centers, pump complications occur in approximately 20% of patients, and although the majority of pumps can be salvaged for use, up to 5–10% of patients who have pumps inserted may have a complication that prevents it from ever being used [65]. Therefore, it is critical to determine if the patient's disease will allow them to safely stay off systemic therapy for this potential duration of time. Accordingly, most protocols for HAI pump insertion (outside of the salvage setting) require patient's CRLM to comprise <70% of liver parenchyma and have stable or responding disease. A critical point to make is that HAI therapy may be useful even in the salvage/chemo-refractory setting, where conversion to complete resection has been demonstrated, and where the risk-benefit ratio may favor HAI pump insertion despite progressive disease or the risks of progressive disease while off treatment for surgery [66, 67].

Patients with liver-predominant disease with low-volume extrahepatic disease, particularly those with asymptomatic, low-volume lung metastases, remain good candidates for insertion of a HAIP. However, high-volume extrahepatic disease, particularly peritoneal or bone metastases, are considered a contraindication for HAI therapy as the efficacy of HAI in this setting remains unclear [48]. In a retrospective review of 219 patients treated at MSKCC who underwent resection of CRLM and the synchronous extrahepatic disease (EHD) (51 of whom received HAI FUDR), the site of EHD affected survival, with portal and retroperitoneal nodes associated with the worst prognoses [68]. Presence of main portal vein thrombosis is also a relative contraindication to the use of HAI FUDR. HAI FUDR may safely be used after failed portal vein embolization or prior liver ablation procedures [68].

Administration of HAI FUDR for Unresectable CRLM

When used for unresectable CRLM, HAI FUDR may be started 2 weeks after insertion of the HAI pump (compared to minimum of 4 weeks after liver surgery for resectable CRLM) [30, 69]. In this setting, HAI FUDR is most commonly delivered by a continuous 14-day infusion, Day 1–14 of a 28-day cycle (Table 12.3). Of note, it is not necessary to wait for the AST or ALT to normalize following insertion of a HAI pump when no liver resection has been performed.

In the setting of unresectable disease, treatment is continued until all visible lesions can be resected and or ablated. In a multicenter, retrospective cohort study of patients with unresectable CRLM treated with HAI FUDR and modern

Table 12.3 Treatment schedule for FUDR following hepatic arterial pump insertion for unresectable of colorectal liver metastases (28-day cycle)

Day 1, Cycle #1 (Day 14 post surgery)	Day 15 (Day 29 post surgery)	Day 29 (Day 1, next cycle)
HAI FUDR + dexamethasone	Systemic chemotherapy + HAI pump emptied and filled with heparinized saline	HAI FUDR + dexamethasone + systemic chemotherapy

HAI Hepatic Arterial Infusion, *FUDR* Floxuridine

Table 12.4 Dosing of systemic FOLFOX, FOLFIRI and panitumumab when used in conjunction with hepatic arterial infusion FUDR

5-Flourouracil	Leucovorin	Irinotecan*/Oxaliplatin	Panitumumab/Cetuximab	FUDR
1000 mg/m^2 (×2 days, for 2000 mg/m^2 total)	400 mg/m^2	Irinotecan:125 mg/m^2 Oxaliplatin: 85 mg/m^2	Panitumumab: 6 mg/kg Cetuximab: 500 mg/m^2	0.12 mg/kg/day

Note: Bolus 5-FU is not given when FOLFOX and FOLFIRI are given concurrent with hepatic arterial infusion FUDR

systemic therapy between 2003 and 2017 at six North American Centers, patients received a median of 5 (interquartile range, 4–7) cycles of FUDR prior to stopping to undergo liver resection, achieving a complete response, or due to toxicity [30].

Assessing the Response to Treatment with HAI FUDR for Unresectable CRLM

Response to treatment is assessed every 8–12 weeks with CT scans. It is our practice to review all imaging at a dedicated hepatobiliary multidisciplinary consensus conference to determine if a patient is a potential candidate for liver resection. For patients who are determined to be potential surgical candidates, MRI imaging is used to evaluate for smaller lesions. MRI and contrast-enhanced intraoperative ultrasound are particularly helpful in patients treated with chemotherapy who have liver metastases which have disappeared ("ghost lesions"), as these modalities have a high negative predictive value for detecting a complete pathological response on histological examination (0.73 and 0.79, respectively) [70]. Therefore, surgical resection may be considered in patients in whom all visible CRLM can be resected even if disappeared liver lesions cannot be technically resected.

Of note, patients with HAI pumps can safely undergo MR Imaging at both 1.5 and 3 T within safety parameters specified by the manufacturers [71]. MR imaging must be done at a center experienced in the care of patients with HAI pumps. The CODMAN® 3000 series pump (now discontinued [72]) and Intera 3000 pump are an MRI conditional propellant-driven pump. During an MRI, a temperature increase of more than 6.5 degrees Celsius may temporarily increase the flow rate by up to 90%, so scans longer than 15 minutes require cooling delay periods of equal length [73]. The Medtronic SynchroMed® series pumps are also considered MRI conditional, but these are motor-driven pumps. While in the MR scanner, the pump is expected to stop operating. Upon completion of the MRI, the pump must be examined to make sure it has not rotated, and it must be electronically interrogated to ensure the pump flow has resumed.

Administration of Systemic Therapy with HAI FUDR

As outlined above, most modern systemic therapies can safely be administered with HAI FUDR with minor dose modifications (Table 12.4). Bevacizumab is the notable exception, and it is not used concurrently with HAI FUDR therapy due to an increased risk of biliary toxicity [32]. In our experience, bevacizumab may be safely used in later lines of therapy when the HAI pump is no longer in use. Similarly, capecitabine is not used with HAI as this drug can lead to drug-related elevations in liver function tests that can complicate dosing of FUDR. Further, FOLFIRINOX and immunotherapy are not used with HAI FUDR as there are no available data confirming acceptable safety profiles with these concurrent regimens.

Dosing Considerations of HAI FUDR

The starting dose of FUDR is calculated based on the predetermined flow rate provided by the manufacturer for each specific HAI pump. Specific dosing guidelines for Intera 3000 Implantable Constant-Flow Infusion Pumps and Medtronic SynchroMed® II Programmable Pumps are provided below:

FUDR Dosing

$$\text{FUDR}: \frac{0.12\text{mg}/\text{kg}/\text{day} \times 14\text{days}}{\text{Pump Flow Rate}}$$

Heparin, Dexamethasone, and Reservoir Volume are Pump Dependent

Intera 3000 Implantable Constant Flow Infusion Pump (total volume 30 ml):

$$\text{FUDR}: \frac{0.12\text{mg}/\text{kg}/\text{day} \times 30\text{ml}}{\text{Pump flow rate}}$$

$$\text{Dexamethasone}(\text{flat dose } 25\text{mg}): \frac{1\text{mg}/\text{day} \times 30\text{ml}}{\text{Pump flow rate}}$$

Heparin: 30,000 units total dose
Normal saline: Quantity sufficient to make total reservoir volume of 30 mL
Note: Flow rate is determined by the manufacturer and is documented at the time of pump placement

Medtronic SynchroMed® II Programmable Pumps (total volume 20 mL):

$$\text{FUDR}: \frac{0.12\text{mg}/\text{kg}/\text{day} \times 20\text{ml} \times 0.9}{\text{Pump flow rate}}$$

$$\text{Dexamethasone}: \frac{1\text{mg}/\text{day} \times 20\text{ml}}{\text{Pump flow rate}}$$

Heparin: 25,000 units total dose
Normal saline: Quantity sufficient to make total reservoir volume of 20 mL
Note: Flow rate is programmed in the operating room at the time of pump placement

Dosing of FUDR for Overweight Patients

If a patient is 35% above ideal weight the dose of FUDR chemotherapy and systemic chemotherapy should be calculated as follows using the *Ideal Average Weight* (kg):

1. *Calculate Ideal Body Weight (kg):*
   Males: 50 kg + (2.3 × height in inches above 5 ft).
   i.e., If patient is 5′10 use 10.
   Females: 45.5 kg + (2.3 × height in inches above 5 ft).
   Example Calculation of Ideal Body Weight:

An overweight male patient who is 100 kg and 5′10.

Ideal Body Weight: 50 kg + (2.3 × 10) = 5 0 kg + 25.3 = 73 kg

$$\frac{\text{Actual Weight} + \text{Ideal Body Weight}}{2}$$

2. *To Calculate Ideal Average Weight:*

Example Calculation of Ideal Average Weight:

An overweight male patient who is 100 kg and 5′10

Ideal Body Weight = 73 kg

Ideal Average Weight = (100 + 73)/2 = 86. 5 kg.

FUDR Dose Modifications for Toxicity

- The major dose-limiting toxicity of FUDR is biliary sclerosis. Aspartate aminotransferase (AST) is usually the first enzyme to rise, followed by a rise in alkaline phosphatase and bilirubin. A study by Kemeny et al. demonstrated that the hyperbilirubinemia occurs in approximately one third of patients treated with FUDR alone and the addition of dexamethasone reduced the incidence from 30% to 9% [24]. There are three main strategies used to limit hepatotoxicity: (1) Holding and dose reducing FUDR in response to elevated AST, ALP, and Bilirubin (Table 12.5 and Table 12.6); (2) Adding dexamethasone to the

Table 12.5 FUDR dose modification schema

Toxicity	Reference value	% FUDR dose
AST At pump emptying (day 14) Or Day of planned Tx (day 28) Whichever is higher	0 to <2 × reference value	100
	2 to <3 × reference value	80
	3 to <4 reference value	50
	>4 × reference value	Hold
ALK PHOS At pump emptying (day 14) Or Day of planned Tx (day 28) Whichever is higher	0 to <1.2 × reference value	100
	1.2 to <1.5 × reference value	50
	>1.5 × reference value	Hold
TOT BILI At pump emptying (day 14) Or Day of planned Tx (day 28) Whichever is higher	0 to <1.2 × reference value	100
	1.2 to <1.5 × reference value	50
	>1.5× reference value	Hold

Notes

- *Reference value* is defined as the value obtained on the first day of the most recent FUDR dose. In order to determine if FUDR dose modification is required the reference value should be compared to either the value obtained on the day the pump was emptied (e.g., day 14) or the day of planned treatment/pump filling (e.g., Day 28) *whichever is higher*. Percentages of the FUDR dose relate to the percentage of the last dose of FUDR administered
- If a patient's alkaline phosphatase or total bilirubin demonstrates a continual rise from Day 1 of treatment then the Day 1 value will be used as the reference value for that patient when determining whether to hold treatment and the time of re-treatment after hold
- If AST > 4 × reference value, alkaline phosphatases >1.5 × reference value, total bilirubin >1.5× reference value treatment will be held and not reinstituted until values return to normal levels
- If patient develops a total bilirubin ≥3.0 mg/dL the pump should be emptied and dexamethasone 23 or 25 (varies with Intera pump based on flow rate) mg plus heparin 2500 units and saline placed in pump every 14 days. Once there is no longer evidence of toxicity dexamethasone should be tapered in increments of 5 mg every 14 days. Tapering will continue unless enzymes increase. FUDR should be permanently discontinued unless there is evidence of disease progression (e.g., rising CEA, radiographic progression, or worsening clinical status) and TOT BILI has returned to ≤1.5 mg/dL. In this situation, FUDR can be restarted as follows: Use 25% of the last FUDR dose given with dexamethasone, heparin, and saline in the pump for 7 days. Pump should be emptied after 7 days and patient should be given a 3-week rest period. The treatment and treatment schedule can continue as long as TOT BILI remains ≤1.5 mg/dl and liver enzymes do not increase

AST Aspartate aminotransferase, *ALK PHOS* Alkaline phosphatase, *TOT BILI* Total Bilirubin

Table 12.6 Dose schema for reintroduction of FUDR after a hold

Toxicity (reason for delay)	Target for resuming treatment	% FUDR dose
AST elevation	3× reference value	25% of last dose
ALK PHOS elevation	1.2× reference value	25% of last dose
TOT BILI elevation	1.2× reference value	25% of last dose

AST Aspartate aminotransferase, *ALK PHOS* Alkaline phosphatase, *TOT BILI* Total Bilirubin

heparinized saline which is put into the pump at the end of each infusion of FUDR when any elevation of AST, ALP, and Bilirubin is noted; (3) Starting oral ursodiol. A recently published manuscript focuses oncologic management of HAI [74] and outlines specific cases of dose adjustments.

Management of Side Effects Commonly Seen with HAI FUDR

Skin Rash, Pruritus

Symptomatically biliary inflammation may manifest as pruritus with/without rash. Symptomatic management is extrapolated from the management of both primary sclerosing cholangitis and primary biliary cholangitis and centers on the use of ursodeoxycholic acid (UCDA) to reduce liver inflammation. UDCA has been shown to markedly reduce serum bilirubin, alkaline phosphatase, GGT and cholesterol in patients with primary biliary cholangitis [75]. Extrapolating from this experience, and the utility in PBC, some recommend UCDA although the optimal dose is not clearly defined [76]. Typically, UCDA is commenced at a dose of 300 mg twice daily and continued throughout treatment.

Abdominal Pain

If a patient presents with abdominal pain HAI FUDR should not be given. If a patient reports pain after pump is filled with FUDR pump should be emptied and heparinized saline or glycerol should be instilled. If abdominal pain is unresponsive to an oral proton pump inhibitor, the clinical concern is for gastroduodenal ulcer or irritation and upper gastrointestinal endoscopy is indicated. If an ulcer or gastroduodenitis is documented FUDR HAI should be held for 1 month. Investigations of abdominal pain should also include a repeat flow scan of pump to rule out extrahepatic perfusion.

HAI Therapy for Unresectable Intrahepatic Cholangiocarcinoma

Based on the decades of experience and success using HAI therapies for advanced CRLM, recent studies have investigated HAI therapies for intrahepatic cholangiocarcinoma (IHCC) [6]. As with CRLM, margin-negative surgical resection offers the only meaningful chance of cure for IHCC [77]. Unfortunately, the vast majority of patients with IHCC, approximately 80% in population-based studies, present with unresectable disease [78, 79]. For patients with locally advanced and unresectable IHCC, systemic therapy with combination chemotherapy and immunotherapy is the current international standard of care [80]. Although there have been several advances in systemic therapy options, median overall survival remains at just over 1 year [81], and very few patients will obtain a response to systemic therapy sufficient to allow curative-intent surgical resection [82]. Moreover, among patients with unresectable IHCC treated with systemic therapy alone, approximately 70% will progress intrahepatically and die of liver failure [83], and improved hepatic disease control is associated with improved overall survival [84]. Thus, intensification of therapy directed towards the liver with HAI therapy, in combination with best available systemic therapy, may improve patient outcomes and is supported as a treatment option by international clinical practice guidelines [80]. HAI therapy offers a particularly attractive treatment option for patients with unresectable IHCC because unlike other locoregional therapies, it is not limited by tumor size, proximity to vascular structures or multi-focality.

In 2009, Jarnagin et al. reported a single-center, phase 2 trial performed at MSKCC which evaluated HAI FUDR and dexamethasone which included 26 patients with unresectable IHCC (and eight patients with hepatocellular carcinoma) [85]. Patients were not treated with concurrent systemic therapy. The enrolled patients had very advanced disease with a median tumor diameter of 9.7 cm, median liver replacement of 45%, and 62% multi-focality. There was a 54% partial response rate, 96% disease control rate, and hepatic PFS was 11.6 months. One patient had a sufficient respond to allow surgical resection from which the pathology showed a complete pathological response. Forty-four percent of patients developed extrahepatic metastases.

In 2020, Cercek et al. reported a phase 2 trial performed at MSKCC and Washington University which evaluated HAI FUDR in combination with systemic gemcitabine and oxaliplatin for 42 patients with unresectable IHCC [86]. Patients received treatment with HAI-FUDR 0.12 mg/kg/day and dexamethasone 30 mg/pump flow rate continuously for 14 days, repeated every 4 weeks. Gemcitabine 800 mg/m^2 and Oxaliplatin 85 mg/m^2 were given on Day 1 and Day 15. Among 38 patients treated at MSKCC, the enrolled patients had a median tumor diameter of 8.3 cm, 66% had bilobar disease and 55% had multifocal disease. There was a 58% partial response rate, 84% disease control rate and four patients had sufficient response to undergo surgical resection wherein the pathology in one patient showed a complete pathological response. The 6-month PFS, the primary study endpoint, was 67% in pretreated patients and 89% in treatment-naïve patients. The median overall survival was 25.0 months (95% CI, 21 to not reached). Four patients (2%) required biliary stents, two related to chemotherapy induced biliary sclerosis and two related to disease progression following discontinuation of treatment. Among ten patients treated in a confirmatory cohort at Washington University, there was a 50% partial response rate and two patients underwent resection.

In 2021, Pietge et al. reported an open-label, prospective, non-randomized, single-arm dose-escalation study of 12 patients with unresectable IHCC treated at the University Hospital Zurich in Switzerland [87]. Patients received treatment with HAI-FUDR 0.2 mg/kg/day and 20 mg of dexamethasone continuously for 14 days, repeated every 4 weeks for 3 cycles with planned evaluation at the end of 3 months. Patients were allowed to continue therapy if effective and well-tolerated. Cisplatin 25 mg/m^2 was given on Days 1 and 8 of a 21-day cycle and Gemcitabine was given according to an assigned dose-level ranging from 600 mg/m^2 to 1000 mg/mg^2 also on Days 1 and 8, for 4 cycles. The maximum tolerated dose of gemcitabine was determined to be 800 mg/m^2. No unexpected serious adverse events were observed. The partial response rate was 27% and the disease control rate was 100%. No patients had a response sufficient to allow surgical resection when evaluated at 3 months. Three-year overall survival was 33% and median overall survival was 24 months (range, 1–49 months).

In 2022, a systemic review and meta-analysis identified nine studies representing 478 patients with unresectable IHCC treated with HAI therapy [6]. The pooled partial response rate was 53% (range, 27–60%) weighted median overall survival was 29.0 months (range, 25–39 months) and the pooled 1-, 3-and 5-year survival rates were 86%, 40%, and 10%, respectively. The presence of long-term survivors is particularly encouraging, as there were no survivors at 3-years in the seminal ABC-02 cholangiocarcinoma clinical trial [88].

At present, HAI therapies for locally advanced cholangiocarcinoma are best offered on a clinical trial so further data on survival and quality of life outcomes can be reported. There is an ongoing randomized phase 2 clinical trial (NCT04891289) evaluating gemcitabine and oxaliplatin with or without HAI FUDR and dexamethasone in patients with advanced cholangiocarcinoma [89].

Duration of HAI and Concurrent Systemic Therapy in the Unresectable Setting

In the unresectable setting, HAI therapy is continued until: (1) A complete response is achieved; (2) A sufficient response is achieved to allow surgical resection and or ablation of all remaining visible lesions; (3) Progression of intrahepatic disease; or (4) Technical or treatment related complications associated with the pump itself, including unacceptable and unsalvageable biliary toxicity that cannot be salvaged by treatment break, use of steroids or intervention. In the setting of asymptomatic extrahepatic disease progression, particularly intrathoracic progression, HAI therapy is generally continued along with a switch of the systemic therapy backbone to the next best available option. In a multicenter, retrospective analysis of six North American HAI programs for unresectable CRLM, the median number of HAI cycles was 5 (IQR, 4–7) until one of the aforementioned events necessitating HAI discontinuation occurred [30].

In one of the most comprehensive reviews of technical issues relating to HAI pumps in the unresectable setting [65], pump failure rate at 2 years was only 16%. Salvage of pump-related complications was more likely if they occurred early (<30 days) after pump insertion and in this series was possible in 45% of the patient cohort. Pump complications were more likely if the surgeon had performed fewer than 25 procedures ($p = 0.002$) underlining the importance of institutional expertise if HAI FUDR is being considered. Notably pump complication rates appear to decrease over time [65, 90] with increasing experience of the treating center.

When a decision is made to cease HAI FUDR, the HAI pump should be left in situ and refilled with glycerin, where available, even when no longer in use. The HAI pump is not usually surgically removed unless there is an absolute indication for its removal, such as infection or wound healing concerns, as there may be opportunity for secondary use later in the patient's disease course.

Conclusion

Over the past four decades, HAI therapy for CRLM has been continually studied, modified, and refined to improve the safety, convenience and efficacy of treatment. HAI therapies have now also successfully been expanded to benefit patients with unresectable IHCC. HAI therapies may be safely combined with most available modern systemic therapies to maximize intrahepatic and extrahepatic responses to treatment. Ongoing and future planned collaborative randomized studies will help further inform the optimal use of HAI therapy in combination with modern systemic therapy for CRLM and IHCC.

References

1. Anteby R, et al. Getting chemotherapy directly to the liver: the historical evolution of hepatic artery chemotherapy. J Am Coll Surg. 2021;232:332–8.
2. Mocellin S, Pilati P, Lise M, Nitti D. Meta-analysis of hepatic arterial infusion for unresectable liver metastases from colorectal cancer: the end of an era? J Clin Oncol. 2007;25:5649–54.
3. Kemeny NE, et al. Hepatic arterial infusion versus systemic therapy for hepatic metastases from colorectal cancer: a randomized trial of efficacy, quality of life, and molecular markers (CALGB 9481). J Clin Oncol. 2006;24:1395–403.
4. Raphael MJ, Karanicolas PJ. Regional therapy for colorectal cancer liver metastases: which modality and when? J Clin Oncol. 2022;21:02505.
5. D'Angelica M, Fong Y, DeMatteo RP, Jarnagin WR. Hepatic arterial infusion chemotherapy for Metatstases from colorectal cancer: is it really the end of an era? J Clin Oncol. 2008;26:2788–9.
6. Holster JJ, et al. Hepatic arterial infusion pump chemotherapy for unresectable intrahepatic cholangiocarcinoma: a systematic review and meta-analysis. Ann Surg Oncol. 2022;29:5528–38.
7. Engstrand J, Nilsson H, Strömberg C, Jonas E, Freedman J. Colorectal cancer liver metastases–a population-based study on incidence, management and survival. BMC Cancer. 2018;18:1–11.
8. Manfredi S, et al. Epidemiology and management of liver metastases from colorectal cancer. Ann Surg. 2006;244:254.
9. Riihimäki M, Hemminki A, Sundquist J, Hemminki K. Patterns of metastasis in colon and rectal cancer. Sci Rep. 2016;6:1–9.

10. Mantke R, Schmidt U, Wolff S, Kube R, Lippert H. Incidence of synchronous liver metastases in patients with colorectal cancer in relationship to clinico-pathologic characteristics. Results of a German prospective multicentre observational study. Eur J Surg Oncol. 2012;38:259–65.
11. Okholm C, Mollerup TK, Schultz NA, Strandby RB, Achiam MP. Synchronous and metachronous liver metastases in patients with colorectal cancer. Dan Med J. 2018;65:A5524.
12. van Gestel YR, et al. Patterns of metachronous metastases after curative treatment of colorectal cancer. Cancer Epidemiol. 2014;38:448–54.
13. Leporrier J, et al. A population-based study of the incidence, management and prognosis of hepatic metastases from colorectal cancer. J Br Surg. 2006;93:465–74.
14. Welch J, Donaldson G. The clinical correlation of an autopsy study of recurrent colorectal cancer. Ann Surg. 1979;189:496.
15. Kerr DJ, et al. Intrahepatic arterial versus intravenous fluorouracil and folinic acid for colorectal cancer liver metastases: a multicentre randomised trial. Lancet. 2003;361:368–73.
16. Power DG, Kemeny NE. The role of floxuridine in metastatic liver disease. Mol Cancer Ther. 2009;8:1015–25.
17. Ensminger WD, et al. A clinical-pharmacological evaluation of hepatic arterial infusions of 5-fluoro-2′-deoxyuridine and 5-fluorouracil. Cancer Res. 1978;38:3784–92.
18. Ensminger W, Gyves J. Semin Oncol. 1983;10:176–82.
19. Archer S, Gray B. Vascularization of small liver metastases. J Br Surg. 1989;76:545–8.
20. Daly JM, Kemeny N, Sigurdson E, Oderman P, Thom A. Regional infusion for colorectal hepatic metastases: a randomized trial comparing the hepatic artery with the portal vein. Arch Surg. 1987;122:1273–7.
21. Ludwig J, Kim CH, Wiesner RH, Krom RA. Floxuridine-induced sclerosing cholangitis: an ischemic cholangiopathy? Hepatology. 1989;9:215–8.
22. Doria JR, Riddell RH, Shepard KV, Levin B. Liver pathology following hepatic arterial infusion chemotherapy: hepatic toxicity with FUDR. Cancer. 1986;58:855–61.
23. Kemeny N, et al. Hepatic artery pump infusion: toxicity and results in patients with metastatic colorectal carcinoma. J Clin Oncol. 1984;2:595–600.
24. Kemeny N, et al. A randomized trial of intrahepatic infusion of fluorodeoxyuridine with dexamethasone versus fluorodeoxyuridine alone in the treatment of metastatic colorectal cancer. Cancer. 1992;69:327–34.
25. Chang AE, et al. A prospective randomized trial of regional versus systemic continuous 5-fluorodeoxyuridine chemotherapy in the treatment of colorectal liver metastases. Ann Surg. 1987;206:685.
26. Kemeny N, et al. Intrahepatic or systemic infusion of fluorodeoxyuridine in patients with liver metastases from colorectal carcinoma: a randomized trial. Ann Intern Med. 1987;107:459–65.
27. Kemeny NE, et al. Conversion to resectability using hepatic artery infusion plus systemic chemotherapy for the treatment of unresectable liver metastases from colorectal carcinoma. J Clin Oncol. 2009;27:3465.
28. D'Angelica MI, et al. Phase II trial of hepatic artery infusional and systemic chemotherapy for patients with unresectable hepatic metastases from colorectal cancer: conversion to resection and long-term outcomes. Ann Surg. 2015;261:353.
29. Pak LM, et al. Prospective phase II trial of combination hepatic artery infusion and systemic chemotherapy for unresectable colorectal liver metastases: long term results and curative potential. J Surg Oncol. 2018;117:634–43.
30. Muaddi H, et al. Safety and feasibility of initiating a hepatic artery infusion pump chemotherapy program for unresectable colorectal liver metastases: a multicenter, retrospective cohort study. J Surg Oncol. 2021;123:252–60.
31. Dekker E, Tanis PJ, Vleugels JLA, Kasi PM, Wallace MB. Colorectal cancer. Lancet. 2019;394:1467–80.
32. Cercek A, et al. Floxuridine hepatic arterial infusion associated biliary toxicity is increased by concurrent administration of systemic bevacizumab. Ann Surg Oncol. 2014;21:479–86.
33. Kemeny NE, et al. A randomized phase II trial of adjuvant hepatic arterial infusion and systemic therapy with or without panitumumab after hepatic resection of KRAS wild-type colorectal cancer. Ann Surg. 2021;274:248.
34. André T, et al. Adjuvant fluorouracil, leucovorin, and oxaliplatin in stage II to III colon cancer: updated 10-year survival and outcomes according to BRAF mutation and mismatch repair status of the MOSAIC study. J Clin Oncol. 2015;33:4176–87.
35. Yothers G, et al. Oxaliplatin as adjuvant therapy for colon cancer: updated results of NSABP C-07 trial, including survival and subset analyses. J Clin Oncol. 2011;29:3768.
36. Kanemitsu Y, et al. Hepatectomy followed by mFOLFOX6 versus hepatectomy alone for liver-only metastatic colorectal cancer (JCOG0603): a phase II or III randomized controlled trial. J Clin Oncol. 2021;21:01032.
37. Bosma NA, et al. Efficacy of perioperative chemotherapy in resected colorectal liver metastasis: a systematic review and meta-analysis. Eur J Surg Oncol. 2021;47:3113.
38. Hallet J, et al. Factors influencing recurrence following initial hepatectomy for colorectal liver metastases. J Br Surg. 2016;103:1366–76.
39. Kemeny N, et al. Hepatic arterial infusion of chemotherapy after resection of hepatic metastases from colorectal cancer. N Engl J Med. 1999;341:2039–48.
40. Kemeny NE, Gonen M. Hepatic arterial infusion after liver resection. N Engl J Med. 2005;352:734–5.
41. Kemeny MM, et al. Combined-modality treatment for resectable metastatic colorectal carcinoma to the

liver: surgical resection of hepatic metastases in combination with continuous infusion of chemotherapy—an intergroup study. J Clin Oncol. 2002;20:1499–505.
42. Alberts SR, et al. Alternating systemic and hepatic artery infusion therapy for resected liver metastases from colorectal cancer: a north central cancer treatment group (NCCTG)/National Surgical Adjuvant Breast and bowel project (NSABP) phase II intergroup trial, N9945/CI-66. J Clin Oncol. 2010;28:853.
43. NSABP. NSABP Clinical Trials Overview—Protocol C-09. <http://www.nsabp.pitt.edu/C-09.asp>.
44. Koerkamp BG, et al. Perioperative hepatic arterial infusion pump chemotherapy is associated with longer survival after resection of colorectal liver metastases: a propensity score analysis. J Clin Oncol. 2017;35:1938.
45. Buisman F, et al. Adjuvant hepatic arterial infusion pump chemotherapy and resection versus resection alone in patients with low-risk resectable colorectal liver metastases–the multicenter randomized controlled PUMP trial. BMC Cancer. 2019;19:1–9.
46. Goéré D, et al. Postoperative hepatic arterial chemotherapy in high-risk patients as adjuvant treatment after resection of colorectal liver metastases-a randomized phase II/III trial–PACHA-01 (NCT02494973). BMC Cancer. 2018;18:1–8.
47. Fong Y, Fortner J, Sun RL, Brennan MF, Blumgart LH. Clinical score for predicting recurrence after hepatic resection for metastatic colorectal cancer: analysis of 1001 consecutive cases. Ann Surg. 1999;230:309.
48. Karanicolas P, et al. Hepatic arterial infusion pump chemotherapy in the management of colorectal liver metastases: expert consensus statement. Curr Oncol. 2014;21:e129.
49. Napier KJ, Lidsky ME, James OG, Wildman-Tobriner B. Hepatic arterial infusion pumps: what the radiologist needs to know. Radiographics. 2021;41:895–908.
50. Kemeny N, Niedzwiecki D, Shurgot B, Oderman P. Prognostic variables in patients with hepatic metastases from colorectal cancer. Importance of medical assessment of liver involvement. Cancer. 1989;63:742–7.
51. Thorn CF, et al. PharmGKB summary: fluoropyrimidine pathways. Pharmacogenet Genomics. 2011;21:237.
52. Lumish M, et al. Precision management of a patient with dihydropyrimidine dehydrogenase deficiency and liver-predominant metastatic rectal cancer using hepatic arterial floxuridine. JCO Precis Oncol. 2023;7:e2200442.
53. Narayan RR, et al. Genomic predictors of recurrence patterns after complete resection of colorectal liver metastases and adjuvant hepatic artery infusion chemotherapy. Ann Surg Oncol. 2022;29:7579–88.
54. Gholami S, et al. Adjuvant hepatic artery infusion chemotherapy is associated with improved survival regardless of KRAS mutation status in patients with resected colorectal liver metastases: a retrospective analysis of 674 patients. Ann Surg. 2020;272:352–6.
55. Lipsyc M, Yaeger R. Impact of somatic mutations on patterns of metastasis in colorectal cancer. J Gastrointest Oncol. 2015;6:645.
56. Bokemeyer C, et al. Addition of cetuximab to chemotherapy as first-line treatment for KRAS wild-type metastatic colorectal cancer: pooled analysis of the CRYSTAL and OPUS randomised clinical trials. Eur J Cancer. 2012;48:1466–75.
57. Venderbosch S, et al. Mismatch repair status and BRAF mutation status in metastatic colorectal cancer patients: a pooled analysis of the CAIRO, CAIRO2, COIN, and FOCUS studies. Clin Cancer Res. 2014;20:5322–30.
58. Margonis GA, et al. Association of BRAF mutations with survival and recurrence in surgically treated patients with metastatic colorectal liver cancer. JAMA Surg. 2018;153:e180996.
59. Schirripa M, et al. BRAF and RAS mutations as prognostic factors in metastatic colorectal cancer patients undergoing liver resection. Br J Cancer. 2015;112:1921–8.
60. Kemeny N, et al. Phase I trial of adjuvant hepatic arterial infusion (HAI) with floxuridine (FUDR) and dexamethasone plus systemic oxaliplatin, 5-fluorouracil and leucovorin in patients with resected liver metastases from colorectal cancer. Ann Oncol. 2009;20:1236–41.
61. Biagi JJ, et al. Association between time to initiation of adjuvant chemotherapy and survival in colorectal cancer: a systematic review and meta-analysis. JAMA. 2011;305:2335–42.
62. Datta J, Narayan RR, Kemeny NE, D'Angelica MI. Role of hepatic artery infusion chemotherapy in treatment of initially unresectable colorectal liver metastases: a review. JAMA Surg. 2019;154:768–76.
63. Van Cutsem E, et al. ESMO consensus guidelines for the management of patients with metastatic colorectal cancer. Ann Oncol. 2016;27:1386–422.
64. Adam R, et al. Managing synchronous liver metastases from colorectal cancer: a multidisciplinary international consensus. Cancer Treat Rev. 2015;41:729–41.
65. Allen PJ, et al. Technical complications and durability of hepatic artery infusion pumps for unresectable colorectal liver metastases: an institutional experience of 544 consecutive cases. J Am Coll Surg. 2005;201:57–65.
66. Cercek A, et al. Response rates of hepatic arterial infusion pump therapy in patients with metastatic colorectal cancer liver metastases refractory to all standard chemotherapies. J Surg Oncol. 2016;114:655–63.
67. Ducreux M, et al. Hepatic arterial oxaliplatin infusion plus intravenous chemotherapy in colorectal cancer with inoperable hepatic metastases: a trial of the gastrointestinal group of the federation Nationale des Centres de Lutte Contre le cancer. J Clin Oncol. 2005;23:4881–7.
68. Leung U, et al. Colorectal cancer liver metastases and concurrent extrahepatic disease treated with resection. Ann Surg. 2017;265:158.

69. Creasy JM, et al. Implementation of a hepatic artery infusion program: initial patient selection and perioperative outcomes of concurrent hepatic artery infusion and systemic chemotherapy for colorectal liver metastases. Ann Surg Oncol. 2020;27:5086–95.
70. Muaddi H, et al. When is a ghost really gone? A systematic review and meta-analysis of the accuracy of imaging modalities to predict complete pathological response of colorectal cancer liver metastases after chemotherapy. Ann Surg Oncol. 2021;28:6805–13.
71. Strnad BS, et al. Contemporary imaging of the surgically placed hepatic arterial infusion chemotherapy pump. Am J Roentgenol. 2021;217:633–43.
72. Ellis RJ, Angelos P, Jarnagin WR, Kemeny NE, Merkow RP. Abrupt discontinuation of the Codman hepatic artery infusion pump: considerations in the era of precision medicine. J Am Coll Surg. 2019;229:217.
73. Johnson J. CODMAN® 3000 Constant Flow Pump MRI Information. https://www.jnjmedtech.com/en-US/codman-pumps/mri-information. 2018.
74. Rao D, Ellis CS, Kemeny N, Cercek A. Case-based clinical guidance on dosing and management of the hepatic artery infusion chemotherapy pump. JCO Oncol Pract. 2023;23:00374.
75. Lindor KD. Ursodiol for primary sclerosing cholangitis. N Engl J Med. 1997;336:691–5.
76. Robles-Díaz M, Nezic L, Vujic-Aleksic V, Björnsson ES. Role of Ursodeoxycholic acid in treating and preventing idiosyncratic drug-induced liver injury. A systematic review. Front Pharmacol. 2021;2722:744488.
77. Mavros MN, Economopoulos KP, Alexiou VG, Pawlik TM. Treatment and prognosis for patients with intrahepatic cholangiocarcinoma: systematic review and meta-analysis. JAMA Surg. 2014;149:565–74.
78. Tan JC, Coburn NG, Baxter NN, Kiss A, Law CH. Surgical management of intrahepatic cholangiocarcinoma-a population-based study. Ann Surg Oncol. 2008;15:600–8.
79. Amini N, et al. Temporal trends in liver-directed therapy of patients with intrahepatic cholangiocarcinoma in the United States: a population-based analysis. J Surg Oncol. 2014;110:163–70.
80. Alvaro D, et al. EASL-ILCA clinical practice guidelines on the management of intrahepatic cholangiocarcinoma. J Hepatol. 2023;79:181–208.
81. Oh D-Y, et al. Durvalumab plus gemcitabine and cisplatin in advanced biliary tract cancer. NEJM Evidence. 2022;1:EVIDoa2200015.
82. Fruscione M, et al. Conversion therapy for intrahepatic cholangiocarcinoma and tumor downsizing to increase resection rates: a systematic review. Curr Probl Cancer. 2021;45:100614.
83. Yamashita S, et al. Local therapy reduces the risk of liver failure and improves survival in patients with intrahepatic cholangiocarcinoma: a comprehensive analysis of 362 consecutive patients. Cancer. 2017;123:1354–62.
84. Soares KC, et al. Hepatic disease control in patients with intrahepatic cholangiocarcinoma correlates with overall survival. Cancer Med. 2023;12:12272.
85. Jarnagin W, et al. Regional chemotherapy for unresectable primary liver cancer: results of a phase II clinical trial and assessment of DCE-MRI as a biomarker of survival. Ann Oncol. 2009;20:1589–95.
86. Cercek A, et al. Assessment of hepatic arterial infusion of floxuridine in combination with systemic gemcitabine and oxaliplatin in patients with unresectable intrahepatic cholangiocarcinoma: a phase 2 clinical trial. JAMA Oncol. 2020;6:60–7.
87. Pietge H, et al. Combination of HAI-FUDR and systemic gemcitabine and cisplatin in unresectable cholangiocarcinoma: a dose finding single center study. Oncology. 2021;99:300–9.
88. Valle J, et al. Cisplatin plus gemcitabine versus gemcitabine for biliary tract cancer. N Engl J Med. 2010;362:1273–81.
89. Rossi AJ, et al. Hepatic artery infusion pump (HAIP) therapy versus chemotherapy in the first-line setting for patients with unresectable intrahepatic cholangiocarcinoma. Ann Surg Oncol. 2022;29:35–6.
90. Doussot A, Kemeny NE, D'Angelica MI. Hepatic arterial infusional chemotherapy in the management of colorectal cancer liver metastases. Hepatic Oncol. 2015;2:275–90.

Hepatic Arterial Infusion Chemotherapy Delivery: Duration, Maintenance, and Secondary Use

13

Agustin Pimentel, Lauren Gallegos, and Namrata Vijayvergia

Duration of HAI Therapy

Colorectal cancer, one of the most common cancers worldwide, and intrahepatic cholangiocarcinoma, a less common cancer, are associated with significant morbidity and mortality. Hepatic arterial infusion (HAI) chemotherapy has been used to treat patients with both diseases. The duration of HAI therapy varies and the optimal duration of FUDR therapy remains controversial. In this section, we will review the recommendations and general considerations around duration of HAI therapy.

Palliative Setting

In the palliative setting when resection is not a feasible option, HAI is typically continued until disease progression or undue toxicities (predominantly biliary). Generally, modern HAI is considered for 6 months, though patients often require dose reduction and/or holds after 3–4 months (typical FUDR cycle = 28 days with FUDR given on days 1–14 and heparinized saline on days 15–28). In different studies, HAI patients received a median of 12 (8–18) 14-day cycles which equates to 6 months [1–4]. If unresectable patients are tolerating HAI FUDR without concern for hepatic or biliary toxicity, then a patient may continue FUDR indefinitely, although this is uncommon.

In other scenarios, response to HAI FUDR may result in conversion of unresectable to resectable disease, at which time the patient may undergo curative-intent hepatectomy. In other unusual circumstances, patients may experience complete radiographic response. In both of these scenarios, it is most common to stop HAI therapy to limit the risk of ongoing cumulative toxicity. The pump, however, typically remains in place and is maintained for potential secondary use in the event of hepatic progression or recurrence, both of which are detailed below.

Adjuvant HAI

There are three prospective randomized studies that explored the role of HAI after resection of colorectal liver metastases. Lorenz et al. performed a randomized trial to determine the impact of adjuvant HAI on survival in patients undergoing radical resection of colorectal liver metastases [5]. The study included patients who underwent liver resec-

A. Pimentel (✉)
Sylvester Comprehensive Cancer Center, Division of Medical Oncology, University of Miami School of Medicine, Miami, FL, USA
e-mail: apimentel@med.miami.edu

L. Gallegos
University of Miami Sylvester Comprehensive Cancer Center, Miami, FL, USA
e-mail: lgallegos@med.miami.edu

N. Vijayvergia
Department of Hematology/Oncology, Fox Chase Cancer Center, Philadelphia, PA, USA
e-mail: Namrata.Vijayvergia@fccc.edu

M. D'Angelica, M. Lidsky (eds.), *Hepatic Arterial Infusion for Malignancy*,
https://doi.org/10.1007/978-3-031-74935-3_13

tion followed by adjuvant HAI with 5FU + folinic acid or liver resection alone. The authors chose the duration of adjuvant HAI to be 6 months. The interim analysis showed that adjuvant HAI had a median survival of 34.5 months compared to 40.8 months in the control group. The treated group trended toward more extrahepatic failures. The Memorial-Sloan Kettering study by Kemeny et al. randomly assigned 156 patients to HAI with FUDR and dexamethasone plus intravenous fluorouracil or to systemic chemotherapy (5FU) alone [6]. Both groups received adjuvant therapy for 6 cycles total (6 months). They concluded that after liver resection, postoperative treatment with a combination of hepatic arterial infusion of floxuridine and intravenous fluorouracil improves the survival outcomes at two years including overall survival (OS) of 86% vs 72% (p=0.03), hepatic progression free survival (PFS) of 90% vs 60%, (p<0.001), and PFS of 57% vs 42% (p=0.07) in favor of the combination group. A subsequent publication update of long-term outcomes from that trial reported greater PFS and hepatic PFS, and a trend toward an improved long-term survival in the combined therapy group, with a survival rate of approximately 40% at 10 years [7]. Finally, the Intergroup trial randomized 75 (of originally planned 109) patients to either resection alone or to HAI with FUDR along with systemic continuous-infusion fluorouracil [8]. Accrual of patients for the study took 9 years. The duration of FUDR in this study was 4 cycles (4 months). Significant differences in recurrence-free survival and hepatic recurrence-free survival were noted between the two groups, but no significant difference was noted in overall survival.

The optimal duration of FUDR therapy in colorectal cancer remains controversial, as indicated by variable adjuvant therapy durations in the above trials. The studies reviewed in this manuscript suggest that 4–6 months of therapy may be associated with improved outcomes. However, longer durations of therapy are also associated with increased toxicity. Therefore, the decision to extend the duration of therapy should be made on an individualized basis, considering the patient's overall health status and the risk of toxicity. Our practice is to aim for 4 months of adjuvant HAI with FUDR in combination with systemic combination chemotherapy. Treatment is further truncated if there is clinical or laboratory evidence of impending biliary toxicities, or if they indeed develop dose limiting toxicity (e.g., require biliary intervention). Given the fact that some of the trials continued adjuvant HAI for 6 months, it is also common to see this duration being standard at some centers. However, it remains important to keep in mind that up to 50% of patients who undergo curative-intent hepatectomy without adjuvant HAI will not recur in the liver, and therefore incur all the potential toxicity of HAI without any benefit. Since we are unable to select those patients who will recur in the liver with accuracy, most centers recommend adjuvant HAI more uniformly, as part of their standard HAI algorithms. Therefore, it remains crucial to avoid hepatic and/or biliary toxicity in these patients, the latter of which is more common in adjuvant HAI patients, compared to those treated with palliative intent.

Maintenance of the HAI Pump

The decision to either conclude or interrupt the delivery of regional hepatic chemotherapy via the HAI pump marks the initiation of the HAI maintenance phase, the purpose of which is to preserve patency of the HAI pump system during periods of HAI therapy inactivity. The care of the HAI pump during this maintenance period differs in the presence of a non-programmable HAI pump (Intera 3000 HAI Pump or CODMAN® 3000 Series Pump) versus a programmable HAI pump (Medtronic SynchroMed™ II Pump).

The reservoir of non-programmable implantable devices can be filled with glycerin which allows for refill periods of 6–8 weeks when patients are not on active treatment. Glycerin is a viscous solution which, given the properties of the compound and mechanics of the device itself (flow restricting microcatheter), infuses at a slower rate and serves to maintain pump catheter patency for extended refill periods while HAI-treated patients are not receiving regional chemotherapy. The actual refill interval may vary based on the concentration of glycerin formulation that typically oscillates between levels of 40–60%, in addition to the sterile dilutant provided by the compounding pharmacy. In our institution, the 50% glycerin injection is the preferred concentration.

The availability of glycerin in health-care facilities requires a collaborative effort with an experienced compounding pharmacy that specializes in preparing personalized and precise drug formulations; thus, serving as a fundamental piece to provide good quality and reliable glycerin compounds to our population of patients carrying an implanted HAI pump. It is one institution's experience that percent glycerin compounded by volume/volume resulted in slower than expected flowrates, prompting several patients to require additional manipulation of the pump to preserve catheter patency. Glycerin formulation prepared in weight/volume prevented any further disruption in glycerin maintenance therapy (Table 13.1).

The formula to calculate the glycerin injection flowrate and the actual refill interval are adapted from the Intera glycerin instruction for use (IFU) [9]:

Formula to calculate the glycerin injection flowrate
(Current flowrate)[a] × (Conversion factor)[b] = Glycerin injection flowrate
Formula to calculate the actual refill interval
[(Reservoir volume) × 0.9[c]]/(Glycerin flowrate) = Refill interval with glycerin injection (days)

[a] Nominal arterial flowrate Nominal arterial flow rate of manufactured pumps (at 100 mmHg with 1000 μ/mL aqueous heparin solution) is indicated on pump labeling
[b] The conversion factor for the three typically formulated glycerin injections is listed in Table 13.1
[c] This factor of 0.9 ensures that the pump will not run dry before the expected refill date by accounting for 90% of the reservoir volume only.

Verification of the actual flowrate at each refill procedure in comparison to the expected flowrate is essential in monitoring pump function. Given the viscosity of the glycerin solution, there is potential for the glycerin residue to build up within the catheter and cause the flowrate to slow down further than expected, which may ultimately lead to catheter occlusion. In the event of a known or suspected catheter occlusion during glycerin maintenance phase, the catheter may be flushed with 2 mg of alteplase when accessed via the special bolus needle pathway. Additionally, it is recommended to rinse the reservoir as described in the procedures for restarting therapy in the Intera Glycerin IFU [9] and maintain the pump with heparinized saline until the flowrate has normalized.

If glycerin injection is not an option for pump maintenance while the patient is off therapy, the implanted non-programmable pump is maintained with heparinized saline on a biweekly schedule.

The Medtronic SynchroMed™ II Programmable Pump is available in two reservoir sizes (20 mL or 40 mL). In general, the 20 mL reservoir pump is preferred for HAI purposes; however, there may be instances where the 40 mL pump is used. For the intent of HAI, it is this institution's experience that all 40 mL pumps were maintained as 20 mL pumps to reduce risk of dosing, refill, and programming error. The Medtronic SynchroMed II Programmable Pump requires a programming system consisting of a Clinician Programmer

Table 13.1 Glycerin injection reference table (Adapted from the Glycerin Infusion Intera 3000 Hepatic Artery Infusion Pump Instruction for Use [9])

	Intera 3000 series (reservoir volume)	Labeled flowrate (intra-arterial) [a]	Approximate refill interval [b]
40% Glycerin injection 0.38 conversion factor[c]	3000 (30 mL)	High	54–60 days
50% Glycerin injection 0.26 conversion factor[c]	3000 (30 mL)	High	79–87 days
60% Glycerin injection[c] 0.17 conversion factor[c]	3000 (30 mL)	High	122–133 days

[a] Nominal arterial flowrate of manufactured pumps (at 100 mmHg with 1000 μ/mL aqueous heparin solution). Individual flowrate may vary, and is indicated on pump labeling
[b] Please refer to the formula below Fig. 13.1 for refill period calculation
[c] Please refer to the glycerin conversion data chart displayed in Fig. 13.1
Adapted from the Glycerin Infusion Intera 3000 Hepatic Artery Infusion Pump Instruction for Use [9]

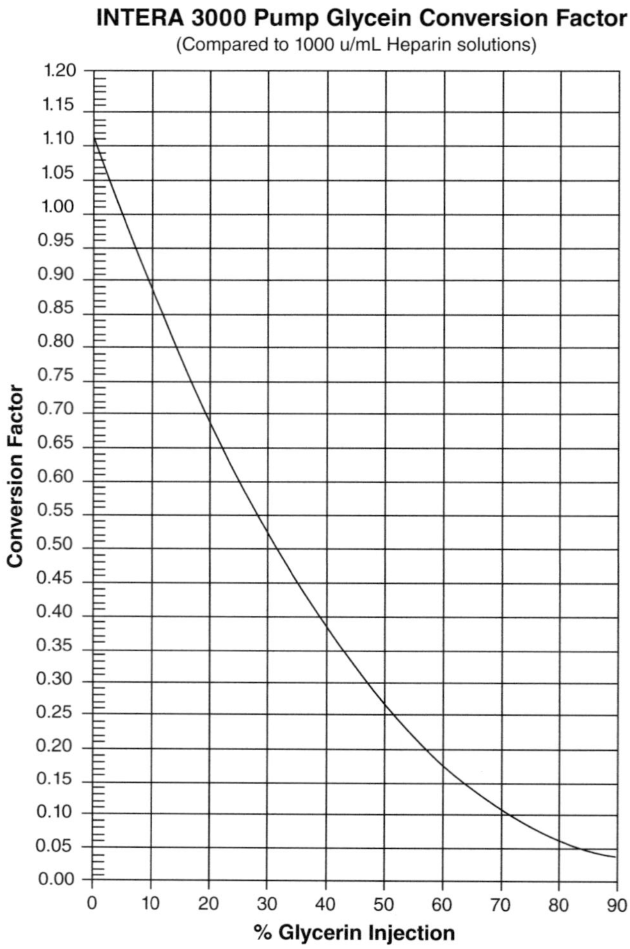

Fig. 13.1 Intera 3000 pump glycerin conversion factor. (Adapted from the Glycerin Infusion Intera 3000 Hepatic Artery Infusion Pump Instruction for Use [9])

Tablet, SynchroMed™ II Clinician Programmer App, and a wireless Communicator which allows the clinician to individualize drug dosing and provide efficient refill intervals in a reliable and consistent fashion. The peristaltic action of the SynchroMed™ II pump moves the drug from the pump reservoir, through the pump tubing, check valve, catheter access port, and implanted catheter, to the infusion site within the hepatic artery [10].

Following a chemotherapy interruption and entering a maintenance phase of the Medtronic Pump system, the programmable pump is refilled with the specified volume of heparinized saline solution and programmed to deliver a constant dose throughout the day.

Various programming options exist with the SynchroMed II pump which can be utilized by the practitioner to slow down the medication infusion rates of the pump. This allows healthcare providers to program dosing intervals that are advantageous to the patients while either on treatment breaks or through their surveillance time as the pump remains implanted.

Practitioners with experience in the use of Medtronic Pumps in these past years would regularly set the programmable pumps for maintenance flowrates ranging between 1 mL/d and 0.7 mL/d. Furthermore, facilities like ours have programmed the pump flowrates as low as 0.5 mL/d which allows patients the convenience of longer refills intervals of up to every 4 weeks. It is imperative to interrogate and program the Medtronic Pump at each refill procedure, including verification of residual volume, and programming of refill volume, drug information, and flowrate for early identification and correction of potential errors. It is our opinion that even during times of maintenance, all nursing safety checks continue to be followed to reduce risk of programming errors.

Access to HAI Pump Centers is limited across the country, often requiring patients to travel long distances for this treatment. During the maintenance phase, oncologists may partner with a patient's local oncologist in the provision of pump refills, allowing patients the flexibility of maintaining their pump closer to home. Direct communication channels to these centers must be established, as well as nursing staff training and necessary supply procurement. It is imperative that the nursing staff are trained and evaluated on the refill procedure, training which is ideally administered by the pump manufacturer representatives. Clinical staff must be trained on potential pump complications, including signs of catheter occlusion, flipped pumps, and variations in flowrates. The center must put in place documentation mechanisms to track the ins and outs of the pump, ensuring proper pump function. It is prudent for the two centers to have contingency plans in place for any pump complications that may arise and determine if the local site is able to manage these occurrences or if the patient is required to travel to an experienced HAI pump center for more thorough investigation and mitigation.

Secondary Use of HAI Pump

When making the decision to restart HAI therapy, there are a few procedures to be mindful of to optimally prepare the non-programmable pump to receive chemotherapy. As noted in the Intera 3000 glycerin IFU [9], when resuming therapy, it is recommended to thoroughly rinse the pump reservoir twice with sterile saline to dilute the concentration of glycerin injection still remaining in the device reservoir. Additionally, it is recommended to flush the bolus pathway to remove any residual glycerin from the bolus channel and silicone catheter. The provider may note that after resuming HAI treatment after a glycerin maintenance period, the pump may continue to run slower, with instances where the pump never returns to its predetermined baseline flowrate. This must be considered as this impacts the calculated and delivered dose of chemotherapy.

The procedural steps described above are limited to pumps where glycerin for injection is used. No additional steps are required when restarting therapy in the Medtronic SynchroMed™ II Programmable Pump other than the required programming adjustments to return the arterial delivery rate to 1 mL/d.

It should also be noted that secondary use of HAI pumps should commence at a dose of FUDR no higher than that of the last cycle given. If patients have had significant durations of systemic therapy since the prior cycle of FUDR, the oncologist may also consider using a starting dose of FUDR that is 50% that of the last dose administered, which can then be titrated back up with reassuring labs.

The determination to explant the HAI pump comes after reaching a minimum number of years of achieving and maintaining a complete hepatic remission as well as being influenced by the presence of any extrahepatic disease, barring no complications involving the HAI device system mandating for an unplanned pump explantation surgery. The decision to remove the HAI pump is a rather sensitive dialogue that takes place between the patient and the HAI center providers through the course of the cancer survivorship. In our experience, we don't consider pump explantation until at least 5 years of continuous remission have been reached, without requiring intermittent rescue with regional hepatic treatment. Other centers consider removal after 2–3 years if there has been no progression in the liver. Hepatic progression in patients who have had no further liver metastases after 3 years is unlikely especially in the adjuvant setting. If the pump is no longer useable due to technical/vascular issues the pump can be removed at any interval.

In those scenarios where the patient develops extrahepatic recurrence only, HAI pump patency is maintained with heparinized saline and/or glycerin subject to the type of device being served, in the event that HAI may be resumed in the future (e.g., after establishing extrahepatic disease control in a patient whose now immediate threat to life is secondary to the hepatic disease burden). Systemic therapy is often reinstituted in a setting where the medical oncologist may select to initiate standard (full) doses of antineoplastic agents, as well as utilize treatment combinations with the addition of antiangiogenic drugs (such as bevacizumab) provided that no regional hepatic chemotherapy is planned during this portion of treatment.

Conclusion

In summary, the duration of HAI FUDR therapy in colorectal cancer and intrahepatic cholangiocarcinoma remains controversial. While longer durations of therapy are typically used in the unresectable/palliative setting to help improve outcomes by providing durable disease control or perhaps convert patients to resection, extended durations of HAI are also associated with increased toxicity. Such dose-dependent toxicity that remains somewhat unpredictable is especially considered in the adjuvant setting where the duration is commonly limited to 4–6 months. The decision to extend the duration of therapy beyond 6 months should be made on an individualized basis. Future research is needed to determine the optimal duration of HAI FUDR therapy, as well as to identify better predictors of tolerance/intolerance to FUDR. In general, after reaching predetermined dosing duration endpoints, or in the setting of conversion or complete clinical response, pumps can be maintained for secondary use in the event of hepatic recurrence. Maintenance strategies are dictated by the device implanted and the treating institution's protocol, most often leveraging glycerin in non-programmable devices to slow the rate of flow thereby extending the interval of time required between pump refills. In the event of hepatic recurrence, standard protocols exist for resuming HAI, the most important consideration being that the treating oncologist restart FUDR at a dose that is no higher than that of the most recent dose given.

References

1. Allen-Mersh T, Earlam S, Fordy C, Abrams K, Houghton J. Quality of life and survival with continuous hepatic-artery floxuridine infusion for colorectal liver metastases. Lancet. 1994;344:1255–60.
2. Chang AE, et al. A prospective randomized trial of regional versus systemic continuous 5-fluorodeoxyuridine chemotherapy in the treatment of colorectal liver metastases. Annal Surg. 1987;206:685.
3. Martin JK, et al. Intra-arterial floxuridine vs systemic fluorouracil for hepatic metastases from colorectal cancer: a randomized trial. Arch Surg. 1990;125:1022–7.
4. Stagg RJ, et al. Alternating hepatic intra-arterial floxuridine and fluorouracil: a less toxic regimen for treatment of liver metastases from colorectal cancer. JNCI J Natl Cancer Inst. 1991;83:423–8.
5. Lorenz M, Müller H-H, Metastases, f. t. G. C. G. o. L. Randomized, multicenter trial of fluorouracil plus Leucovorin administered either via hepatic arterial or intravenous infusion versus Fluorodeoxyuridine administered via hepatic arterial infusion in patients with Nonresectable liver metastases from colorectal carcinoma. J Clin Oncol. 2000;18:243. https://doi.org/10.1200/jco.2000.18.2.243.
6. Kemeny N, et al. Hepatic arterial infusion of chemotherapy after resection of hepatic metastases from colorectal cancer. N Engl J Med. 1999;341:2039–48.
7. Kemeny NE, Gonen M. Hepatic arterial infusion after liver resection. N Engl J Med. 2005;352:734–735.
8. Kemeny MM, et al. Combined-modality treatment for resectable metastatic colorectal carcinoma to the liver: surgical resection of hepatic metastases in combination with continuous infusion of chemotherapy—an intergroup study. J Clin Oncol. 2002;20:1499–505.
9. Anon. Instruction for use: glycerin infusion Intera 3000 hepatic artery infusion pump. Wellesley, MA: Intera Oncology; 2019. Accessed 3 Aug 2023. https://www.interaoncology.com/files/6e4aef4a.pdf.
10. Medtronic. Drug infusion systems—synchromedTM II. Medtronic. 2022. Accessed 3 Aug 2023. https://www.medtronic.com/us-en/healthcare-professionals/products/neurological/drug-infusion-systems/synchromed-ii.html.

Part IV

Patient Selection and Efficacy

14 HAI for Unresectable Colorectal Liver Metastases

Kelly M. Mahuron, Vikram C. Gorantla, Moh'd M. Khushman, and Laleh G. Melstrom

Introduction

Up to half of patients with colorectal cancer will develop liver metastasis during their disease course, and one-quarter will have liver metastases at the time of diagnosis [1]. In well-selected patients, complete resection is potentially curative with a 5-year survival up to 50% [2]. However, fewer than 25% of patients with colorectal liver metastases (CRLM) have resectable disease at the time their metastases are diagnosed [3].

For these unresectable CRLM patients, systemic chemotherapy is the standard of care (SOC). Even with advances in modern-day systemic therapy, treatment resistance is common and response rates to second and third line regimens are poor [4]. For example, response rates to third-line therapy such as TAS-102 are only 1.6% with median improvements in overall survival of 7–8 weeks [5].

K. M. Mahuron · L. G. Melstrom (✉)
Department of Surgery, City of Hope National Medical Center, Duarte, CA, USA
e-mail: kmahuron@coh.org; lmelstrom@coh.org

V. C. Gorantla
Division of Medical Oncology, University of Pittsburgh Medical Center, Pittsburgh, PA, USA
e-mail: gorantlavc2@upmc.edu

M. M. Khushman
Department of Medicine, Washington University in St. Louis, St. Louis, MO, USA
e-mail: mkushman@wustl.edu

As liver disease is often a determinant of patient survival and resection is the main potential modality for cure, converting these initially unresectable patients to surgical candidates is an important treatment goal. Although a proportion of CRLM patients may have significant response to systemic therapy with downstaging of their liver involvement to resectable disease, the conversion rate is extremely variable ranging from 12.5% to 61% in different trials depending on patient factors and the systemic regimen received [6, 7]. Additionally, there is extreme heterogeneity in the definition of resectable disease.

Outside of systemic therapies, regional liver-directed therapies are of interest, and the utility of hepatic artery infusion pump therapy has been evaluated in the context of unresectable disease. For patients with unresectable CRLM, HAI therapy has been associated with high rates of response and conversion to resectable disease. There are multiple, key considerations for the use and timing of this modality that take into context a patient's disease status and the potential risks and benefits of a surgical intervention.

Patient Selection

Appropriate patient selection is crucial to identify appropriate candidates for HAIP therapy in the setting of unresectable CRLM. The criteria used to define unresectable liver disease has

M. D'Angelica, M. Lidsky (eds.), *Hepatic Arterial Infusion for Malignancy*,
https://doi.org/10.1007/978-3-031-74935-3_14

evolved over the past two decades but remains highly variable and is institutional- and surgeon-dependent. Additionally, combining resection with ablation, two-stage resection and utilization of portal vein embolization to remedy anticipated small liver remnants are strategies that allow for more extensive resections and expanded indications. All definitions follow the general principle that after complete resection, an adequate functional liver remnant must be maintained (Table 14.1). The determination of which unresectable CRLM patients might benefit from HAI therapy depends on multiple factors (Fig. 14.1).

Patient Characteristics

Patients must be screened for their general surgical candidacy as well as underlying hepatic function. Regarding general surgical candidacy, patients should have an adequate performance status (ECOG 0–1/Karnofsky > = 70%). Previous history of abdominal surgery must be evaluated to ensure that extensive adhesive disease or inflammation and fibrosis does not preclude catheter placement. Additionally, patients must be able to tolerate general anesthesia with sufficient cardiopulmonary reserve. The majority of HAI pump (HAIP) placements are performed with laparotomy, which requires recovery prior to resumption of systemic chemotherapy; however, HAIP therapy can be instituted early as there is no significant systemic exposure to the drug. More centers are beginning to perform robotic HAIP placement with the intention of shortening recovery time [8]. Patients must also have access to medical institutions with established, experienced, high-volume HAIP programs as HAI pump maintenance requires frequent visits. While HAI chemotherapy (HAIC) was initially only administered at few high-volume centers, the initiation of new HAIP programs is expanding access to more patients [9].

In addition to a patient's surgical candidacy, evaluation of their baseline hepatic function is of upmost importance as patients with unresectable CRLM may have extensive hepatic replacement by their tumor and are at high risk for chemotherapy-associated steatohepatitis (CASH) due to prolonged systemic chemotherapy [10]. Therefore, the number of prior chemotherapy cycles and regimens needs to be well-documented, and a complete laboratory and imaging assess-

Table 14.1 Principles defining CRLM not amenable to resection and/or ablation

Unresectable liver disease
Diffuse, bilobar liver involvement
Anticipated insufficient future liver remnant due to high tumor burden (>70%) or poor hepatic function that cannot be remedied with PVE, ALPPS, and/or a two-stage approach
Critical vascular involvement of inflow (both portal veins) and/or outflow (three hepatic veins or retro-hepatic vena cava) structures
Inability to preserve two continuous anatomic liver segments

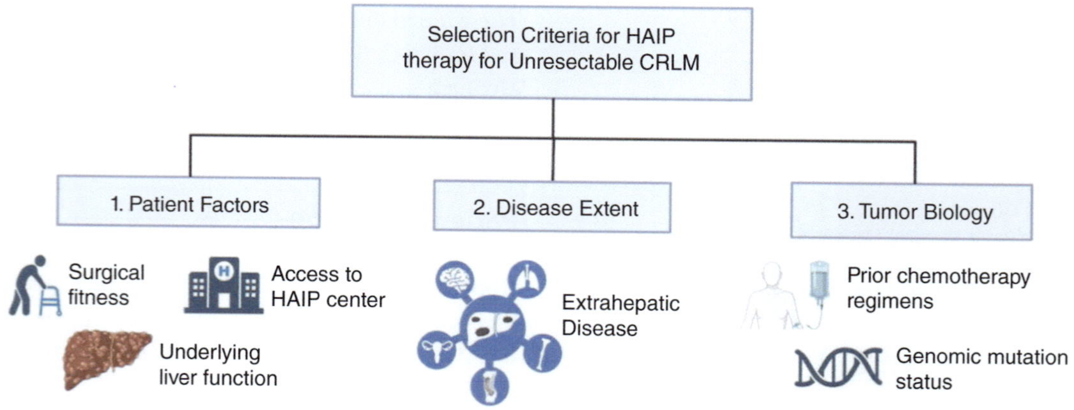

Fig. 14.1 Factors to consider when selecting CRLM patients for HAIP candidacy

ment must be performed to assess for signs of hepatic insufficiency, portal hypertension, and cirrhosis. Laboratory studies should include liver function tests such as serum bilirubin and alkaline phosphatase, as well as coagulation panels and platelet counts to evaluate for thrombocytopenia. Imaging should be examined for signs of portal hypertension (splenomegaly, varices, ascites) as well as steatohepatitis which can be seen as hepatic attenuation lower than the spleen [11]. Additionally, patients should be screened for other conditions that impact liver function such as viral-hepatitis, NASH, and alcohol-induced cirrhosis. Significant hepatic insufficiency is a contraindication for HAIP placement as it places patients at higher risk for liver failure postoperatively which precludes HAIP therapy.

Extrahepatic Disease

In addition to patient factors including underlying hepatic function, extrahepatic disease (EHD) develops in up to 50% of patients with CRLM and has historically been considered a contraindication for both liver resection and HAIP placement. However, studies have shown promising outcomes and the potential for cure with complete resection of both the hepatic and extrahepatic metastases in the setting of CRLM with limited EHD [12]. Furthermore, the site of EHD and extent of its resection have been shown to impact survival. Among resectable patients, metastases to portal or retroperitoneal lymph nodes, multiple sites of EHD, and incomplete resection of EHD are associated with worse prognosis [13].

These same principles are applied for selection of HAIP candidates in the context of EHD. As initial HAI chemotherapy (HAIC) studies such as the CALGB (Cancer Leukemia Group B) 9481 trial did not include concurrent systemic chemotherapy in the HAI treatment arm, hepatic disease control was observed at the cost of EHD progression [14]. Combining HAIC with systemic chemotherapy is now a standard protocol, and EHD is now only considered a relative contraindication for HAIC at many centers with careful patient selection. Appropriate HAIP candidates should have stable EHD that is not immediately life-threatening, and mortality should be driven by the hepatic involvement rather than EHD. Prospective trials have shown good results with HAIC with inclusion of patients that have limited and resectable EHD [15].

Tumor Biology and Mutational Status

The biology of a patient's disease and their tumor mutational status should be taken into consideration for HAIP therapy. Response to systemic therapy and disease progression should be considered as patients with rapid progression of their hepatic or extrahepatic metastases may not benefit from HAIP therapy. Additionally, genomic sequencing of tumors is becoming interestingly more common as specific mutations have been associated with worse prognoses. KRAS and BRAF mutations are negatively associated with survival in CRLM patients who undergo hepatectomy, and they can be considered in the evaluation of patients undergoing resection [16]. Similarly, potential HAIP candidates should undergo genomic sequencing as mutations such as KRAS G12C, BRAFV600E, and HER2 amplification may influence treatment decisions given both their predictive and prognostic significance.

Therefore, a thorough evaluation to appropriately select unresectable CRLM patients for HAIP therapy includes a multitude of factors including a patient's fitness and ability to recover from surgery, their underlying hepatic function and reserve, the extent of their liver disease and the presence of EHD, as well as the biology of their disease and mutational status. Once a patient is determined to be a good candidate for HAIP therapy, the goals of therapy and whether they may be converted into surgical candidates will determine the remainder of their care.

HAIP for Palliation and Salvage Therapy

Patients with unresectable CRLM can be conceptually divided into those who may be converted into surgical candidates with HAIP therapy and those who will never have surgery.

As the majority of unresectable CRLM patients will not be candidates for resection, the treatment goal for this group is durable disease control to prolong survival.

Initial studies for this patient population looked at the response and survival rates of HAIP chemotherapy compared to standard systemic therapy. The HAIP arms of these trials did not include systemic therapy, and at least ten randomized controlled trials were performed [17–26] (Table 14.2). The results from these trials were mixed, with six (60%) demonstrating a significantly higher response rate for HAIP compared to systemic therapy, and only three (30%) trials showed improved median OS. A meta-analysis which included these studies found that although the response rate was higher for HAIP compared to systemic therapy (42.9% versus 18.4%, $p < 0.0001$), there was no difference in mOS [27]. Criticisms of these trials include that they are small single-institution studies, many allowed crossover, and some used HAIP FU rather than FUDR, the latter having a higher hepatic extraction rate. Additionally, the rate of extrahepatic progression was much higher in the HAIP treatment arms compared to the patients receiving systemic therapy, as these patients didn't receive any systemic chemotherapy on trial. Therefore, HAIP therapy for CRLM in the modern era now includes concurrent systemic chemotherapy as standard practice.

As unresectable CRLM patients typically receive multiple lines of chemotherapy and have limited systemic options, HAIP in combination with systemic chemotherapy can be considered as a form of salvage therapy for hepatic disease control. A retrospective review of 110 patients who progressed on at least three lines of systemic therapy at MSKCC demonstrated an response rate of 33%, disease control in 87%, and a median survival of 20 months from the time of pump placement [28]. In line with this study, another

Table 14.2 Randomized controlled trials of HAIP therapy compared to systemic chemotherapy or best supportive care for unresectable CRLM

Trial	Institution	Year	Treatment arms	Number of patients	Response rate[a] (%)	Median OS[a] (months)
Chang et al. [17]	NCI	1987	HAI: FUDR	32	**62**	17
			Sys: FUDR	32	**17**	12
Kemeny et al. [18]	MSKCC	1987	HAI: FUDR	48	**50**	17
			Sys: FUDR	51	**20**	12
Hohn et al. [19]	NCOG	1989	HAI: FUDR	67	**42**	16.5
			Sys: FUDR	76	**9**	15.8
Martin et al. [20]	Mayo	1990	HAI: FUDR	39	**48**	12.6
			Sys: FU/LV	35	**21**	10.5
Wagman et al. [21]	COH	1990	HAI: FUDR	31	55	13.8
			Sys: FU	10	20	11.6
Rougier et al. [22]	France	1992	HAI: FUDR	81	**41**	**15**
			Sys: FU or BSC	82	**9**	**11**
Allen-Mersh et al. [23]	England	1994	HAI: FUDR	51	NR	**13.5**
			Sys: FU or BSC	49		**7.5**
Lorenz and Muller [24]	Germany	2000	HAI: FUDR	54	43	12.7
			HAI: FU/LV	57	45	18.7
			Sys: FU/LV	57	27	17.6
Kerr et al. [25]	EORTC	2003	HAI: FU/LV	145	22	14.7
			Sys: FU/LV	145	19	14.8
Kemeny et al. [26] (CALBG 9481)	MSKCC	2006	HAI: FUDR	68	**47**	**24.4**
			Sys: FU/LV	67	**24**	**20**

OS overall survival, *HAI* hepatic artery infusion, *Sys* systemic chemotherapy, *BSC* best supportive care, *NR* not reported, *FUDR* floxuridine, *FU* fluorouracil, *LV* leucovorin

[a]Numbers in bold refer to statistically significant differences for response rates and median OS

single-institution retrospective study of 25 heavily pretreated CRLM patients demonstrated an response rate of 40% and 6-month median PFS with HAIP therapy [29]. Both studies reported encouraging results with HAIP for liver-confined disease as well as for patients with low-volume extrahepatic disease.

However, while HAIP therapy may provide disease palliation for unresectable CRLM, there are unique considerations for this group of patients. Postoperative complications including pump-related complications may delay resumption of chemotherapy and result in disease progression although this occurs at a relatively low rate. Additionally, patients may lose candidacy for enrollment in novel clinical trials if they undergo HAIP placement. If hepatic function is maintained, some patients may derive more benefit from additional systemic therapy prior to HAIC.

HAI with Goal of Conversion to Resection

A proportion of initially unresectable CRLM patients, such as a patient with liver-dominant disease primarily limited to one lobe of the liver with inflow involvement, may become a hepatectomy or ablation candidate depending on their response to chemotherapy. As liver-disease clearance is the only potential for cure, the likelihood of a patient's conversion to resectable disease may dictate how aggressive treatment measures should be.

Conversion to resection (CTR) is therefore the ultimate treatment goal, and it has been the endpoint of many prospective clinicals trials. One of the first prospective trials was a phase II study performed at MSKCC, published in 2009, that measured the rates of CTR as a secondary otucome in 49 patients receiving combination HAI FUDR and systemic chemotherapy. The overall response rate (ORR) was 92%, and the rate of CTR was 47%. CTR rate increased to 57% for patients that were chemotherapy naïve [30].

Another prospective trial from MSKCC was a 2015 phase II trial that investigated rates of CTR with combination HAI FUDR and modern systemic chemotherapy in 49 initially unresectable CRLM patients. The ORR was 76%, and 47% of patients had CTR [31]. An update of long-term outcomes of the trial was published with an expansion cohort including 64 patients; ORR was 73% and CTR was achieved in 52%. Patients with EHD were excluded from the trial, and 34% of patients had KRAS-mutated tumors. Improved ORR was seen for KRAS-WT versus KRAS-mutated tumors (68% versus 56%, $p = 0.009$), as well as for chemotherapy-naïve patients versus those that were pretreated (86% versus 61%). Of the 33 patients who underwent resection, 12 (36%) had preoperative PVE to increase the volume of their anticipated future liver remnant to an adequate size. Of all factors in this trial, only CTR was significantly associated with improved OS [32].

Of note, all patients received HAI FUDR along with best systemic chemotherapy and Bevacizumab (Bev) in the initial protocol of this phase II trial. While similar ORR was seen with and without Bev, it was discontinued after the initial 24 patients due to high rates of biliary toxicity requiring biliary stent placement (13% of patients with Bev required biliary stents versus 2.5% without Bev).

Non-FUDR HAI drug regimens have also been studied. The prospective phase II European multicenter OPTILIV (Optimal Control of Liver Metastases from Colorectal Cancer with Cetuximab and Hepatic Artery Infusion of Chemotherapy) trial studied CTR rates with triplet HAIC (irinotecan, 5-FU, and oxaliplatin) and intravenous cetuximab for 64 patients with wild-type (WT)-*KRAS* who had received 1–3 previous lines of systemic chemotherapy. A total of 41% had limited extrahepatic disease, and 44% of patients had received one previous line of chemotherapy while 56% had received 2–3 lines. The ORR was 41%, and the rate of CTR was 30% in the intent-to-treat population. CTR rates were higher for patients on their second line of therapy compared to third or subsequent lines (46% versus 17%, $p = 0.01$). While no biliary toxicity was observed with HAI FUDR, hepatic artery thrombosis or arteritis led to interruption of HAIP therapy for nearly half of patients [15].

While these trials demonstrate encouraging rates of CTR for HAIC and systemic chemotherapy compared to systemic chemotherapy alone [33], randomized trials are needed to directly compare CTR rates with the two approaches. Currently, the randomized phase II SULTAN study (NCT03164655) is underway and compares combination HAI oxaliplatin and systemic therapy to conventional systemic therapy. This trial includes unresectable CRLM patients without EHD who have previously received 2 months of systemic therapy, and the primary endpoint is conversion to complete resection or ablation [34]. The study has completed enrollment and results are pending, and additional trials in this area are in active recruitment (NCT05103020, NCT02102789). Another study in the United States, EA2222, activated in late 2023 and is randomizing patients with persistently unresectable CRLM after 3–6 months of chemotherapy to standard of care chemotherapy with or without HAI FUDR. The primary endpoint of EA2222 is overall survival and it has been designed to definitively answer the question of whether HAI improves survival for this patient population.

Conclusion

Unresectable CRLM, which is often a driver of patient mortality in the setting of metastatic CRC, eventually progresses on several lines of systemic therapy without effective standard-of-care treatment options remaining. HAIP chemotherapy is a regional option that has demonstrated high rates of disease control as a palliative approach as well as high rates of conversion to resection and survival benefit with appropriate patient selection, though modern-day randomized trials are needed to define the role of HAI in patients with unresectable CRLM. Surgical candidacy should be based upon factors including patient fitness and underlying liver health, extent of extrahepatic disease, and disease biology. As the use of HAIP therapy for unresectable CRLM continues to expand to more patients, the goal of treatment should be clearly defined, and its benefits must be weighed heavily with its risks to optimize patient outcomes.

References

1. Pan Z, Peng J, Lin J, et al. Is there a survival benefit from adjuvant chemotherapy for patients with liver oligometastases from colorectal cancer after curative resection? Cancer Commun (Lond). 2018;38(1):29.
2. Sadot E, Groot Koerkamp B, Fau-Leal JN, Leal JN, Fau-Shia J, et al. Resection margin and survival in 2368 patients undergoing hepatic resection for metastatic colorectal cancer: surgical technique or biologic surrogate? (1528–1140 (Electronic)).
3. Devaud N, Kanji ZS, Fau-Dhani N, Dhani N, Fau-Grant RC, et al. Liver resection after chemotherapy and tumour downsizing in patients with initially unresectable colorectal cancer liver metastases. (1477–2574 (Electronic)).
4. Grothey A, Van Cutsem E, Sobrero A, et al. Regorafenib monotherapy for previously treated metastatic colorectal cancer (CORRECT): an international, multicentre, randomised, placebo-controlled, phase 3 trial. Lancet. 2013;381(9863):303–12.
5. Mayer RJ, Van Cutsem E, Falcone A, et al. Randomized trial of TAS-102 for refractory metastatic colorectal cancer. N Engl J Med. 2015;372(20):1909–19.
6. Adam R, Delvart V Fau-Pascal G, Pascal G, Fau-Valeanu A, et al. Rescue surgery for unresectable colorectal liver metastases downstaged by chemotherapy: a model to predict long-term survival. (0003–4932 (Print)).
7. Gruenberger T, Bridgewater J, Chau I, et al. Bevacizumab plus mFOLFOX-6 or FOLFOXIRI in patients with initially unresectable liver metastases from colorectal cancer: the OLIVIA multinational randomised phase II trial. Ann Oncol. 2015;26(4):702–8. https://doi.org/10.1093/annonc/mdu580.
8. Qadan M, D'Angelica MI, Kemeny NE, Cercek A, Kingham TP. Robotic hepatic arterial infusion pump placement. (1477–2574 (Electronic)).
9. Muaddi H, D'Angelica M, Wiseman JT, et al. Safety and feasibility of initiating a hepatic artery infusion pump chemotherapy program for unresectable colorectal liver metastases: a multicenter, retrospective cohort study. J Surg Oncol. 2022;123(1):252–60.
10. Meunier L, Larrey D. Chemotherapy-associated steatohepatitis. (1665–2681 (Print)).
11. Fong Y Fau-Bentrem DJ, Bentrem DJ. CASH (Chemotherapy-Associated Steatohepatitis) costs. (0003–4932 (Print)).

12. Hadden WJ, de Reuver PR, Brown K, Mittal A, Samra JS, Hugh TJ. Resection of colorectal liver metastases and extra-hepatic disease: a systematic review and proportional meta-analysis of survival outcomes. (1477–2574 (Electronic)).
13. Leung U, Gönen M Fau-Allen PJ, Allen PJ, Fau-Kingham TP, et al. Colorectal Cancer Liver Metastases and Concurrent Extrahepatic Disease Treated With Resection. (1528–1140 (Electronic)).
14. Kemeny NE, Niedzwiecki D Fau-Hollis DR, Hollis DR, Fau-Lenz H-J, et al. Hepatic arterial infusion versus systemic therapy for hepatic metastases from colorectal cancer: a randomized trial of efficacy, quality of life, and molecular markers (CALGB 9481). (1527–7755 (Electronic)).
15. Lévi FA, Boige V, Hebbar M, et al. Conversion to resection of liver metastases from colorectal cancer with hepatic artery infusion of combined chemotherapy and systemic cetuximab in multicenter trial OPTILIV. (1569–8041 (Electronic)).
16. Tosi F, Magni E, Amatu A, et al. Effect of KRAS and BRAF Mutations on Survival of Metastatic Colorectal Cancer After Liver Resection: A Systematic Review and Meta-Analysis. (1938–0674 (Electronic)).
17. Chang AE, Schneider PD, Fau-Sugarbaker PH, Sugarbaker PH, Fau-Simpson C, Simpson C, Fau-Culnane M, M Culnane, Fau-Steinberg SM, Steinberg SM. A prospective randomized trial of regional versus systemic continuous 5-fluorodeoxyuridine chemotherapy in the treatment of colorectal liver metastases. (0003–4932 (Print)).
18. Kemeny N, Daly J, Reichman B, Geller N, Botet J, Oderman P. Intrahepatic or systemic infusion of fluorodeoxyuridine in patients with liver metastases from colorectal carcinoma. A randomized trial. Ann Intern Med. 1987;107(4):459–65. https://doi.org/10.7326/0003-4819-107-4-459.
19. Hohn DC, Stagg RJ, Friedman MA, et al. A randomized trial of continuous intravenous versus hepatic intra-arterial floxuridine in patients with colorectal cancer metastatic to the liver: the northern California oncology group trial. J Clin Oncol. 1989;7(11):1646–54. https://doi.org/10.1200/JCO.1989.7.11.1646.
20. Martin JK, O'Connell MJ, Wieand HS, et al. Intra-arterial floxuridine vs systemic fluorouracil for hepatic metastases from colorectal cancer. A randomized trial. Arch Surg. 1990;125(8):1022–7. https://doi.org/10.1001/archsurg.1990.01410200086013.
21. Wagman LD, Kemeny MM, Leong L, et al. A prospective, randomized evaluation of the treatment of colorectal cancer metastatic to the liver. J Clin Oncol. 1990;8(11):1885–93. https://doi.org/10.1200/JCO.1990.8.11.1885.
22. Rougier P, Laplanche A, Huguier M, et al. Hepatic arterial infusion of floxuridine in patients with liver metastases from colorectal carcinoma: long-term results of a prospective randomized trial. J Clin Oncol. 1992;10(7):1112–8. https://doi.org/10.1200/JCO.1992.10.7.1112.
23. Allen-Mersh TG, Earlam S, Fordy C, Abrams K, Houghton J. Quality of life and survival with continuous hepatic-artery floxuridine infusion for colorectal liver metastases. Lancet. 1994;344(8932):1255–60. https://doi.org/10.1016/s0140-6736(94)90750-1.
24. Lorenz M, Müller HH. Randomized, multicenter trial of fluorouracil plus leucovorin administered either via hepatic arterial or intravenous infusion versus fluorodeoxyuridine administered via hepatic arterial infusion in patients with nonresectable liver metastases from colorectal carcinoma. J Clin Oncol. 2000;18(2):243–54. https://doi.org/10.1200/JCO.2000.18.2.243.
25. Kerr DJ, McArdle CS, Ledermann J, et al. Intrahepatic arterial versus intravenous fluorouracil and folinic acid for colorectal cancer liver metastases: a multicentre randomised trial. Lancet. 2003;361(9355):368–73. https://doi.org/10.1016/S0140-6736(03)12388-4.
26. Kemeny NE, Niedzwiecki D, Hollis DR, et al. Hepatic arterial infusion versus systemic therapy for hepatic metastases from colorectal cancer: a randomized trial of efficacy, quality of life, and molecular markers (CALGB 9481). J Clin Oncol. 2006;24(9):1395–403. https://doi.org/10.1200/JCO.2005.03.8166.
27. Mocellin S, Pilati P, Lise M, Nitti D. Meta-analysis of hepatic arterial infusion for unresectable liver metastases from colorectal cancer: the end of an era? J Clin Oncol. 2007;25(35):5649–54. https://doi.org/10.1200/JCO.2007.12.1764.
28. Cercek A, Boucher TM, Gluskin JS, et al. Response rates of hepatic arterial infusion pump therapy in patients with metastatic colorectal cancer liver metastases refractory to all standard chemotherapies. (1096–9098 (Electronic)).
29. O'Leary MP, Wang C, Sandhu J, et al. Salvage regional therapy using hepatic artery infusion pump in unresectable chemotherapy resistant colorectal liver metastases. (1879–1883 (Electronic)).
30. Kemeny NE, Melendez FD Fau-Capanu M, Capanu M, Fau-Paty PB, et al. Conversion to resectability using hepatic artery infusion plus systemic chemotherapy for the treatment of unresectable liver metastases from colorectal carcinoma. (1527–7755 (Electronic)).
31. D'Angelica MI, Correa-Gallego C Fau-Paty PB, Paty Pb Fau-Cercek A, et al. Phase II trial of hepatic artery infusional and systemic chemotherapy for patients with unresectable hepatic metastases from colorectal cancer: conversion to resection and long-term outcomes. (1528–1140 (Electronic)).
32. Pak LA-O, Kemeny NE, Capanu M, et al. Prospective phase II trial of combination hepatic artery infusion and systemic chemotherapy for unresectable colorectal liver metastases: Long term results and curative potential. (1096–9098 (Electronic)).
33. Lam VW, Spiro C Fau-Laurence JM, Laurence Jm Fau-Johnston E, et al. A systematic review of clinical response and survival outcomes of downsizing systemic chemotherapy and rescue liver surgery in

patients with initially unresectable colorectal liver metastases. (1534–4681 (Electronic)).
34. Boilève AA-O, Maillard A, Wagner M, et al. Treatment intensification with hepatic arterial infusion chemotherapy in patients with liver-only colorectal metastases still unresectable after systemic induction chemotherapy—a randomized phase II study—SULTAN UCGI 30/PRODIGE 53 (NCT03164655)—study protocol. (1471–2407 (Electronic)).

Adjuvant Hepatic Arterial Infusion Chemotherapy for Resectable Colorectal Liver Metastases

15

Hakan Bokhoven, Marwan G. Fakih, Celina Ang, and Bas Groot Koerkamp

Abbreviations

ASCO	American Society of Clinical Oncology
CRLM	Colorectal Liver Metastases
CRS	Clinical Risk Score
DFS	Disease-Free Survival
ESMO	European Society for Medical Oncology
HAI	Hepatic Arterial Infusion
HAIC	Hepatic Arterial Infusion Chemotherapy
hDFS	Hepatic Disease-Free Survival
hPFS	Hepatic Progression-Free Survival
HR	Hazard Ratio
hRFS	Hepatic Recurrence-Free Survival
MSKCC	Memorial Sloan Kettering Cancer Center
MUT	Mutated/Mutant
NCCN	National Comprehensive Cancer Network
OS	Overall Survival
PFS	Progression-Free Survival
Pmab	Panitumumab
PVI	Portal Vein Infusion
RCT	Randomized Controlled Trial
RFS	Recurrence-Free Survival
WT	Wild-Type

H. Bokhoven
Department of Surgery, Erasmus University Medical Center, Rotterdam, The Netherlands
e-mail: h.bokhoven.1@erasmusmc.nl

M. G. Fakih
Department of Medicine, Hematology and Medical Oncology, City of Hope Helford Clinical Research Hospital, Duarte, CA, USA
e-mail: mfakih@coh.org

C. Ang
Department of Medical Oncology, Mount Sinai Hospital, New York, NY, USA
e-mail: celina.ang@mssm.edu

B. G. Koerkamp (✉)
Surgical Oncologist and Epidemiologist, Department of Surgery, Erasmus University Medical Center, Rotterdam, The Netherlands
e-mail: b.grootkoerkamp@erasmusmc.nl

Background

Colorectal cancer is the third most common cancer worldwide, with an estimated incidence of 1.9 million patients in 2020 [1]. Over the course of their disease, about 50% of patients with colorectal cancer will develop liver metastases, of whom about 50% have liver-confined metastases. Resection of colorectal liver metastases (CRLM) is the only potentially curative treatment option, achievable in approximately 20% of resected patients, with an overall 10-year survival of approximately 25% [2, 3]. However, depending on selection, at least two-thirds of patients develop recurrent disease after resection of CRLM, which in up to 50% of patients is con-

M. D'Angelica, M. Lidsky (eds.), *Hepatic Arterial Infusion for Malignancy*,
https://doi.org/10.1007/978-3-031-74935-3_15

fined to the liver [4–6]. This raises the demand for an effective adjuvant therapy to lower hepatic recurrence and increase cure rates.

Over the last few decades, systemic chemotherapy has been the cornerstone of adjuvant treatment after resection of CRLM. However, several large randomized controlled trials (RCTs) have failed to prove that perioperative or adjuvant systemic chemotherapy increases overall survival (OS) after resection of CRLM [7–9].

Rationale for Adjuvant Hepatic Arterial Infusion Chemotherapy

Hepatic arterial infusion chemotherapy (HAIC) has gained renewed interest for postponing or preventing intrahepatic recurrence of CRLM. The rationale for intra-arterial liver-directed therapy is based on two principles. First, as opposed to normal liver parenchyma, the blood supply of CRLM is primarily derived from the hepatic artery rather than the portal vein [10, 11]. Second, due to the high first-pass effect in the liver of certain drugs (e.g., floxuridine), HAIC has limited systemic side effects. For floxuridine, this allows for a 400-fold increase in hepatic exposure compared to systemic administration [12–15].

After complete resection of CRLM, approximately 20% of patients are cured and therefore will not benefit from adjuvant chemotherapy [2–4]. Patients who quickly progress with extrahepatic recurrence are also unlikely to gain an advantage from HAIC. About a third of all resected patients, however, will develop recurrence confined to the liver. The rationale of adjuvant HAIC for these patients is to target micrometastases in the liver to delay or prevent intrahepatic recurrence after complete resection of CRLM. Unfortunately, existing clinical risk scores (CRS) and other biomarkers are inadequate to predict which patients are most likely to have recurrent disease confined to the liver or to be cured by surgery alone.

Approaches to Adjuvant Hepatic Arterial Infusion Chemotherapy

Pump Versus Percutaneous Catheterization

Adjuvant HAIC approaches vary widely across trials and hospitals. Most commonly, chemotherapy is administered continuously through the hepatic artery via a surgically implantable subcutaneous pump or port with a catheter in the gastroduodenal artery [16–19]. An advantage of HAIC in the adjuvant setting compared to neoadjuvant/induction setting is that pump placement can be combined with resection of the CRLM. The additional surgical risk due to pump placement is limited. Robot-assisted approaches have further reduced the morbidity by allowing for simultaneous minimally-invasive partial hepatectomy and pump-placement [20, 21]. An alternative to surgical placement of a catheter and pump is percutaneous catheterization of the hepatic artery to administer chemotherapy either intermittently or as a single bolus [22, 23]. High complication rates have been reported after percutaneous catheter placement, in particular hepatic artery thrombosis and catheter dislodgement with extrahepatic perfusion [24–27]. However, technical advancements in percutaneous catheter placement may improve these outcomes [28].

In a systematic review, separate pooled analyses were performed for studies in which the catheter was placed surgically versus percutaneously [29]. A surgically placed catheter was used in 13 studies, representing 1324 patients treated with adjuvant HAIC (regardless of the drug used) and 2125 without [16–18, 24, 30–38]. In these studies, the pooled hazard ratio (HR) for OS was 0.71 (95% CI 0.61–0.84, $P < 0.001$) in favor of HAIC. Two RCTs used percutaneous intra-arterial catheter placement, representing a total of 67 patients treated with adjuvant HAIC and 68 patients without [22, 23]. The pooled HR for OS for HAIC in these studies was 1.48 (95% CI

0.86–2.57). Based on the existing literature, the most common and reliable approach to deliver HAIC is a surgically implanted subcutaneous infusion pump connected to a catheter with the tip in the gastroduodenal artery, just outside the flow of the hepatic artery.

Floxuridine Versus Other Drugs

Floxuridine has been used as the primary chemotherapeutic agent for HAIC in most centers due to its short half-life and 95–99% hepatic extraction. Floxuridine is a prodrug of 5-FU. Systemic effects are rare because of the high first-pass effect with minimal systemic exposure [12, 16, 18, 19]. Other chemotherapeutic agents have also been used for HAIC. In some studies, patients received adjuvant HAIC with oxaliplatin, 5-FU, irinotecan, or mitomycin-C, either as monotherapy or as doublet therapy [17, 31, 33]. Compared to floxuridine, these drugs have much lower first-pass hepatic extraction rates with increased risk of systemic toxicity [39, 40]. For example, while HAIC with floxuridine allows for a 400-fold increased intra-tumoral exposure, this is only four-fold with cisplatin and 100-fold with 5-FU (Table 15.1) [41, 42].

In a meta-analysis of adjuvant HAIC consisting of seven studies including three RCTs in which floxuridine was the primary HAIC agent, a pooled HR for OS of 0.76 (95% CI 0.62–0.94) was found in favor of HAIC [16, 18, 19, 34, 35, 37, 38]. This analysis represented 1036 patients treated with HAIC versus 1838 patients without. In the same meta-analysis, the pooled HR for OS for HAIC of 5-FU or oxaliplatin was 0.74 (95% CI 0.52–1.06). This analysis included five RCTs and three non-randomized trials together representing 355 HAIC patients and 355 non-HAIC patients [29].

Dosage and Duration of HAIC

In most studies with *adjuvant* HAIC using floxuridine, patients have been scheduled for six cycles. Each cycle consisted of 14 days of HAIC followed by 14 days of normal saline with heparin. Intra-arterial floxuridine was historically administered at a dosage of 0.05–0.5 mg/kg/day [16, 18, 35, 37, 43], though the dose used in the modern era is a maximum dose of 0.12 mg/kg/day. Patients who have undergone major liver resection or neo-adjuvant chemotherapy are typically treated with a lower dosage. Most patients require dose reductions due to hepatic toxicity which can result in biliary sclerosis, a complication more frequent in the adjuvant setting compared with HAIC given in unresectable patients. Usually, development of biliary strictures can be prevented by dose reduction or (temporarily) discontinuing HAIC [44]. An algorithm developed at Memorial Sloan Kettering Cancer Center (MSKCC) can be used as a guideline for dose reductions (Table 15.2), and the full details of FUDR dosing can be found in Chap. 11 [45]. Dose reductions are based on increased values of alkaline phosphatase, aspartate aminotransferase, and total bilirubin. For this reason, it is important to monitor these blood values biweekly during therapy.

Concomitant HAI administration of dexamethasone at 1 mg/day (25 mg flat dose loaded into pump) during cycles of floxuridine reduces the risk of liver toxicity. A trial randomly allo-

Table 15.1 Pharmacokinetics of chemotherapeutic agents used for HAI [41]

Drug	$T_{1/2}$ (min)	Total body drug clearance (l/min)	Increased exposure with HAI
Floxuridine	<10	5–15	400 fold
5-FU	10	5	100 fold
Mitomycin-C	<10	0.6	3–4 fold
Cisplatin	20–30	Not reported	4–7 fold

Table 15.2 Dose adjustment schedule for HAIC of floxuridine, developed at MSKCC [45]

	Reference value (RV) Defined as the value obtained on D1 of previous cycle (CX-1)	% FUDR dose Relative to the dose administered in the most recent FUDR cycle
AST	2 to <3 × RV	80%
	3 to ≤4 × RV	50%
	> 4 × RV	**Hold**
ALK Phos	1.2 to ≤1.5 × RV	50%
	> 1.5 × RV	**Hold**
*Total bilirubin	1.2 to ≤1.5 × RV	50%
	> 1.5 × RV	**Hold**

If treatment is held for any of the above situations, treatment will not be reinstituted until values come down to 3X RV (for SGOT) or 1.2X RV (for Alk Phos, Tot Bili), at which time treatment will resume at 25% of the last dose received.

cated patients with unresectable CRLM to HAIC with or without dexamethasone. Patients treated with concomitant dexamethasone developed less hyperbilirubinemia (9% vs 30%; $P = 0.07$). Moreover, this study found superior response rates for patients treated with additional dexamethasone (complete response 8% vs 4%, partial response 63% vs 36%, $P = 0.03$) [46] In patients with hepatic or biliary toxicity, HAI with dexamethasone is typically continued after withholding floxuridine, until toxicity is resolved.

To determine the dose of FUDR to be given on CXD1, the labs on CXD1 and CX-1D15 must be compared to labs on CX-1D1 (reference value, RV). FUDR dose modification is required if the labs on CXD1 or CX-1D15 are elevated beyond the above thresholds compared to CX-1D1 (RV). The reference value is always D1 of the last cycle (CX-1) that the FUDR was administered. Full details can be found in Chap. 11.

Toxicity of HAIC

HAIC with floxuridine rarely results in systemic toxicity due to the high hepatic extraction [12]. Toxicity of HAIC with floxuridine mainly consists of biliary sclerosis and gastroduodenal ulceration related to extrahepatic perfusion. Extrahepatic perfusion can also result in pancreatitis or cholecystitis. For this reason, a cholecystectomy is performed and all non-hepatic branches of the hepatic artery are ligated during catheter placement. Moreover, a nuclear scan (see Chap. 9) is performed postoperatively to rule out extrahepatic perfusion of the pump prior to initiating HAIC.

Biliary sclerosis is the most common serious complication of HAIC with floxuridine. In a series of 293 patients treated with adjuvant HAIC at MSKCC, 5.5% of the patients developed biliary sclerosis requiring stenting [44]. Early signs of biliary toxicity are elevated alkaline phosphatase, aspartate aminotransferase, and bilirubin [47]. Dose reductions are effective at preventing biliary toxicity from developing into biliary sclerosis (Table 15.1 and Chap. 11) [45]. The risk of developing biliary sclerosis increases with the cumulative dose of HAIC, and is most common when used as adjuvant therapy. Consequently, many centers have limited HAIC in the adjuvant setting to 3–4 cycles. Future studies and guidelines should investigate risk factors associated with biliary sclerosis for a tailored algorithm for dosage and duration of HAIC with floxuridine.

Randomized Controlled Trials with Adjuvant HAIC

The first RCT for *adjuvant* HAIC was published in 1990 by Wagman et al. and included only 35 patients. Patients with resectable CRLM were randomly allocated to resection plus HAIC with floxuridine or resection alone. Patients with a solitary CRLM had superior progression-free survival (PFS) with HAIC versus without HAIC (30.7 vs 8.7 months, $P = 0.03$). For patients with multiple CRLM, a benefit in PFS could not be demonstrated (15.6 vs 9.4 months, $P = 0.18$). This trial, however, was inadequately powered to detect differences in the measured outcomes [16].

In 1998, Lorenz et al. published the results of a German RCT in which patients with resectable CRLM were randomly assigned to resection with or without adjuvant HAIC with 5-FU and leucovorin. The first intention-to-treat interim analysis after inclusion of 226 patients showed inferior median OS for patients treated with adjuvant HAIC. Therefore, patient accrual was terminated prematurely. This can partly be attributed to technical complications in up 10% of patients treated with HAIC. Also, 30-day mortality after surgery was 7.5% in the HAIC-group versus 2.7% in the control-group. Moreover, 24 patients (22%) in the HAIC group were not treated per protocol [17]. Finally, HAIC with 5-FU rather than floxuridine was used.

An RCT including 156 patients performed by N. Kemeny et al. in 1999 demonstrated superior 2-year OS rates for patients treated with combined adjuvant chemotherapy (HAIC with floxuridine and systemic 5-FU +/− leucovorin) versus systemic 5-FU alone [43]. Two-year hepatic progression-free survival (hPFS) was 90% for patients treated with HAIC vs 60% without ($P = 0.001$). Patients treated with adjuvant HAIC also had significantly longer overall progression free intervals (37.4 months with HAIC vs 17.2 months without, $P = 0.01$). Thus far, this has been the only RCT that has shown a statistically significant benefit in terms of OS for adjuvant HAIC after resection of CRLM. In fact, it is the only RCT that has found a statistically significant benefit in OS for *any* adjuvant treatment after resection of CRLM. In 2005, an update of this RCT with extended median follow-up of 10.3 years was published [19]. Overall PFS remained superior for patients treated with HAIC (31.2 vs 17.2 months, $P = 0.02$). Ten-year OS was 41.1% for patients treated with HAIC and 27.2% without. OS was superior even in patients with the highest risk of recurrence (Fong CRS 3–5; 38.7% with HAIC vs 16.3% without). The difference in median OS, however, was not definitively demonstrated (68.4 months with HAIC vs 58.8 months without HAIC, $P = 0.10$). Nonetheless, the significant and clinically meaningful differences in long-term overall disease-free survival definitively demonstrated clinical benefit.

Additional studies include a small trial that was published in 1999 that randomly allocated 30 patients with resectable CRLM and mesenteric lymph-node metastases into two groups: adjuvant HAIC with mitomycin-C plus 5-FU versus resection alone. No significant difference in either disease-free survival (DFS; 23% with HAIC vs 15% without, $P = 0.79$) or 5-year OS (31% with HAIC vs without 25%, $P = 0.92$) was detected between these groups [31].

A small Japanese trial by Tono et al. from 2000 randomly assigned 19 patients to undergo resection with or without adjuvant HAIC with 5-FU. Median DFS was significantly better for patients treated with adjuvant HAIC (62.6 vs 13.8 months; $P = 0.045$) [33].

The trial by M. Kemeny et al. from 2002 randomized 109 patients with resectable CRLM between resection with or without systemic 5-FU and HAIC with floxuridine. Due to the timing of randomization, 34 patients did not meet eligibility criteria at the time of surgery and were therefore excluded. Seventy-five patients (30 adjuvant HAIC, 45 without) were analyzed. At a median follow-up of 51 months, the 4-year RFS (45.7% vs 25.2%; $P = 0.04$) and hepatic recurrence-free survival (hRFS) (66.9% vs 43.0%, $P = 0.03$) were significantly better in patients treated with adjuvant chemotherapy. The 4-year OS rate, however, was similar in both groups (61.5% vs 52.7%, $P = 0.6$) [18].

The RCT from Kusano et al. (2017) randomly allocated 91 patients to adjuvant systemic 5-FU or HAIC with 5-FU. Five-year OS rates were similar between both groups (59.0% with systemic chemotherapy vs 34.9% with HAIC; $P = 0.15$) [22]. Another RCT from Kusano et al. (2018, $n = 44$) compared adjuvant HAIC (5-FU) and subsequent systemic chemotherapy with systemic chemotherapy alone (5-FU and leucovorin). This trial was prematurely discontinued due to slow accrual. No significant differences in 3-year OS (80% vs 85%, $P = 0.19$) and DFS

Table 15.3 Summary of randomized trials with adjuvant HAIC

Author, year	Sample size	HAI catheter implantation	Infusion rate	HAIC regimen	Concomitant systemic treatment	Control-arm adjuvant treatment	Primary outcome (HAI vs no HAI)
Wagman, 1990 [16]	35	Surgical	Continuous	FUDR	None	None	Median PFS 30.7 vs 8.7 months ($p = 0.03$)
Lorenz, 1998 [17]	226	Surgical	Continuous 5 days	5-FU + LV	None	None	Median OS 34.5 vs 40.8 months HR 0.76 (95% CI 0.50–1.15, $p = 0.15$)
Rudroff, 1999 [31]	30	Surgical	Bolus 4 h	5-FU + MMC	None	None	5-year OS 31% vs 25% ($p = 0.92$)
Tono, 2000 [33]	19	Surgical	Continuous 5 days	5-FU	5-FU	5-FU	Median DFS 62.6 vs 13.8 months ($p = 0.045$)
M Kemeny, 2002 [18]	109	Surgical	Continuous 14 days	FUDR	5-FU	None	4-year RFS 46% vs 25% ($p = 0.04$)
N Kemeny, 2005 [19, 43]	156	Surgical	Continuous 14 days	FUDR	5-FU + LV	5-FU + LV	Median OS 68.4 vs 58.8 months ($p = 0.1$)
Kusano 2017 [22]	91	Percutaneous	Bolus 24 h	5-FU	None	5-FU	5-year OS 34.9% vs 59.0% ($p = 0.15$)
Kusano, 2018 [23]	44	Percutaneous	Bolus 24 h	5-FU	UFT + LV	UFT + LV	3-year OS (80% vs 85%, $p = 0.19$)
N Kemeny 2021 [48]	75	Surgical	Continuous 14 days	FUDR	FOLFIRI + Pmab	FOLFIRI	15-month DFS 69% (95% CI 53–82) vs 47% (95% CI 32–63)

(44% vs 58%, $P = 0.53$) were found between both groups [23].

In a meta-analysis by Buisman et al., a pooled analysis was done for the above-mentioned eight RCTs, representing 312 HAIC- and 340 non-HAIC patients [16–19, 22, 23, 31, 43]. The pooled HR for OS with HAIC was 0.91 (95% CI 0.72–1.14) [29].

In 2021, N. Kemeny et al. published a phase II RCT in which patients with KRAS wild-type resected CRLM were randomly allocated to adjuvant HAIC (Table 15.3) with floxuridine and systemic FOLFIRI with or without panitumumab (Pmab) [48]. In total, 75 patients were randomized and the median follow-up was 56.6 months. The 15-month DFS was 69% (95% CI 53–82) with Pmab and 49% (95% CI 32–63) without. The 3-year DFS was 57% (95% CI 43–76) with Pmab and 42% (95% CI 29–61) without Pmab, while 3-year OS was 97% (95% CI 90–99) and 91% (95% CI 83–100). Toxicity was similar in both groups. This met the prespecified primary endpoint of the trial.

Non-Randomized Evidence for Adjuvant HAIC

The 1999 three-armed study from Ambiru et al. retrospectively compared adjuvant HAIC versus portal vein infusion (PVI) with 5-FU, aclarubicin, and mitomycin C versus resection of CRLM alone [30]. Five-year DFS was significantly better in the HAIC group than in the PVI group (35% vs 13%, $P = 0.01$) and the control group (35% vs 9%, $P = 0.0001$). Moreover, patients in the HAIC group also had superior 5-year OS rates compared to the PVI group (40% vs 17%, $P = 0.02$) and the control group (40% vs 20%, $P = 0.001$).

A study including 287 patients from four non-randomized clinical trials undergoing HAIC with floxuridine after resection of CRLM showed 5- and 10-year OS of respectively 78% and 61% when combined with modern systemic chemotherapy (FOLFOX/FOLFIRI +/− bevacizumab) [49].

A propensity score matched analysis of 2368 patients who underwent complete resection of CRLM at MSKCC showed a median OS of 67 months for patients that received adjuvant HAIC and systemic chemotherapy ($n = 785$), vs 44 months with systemic chemotherapy alone ($n = 1583$). A variety of systemic chemotherapy regimens was used over time and consisted of oxaliplatin or irinotecan. All patients undergoing HAIC were scheduled to receive 5-FU with or without additional systemic chemotherapy. An increased benefit in median OS was found for patients with node-negative status of the primary tumor (129 months with HAIC vs 51 months without; $P < 0.001$) and a low (0–2 points) Fong CRS (89 months with HAIC vs 53 months without; $P < 0.001$) [38].

In 2020, Buisman et al. published a retrospective study from MSKCC and Erasmus MC on the impact of adjuvant HAIC on patterns of recurrence after resection of CRLM. All 2128 patients received preoperative and/or postoperative systemic chemotherapy, of which 601 patients (28.2%) were treated with additional HAIC (floxuridine). The majority (>75%) of all patients received oxaliplatin or irinotecan based systemic chemotherapy regimens, with 25% of patients receiving additional bevacizumab. Patients treated with HAIC were more likely to have multiple CRLM (68% vs 56%, $P < 0.001$) and a high CRS (47% vs 40%, $P = 0.005$) at baseline. In a competing risk analysis of this dataset, the 5-year risk of intrahepatic recurrence was 22.9% with adjuvant HAIC versus 38.4% without ($P < 0.001$). This difference was largely explained by a lower rate of intrahepatic recurrence within the first year after resection of CRLM for patients treated with both HAIC and systemic chemotherapy (11.2% vs 24.4%, $P < 0.001$). Both DFS (20 vs 14 months, $P < 0.001$) and OS (84 vs 57 months, $P < 0.001$) were superior after HAIC [50].

In another retrospective study of MSKCC and Erasmus MC, adjuvant HAIC was investigated in patients with *recurrent* CRLM [51]. The majority of patients (77%) received perioperative systemic chemotherapy, with varying regimens over time. Patients treated with additional adjuvant HAIC after resection or ablation of recurrent CRLM had superior hDFS of 46 months versus 19 months ($P = 0.001$) and superior OS of 92 versus 57 months ($P = 0.002$).

Combined HAIC and Systemic Treatment

In a meta-analysis, concomitant adjuvant systemic chemotherapy with adjuvant HAIC was administered in 11 studies representing 1174 HAIC- and 2020 non-HAIC patients [18, 23, 24, 30, 32, 33, 35–38]. Various systemic regimens such as 5-FU/leucovorin, irinotecan alone, FOLFOX or FOLFIRI +/− bevacizumab, and FOLFIRI + panitumumab have been combined with HAIC. However, bevacizumab is no longer used in combination with HAIC since a study demonstrated it increased the risk of biliary sclerosis [52]. When combined with HAIC, the dosage of systemic chemotherapy has to be reduced to limit hepatic toxicity. At MSKCC, the following dosage has been used for FOLFOX when combined with HAIC; no 5-FU bolus, oxaliplatin 85 mg/m^2 (2-hour infusion) concurrently with leucovorin 400 mg/m^2, followed by a 48-h infusion of 5-FU 2000 mg/m^2. Patients previously treated with oxaliplatin received irinotecan 125–150 mg/m^2 over 30 min instead [48, 52].

While there is no RCT comparing a contemporary systemic regiment with or without HAIC, retrospective series indicate that HAIC still confers benefit over contemporary systemic regimens alone [38, 49]. In the absence of definitive evidence to guide choice of systemic regimen to combine with HAIC, clinicians make decisions based on patients' prior therapy history, response and lingering toxicities (see Chap. 12 for full details on concurrent systemic therapy).

Guideline Recommendations

Adjuvant HAIC is included in the 2022 National Comprehensive Cancer Network (NCCN) guidelines [53]. Due to limitations of HAIC such as the risk of biliary toxicity and the need for specific expertise, the NCCN panel consensus is that HAIC should be considered selectively and only at institutions with extensive experience in the surgical and medical oncological procedures of this treatment [53]. The 2020 American Society of Clinical Oncology (ASCO) guidelines for treatment of late-stage colorectal cancer recommends HAIC to be used in centers with a high level of expertise only [54]. The 2022 guidelines for metastatic colorectal cancer of the European Society for Medical Oncology (ESMO) recommend HAIC to be "considered as a non-curative intent treatment option" [55].

Ongoing Clinical Trials with Adjuvant HAIC

In France, Goeré et al. have designed the phase II/III randomized PACHA-01 trial (NCT02494973) for patients with high risk of recurrence after local treatment of CRLM. In this trial, patients with at least four resectable CRLM are randomly assigned to adjuvant systemic FOLFOX or adjuvant HAIC with oxaliplatin plus systemic 5-FU and leucovorin. Primary outcome in the phase II trial is 18-month hDFS. If the 18-month hDFS is greater than 50% in the phase II trial, this study will be continued in a phase III trial with a sample size of 114 patients. In 2018, after inclusion of 55 patients, this prespecified endpoint was reached and the phase III trial was started. The primary outcome in the phase III trial is DFS. Secondary outcomes are feasibility of delivering at least four cycles of oxaliplatin, toxicity, and OS [56].

Since 2018, the PUMP-trial has been open for accrual in the Netherlands (NTR7493) [45]. Patients with resectable CRLM and a low clinical risk of recurrence (Fong score of 0–2) are eligible for this multicenter phase 3 RCT. Patients with (a history of) extrahepatic metastases are ineligible. Patients are randomly allocated to resection with or without six cycles of HAIC with floxuridine (0.12 mg/kg/day) without any systemic chemotherapy. As of November 2022, a total of 140/230 patients (61%) have been included. The primary outcome is PFS, but the study is also powered to detect a clinically relevant difference in OS with an additional 3 years of follow-up [45].

Another study on adjuvant HAIC from the Netherlands is the PUMP-III trial (NL9294) [57]. This is a single arm prospective study for patients with liver-only recurrent CRLM after previous resection of CRLM. Patients with (a history of) extrahepatic metastases are ineligible for this trial. All patients undergo complete resection or ablation of all CRLM followed by up to six cycles of adjuvant HAIC with floxuridine monotherapy (0.12 mg/kg/day). Primary outcome is hepatic disease-free survival. As of November 2022, 38/45 patients (84%) have been included.

Patient Selection and Biomarkers

In subgroup analyses of the largest cohort of MSKCC with almost 800 patients receiving adjuvant HAIC for CRLM, HAIC was associated with superior OS in all subgroups, except for patients with extrahepatic metastases [38]. In general, the benefit of HAIC was smaller in subgroups with more advanced disease. The rationale is that patients with more advanced disease (i.e., more lesions, node-positive CRC, larger lesions) are more likely to succumb to extrahepatic disease progression. The most pronounced association of HAIC with OS was found in subgroups with a low Fong CRS of 0–2 (89 months with HAIC vs 53 months without, $P < 0.001$) or node-negative primary tumor status (129 months with HAIC vs 51 months without, $P < 0.001$) [38]. However, in the 1999 RCT by Kemeny et al., high-risk patients benefitted from adjuvant HAIC whereas low-risk patients did not [19].

The impact of KRAS mutational status on the prognosis after resection of CRLM with adjuvant HAIC has been investigated by Kemeny et al. in 2014 [58]. A total of 169 patients were retrospectively evaluated, of whom 118 patients with KRAS wild-type (WT) and 51 patients with KRAS mutated (MUT) tumors. The 3-year OS rate was 95% (95% CI 97%–98%) with KRAS WT and 81% (95% CI 62%–95%) with KRAS MUT (P = 0.07). Patients with KRAS MUT developed significantly more recurrences in the bones, brain, and lungs than patients with KRAS WT. These findings are supported by the results of the study by Vauthey et al. from 2013, in which patients with KRAS MUT had significantly more recurrences in the lungs after resection of CRLM (3-year lung DFS 34.6% vs 59.3%, $P < 0.001$) [59]. Based on the results of these studies one could argue that KRAS mutant patients benefit less of HAIC due to their increased risk of extrahepatic metastases. However, another study from MSKCC found that KRAS status was not a predictive factor for the benefit of HAIC [60]. This retrospective study representing 674 patients (418 WT, 256 MUT, 54% adjuvant HAIC) found an association with improved outcome with adjuvant HAIC regardless of KRAS mutational status. Five-year OS was significantly better for patients treated with adjuvant HAIC, both for KRAS WT patients (78% vs 57%, $P < 0.001$) and KRAS MUT patients (59% vs 40%, $P < 0.001$).

BRAF mutations (BRAF-MUT) are found in 5–15% of all CRC patients [61–63]. In patients undergoing resection of CRLM, however, these mutations are only seen in about 0.6–5% [59, 64–67]. BRAF mutation in patients with resected CRLM is associated with inferior outcomes in terms of median OS and DFS. Nevertheless, 5-year OS is possible and associated with node-negative primary status, a Fong CRS < 4 and CEA ≤ 200 μg/L [67]. However, the clinical relevance of BRAF as a biomarker in the adjuvant setting is limited because most patients with BRAF-MUT CRC typically present with more advanced disease, with multiple, unresectable and/or extrahepatic metastases, and are therefore not considered for curative-intent hepatectomy.

Patients with right-sided CRC usually present with more advanced disease compared to patients with left-sided CRC [68]. Several studies demonstrated inferior outcomes in terms of median OS after resection of CRLM for patients with right-sided CRC. However, no significant difference in long-term OS was found [69–71]. The retrospective study by Gholami et al. evaluated patients treated with or without adjuvant HAIC after resection of CRLM [72]. Adjuvant HAIC was associated with superior 5-year OS for right-sided CRC patients (68% with HAIC vs 45% without, $P < 0.01$) and left-sided CRC patients (73% vs 55%, $P < 0.01$). HAIC was independently associated with improved OS (HR 0.52, 95% CI 0.38–0.69, $P < 0.01$) in multivariable analysis, whereas location of primary tumor was not (HR 0.83, 95% CI 0.63–1.11, $P = 0.21$).

To improve patient selection for *adjuvant* HAIC, better predictive biomarkers are needed. Solid tumors release fragments of isolated tumor DNA into the circulation due to tumor apoptosis or lysis. CRC has the tendency to shed high amounts of circulating tumor DNA (ctDNA) compared to other solid tumors. There have been no trials investigating the prognostic or predictive value of ctDNA in patients treated with HAIC. Multiple trials, however, investigated ctDNA after resection of CRLM. In the cohort study of Tie et al., patients with detectable ctDNA after curative-intent surgery of CRLM had a 5-year DFS of 0%, compared to 75.6% for patients without detectable ctDNA [73, 74]. Patients with elevated ctDNA are more likely to progress outside the liver and therefore may be less likely to benefit from HAIC. Blood samples for ctDNA should be drawn before systemic treatment, because ctDNA normalizes with systemic chemotherapy in 34% of patients with stage IV disease [75]. Furthermore, to detect ctDNA, highly sensitive tests are required which are expensive, though are becoming more widely available. Future trials should investigate whether ctDNA at baseline is a predictive factor for the effectiveness of HAIC.

Discussion

Several RCTs demonstrated superior hDFS and overall DFS with adjuvant HAIC floxuridine after resection of CRLM. Only the 1999 RCT by N. Kemeny et al. demonstrated superior 2-year OS [43]. Future RCTs should be powered to detect a clinically relevant difference in OS with adjuvant HAIC using floxuridine following resection of CRLM compared to the current standard of care [48]. Future research should investigate if combined HAIC and modern systemic chemotherapy have a synergistic effect resulting in improved survival.

As HAIC is a liver-directed therapy, it seems important to select patients that do not (quickly) progress beyond the liver. To identify patients that benefit the most from adjuvant HAIC, biomarkers such as ctDNA, and clinical parameters should be evaluated and combined into a prediction tool. It is unclear which patients benefit (the most) from HAIC. The RCT by Kemeny et al. demonstrated superior 10-year survival for patients with a high risk of recurrence [19]. This is contradictory to the results of the propensity matched analysis from MSKCC, in which HAIC was associated with superior OS particularly in patients with a low risk of recurrence [38]. Limitations of this retrospective study design are a possible explanation for this discrepancy. Further prospective research should aim to determine whether adjuvant HAIC is beneficial for all patients with resectable CRLM, or only a subgroup.

Reluctance to treating all patients with resected CRLM with adjuvant HAIC, even at centers using HAI routinely, can likely be attributed to biliary sclerosis, the most significant complication of HAIC, because it requires biliary stenting in about 5.5% of patients [44]. The risk for biliary sclerosis is higher in the adjuvant setting and increases with the number of cycles. For that reason, many centers now limit the number of adjuvant cycles to 4. Future research should also investigate known and unknown risk factors for biliary sclerosis, such as the duration of prior chemotherapy, the extent of hepatectomy, and the presence of hepatic steatosis. An algorithm that doses patients according to these factors could decrease biliary toxicity.

The majority of the evidence that supports HAIC is from a single center, MSKCC [19, 38]. This may have resulted in potential single center bias. Future studies outside MSKCC, such as the PUMP-trials in the Netherlands, are ongoing and several other clinical trials are in the design phase, including trials in development within the HAI Consortium Research Network (HCRN) [45].

Recommendations

The authors recommend that *adjuvant* HAIC should be limited to centers with extensive multidisciplinary experience and/or in clinical trials. Patients with a high risk of intrahepatic recurrence are most likely to benefit from adjuvant HAIC, although it is unclear how to best select these patients. No consensus exists on the benefit, type, duration, and dosage of HAIC and concurrent systemic chemotherapy for patients with resected CRLM. Adjuvant strategies vary widely within and across countries. The available evidence for adjuvant HAIC with floxuridine should be validated in well-designed and adequately powered multicenter RCTs.

Acknowledgments None.

Funding None.

Conflicts of Interest None.

References

1. Cancer IAfRo. Cancer Today: Estimated number of new cases in 2020, worldwide, both sexes, all ages (excl. NMSC) 2020. https://gco.iarc.fr/today/online-analysis-table?v=2020&mode=cancer&mode_population=continents&population=900&populations=900&key=asr&sex=0&cancer=39&type=0&statistic=5&prevalence=0&population_group=0&ages_group%5B%5D=0&ages_group%5B%5D=17&group_cancer=1&include_nmsc=0&include_nmsc_other=1.

2. Engstrand J, Nilsson H, Strömberg C, Jonas E, Freedman J. Colorectal cancer liver metastases—a population-based study on incidence, management and survival. BMC Cancer. 2018;18(1):78.
3. Creasy JM, Sadot E, Koerkamp BG, Chou JF, Gonen M, Kemeny NE, et al. Actual 10-year survival after hepatic resection of colorectal liver metastases: what factors preclude cure? Surgery. 2018;163(6):1238–44.
4. Tomlinson JS, Jarnagin WR, DeMatteo RP, Fong Y, Kornprat P, Gonen M, et al. Actual 10-year survival after resection of colorectal liver metastases defines cure. J Clin Oncol. 2007;25(29):4575–80.
5. Buisman FE, Galjart B, van der Stok EP, Balachandran VP, Boerner T, Drebin JA, et al. Recurrence patterns after resection of colorectal liver metastasis are modified by perioperative systemic chemotherapy. World J Surg. 2020;44(3):876–86.
6. de Jong MC, Pulitano C, Ribero D, Strub J, Mentha G, Schulick RD, et al. Rates and patterns of recurrence following curative intent surgery for colorectal liver metastasis: an international multi-institutional analysis of 1669 patients. Ann Surg. 2009;250(3):440–8.
7. Nordlinger B, Sorbye H, Glimelius B, Poston GJ, Schlag PM, Rougier P, et al. Perioperative FOLFOX4 chemotherapy and surgery versus surgery alone for resectable liver metastases from colorectal cancer (EORTC 40983): long-term results of a randomised, controlled, phase 3 trial. Lancet Oncol. 2013;14(12):1208–15.
8. Portier G, Elias D, Bouche O, Rougier P, Bosset JF, Saric J, et al. Multicenter randomized trial of adjuvant fluorouracil and folinic acid compared with surgery alone after resection of colorectal liver metastases: FFCD ACHBTH AURC 9002 trial. J Clin Oncol. 2006;24(31):4976–82.
9. Kanemitsu Y, Shimizu Y, Mizusawa J, Inaba Y, Hamaguchi T, Shida D, et al. Hepatectomy followed by mFOLFOX6 versus hepatectomy alone for liver-only metastatic colorectal cancer (JCOG0603): a phase II or III randomized controlled trial. J Clin Oncol. 2021;39(34):3789–99.
10. Breedis C, Young G. The blood supply of neoplasms in the liver. Am J Pathol. 1954;30(5):969–77.
11. Ackerman NB. The blood supply of experimental liver metastases. IV. Changes in vascularity with increasing tumor growth. Surgery. 1974;75(4):589–96.
12. Ensminger WD, Gyves JW. Clinical pharmacology of hepatic arterial chemotherapy. Semin Oncol. 1983;10(2):176–82.
13. Guthoff I, Lotspeich E, Fester C, Wallin I, Schatz M, Ehrsson H, et al. Hepatic artery infusion using oxaliplatin in combination with 5-fluorouracil, folinic acid and mitomycin C: oxaliplatin pharmacokinetics and feasibility. Anticancer Res. 2003;23(6D):5203–8.
14. Dzodic R, Gomez-Abuin G, Rougier P, Bonnay M, Ardouin P, Gouyette A, et al. Pharmacokinetic advantage of intra-arterial hepatic oxaliplatin administration: comparative results with cisplatin using a rabbit VX2 tumor model. Anti-Cancer Drugs. 2004;15(6):647–50.
15. Dizon DS, Schwartz J, Kemeny N. Regional chemotherapy: a focus on hepatic artery infusion for colorectal cancer liver metastases. Surg Oncol Clin N Am. 2008;17(4):759–71. viii
16. Wagman LD, Kemeny MM, Leong L, Terz JJ, Hill LR, Beatty JD, et al. A prospective, randomized evaluation of the treatment of colorectal cancer metastatic to the liver. J Clin Oncol. 1990;8(11):1885–93.
17. Lorenz M, Müller HH, Schramm H, Gassel HJ, Rau HG, Ridwelski K, et al. Randomized trial of surgery versus surgery followed by adjuvant hepatic arterial infusion with 5-fluorouracil and folinic acid for liver metastases of colorectal cancer. German cooperative on liver metastases (Arbeitsgruppe Lebermetastasen). Ann Surg. 1998;228(6):756–62.
18. Kemeny MM, Adak S, Gray B, Macdonald JS, Smith T, Lipsitz S, et al. Combined-modality treatment for resectable metastatic colorectal carcinoma to the liver: surgical resection of hepatic metastases in combination with continuous infusion of chemotherapy--an intergroup study. J Clin Oncol. 2002;20(6):1499–505.
19. Kemeny NE, Gonen M. Hepatic arterial infusion after liver resection. N Engl J Med. 2005;352(7):734–5.
20. Dhir M, Zenati MS, Padussis JC, Jones HL, Perkins S, Clifford AK, et al. Robotic assisted placement of hepatic artery infusion pump is a safe and feasible approach. J Surg Oncol. 2016;114(3):342–7.
21. Qadan M, D'Angelica MI, Kemeny NE, Cercek A, Kingham TP. Robotic hepatic arterial infusion pump placement. HPB (Oxford). 2017;19(5):429–35.
22. Kusano M, Honda M, Okabayashi K, Akimaru K, Kino S, Tsuji Y, et al. Randomized controlled phase III study comparing hepatic arterial infusion with systemic chemotherapy after curative resection for liver metastasis of colorectal carcinoma: JFMC 29-0003. J Cancer Res Ther. 2017;13(1):84–90.
23. Kusano M, Aoyama T, Okabayashi K, Hirata K, Tsuji Y, Nakamori S, et al. A randomized phase III study of hepatic arterial infusion chemotherapy with 5-fluorouracil and subsequent systemic chemotherapy versus systemic chemotherapy alone for colorectal cancer patients with curatively resected liver metastases (Japanese Foundation for Multidisciplinary Treatment of cancer 32). J Cancer Res Ther. 2018;14(Supplement):S761–S6.
24. Goéré D, Benhaim L, Bonnet S, Malka D, Faron M, Elias D, et al. Adjuvant chemotherapy after resection of colorectal liver metastases in patients at high risk of hepatic recurrence: a comparative study between hepatic arterial infusion of oxaliplatin and modern systemic chemotherapy. Ann Surg. 2013;257(1):114–20.
25. Herrmann KA, Waggershauser T, Sittek H, Reiser MF. Liver intraarterial chemotherapy: use of the femoral artery for percutaneous implantation of catheter-port systems. Radiology. 2000;215(1):294–9.

26. Oi H, Kishimoto H, Matsushita M, Hori M, Nakamura H. Percutaneous implantation of hepatic artery infusion reservoir by sonographically guided left subclavian artery puncture. AJR Am J Roentgenol. 1996;166(4):821–2.
27. Petrek JA, Minton JP. Treatment of hepatic metastases by percutaneous hepatic arterial infusion. Cancer. 1979;43(6):2182–8.
28. Deschamps F, Rao P, Teriitehau C, Hakime A, Malka D, Boige V, et al. Percutaneous femoral implantation of an arterial port catheter for intraarterial chemotherapy: feasibility and predictive factors of long-term functionality. J Vasc Interv Radiol. 2010;21(11):1681–8.
29. Buisman FE, Filipe WF, Galjart B, Grünhagen DJ, Homs MYV, Moelker A, et al. Adjuvant intra-arterial chemotherapy for patients with resected colorectal liver metastases: a systematic review and meta-analysis. HPB (Oxford). 2022;24(3):299–308.
30. Ambiru S, Miyazaki M, Ito H, Nakagawa K, Shimizu H, Nakajima N. Adjuvant regional chemotherapy after hepatic resection for colorectal metastases. Br J Surg. 1999;86(8):1025–31.
31. Rudroff C, Altendorf-Hoffmann A, Stangl R, Scheele J. Prospective randomised trial on adjuvant hepatic-artery infusion chemotherapy after R0 resection of colorectal liver metastases. Langenbeck's Arch Surg. 1999;384(3):243–9.
32. Kusunoki M, Yanagi H, Noda M, Yoshikawa R, Yamamura T. Results of pharmacokinetic modulating chemotherapy in combination with hepatic arterial 5-fluorouracil infusion and oral UFT after resection of hepatic colorectal metastases. Cancer. 2000;89(6):1228–35.
33. Tono T, Hasuike Y, Ohzato H, Takatsuka Y, Kikkawa N. Limited but definite efficacy of prophylactic hepatic arterial infusion chemotherapy after curative resection of colorectal liver metastases: a randomized study. Cancer. 2000;88(7):1549–56.
34. Moroz P, Salama PR, Gray BN. Resecting large numbers of hepatic colorectal metastases. ANZ J Surg. 2002;72(1):5–10.
35. Onaitis M, Morse M, Hurwitz H, Cotton P, Tyler D, Clavien P, et al. Adjuvant hepatic arterial chemotherapy following metastasectomy in patients with isolated liver metastases. Ann Surg. 2003;237(6):782–8; discussion 8–9.
36. Martin RC, Edwards MJ, McMasters KM. Morbidity of adjuvant hepatic arterial infusion pump chemotherapy in the management of colorectal cancer metastatic to the liver. Am J Surg. 2004;188(6):714–21.
37. Bolton JS, O'Connell MJ, Mahoney MR, Farr GH Jr, Fitch TR, Maples WJ, et al. Hepatic arterial infusion and systemic chemotherapy after multiple metastasectomy in patients with colorectal carcinoma metastatic to the liver: a north central cancer treatment group (NCCTG) phase II study, 92-46-52. Clin Colorectal Cancer. 2012;11(1):31–7.
38. Groot Koerkamp B, Sadot E, Kemeny NE, Gönen M, Leal JN, Allen PJ, et al. Perioperative hepatic arterial infusion pump chemotherapy is associated with longer survival after resection of colorectal liver metastases: a propensity score analysis. J Clin Oncol. 2017;35(17):1938–44.
39. van Riel JM, van Groeningen CJ, de Greve J, Gruia G, Pinedo HM, Giaccone G. Continuous infusion of hepatic arterial irinotecan in pretreated patients with colorectal cancer metastatic to the liver. Ann Oncol. 2004;15(1):59–63.
40. Fiorentini G, Rossi S, Dentico P, Bernardeschi P, Calcinai A, Bonechi F, et al. Irinotecan hepatic arterial infusion chemotherapy for hepatic metastases from colorectal cancer: a phase II clinical study. Tumori. 2003;89(4):382–4.
41. Ensminger WD, Gyves JW. Regional chemotherapy of neoplastic diseases. Pharmacol Ther. 1983;21(2):277–93.
42. Ensminger WD, Gyves JW. Regional cancer chemotherapy. Cancer Treat Rep. 1984;68(1):101–15.
43. Kemeny N, Huang Y, Cohen AM, Shi W, Conti JA, Brennan MF, et al. Hepatic arterial infusion of chemotherapy after resection of hepatic metastases from colorectal cancer. N Engl J Med. 1999;341(27):2039–48.
44. Ito K, Ito H, Kemeny NE, Gonen M, Allen PJ, Paty PB, et al. Biliary sclerosis after hepatic arterial infusion pump chemotherapy for patients with colorectal cancer liver metastasis: incidence, clinical features, and risk factors. Ann Surg Oncol. 2012;19(5):1609–17.
45. Buisman FE, Homs MYV, Grünhagen DJ, Filipe WF, Bennink RJ, Besselink MGH, et al. Adjuvant hepatic arterial infusion pump chemotherapy and resection versus resection alone in patients with low-risk resectable colorectal liver metastases—the multicenter randomized controlled PUMP trial. BMC Cancer. 2019;19(1):327.
46. Kemeny N, Seiter K, Niedzwiecki D, Chapman D, Sigurdson E, Cohen A, et al. A randomized trial of intrahepatic infusion of fluorodeoxyuridine with dexamethasone versus fluorodeoxyuridine alone in the treatment of metastatic colorectal cancer. Cancer. 1992;69(2):327–34.
47. Cohen AD, Kemeny NE. An update on hepatic arterial infusion chemotherapy for colorectal cancer. Oncologist. 2003;8(6):553–66.
48. Kemeny NE, Chou JF, Capanu M, Chatila WK, Shi H, Sanchez-Vega F, et al. A randomized phase II trial of adjuvant hepatic arterial infusion and systemic therapy with or without Panitumumab after hepatic resection of KRAS wild-type colorectal cancer. Ann Surg. 2021;274(2):248–54.
49. Kemeny NE, Chou JF, Boucher TM, Capanu M, DeMatteo RP, Jarnagin WR, et al. Updated long-term survival for patients with metastatic colorectal cancer treated with liver resection followed by hepatic

arterial infusion and systemic chemotherapy. J Surg Oncol. 2016;113(5):477–84.
50. Buisman FE, Galjart B, van der Stok EP, Kemeny NE, Balachandran VP, Boerner T, et al. The impact of hepatic arterial infusion pump chemotherapy on hepatic recurrences and survival in patients with resected colorectal liver metastases. HPB (Oxford). 2020;22(9):1271–9.
51. Buisman FE, Filipe WF, Kemeny NE, Narayan RR, Srouji RM, Balachandran VP, et al. Recurrence after liver resection of colorectal liver metastases: repeat resection or ablation followed by hepatic arterial infusion pump chemotherapy. Ann Surg Oncol. 2021;28(2):808–16.
52. Kemeny NE, Jarnagin WR, Capanu M, Fong Y, Gewirtz AN, Dematteo RP, et al. Randomized phase II trial of adjuvant hepatic arterial infusion and systemic chemotherapy with or without bevacizumab in patients with resected hepatic metastases from colorectal cancer. J Clin Oncol. 2011;29(7):884–9.
53. Benson AB, 3rd. NCCN Guidelines Version 1.2022 Colon Cancer. National Comprehensive Cancer Network. 2022.
54. Chiorean EG, Nandakumar G, Fadelu T, Temin S, Alarcon-Rozas AE, Bejarano S, et al. Treatment of patients with late-stage colorectal cancer: ASCO resource-stratified guideline. JCO Glob Oncol. 2020;6:414–38.
55. Cervantes A. Metastatic colorectal cancer: ESMO clinical practice guideline for diagnosis, treatment and follow-up. European Society of Medical Oncology; 2022.
56. Goéré D, Pignon JP, Gelli M, Elias D, Benhaim L, Deschamps F, et al. Postoperative hepatic arterial chemotherapy in high-risk patients as adjuvant treatment after resection of colorectal liver metastases—a randomized phase II/III trial—PACHA-01 (NCT02494973). BMC Cancer. 2018;18(1):787.
57. Grünhagen D. Adjuvant hepatic arterial infusion pump chemotherapy after repeat hepatectomy for patients with liver confined recurrence of colorectal cancer—a phase II study: Trialsearch; 2021. https://trialsearch.who.int/Trial2.aspx?TrialID=NL9294.
58. Kemeny NE, Chou JF, Capanu M, Gewirtz AN, Cercek A, Kingham TP, et al. KRAS mutation influences recurrence patterns in patients undergoing hepatic resection of colorectal metastases. Cancer. 2014;120(24):3965–71.
59. Vauthey JN, Zimmitti G, Kopetz SE, Shindoh J, Chen SS, Andreou A, et al. RAS mutation status predicts survival and patterns of recurrence in patients undergoing hepatectomy for colorectal liver metastases. Ann Surg. 2013;258(4):619–26; discussion 26–7.
60. Gholami S, Kemeny NE, Boucher TM, Gönen M, Cercek A, Kingham TP, et al. Adjuvant hepatic artery infusion chemotherapy is associated with improved survival regardless of KRAS mutation status in patients with resected colorectal liver metastases: a retrospective analysis of 674 patients. Ann Surg. 2020;272(2):352–6.
61. Davies H, Bignell GR, Cox C, Stephens P, Edkins S, Clegg S, et al. Mutations of the BRAF gene in human cancer. Nature. 2002;417(6892):949–54.
62. Nagasaka T, Koi M, Kloor M, Gebert J, Vilkin A, Nishida N, et al. Mutations in both KRAS and BRAF may contribute to the methylator phenotype in colon cancer. Gastroenterology. 2008;134(7):1950–60, 60 e1.
63. Nagasaka T, Sasamoto H, Notohara K, Cullings HM, Takeda M, Kimura K, et al. Colorectal cancer with mutation in BRAF, KRAS, and wild-type with respect to both oncogenes showing different patterns of DNA methylation. J Clin Oncol. 2004;22(22):4584–94.
64. Frankel TL, Vakiani E, Nathan H, DeMatteo RP, Kingham TP, Allen PJ, et al. Mutation location on the RAS oncogene affects pathologic features and survival after resection of colorectal liver metastases. Cancer. 2017;123(4):568–75.
65. Karagkounis G, Torbenson MS, Daniel HD, Azad NS, Diaz LA Jr, Donehower RC, et al. Incidence and prognostic impact of KRAS and BRAF mutation in patients undergoing liver surgery for colorectal metastases. Cancer. 2013;119(23):4137–44.
66. Schirripa M, Bergamo F, Cremolini C, Casagrande M, Lonardi S, Aprile G, et al. BRAF and RAS mutations as prognostic factors in metastatic colorectal cancer patients undergoing liver resection. Br J Cancer. 2015;112(12):1921–8.
67. Gagnière J, Dupré A, Gholami SS, Pezet D, Boerner T, Gönen M, et al. Is hepatectomy justified for BRAF mutant colorectal liver metastases?: a multi-institutional analysis of 1497 patients. Ann Surg. 2020;271(1):147–54.
68. Weiss JM, Pfau PR, O'Connor ES, King J, LoConte N, Kennedy G, et al. Mortality by stage for right- versus left-sided colon cancer: analysis of surveillance, epidemiology, and end results--Medicare data. J Clin Oncol. 2011;29(33):4401–9.
69. Sasaki K, Andreatos N, Margonis GA, He J, Weiss M, Johnston F, et al. The prognostic implications of primary colorectal tumor location on recurrence and overall survival in patients undergoing resection for colorectal liver metastasis. J Surg Oncol. 2016;114(7):803–9.
70. Creasy JM, Sadot E, Koerkamp BG, Chou JF, Gonen M, Kemeny NE, et al. The impact of primary tumor location on long-term survival in patients undergoing hepatic resection for metastatic colon cancer. Ann Surg Oncol. 2018;25(2):431–8.
71. Wang K, Xu D, Yan XL, Poston G, Xing BC. The impact of primary tumour location in patients undergoing hepatic resection for colorectal liver metastasis. Eur J Surg Oncol. 2018;44(6):771–7.
72. Gholami S, Stewart S, Kemeny N, Gönen M, Groot Koerkamp B, Cercek A, et al. Impact of primary tumor laterality on adjuvant hepatic artery infusion

pump chemotherapy in resected colon cancer liver metastases: analysis of 487 patients. Ann Surg Oncol. 2021;28(7):3685–94.
73. Mason MC, Tzeng CD, Tran Cao HS, Aloia TA, Newhook TE, Overman MJ, et al. Preliminary analysis of liquid biopsy after hepatectomy for colorectal liver metastases. J Am Coll Surg. 2021;233(1):82–9 e1.
74. Tie J, Wang Y, Cohen J, Li L, Hong W, Christie M, et al. Circulating tumor DNA dynamics and recurrence risk in patients undergoing curative intent resection of colorectal cancer liver metastases: a prospective cohort study. PLoS Med. 2021;18(5):e1003620.
75. Vidal J, Fernández-Rodríguez MC, Casadevall D, Garcia-Alfonso P, Páez D, Guix M, et al. Liquid biopsy detects early molecular response and predicts benefit to first-line chemotherapy plus cetuximab in metastatic colorectal cancer: PLATFORM-B study. Clin Cancer Res. 2022;29:379–88.

16 Hepatic Arterial Infusion Chemotherapy for Intrahepatic Cholangiocarcinoma

Roheena Z. Panni and William R. Jarnagin

Introduction and Rationale

The incidence of intrahepatic cholangiocarcinoma (ICC) has increased over the recent years, and complete resection remains the only potentially curative treatment. However, due to the advanced stage of disease at the time of diagnosis, including multifocal liver disease, lymph node, or distant metastases, most patients do not qualify for curative-intent resection. Systemic therapy, specifically gemcitabine/cisplatin, has been indicated to prolong survival in patients with advanced biliary tract malignancies, including ICC, and is accepted as the first-line treatment based on the results of ABC-02 (advanced biliary cancer) phase III trial [1]. This remained the standard of care for more than a decade until the results of TOPAZ-1 trial demonstrated a significant improvement in overall survival (OS) and progression-free survival (PFS) with durvalumab plus gemcitabine/cisplatin compared to cytotoxic chemotherapy alone, supporting the role of immunotherapy in ICC and making it a first-line regimen [2].

Recent advances in the understanding of molecular and genetic features of ICC has led to identification of several actionable targets for specific genetic alterations, including IDH1 mutations and FGFR2 fusions; KRAS and microsatellite instability are also potentially targetable alterations [3–5]. Targeted therapies such as inhibitors of isocitrate dehydrogenase 1 (IDH1) [6], fibroblast growth factor receptor (FGFR) [7, 8], and tropomyosin receptor kinases (TRK) [9] or WNT [10] pathway alterations have recently been or are currently being tested in patients with ICC. The final results from ClarIDHy, a phase III study, demonstrated a small but measurable clinical benefit in progression-free survival (HR 0.37) and median OS (HR 0.69) with ivosidenib (a small-molecule targeted inhibitor of mutated isocitrate dehydrogenase 1) versus placebo in patients with previously treated ICC and IDH1 mutation [6]. Despite the recent trials evaluating several additional targeted therapies and showing promising results, the standard of care for advanced ICC has remained a systemic gemcitabine and cisplatin backbone, unchanged for the past decade and associated with a median OS of 11.7–12.8 months [11, 12]. The benefit of second-line systemic therapy is limited.

R. Z. Panni
Division of Hepatopancreatobiliary Surgery, Department of Surgery, Washington University School of Medicine, St. Louis, MO, USA
e-mail: roheenazpanni@wustl.edu

W. R. Jarnagin (✉)
Department of Surgery, Hepatopancreatobiliary Service, Memorial Sloan Kettering Cancer Center, New York, NY, USA

Cornell University, Weill Medical College, Memorial Sloan Kettering Cancer Center, New York, NY, USA
e-mail: jarnagiw@mskcc.org

M. D'Angelica, M. Lidsky (eds.), *Hepatic Arterial Infusion for Malignancy*,
https://doi.org/10.1007/978-3-031-74935-3_16

Most patients with advanced/unresectable tumors have liver confined disease with vascular infiltration and/or multifocality and are eligible for liver-directed therapies, including transarterial chemoembolization (TACE) and transarterial radioembolization with Yttrium-90 (TARE), stereotactic body radiotherapy (SBRT), and hepatic arterial infusion (HAI) chemotherapy [13]. TARE is the most developed approach but robust evidence to support its use is still lacking. Overall, TARE is a well-tolerated treatment with few significant adverse events. Key studies on TARE in ICC, including the phase II single-arm MISPHEC trial, reveal a median OS of 14.2–29 months, with objective response rates and adverse events reported at 25–39% and 38.4%, respectively [14–20]. Mouli et al. and Hoffman et al. have reported favorable outcomes with TARE, underscoring the importance of factors such as ECOG status, tumor location, and tumor response in determining survival rates [21, 22]. A meta-regression analysis concluded that TARE yields the best results in patients with mass-forming disease (vs. infiltrative, 20 vs. 8 months), those who are treatment-naive (vs. previously treated, 24 vs. 12 months), and when given with concurrent systemic chemotherapy (vs. TARE alone, 20 vs. 6 months) [23]. While there are no randomized trials evaluating the role of TARE specifically, there are also no randomized trials comparing TACE and TARE in the treatment of inoperable ICC. However, meta-analyses have compared their effectiveness and revealed similar median OS rates among TARE, conventional chemoembolization, and drug eluting bead chemoembolization [24], though these studies carry a high risk of selection bias arising from diverse inclusion criteria applied to different patient groups.

HAI chemotherapy was initially developed and used for the treatment of colorectal liver metastasis, but in the last two decades, multiple studies have been published for its use in ICC. The dual blood supply of liver vasculature allows delivery of higher doses of chemotherapy directly into the tumors (400-fold with floxuridine), compared to systemic chemotherapy, through the hepatic artery. Selective drug delivery to the tumor and the first-pass metabolism also minimizes the systemic side effects, making hepatic arterial infusion pump (HAIP) chemotherapy a favorable option for liver confined disease (see Chaps. 1–4).

At Memorial Sloan Kettering Cancer Center, investigations into the use of HAI FUDR for advanced liver confined ICC began in earnest in the late 1990s (Fig. 16.1). This initial experience, summarized in Table 16.1, showed the potential advantage of HAIP chemotherapy over systemic therapy alone and led to the initiation of several clinical trials.

The current NCCN (National Comprehensive Cancer Network) guidelines (v.1.2022) recommend the use of liver-directed therapies including HAI chemotherapy for patients with unresectable or metastatic ICC without extrahepatic disease [25]. HAI chemotherapy is only recommended in the context of a clinical trial or in tertiary referral hepatopancreatobiliary (HPB) centers for patients with advanced disease confined to the liver. In this chapter, we will review and summarize the results of studies using HAI chemotherapy for unresectable ICC.

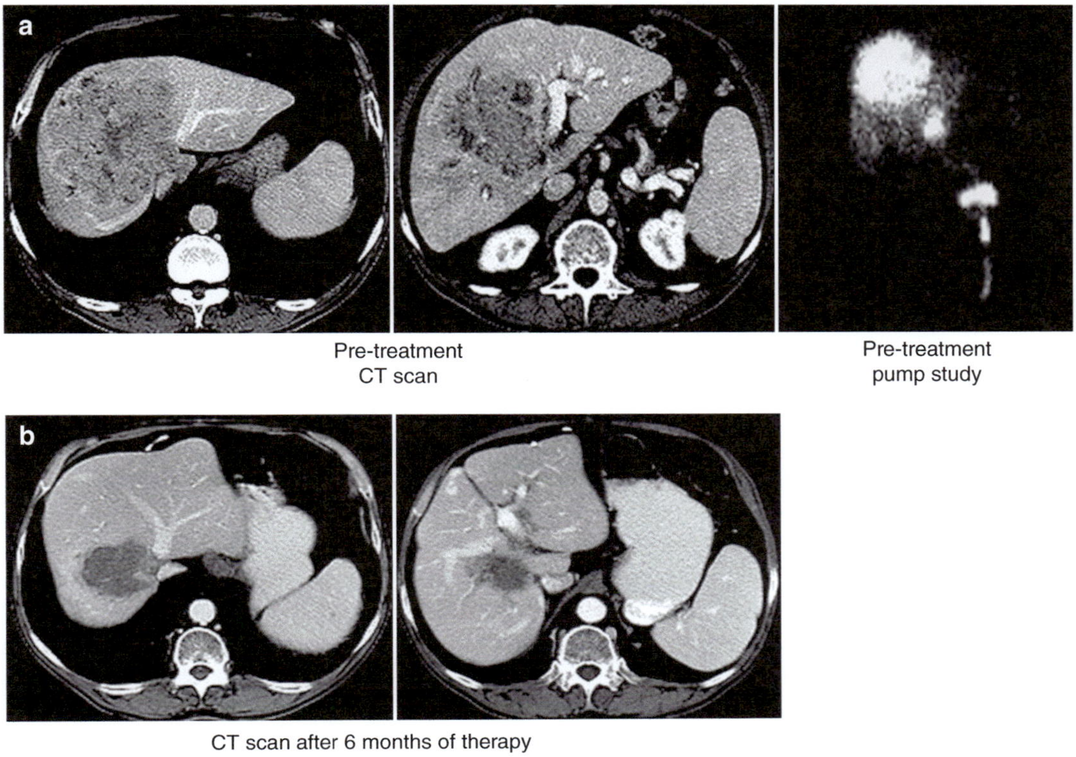

Fig. 16.1 (**a**) Initial ICC patient treated with HAI FUDR. At left, CT scan showing a large tumor with extensive vascular involvement. At right, a nuclear flow study through the HAI pump showing intense uptake in the tumor. (**b**) CT scan images showing significant tumor regression after 6 months of treatment

Table 16.1 Initial results in patients with unresectable disease (MSKCC, unpublished data)

Chemotherapy Type	N	Median Survival (months)	*p*
HAI Pump FUDR*	28	22	<0.001
Systemic Alone	75	9	
Systemic Therapy for Liver-Only Disease	52	10	–

Literature Review

The role of HAI chemotherapy has evolved over the last two decades and several prospective and retrospective studies have compared the results of different HAI chemotherapy regimens to systemic chemotherapy. In 2005, a phase II study by Cantore et al. reported results of 30 patients with unresectable ICC ($n = 25$) or gallbladder adenocarcinoma ($n = 5$) treated with epirubicin and cisplatin HAI as a bolus in combination with systemic continuous infusion of 5-fluorouracil (5-FU). The overall response rate in this study was 40%. The median PFS and OS were 7.1 and 13.2 months, respectively, and the 1-and 2-year survival rates were 54% and 20%, respectively [26].

In 2009, Jarnagin and Kemeny et al. investigated the efficacy of HAI with floxuridine (FUDR) and dexamethasone in 34 patients with unresectable primary liver cancer (ICC: $n = 26$ and HCC: $n = 8$). This trial used liver-directed chemotherapy only, with no systemic component, and results showed a response rate of 47.1%, with a median OS of 29.5 months. Patients with ICC had a higher response rate (53.8%) compared to those with HCC (25%). Median PFS in ICC patients was 11.3 months and one patient was downstaged to resection. All patients ultimately developed disease progression, and nearly all ultimately required treatment with systemic chemotherapy. The 1-, 2-, and 3-year survival rates were 88%, 67%, and 29%, respectively. This was the first study to suggest a role of HAI chemotherapy in ICC in the absence of any concomitant systemic chemotherapy [27].

The advent of vascular endothelial growth factor (VEGF) and other angiogenesis inhibitors led to a flurry of clinical trials in several primary and secondary liver malignancies, and ICC was no exception; however, a clear role for these agents in ICC remains to be established. In a follow-up to the original study using HAIP for unresectable ICC, Kemeny et al. reported the results of adding bevacizumab (Avastin, angiogenesis inhibitor) in combination with HAI FUDR. A total of 22 patients (ICC = 18, HCC = 4) were treated with HAI chemotherapy in addition to systemic bevacizumab. While a similar level of activity with HAIP was noted, the trial was prematurely terminated due to increased biliary toxicity; 24% patients experienced bilirubin elevation and 13.6% required biliary stents [28]. The results also found no significant improvement in response rate or survival, which was reported as median OS = 31.1 months (CI 14.14–33.59), PFS was 8.45 months (CI 5.53–11.05) in the combination group compared to HAI alone.

A follow-up study examined the long-term outcomes of patients in these two study cohorts was reported in 2013, inclusive of 44 patients. The PR rate was 50%, and median OS was 29 months. Of interest, 10 patients in this study (23%) survived beyond 3 years and 11% beyond 5 years. The only notable difference in the long-term (>3 years) survivors compared with short-term (<3 years) survivors was a longer hepatic progression-free survival. These results suggested that a relationship between control of the hepatic disease and overall survival exists, an observation that was made in subsequent reports [29].

In 2016, Konstantinidis et al. reported the largest series to date of patients with advanced ICC treated with HAI chemotherapy. This study was comprised of 104 patients with liver-only, unresectable ICC treated with HAI with or without systemic chemotherapy (n = 78) or systemic chemotherapy alone (n = 26), and showed a better response rate for patients treated with HAI chemotherapy compared to those who received systemic chemotherapy alone [30]. Progression-free survival was 12 vs. 7 months for HAI plus systemic chemotherapy group vs. systemic chemotherapy alone, respectively, and OS was similarly greater at 30.8 vs. 18.4 months, respectively. In the cohort of HAIP-treated patients, 8/104 patients were converted to resection, which is still far below the rates of resectability achieved for colorectal liver metastasis, emphasizing the differences in underlying biology of the two diseases.

Several other groups have published results with different HAI and systemic chemotherapy regimens. In 2014, a French retrospective study by Ghiringhelli et al. analyzed the outcomes of 12 consecutive patients with unresectable ICC treated with HAI (percutaneously placed catheter-port system) of Gemcitabine (1000 mg/m^2) followed by systemic oxaliplatin (100 mg/m^2) as second-line treatment. The overall response rate was 66% and the disease control rate was 91%. In this study, the median PFS was 9.2 months (CI 5.1–29.4) and the median OS was 20.3 months (CI 13.2–49.7) [31]. Similarly, Massani et al. published their retrospective experience with HAI treatment alone (fluorouracil and oxaliplatin) in 11 unresectable ICC patients. A CT scan performed after the sixth cycle of therapy revealed that 5 of them had partial hepatic response, 2 had stable disease, and 4 had disease progression. The median OS was 17.6 months. Three of the patients with partial hepatic response underwent resection and two had more than 70% tumor necrosis. The median survival of patients with liver-only disease treated with systemic chemotherapy, who did not qualify for resection, was 15.3 months [32].

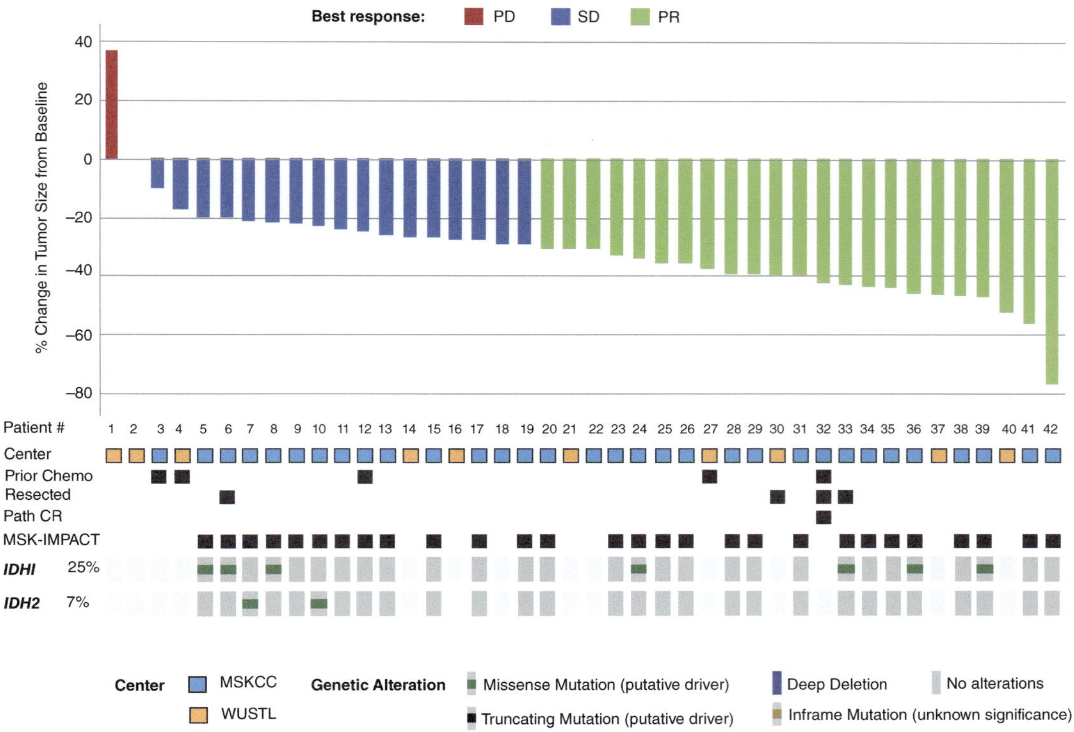

Fig. 16.2 Waterfall plot taken from Cercek et al (JAMA Oncol 2020;6:60) showing disease responses in 42 patients with advanced IHC treated with HAI FUDR and systemic GEMOX

In 2019, Cercek et al. published a phase II clinical trial, which included 42 unresectable ICC patients treated with HAI FUDR chemotherapy combined with systemic gemcitabine and oxaliplatin (GEMOX). This trial included patients with advanced ICC: 71% had multifocal disease, median tumor size was 8.2 cm and 41% had metastatic disease to regional lymph nodes. Despite these unfavorable characteristics, HAI provided a disease control rate of 97%, with a partial response of 52%, and four patients (7%) converted to resection [33] (Fig. 16.2). Of note, in the subgroup analysis, patients with node positive disease had similar outcomes as patients with node negative disease, which stands in contrast to the results in patients submitted to resection. The median PFS, which was the primary endpoint in this study, was 11.8 months. The median OS was 25.0 months, and the 1-year OS rate was 89.5%. The results of the study highlight the importance of combination approach in the management of ICC with improvements in PFS compared to systemic chemotherapy alone [33]. These encouraging results have prompted a multicenter, randomized trial (ClinicalTrials.gov identifier NCT04891289), evaluating HAI with concurrent GEMOX in treatment-naive patients with unresectable, liver predominant ICC with or without resectable lymph node metastases using PFS as the primary end point. The current ongoing HAI trials in unresectable-liver confined ICC are summarized in Table 16.2.

The impact of lymph node disease and treatment approach on outcome was delineated in a recent study by Jolissaint et al. This retrospective analysis included 573 patients with liver dominant ICC with or without regional lymph node metastases managed with resection (n = 237), HAI, (n = 196), or systemic chemotherapy (n = 140), and also investigated prognostic genetic alterations. In patients with N0 disease, resection was associated with the best long-term survival, followed by HAIP chemotherapy and systemic therapy alone (median OS = 59.9 months

Table 16.2 Ongoing HAI trials in unresectable liver confined ICC

Ongoing HAI trials in unresectable liver confined ICC (*clinicaltrials.gov*)			
Clinical trial		Comparison groups	Primary outcome
Phase 2	NCT04891289	HAI with concurrent GEMOX in treatment-naive patients	PFS
Phase 1	NCT01525069	HAI of FUDR alone or in combination with oxaliplatin and/or gemcitabine	Dose limiting toxicity
Phase 3	NCT03771846	HAI of irinotecan, oxaliplatin, 5-fluorouracil, and leucovorin compared to systemic chemotherapy of gemcitabine and oxaliplatin	OS
Phase 2	NCT03364530	HAI of gemcitabine/oxaliplatin administered as second-line treatment	ORR
Phase 2	NCT04251715	mFOLFIRINOX, followed by HAI of FUDR plus dexamethasone administered concurrently with systemic mFOLFIRI	Disease control rate, incidence of abnormal liver function

HAI Hepatic artery infusion, *FUDR* floxuridine, *GEMOX* gemcitabine/oxaliplatin, *mFOLFIRINOX* modified fluorouracil, irinotecan, oxaliplatin, leucovorin, *mFOLFIRI* modified 5-FU, irinotecan, leucovorin

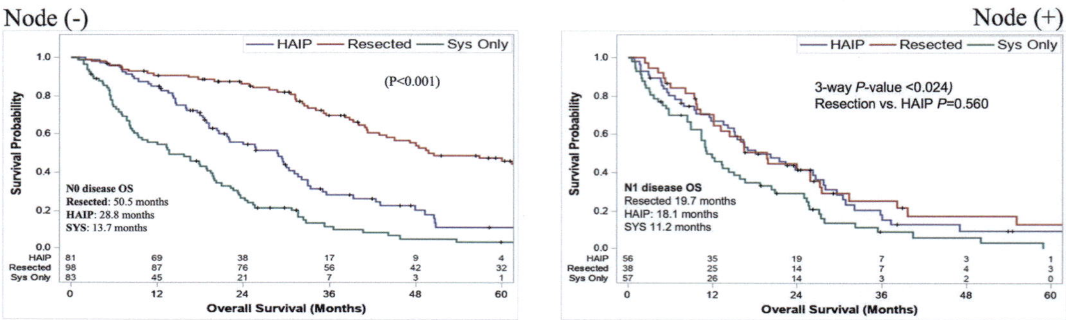

Fig. 16.3 Overall survival curves of patients with unresectable IHC (with or without lymph node metastases) treated with resection, HAI chemotherapy or systemic chemotherapy. Node (−) patients shown at left, Node (+) patients show at right. (Adapted From Jolissaint JS et al *Clin Cancer Res* 2021)

(95% CI = 47.2–74.3); 24.9 months (95% CI = 20.3–29.6); 13.7 months (95% CI = 8.9–15.9), respectively; $P < 0.001$) (Fig. 16.3 (left)). However, this benefit of resection disappeared in the presence of lymph node disease, with no difference in survival for node-positive patients treated with resection (median OS = 19.7 months; 95% CI = 12.1–27.2) or HAI (18.1 months; 95% CI = 14.1–26.6; $P = 0.560$), although survival in both groups was greater than that for systemic chemotherapy alone (11.2 months; 95% CI = 14.1–26.6; $P = 0.024$) [34]. Furthermore, in this analysis, node-positive patients with at least one high-risk genetic alteration (*TP53* mutation, *KRAS* mutation, *CDKN2A/B* deletion) had worse survival compared to wild-type patients, regardless of treatment. Conversely, mutations in IDH1 and IDH2 as well as FGFR2 fusion events had no association with survival. Overall, these results support the routine use of next-generation sequencing in all patients with ICC, which may provide valuable insights into which patients are unlikely to derive benefit from any form of liver-directed therapy.

Conclusions

The weight of data from several retrospective and prospective studies suggests that treatment with the combination approach of HAI FUDR and systemic chemotherapy is associated with favorable PFS and OS compared to systemic chemotherapy alone in patients with unresectable ICC. Despite the overall promising results achieved with HAI therapy, conversion to resectability is far below those achieved for colorectal liver metastases, almost certainly reflecting differences in tumor biology and limited effective systemic therapies for ICC. One of the major limitations of HAI chemotherapy has been the limited availability of surgeons and medical oncologists experienced with its use outside of a few high volume HPB centers worldwide; however, this is evolving, with more centers adapting the technique and establishing multi-institutional collaborations. The ongoing clinical trials evaluating the role of HAI in combination with chemotherapy regimens in unresectable ICC will provide more information regarding the long-term follow-up. Therefore, rigorous evaluation and individualization of locoregional (HAI) and chemotherapy regimen based on selective mutations in clinical trials is essential.

References

1. Valle J, Wasan H, Palmer DH, Cunningham D, Anthoney A, Maraveyas A, et al. Cisplatin plus gemcitabine versus gemcitabine for biliary tract cancer. N Engl J Med. 2010;362(14):1273–81.
2. Oh DY, Lee KH, Lee DW, Yoon J, Kim TY, Bang JH, et al. Gemcitabine and cisplatin plus durvalumab with or without tremelimumab in chemotherapy-naive patients with advanced biliary tract cancer: an open-label, single-Centre, phase 2 study. Lancet Gastroenterol Hepatol. 2022;7(6):522–32.
3. Cloyd JM, Chun YS, Ikoma N, Vauthey JN, Aloia TA, Cuddy A, et al. Clinical and genetic implications of DNA mismatch repair deficiency in biliary tract Cancers associated with lynch syndrome. J Gastrointest Cancer. 2018;49(1):93–6.
4. Nakamura H, Arai Y, Totoki Y, Shirota T, Elzawahry A, Kato M, et al. Genomic spectra of biliary tract cancer. Nat Genet. 2015;47(9):1003–10.
5. Zhu AX, Borger DR, Kim Y, Cosgrove D, Ejaz A, Alexandrescu S, et al. Genomic profiling of intrahepatic cholangiocarcinoma: refining prognosis and identifying therapeutic targets. Ann Surg Oncol. 2014;21(12):3827–34.
6. Zhu AX, Macarulla T, Javle MM, Kelley RK, Lubner SJ, Adeva J, et al. Final overall survival efficacy results of Ivosidenib for patients with advanced cholangiocarcinoma with IDH1 mutation: the phase 3 randomized clinical ClarIDHy trial. JAMA Oncol. 2021;7(11):1669–77.
7. Javle M, Lowery M, Shroff RT, Weiss KH, Springfeld C, Borad MJ, et al. Phase II study of BGJ398 in patients with FGFR-altered advanced cholangiocarcinoma. J Clin Oncol. 2018;36(3):276–82.
8. Vogel A, Segatto O, Stenzinger A, Saborowski A. FGFR2 inhibition in cholangiocarcinoma. Annu Rev Med. 2023;74:293–306.
9. Drilon A, Siena S, Ou SI, Patel M, Ahn MJ, Lee J, et al. Safety and antitumor activity of the multitargeted pan-TRK, ROS1, and ALK inhibitor Entrectinib: combined results from two phase I trials (ALKA-372-001 and STARTRK-1). Cancer Discov. 2017;7(4):400–9.
10. Ong CK, Subimerb C, Pairojkul C, Wongkham S, Cutcutache I, Yu W, et al. Exome sequencing of liver fluke-associated cholangiocarcinoma. Nat Genet. 2012;44(6):690–3.
11. Boileve A, Hilmi M, Smolenschi C, Ducreux M, Hollebecque A, Malka D. Immunotherapy in advanced biliary tract cancers. Cancers (Basel). 2021;13(7):1569.
12. Brindley PJ, Bachini M, Ilyas SI, Khan SA, Loukas A, Sirica AE, et al. Cholangiocarcinoma. Nat Rev Dis Primers. 2021;7(1):65.
13. Koay EJ, Odisio BC, Javle M, Vauthey JN, Crane CH. Management of unresectable intrahepatic cholangiocarcinoma: how do we decide among the various liver-directed treatments? Hepatobiliary Surg Nutr. 2017;6(2):105–16.
14. Buettner S, Braat A, Margonis GA, Brown DB, Taylor KB, Borgmann AJ, et al. Yttrium-90 Radioembolization in intrahepatic cholangiocarcinoma: a multicenter retrospective analysis. J Vasc Interv Radiol. 2020;31(7):1035–43 e2.
15. Edeline J, Lamarca A, McNamara MG, Jacobs T, Hubner RA, Palmer D, et al. Locoregional therapies in patients with intrahepatic cholangiocarcinoma: a systematic review and pooled analysis. Cancer Treat Rev. 2021;99:102258.
16. Gupta AN, Gordon AC, Gabr A, Kalyan A, Kircher SM, Mahalingam D, et al. Yttrium-90 Radioembolization of Unresectable intrahepatic cholangiocarcinoma: long-term follow-up for a 136-patient cohort. Cardiovasc Intervent Radiol. 2022;45(8):1117–28.
17. Mosconi C, Cacioppa LM, Cappelli A, Gramenzi AG, Vara G, Modestino F, et al. Update of the Bologna experience in Radioembolization of intrahepatic cholangiocarcinoma. Technol Cancer Res Treat. 2023;22:15330338231155690.
18. Robinson TJ, Du L, Matsuoka L, Sze DY, Kennedy AS, Gandhi RT, et al. Survival and toxicities after Yttrium-90 Transarterial Radioembolization of cholangiocarcinoma in the RESiN registry. J Vasc Interv Radiol. 2023;34(4):694–701 e3.
19. Al-Adra DP, Gill RS, Axford SJ, Shi X, Kneteman N, Liau SS. Treatment of unresectable intrahepatic cholangiocarcinoma with yttrium-90 radioembolization: a systematic review and pooled analysis. Eur J Surg Oncol. 2015;41(1):120–7.
20. Edeline J, Touchefeu Y, Guiu B, Farge O, Tougeron D, Baumgaertner I, et al. Radioembolization plus chemotherapy for first-line treatment of locally advanced

intrahepatic cholangiocarcinoma: a phase 2 clinical trial. JAMA Oncol. 2020;6(1):51–9.
21. Hoffmann RT, Paprottka PM, Schon A, Bamberg F, Haug A, Durr EM, et al. Transarterial hepatic yttrium-90 radioembolization in patients with unresectable intrahepatic cholangiocarcinoma: factors associated with prolonged survival. Cardiovasc Intervent Radiol. 2012;35(1):105–16.
22. Mouli S, Memon K, Baker T, Benson AB 3rd, Mulcahy MF, Gupta R, et al. Yttrium-90 radioembolization for intrahepatic cholangiocarcinoma: safety, response, and survival analysis. J Vasc Interv Radiol. 2013;24(8):1227–34.
23. Cucchetti A, Zhong J, Berhane S, Toyoda H, Shi K, Tada T, et al. The chances of hepatic resection curing hepatocellular carcinoma. J Hepatol. 2020;72(4):711–7.
24. Boehm LM, Jayakrishnan TT, Miura JT, Zacharias AJ, Johnston FM, Turaga KK, et al. Comparative effectiveness of hepatic artery based therapies for unresectable intrahepatic cholangiocarcinoma. J Surg Oncol. 2015;111(2):213–20.
25. Hepatobiliary Cancers. Version 1.2022 NCCNN.
26. Cantore M, Mambrini A, Fiorentini G, Rabbi C, Zamagni D, Caudana R, et al. Phase II study of hepatic intraarterial epirubicin and cisplatin, with systemic 5-fluorouracil in patients with unresectable biliary tract tumors. Cancer. 2005;103(7):1402–7.
27. Jarnagin WR, Schwartz LH, Gultekin DH, Gonen M, Haviland D, Shia J, et al. Regional chemotherapy for unresectable primary liver cancer: results of a phase II clinical trial and assessment of DCE-MRI as a biomarker of survival. Ann Oncol. 2009;20(9):1589–95.
28. Kemeny NE, Schwartz L, Gonen M, Yopp A, Gultekin D, D'Angelica MI, et al. Treating primary liver cancer with hepatic arterial infusion of floxuridine and dexamethasone: does the addition of systemic bevacizumab improve results? Oncology. 2011;80(3–4):153–9.
29. Yamashita S, Koay EJ, Passot G, Shroff R, Raghav KP, Conrad C, et al. Local therapy reduces the risk of liver failure and improves survival in patients with intrahepatic cholangiocarcinoma: a comprehensive analysis of 362 consecutive patients. Cancer. 2017;123(8):1354–62.
30. Konstantinidis IT, Groot Koerkamp B, Do RK, Gonen M, Fong Y, Allen PJ, et al. Unresectable intrahepatic cholangiocarcinoma: systemic plus hepatic arterial infusion chemotherapy is associated with longer survival in comparison with systemic chemotherapy alone. Cancer. 2016;122(5):758–65.
31. Ghiringhelli F, Lorgis V, Vincent J, Ladoire S, Guiu B. Hepatic arterial infusion of gemcitabine plus oxaliplatin as second-line treatment for locally advanced intrahepatic cholangiocarcinoma: preliminary experience. Chemotherapy. 2013;59(5):354–60.
32. Massani M, Nistri C, Ruffolo C, Bonariol R, Pauletti B, Bonariol L, et al. Intrahepatic chemotherapy for unresectable cholangiocarcinoma: review of literature and personal experience. Updat Surg. 2015;67(4):389–400.
33. Cercek A, Boerner T, Tan BR, Chou JF, Gonen M, Boucher TM, et al. Assessment of hepatic arterial infusion of Floxuridine in combination with systemic gemcitabine and Oxaliplatin in patients with Unresectable intrahepatic cholangiocarcinoma: a phase 2 clinical trial. JAMA Oncol. 2020;6(1):60–7.
34. Jolissaint JS, Soares KC, Seier KP, Kundra R, Gonen M, Shin PJ, et al. Intrahepatic cholangiocarcinoma with lymph node metastasis: treatment-related outcomes and the role of tumor genomics in patient selection. Clin Cancer Res. 2021;27(14):4101–8.

HAI for Indications Beyond Colorectal Liver Metastases and Intrahepatic Cholangiocarcinoma

17

Jesse Kelley, G. Paul Wright, and Yuman Fong

Introduction

As mentioned in previous chapters, hepatic arterial infusion (HAI) therapy can be used for treatment of unresectable colorectal liver metastases (CRLM, Chap. 14), adjuvant treatment for resected CRLM (Chap. 15), or treatment of intrahepatic cholangiocarcinoma (ICC, Chap. 16). Other malignant processes for which HAI therapy is being investigated include hepatocellular carcinoma (HCC), neuroendocrine tumor liver metastases, breast cancer liver metastases, and pancreatic cancer liver metastases. In this chapter we will review patient selection and efficacy of HAI therapy for each of the remaining malignant processes.

Hepatocellular Carcinoma (HCC)

Hepatocellular carcinoma is the sixth most common cancer worldwide and the fourth leading cause of cancer-related death. The reported median overall survival for all HCC is 4–8 months; however, many patients present with advanced disease. Surgical management via either resection or transplant is the treatment of choice, but most patients are not appropriate candidates. Reasons for surgical exclusion include both patient-related and tumor-related characteristics. Scoring systems, such as the Barcelona-Clinic Liver Cancer (BCLC) staging system , have allowed surgeons to stratify patients with HCC into operative versus nonoperative groups.

For liver-limited or dominant but unresectable cases, arterial-based therapies are a key option for HCC treatment. These include transarterial radioembolization (TARE), transarterial chemoembolization (TACE), and hepatic arterial infusion (HAI) chemotherapy. There is a paucity of high-quality comparative data for these treatments. While HAI treatment for colorectal liver metastases (CRLM) and intrahepatic cholangiocarcinoma (ICC) have more commonly been delivered via implanted subcutaneous pumps, contemporary studies in HCC have more commonly utilized percutaneous catheters, perhaps owing to practice pattern variation in Asian countries where HAI chemotherapy for HCC is almost exclusively used.

Systemic therapy for advanced HCC was predominantly centered around sorafenib, an oral multikinase inhibitor, until recent studies have demonstrated improved survival with newer combination immunotherapy regimens [1, 2]. The IMbrave150 trial compared the combination atezolizumab, a drug that binds the PD-L1 ligand,

J. Kelley · G. P. Wright (✉)
Corewell Health/Michigan State University College of Human Medicine, Grand Rapids, MI, USA
e-mail: paul.wright@corewellhealth.org

Y. Fong
Department of Surgery, City of Hope Medical Center, Duarte, CA, USA

M. D'Angelica, M. Lidsky (eds.), *Hepatic Arterial Infusion for Malignancy*,
https://doi.org/10.1007/978-3-031-74935-3_17

and bevacizumab, a vascular endothelial growth factor inhibitor, against sorafenib monotherapy and demonstrated an overall survival benefit of 6 months [3]. Similarly, the HIMALAYA study compared a combination of two immune checkpoint inhibitors, tremelimumab and durvalumab, against sorafenib monotherapy and found a 3-month overall survival benefit [4]. Both regimens are currently available as first-line options in the treatment of advanced HCC and represent progress in the understanding and treatment of this disease.

Recently, studies have focused on using HAI therapy, either alone or in combination with sorafenib, to improve patient outcomes. To be a candidate for HAI therapy, patients must have advanced HCC, be a candidate for surgery, and have adequate anatomy and liver function amenable to HAI catheter/pump placement and eventual locoregional therapy. In our practice, we prefer ANC >1500/mcL, PLT >100,000/mcL, total bilirubin <1.5 mg/dL, alkaline phosphatase <300 IU/L, AST <120 IU/L, and serum creatinine <2.0 mg/dL. In addition, it is important to consider the comorbidities of the patients relative to the therapeutic agents being administered via HAI therapy to ensure there is not a higher-than-acceptable risk.

Several HAI chemotherapy regimens have been trialed for patients with unresectable HCC, such as oxaliplatin, cisplatin, epirubicin, mitomycin-c, and 5-fluorouracil (Table 17.1). In recent studies, liver-directed fluorouracil, leucovorin, and oxaliplatin (FOLFOX) have been shown to significantly increase the progression-free survival and overall survival in patients with unresectable HCC compared to patients who took sorafenib alone [1, 5–7]. HAI has also been researched in the adjuvant setting for patients who had portal venous infiltration, particularly with a cisplatin regimen [8]. There continues to be ongoing research of HAI therapy for patients with HCC. A multidisciplinary approach is critical for selecting the best treatment for these patients.

Table 17.1 Studies evaluating hepatic artery infusion therapy in patients with hepatocellular carcinoma

First author (year)	Study title	Study design	Findings
Lyu (2018) [1]	Hepatic arterial infusion of oxaliplatin plus fluorouracil/leucovorin vs. sorafenib for advanced hepatocellular carcinoma	Propensity-matched retrospective study comparing OS and PFS for patients receiving sorafenib alone ($n = 147$) vs. HAI-FOLFOX ($n = 147$)	OS (14.5 vs. 7.0 months) and PFS (7.1 vs. 3.3 months) are significantly longer in patients treated with HAI-FOLFOX vs. sorafenib
He (2018) [5]	Phase II study of sorafenib combined with concurrent hepatic arterial infusion of oxaliplatin, 5-fluorouracil, and leucovorin for unresectable hepatocellular carcinoma with major portal vein thrombosis	Prospective single-arm study evaluating addition of HAI-FOLFOX to sorafenib and its effect on PFS in patients with HCC and major portal vein tumor thrombosis	PFS at 3-, 6-, and 12 months were 82.9%, 51.4%, and 22.9%, respectively, with five patients converting to complete resection, and one patient having complete pathologic response
He (2019) [6]	Sorafenib plus hepatic arterial infusion of oxaliplatin, fluorouracil, and leucovorin vs. sorafenib alone for hepatocellular carcinoma with portal vein invasion: a randomized clinical trial	Randomized, multi-institutional clinical trial of 247 patients randomized 1:1 to either receive sorafenib alone or sorafenib + HAI-FOLFOX with comparison of OS	Patients receiving sorafenib + HAI-FOLFOX had a longer OS than those taking sorafenib alone (13.4 vs. 7.1 months)
Kim (2020) [7]	Efficacy and safety of liver-directed concurrent chemoradiotherapy and sequential sorafenib for advanced hepatocellular carcinoma: a prospective phase 2 trial	Prospective single-arm study phase II trial in which 47 patients with unresectable HCC received concurrent liver-directed fluorouracil, leucovorin, and radiation, followed by sorafenib	Objective response rates 4 weeks after LD-CCRT and during sorafenib maintenance was 44.7%, with nine patients able to undergo curative resection or transplantation due to downstaging. The overall survival was 24.6 months
Hamada (2020) [8]	Increased survival benefit of adjuvant intra-arterial infusion chemotherapy in HCC patients with portal vein infiltration after hepatectomy	Retrospective study comparing treatment effects of adjuvant HAI therapy in patients with HCC and PVI following hepatectomy ($n = 37$) relative to patients who underwent hepatectomy without adjuvant HAI therapy ($n = 85$)	Patients who received adjuvant HAI-cisplatin tended to have better PFS and OS than those who did not receive adjuvant therapy

OS overall survival, *PFS* progression-free survival, *HAI* hepatic artery infusion, *FOLFOX* fluorouracil, oxaliplatin, and leucovorin, *HCC* hepatocellular carcinoma, *PVI* portal vein invasion, *LD-CCRT* liver-directed concurrent chemoradiotherapy

Neuroendocrine Tumor Liver Metastases

Liver metastases are estimated to occur in approximately 80% of patients with neuroendocrine tumors [9]. For these patients, resection provides the only curative option; however, this requires that the tumor deposits be in a location amenable to resection. If complete resection cannot be achieved, cytoreductive surgery can be considered. Another potential option is liver transplantation; however, this is reserved for a select group of patients. For patients who are not appropriate for the surgeries discussed, liver-directed therapy options, such as TARE, TACE, and HAI chemotherapy, have been explored with the goal to control symptoms, slow progression, and increase survival.

With a paucity of data in the literature on HAI use in this population, no formal recommendations can be made at this time. There is currently an ongoing phase II clinical trial (NCT04837885)

researching HAI somatostatin analogue treatment in neuroendocrine tumors with estimated completion in 2024.

Breast Cancer Liver Metastases

Patients with metastatic breast cancer have a reported median survival of 24–30 months, with the primary treatment being systemic chemotherapy. Within this population, approximately 25% have liver involvement that portends an even worse survival of 5–13 months [10, 11]. Given the unfavorable prognosis associated with breast cancer liver metastases (BCLM), studies have analyzed whether HAI therapies may provide clinically meaningful benefit, especially in patients who have had disease progression on chemotherapy, hormonal therapy, and biologic therapy. Several retrospective and small prospective studies have shown an increase in median overall survival in patients treated with HAI therapy in combination with systemic therapies (Table 17.2). Initial regimens included vinblastine, cisplatin, or both in combination [12–14]. More recently, liver-directed paclitaxel, floxuridine (FUDR)/gemcitabine, and FUDR/dexamethasone regimens have been evaluated for their effects on BCLM [15–17]. Of note, these studies pre-date the emergence of immunotherapy for triple negative breast cancer (KEYNOTE-012) and targeted therapies for

Table 17.2 Studies evaluating hepatic artery infusion therapy in patients with breast cancer liver metastases

First author (year)	Study title	Study design	Findings
Fraschini (1987) [12]	Percutaneous hepatic arterial infusion of cisplatin for metastatic breast cancer	HAI-cisplatin was administered to 31 patients with chemotherapy-refractory BCLM	PR occurred in 19% of patients. The PFS was 15 weeks and the OS was 11 months. The toxicity of the treatment was acceptable
Fraschini (1987) [13]	Continuous 5-day infusion of vinblastine for percutaneous hepatic arterial chemotherapy for metastatic breast cancer	HAI-vinblastine was administered to 26 patients with chemotherapy-refractory BCLM	PR occurred in 36% of patients and MR in 16%. The PFS was 21 weeks and the OS was 11 months. The toxicity of the treatment was acceptable
Fraschini (1988) [14]	Percutaneous hepatic arterial infusion of cisplatin–vinblastine for refractory breast carcinoma metastatic to the liver	Sequential HAI-cisplatin/vinblastine was administered to 34 patients with chemotherapy-refractory BCLM	PR was achieved in 33% of patients and MR in 24%. The PFS was 31 weeks and the OS was 11 months. Seven treatment failures were related to treatment intolerance or major toxicity
Camacho (2007) [15]	Pilot study of regional, hepatic intra-arterial paclitaxel in patients with breast carcinoma metastatic to the liver	Prospective pilot study of HAI-paclitaxel in 10 female patients with chemotherapy-refractory BCLM	Four patients experienced disease progression during the HAI treatment course. The PFS was 5.7 months
Ang (2013) [16]	Hepatic arterial infusion and systemic chemotherapy for breast cancer liver metastases	Retrospective review of 9 patients with refractory BCLM who received HAI-FUDR/dex in combination with systemic chemotherapy	The PFS was 6 months and the OS was 17 months from starting HAI (110 months from diagnosis)
Shi (2021) [17]	Hepatic artery infusion pump combined with systemic chemotherapy for patients with liver metastases from breast carcinoma	Retrospective review of 19 female patients with BCLM who received HAI-FUDR/gemcitabine in combination with systemic chemotherapy	An ORR was 73.3%, with 10.5% of patients having CR, 63.2% having PR, and 15.8% having SD. The OS was 13.1 months

HAI hepatic artery infusion, *BCLM* breast cancer liver metastases, *FUDR* floxuridine, *dex* dexamethasone, *OS* overall survival, *PFS* progression-free survival, *ORR* overall response rate, *CR* complete response, *PR* partial response, *MR* minor response, *SD* stable disease

HER2 overexpressing or hormone receptor-positive breast cancer [18–23]. As such, the decision to treat patients who have unresectable BCLM with liver-directed therapy should be made in multidisciplinary fashion as systemic therapy remains the accepted standard.

Pancreatic Cancer Liver Metastases

Pancreatic ductal adenocarcinoma is often diagnosed at an advanced stage, resulting in a very bleak prognosis. Traditionally, metastatic pancreatic cancer was treated with gemcitabine monotherapy. More recent studies have demonstrated an increased survival with either fluorouracil, leucovorin, oxaliplatin, and irinotecan (FOLFIRINOX) or nab-paclitaxel and gemcitabine [24, 25]. With the most common site of metastases being the liver, even after curative pancreatectomy, and liver metastases commonly being responsible for patient demise, liver-directed therapies became an intriguing consideration. In 2009, a study by Ohigashi et al. demonstrated that patients with T3-pancreatic cancer who received adjuvant liver-perfusion chemotherapy had better 5-year survival after pancreatectomy compared to historic data, with low incidences of local recurrence (9%) and liver metastasis (7%) [26]. Since that time, additional studies have shown HAI chemotherapy to be both effective at preventing development of liver metastases after curative pancreatectomy and after hepatic metastasectomy for metastases that have already developed (Table 17.3) [27–29].

In 2021, a propensity-matched retrospective study of patients with unresectable pancreatic cancer liver metastases reported that administration of HAI floxuridine (FUDR) in combination with systemic chemotherapy yielded an increase in overall survival by 3 months relative to patients treated with systemic chemotherapy alone [30]. Currently, there are no data regarding combined HAI and systemic chemotherapies in treatment of unresectable pancreatic liver metastases; however, there is one ongoing clinical trial called "A Phase II Trial of Hepatic Artery Infusional Floxuridine with Systemic Chemotherapy in the Treatment of Pancreatic Cancer Liver Metastases" (NCT03856658) that aims to study its effects. In this single-arm study, adult patients with good liver function who have received a minimum of 2 months of systemic chemotherapy undergo hepatic artery infusion pump placement followed by infusion of floxuridine in 28-day cycles for a maximum of six cycles. The estimated study completion date is April 2023. With improvements in systemic therapy, further investigation to identify opportunities for liver-directed therapies to have meaningful impact on patients with PDAC is needed.

Table 17.3 Studies evaluating hepatic artery infusion therapy in patients with pancreatic cancer liver metastases

First author (year)	Study title	Study design	Findings
Ohigashi (2009) [26]	Feasibility and efficacy of combination therapy with preoperative full-dose gemcitabine, concurrent three-dimensional conformal radiation, surgery, and postoperative liver perfusion chemotherapy for T3-pancreatic cancer	Retrospective review of 38 patients with T3-pancreatic cancer who received either chemoradiation alone ($n = 7$) or chemoradiation and surgery followed by adjuvant HAI-5-FU ($n = 31$)	The OS in those who received chemoradiation alone was 13 months with a 2-year survival rate of 14%. For patients who received chemoradiation followed by surgery and adjuvant HAI-5-FU, the 2- and 5-year survival rates were 72% and 59%, respectively
Tajima (2011) [27]	Pilot study of hepatic arterial infusion chemotherapy with gemcitabine and 5-fluorouracil for patients with postoperative liver metastases from pancreatic cancer	Pilot study in which 5 patients with pancreatic cancer received adjuvant HAI-gemcitabine/5-FU	ORR was 100%, with 40% of patients having PR and 60% having SD. The PFS was 10 months and the OS was 22.4 months
Tajima (2013) [28]	Hepatic arterial infusion chemotherapy with gemcitabine and 5-fluorouracil or oral S-1 improves the prognosis of patients with postoperative liver metastases from pancreatic cancer	Seven patients who underwent surgical resection of their pancreatic cancer received either HAI-gemcitabine/5-FU alone if they had an R0 resection ($n = 5$) or in combination with S-1[a] if they had R1/R2 resection ($n = 2$)	ORR was 85.7%, with PR in 28.6%, SD in 57%, and PD in 14%. The PFS was 8 months and the OS was 17.4 months
Zheng (2014) [29]	Hepatic arterial infusion chemotherapy reduced hepatic metastases from pancreatic cancer after pancreatectomy	Prospective RCT in which 106 patients with pancreatic cancer were randomized to receive systemic chemotherapy alone or in combination with HAI-gemcitabine/5-FU	The 3-year OS and liver metastases-free survival were significantly higher in the patients who received HAI therapy relative to their counterparts who received chemotherapy alone (23.1% vs. 14.8% and 80.8% vs. 55.6%, respectively)
Peng (2021) [30]	Hepatic artery infusion of floxuridine in combination with systemic chemotherapy for pancreatic cancer liver metastasis: a propensity score-matched analysis in two centers	Multi-institutional 1:1 propensity-matched retrospective review of patients with PCLM who received first-line chemotherapy alone ($n = 62$) and with HAI-FUDR ($n = 62$)	The intra-hepatic ORR was higher in the HAI group than in the non-HAI group (66.1% vs. 22.6%). There was no significant difference in the extrahepatic ORR. The OS was significantly longer in the HAI group (14.0 vs. 10.8 months)

HAI hepatic artery infusion, *5-FU* 5-fluorouracil, *OS* overall survival, *PFS* progression-free survival, *ORR* overall response rate, *PR* partial response, *SD* stable disease, *PD* progression of disease, *RCT* randomized control trial, *PCLM* pancreatic cancer liver metastases, *FUDR* floxuridine

[a]S-1 is an oral fluorinated pyrimidine compound developed by Taiho Pharmaceutical Co., Ltd., (Tokyo, Japan)

Conclusion

HAI for diseases beyond CRLM and ICC has been studied, though data remain sparse and inconclusive. For patients with liver-confined disease and in the context of extent of systemic therapy already given, multidisciplinary teams may consider HAI for highly selected patients, though it remains important to acknowledge the paucity of data supporting its use, and risk of pump placement and HAI chemotherapy must be weighed against perceived benefit. There is an obvious need for well-designed clinical trials evaluating HAI for these diseases.

References

1. Lyu N, Kong Y, Mu L, Lin Y, Li J, Liu Y, Zhang Z, Zheng L, Deng H, Li S, Xie Q, Guo R, Shi M, Xu L, Cai X, Wu P, Zhao M. Hepatic arterial infusion of oxaliplatin plus fluorouracil/leucovorin vs. sorafenib for advanced hepatocellular carcinoma. J Hepatol. 2018;69(1):60–9. https://doi.org/10.1016/j.jhep.2018.02.008. Epub 2018 Feb 20.
2. Llovet JM, Ricci S, Mazzaferro V, Hilgard P, Gane E, Blanc JF, et al. Sorafenib in advanced hepatocellular carcinoma. N Engl J Med. 2008;359:378–90.
3. Finn RS, Qin S, Ikeda M, Galle PR, Ducreux M, Kim TY, Kudo M, Breder V, Merle P, Kaseb AO, Li D, Verret W, Xu DZ, Hernandez S, Liu J, Huang C, Mulla S, Wang Y, Lim HY, Zhu AX, Cheng AL. Atezolizumab plus Bevacizumab in Unresectable Hepatocellular Carcinoma. N Engl J Med. 2020;382(20):1894–905.
4. Abou-Alfa GK, Lau G, Kudo M, Chan SL, Kelley RK, Furuse J, Sukeepaisarnjaroen W, Kang YK, Dao TV, De Toni EN, Rimassa L, Breder V, Vasilyev A, Heurgue A, Tam VC, Mody K, Thungappa SC, Ostapenko Y, Yau T, Azevedo S, Varela M, Cheng AL, Qin S, Galle PR, Ali S, Marcovitz M, Makowsky M, He P, Kurland JF, Negro A, Sangro B. Tremelimumab plus Durvalumab in Unresectable Hepatocellular Carcinoma. NEJM Evid. 2022;1(8):EVIDoa2100070. https://doi.org/10.1056/EVIDoa2100070.
5. He M-K, Zou R-H, Li Q-J, Zhou Z-G, Shen J-X, Zhang Y-F, et al. Phase II study of Sorafenib combined with concurrent hepatic arterial infusion of Oxaliplatin, 5-fluorouracil and Leucovorin for Unresectable hepatocellular carcinoma with major portal vein thrombosis. Cardiovasc Intervent Radiol. 2018;41:734–43. https://doi.org/10.1007/s00270-017-1874-z.
6. He M, Li Q, Zou R, Shen J, Fang W, Tan G, et al. Sorafenib plus hepatic arterial infusion of Oxaliplatin, fluorouracil, and Leucovorin vs Sorafenib alone for hepatocellular carcinoma with portal vein invasion: a randomized clinical trial. JAMA Oncol. 2019;5:953. https://doi.org/10.1001/jamaoncol.2019.0250.
7. Kim BK, Kim DY, Byun HK, Choi HJ, Beom SH, Lee HW, Kim SU, Park JY, Ahn SH, Seong J, Han KH. Efficacy and safety of liver-directed concurrent Chemoradiotherapy and sequential Sorafenib for advanced hepatocellular carcinoma: a prospective phase 2 trial. Int J Radiat Oncol Biol Phys. 2020;107(1):106–15. https://doi.org/10.1016/j.ijrobp.2020.01.027. Epub 2020 Feb 19.
8. Hamada T, Yano K, Wada T, Imamura N, Hiyoshi M, Kondo K, Nanashima A. Increased survival benefit of adjuvant intra-arterial infusion chemotherapy in HCC patients with portal vein infiltration after hepatectomy. World J Surg. 2020;44(8):2770–6. https://doi.org/10.1007/s00268-020-05527-w.
9. Cazzato RL, Hubelé F, De Marini P, Ouvrard E, Salvadori J, Addeo P, Garnon J, Kurtz JE, Greget M, Mertz L, Goichot B, Gangi A, Imperiale A. Liver-directed therapy for neuroendocrine metastases: from interventional radiology to nuclear medicine procedures. Cancers (Basel). 2021;13(24):6368. https://doi.org/10.3390/cancers13246368. PMID: 34944988; PMCID: PMC8699378.
10. Chia SK, Speers CH, D'Yachkova Y, et al. The impact of new chemotherapeutic and hormone agents on survival in a population-based cohort of women with metastatic breast cancer. Cancer. 2007;110(973–9):2.
11. Largillier R, Ferrero JM, Doyen J, et al. Prognostic factors in 1038 women with metastatic breast cancer. Ann Oncol. 2008;19:2012–9.
12. Fraschini G, Fleishman G, Yap HY, Carrasco CH, Charnsangavej C, Patt YZ, Hortobagyi GN. Percutaneous hepatic arterial infusion of cisplatin for metastatic breast cancer. Cancer Treat Rep. 1987;71(3):313–5.
13. Fraschini G, Fleishman G, Charnsangavej C, Carrasco CH, Hortobagyi GN. Continuous 5-day infusion of vinblastine for percutaneous hepatic arterial chemotherapy for metastatic breast cancer. Cancer Treat Rep. 1987;71(11):1001–5.
14. Fraschini G, Charnsangavej C, Carrasco CH, Buzdar AU, Jabboury KW, Hortobagyi GN. Percutaneous hepatic arterial infusion of cisplatin-vinblastine for refractory breast carcinoma metastatic to the liver. Am J Clin Oncol. 1988;11(1):34–8. https://doi.org/10.1097/00000421-198802000-00008.
15. Camacho LH, Kurzrock R, Cheung A, Barber DF, Gupta S, Madoff DC, Wallace MJ, Kim EE, Curley SA, Hortobagyi GN, Mavligit G. Pilot study of regional, hepatic intra-arterial paclitaxel in patients with breast carcinoma metastatic to the liver. Cancer. 2007;109(11):2190–6. https://doi.org/10.1002/cncr.22672.
16. Ang C, Jhaveri K, Patel D, Gewirtz A, Seidman A, Kemeny N. Hepatic arterial infusion and systemic chemotherapy for breast cancer liver metastases. Breast J. 2013;19(1):96–9. https://doi.org/10.1111/tbj.12050. Epub 2012 Nov 23.
17. Shi HB, Qiang WG, Zhu WL, Yuan Y, Wang JJ, Zhao JM, Hu WW. Hepatic artery infusion pump combined with systemic chemotherapy for patients with liver metastases from breast carcinoma. Technol Cancer Res Treat. 2021;20:15330338211051552. https://doi.org/10.1177/15330338211051552. PMID: 34657511; PMCID: PMC8524696.
18. Nanda R, Chow LQ, Dees EC, Berger R, Gupta S, Geva R, Pusztai L, Pathiraja K, Aktan G, Cheng JD, Karantza V, Buisseret L. Pembrolizumab in patients with advanced triple-negative breast cancer: phase Ib KEYNOTE-012 study. J Clin Oncol. 2016;34(21):2460–7. https://doi.org/10.1200/JCO.2015.64.8931. Epub 2016 May 2. PMID: 27138582; PMCID: PMC6816000.
19. Gianni L, Eiermann W, Semiglazov V, Manikhas A, Lluch A, Tjulandin S, Zambetti M, Vazquez F, Byakhow M, Lichinitser M, Climent MA, Ciruelos E, Ojeda B, Mansutti M, Bozhok A, Baronio R, Feyereislova A, Barton C, Valagussa P, Baselga J. Neoadjuvant chemotherapy with trastuzumab

followed by adjuvant trastuzumab versus neo-adjuvant chemotherapy alone, in patients with HER2-positive locally advanced breast cancer (the NOAH trial): a randomised controlled superiority trial with a parallel HER2-negative cohort. Lancet. 2010;375(9712):377–84. https://doi.org/10.1016/S0140-6736(09)61964-4.
20. Slamon DJ, Leyland-Jones B, Shak S, Fuchs H, Paton V, Bajamonde A, Fleming T, Eiermann W, Wolter J, Pegram M, Baselga J, Norton L. Use of chemotherapy plus a monoclonal antibody against HER2 for metastatic breast cancer that overexpresses HER2. N Engl J Med. 2001;344(11):783–92. https://doi.org/10.1056/NEJM200103153441101.
21. Turner NC, Ro J, André F, Loi S, Verma S, Iwata H, Harbeck N, Loibl S, Huang Bartlett C, Zhang K, Giorgetti C, Randolph S, Koehler M, Cristofanilli M, PALOMA3 Study Group. Palbociclib in hormone-receptor-positive advanced breast cancer. N Engl J Med. 2015;373(3):209–19. https://doi.org/10.1056/NEJMoa1505270. Epub 2015 Jun 1.
22. Hortobagyi GN, Stemmer SM, Burris HA, Yap YS, Sonke GS, Paluch-Shimon S, Campone M, Blackwell KL, André F, Winer EP, Janni W, Verma S, Conte P, Arteaga CL, Cameron DA, Petrakova K, Hart LL, Villanueva C, Chan A, Jakobsen E, Nusch A, Burdaeva O, Grischke EM, Alba E, Wist E, Marschner N, Favret AM, Yardley D, Bachelot T, Tseng LM, Blau S, Xuan F, Souami F, Miller M, Germa C, Hirawat S, O'Shaughnessy J. Ribociclib as first-line therapy for HR-positive, advanced breast cancer. N Engl J Med. 2016;375(18):1738–48. https://doi.org/10.1056/NEJMoa1609709. Epub 2016 Oct 7. Erratum in: N Engl J Med 2018 Dec 27;379(26):2582.
23. Sledge GW Jr, Toi M, Neven P, Sohn J, Inoue K, Pivot X, Burdaeva O, Okera M, Masuda N, Kaufman PA, Koh H, Grischke EM, Conte P, Lu Y, Barriga S, Hurt K, Frenzel M, Johnston S, Llombart-Cussac A. The effect of Abemaciclib plus Fulvestrant on overall survival in hormone receptor-positive, ERBB2-negative breast cancer that progressed on endocrine therapy-MONARCH 2: a randomized clinical trial. JAMA Oncol. 2020;6(1):116–24. https://doi.org/10.1001/jamaoncol.2019.4782. PMID: 31563959; PMCID: PMC6777264.
24. Conroy T, Desseigne F, Ychou M, et al. FOLFIRINOX versus gemcitabine for metastatic pancreatic cancer. N Engl J Med. 2011;364:1817–25.
25. Von Hoff DD, Ervin T, Arena FP, et al. Increased survival in pancreatic cancer with nab-paclitaxel plus gemcitabine. N Engl J Med. 2013;369:1691–703.
26. Ohigashi H, Ishikawa O, Eguchi H, Takahashi H, Gotoh K, Yamada T, Yano M, Nakaizumi A, Uehara H, Tomita Y, Nishiyama K. Feasibility and efficacy of combination therapy with preoperative full-dose gemcitabine, concurrent three-dimensional conformal radiation, surgery, and postoperative liver perfusion chemotherapy for T3-pancreatic cancer. Ann Surg. 2009;250(1):88–95. https://doi.org/10.1097/SLA.0b013e3181ad65cc.
27. Tajima H, Ohta T, Kitagawa H, Sakai S, Makino I, Hayashi H, Oyama K, Nakagawara H, Fujita H, Onishi I, Takamura H, Ninomiya I, Fushida S, Tani T, Fujimura T, Koda W, Minami T, Ryu Y, Sanada J, Gabata T, Matsui O. Pilot study of hepatic arterial infusion chemotherapy with gemcitabine and 5-fluorouracil for patients with postoperative liver metastases from pancreatic cancer. Exp Ther Med. 2011;2(2):265–9. https://doi.org/10.3892/etm.2011.190. Epub 2011 Jan 12. PMID: 22977495; PMCID: PMC3440666.
28. Tajima H, Kitagawa H, Tsukada T, Okamoto K, Nakanuma SI, Sakai S, Makino I, Furukawa H, Hayashi H, Oyama K, Inokuchi M, Nakagawara H, Miyashita T, Itoh H, Fujita H, Takamura H, Ninomiya I, Fushida S, Fujimura T, Ohta T, Koda W, Minami T, Ryu Y, Sanada J, Gabata T, Matsui O, Sai Y. Hepatic arterial infusion chemotherapy with gemcitabine and 5-fluorouracil or oral S-1 improves the prognosis of patients with postoperative liver metastases from pancreatic cancer. Mol Clin Oncol. 2013;1(5):869–74. https://doi.org/10.3892/mco.2013.152. Epub 2013 Jul 23. PMID: 24649263; PMCID: PMC3916203.
29. Zheng YY, Tang CW, Xu YQ, Feng WM, Bao Y, Fei MY. Hepatic arterial infusion chemotherapy reduced hepatic metastases from pancreatic cancer after pancreatectomy. Hepato-Gastroenterology. 2014;61(133):1415–20.
30. Peng C, Xu B, Xiao J, Zhou C, Li X, Shi H, Qiang W, Wang T, Zhao J, Liu F, Li G, Li H, Chen C, Shi L. Hepatic artery infusion of Floxuridine in combination with systemic chemotherapy for pancreatic cancer liver metastasis: a propensity score-matched analysis in two centers. Front Oncol. 2021;11:652426. https://doi.org/10.3389/fonc.2021.652426. PMID: 33996572; PMCID: PMC8113695.

Part V

Long-Term Consequences of Hepatic Arterial Infusion

18 Hepatic Arterial Infusion Pump Chemotherapy-Induced Biliary Sclerosis

Lynn A. Brody and Anne M. Covey

History and Pathophysiology

Hepatic arterial infusion pumps (HAIP) were first introduced in the 1980s to treat patients with metastatic disease to the liver. The rationale behind arterially directed therapy to treat liver metastases is based on the fact that liver metastases are preferentially supplied by the hepatic artery, whereas the nutrient flow to the non-tumor-bearing liver is predominantly derived from the portal vein. HAIP catheters are typically placed in the gastroduodenal artery, which is ligated distally to isolate the flow from the pump into the hepatic artery where a high first-pass extraction allows administration of high doses of chemotherapy to the liver that would not be tolerated systemically. Adoption of this practice has been relatively slow due in part to the complexity of managing these patients and the associated complications. Complications may be postoperative (e.g., postoperative collection in the pump pocket, infection, non-hepatic perfusion) or related to the treatment itself. The most common treatment-related complication is chemotherapy-induced biliary sclerosis (CIBS).

Ideally, every patient in whom a hepatic arterial infusion pump (HAIP) is placed would complete their planned course of intra-arterial chemotherapy. Unfortunately, in some patients, HAIP induced CIBS may require dose reduction or cessation of pump therapy due to rising liver function tests (LFTs), particularly alkaline phosphatase (ALK) and bilirubin. Some of these patients ultimately require endoscopic or percutaneous biliary intervention to treat biliary obstruction.

Early reports of HAIP therapy noted a high percentage of patients with elevated ALK and jaundice. In 1983, Balch et al., reported that "transient jaundice" occurred in one-third of the patients receiving HAIP, more commonly after 4 or more months of floxuridine exposure [1]. "Anicteric chemical hepatitis" was seen in 30 of 93 (30%) patients with metastatic colon cancer treated in a Phase I–II study of HAIP FUDR, and 22 (24%) patients went on to develop jaundice [2]. Similarly, Kemeny et al. described hepatic enzyme abnormalities in 71% of patients with hyperbilirubinemia in 22% [3]. A review of HAIP morbidity by Martin et al. in 2004 lists the rate of reported CIBS from 1983 to 2003 between 0 and 26% and noted an incidence of 18% in their own cohort of 34 patients. In this study, only 47% of their patients received all planned cycles of FUDR, with more than one-third requiring some form of dose reduction [4].

Various modifications to FUDR pump chemotherapy have been shown to impact the occurrence of biliary complications as well as oncologic outcomes. In 1992, Kemeny et al.

L. A. Brody · A. M. Covey (✉)
Interventional Radiology Service, Department of Radiology, Memorial Sloan Kettering Cancer Center, New York, NY, USA
e-mail: brodyl@mskcc.org; coveya@mskcc.org

M. D'Angelica, M. Lidsky (eds.), *Hepatic Arterial Infusion for Malignancy*,
https://doi.org/10.1007/978-3-031-74935-3_18

reported a randomized trial of 50 patients treated with FUDR HAIP therapy with or without hepatic arterial dexamethasone [5]. There was a trend toward decreased incidence of hyperbilirubinemia more than 200% of baseline (30% vs. 9%, $p = 0.07$) in patients who received dexamethasone. The patients treated with intra-arterial dexamethasone also received higher doses of FUDR at most time points and were less likely to require dose reduction and any point. In addition, the complete and partial response rates were significantly better in patients receiving FUDR plus dexamethasone and the survival in patients receiving dexamethasone was 23 months compared to 15 months for those in which dexamethasone was omitted ($p = 0.06$). The protective value of dexamethasone was later validated in a canine model; mitigating effects were seen both radiographically and pathologically [6].

Also in 1992, a meta-analysis of nine HAIP randomized trials reported that fluorouracil (5-FU) plus leucovorin (LV) resulted in significantly higher tumor response rates, though without improvement in survival [7]. However, in 1994, Kemeny et al. evaluated various dose schedules of FUDR and LV and showed that while response rates were good, biliary toxicity was higher in patients given combination therapy, producing elevated liver enzymes in 60% of patients and documented CIBS in 21% [8]. This led to a randomized trial adding dexamethasone to FUDR and LV, where only 2 of 62 (3%) of patients developed CIBS while high response rates were maintained [9]. There was also a suggestion that biliary toxicity could be mitigated by alternating FUDR and 5-FU [10].

Combining Mitomycin C (Mit-C) with FUDR showed increased response rates in animal studies [11] and some human studies suggested a role for combination therapy [12, 13]. However, a phase II trial published in 2005 by Kemeny et al. found higher than expected biliary toxicity, including CIBS in 9.5% of patients and liver bilomas in 7.9% [14]. They concluded that alternatives to high-dose Mit-C should be investigated when exploring additions to FUDR pump therapy.

Systemic regimens may also impact the incidence and extent of HAIP-related CIBS. Cercek et al. found increased biliary toxicity in patients who received systemic bevacizumab (BEV) concurrently with HAIP FUDR [15]. They analyzed a total of 203 patients enrolled in three different prospective studies and found that in each study group the addition of BEV was associated with an increased incidence of hyperbilirubinemia and biliary stent placement within 1 year of treatment. Further, they failed to demonstrate any survival advantage with the addition of BEV in these trials. The authors proposed two hypotheses for the increased incidence of CIBS with systemic BEV: one, that the effect of BEV on vascular permeability may lead to a greater influx of chemotherapy and result in greater biliary injury. The other hypothesis was that inhibition of angiogenesis impairs healing of injury and inflammation of the bile ducts. Regardless of the mechanism, the authors recommended that BEV should not be combined with HAIP FUDR therapy.

In an interesting paper, Ito et al. assessed the incidence, clinical features, and risk factors for CIBS in 475 consecutive patients treated with HAIP therapy from 1991 to 2008 [16]. They reported an incidence of CIBS of 5.5% in patients treated with HAIP chemotherapy as an adjuvant treatment after hepatectomy and 2% of patients treated with HAIP for unresectable disease. In postresection adjuvant HAIP, they found significantly higher rates of CIBS in patients who had abnormal postoperative nuclear flow scans, postoperative infectious complications, and larger dose/cycle/weight of FUDR. Of note, 82 of the 475 patients received HAIP with FUDR and Mit-C, and 11 (13.4%) of these developed CIBS. It is not explicitly stated, but from prior publications, it seems that the Mit-C patients did not also undergo resection [12, 14]. They note that CIBS resulting from HAIP treatment can be treated with dilation or stenting, though the specific management of patients requiring endoscopic or percutaneous management is not detailed.

The etiology of CIBS is thought to be both ischemic and inflammatory. Pathologic studies have shown replacement of the bile duct wall with sclerotic collagenous tissue [17], portal triad fibrosis, central vein sclerosis, cirrhosis related to dose and duration of therapy [18], canalicular cholestasis, focal ductal proliferation, and "pericholangitis," as well as fibrosis involving the porta hepatis [19–21]. Interestingly, these findings occurred in the setting of minimal hepatocyte damage [22]. The principal site of injury related to HAIP is the biliary epithelium and not the hepatocytes and has also been shown in a canine model of HAIP [6].

It remains unclear whether the injury is predominantly ischemic or inflammatory. In 1989, Ludwig et al. questioned whether the cholangiopathy associated with floxuridine-induced sclerosing cholangitis was ischemic in nature [23]. They noted that prior to that time, most authors thought that FUDR-associated cholangiopathy was caused by the toxicity of the drug. Like liver metastases, the bile ducts receive most of their blood supply from the hepatic arteries, and we now have several decades of data that showing that delivery of high doses of FUDR or mitomycin into the hepatic arteries can result in biliary sclerosis.

The blood supply to the bile ducts was elegantly shown by Northover and Terblanche in 1979 [24]. They created resin casts from fresh human cadavers and subdivided blood supply to the bile duct into three segments: a *hilar* segment supplying the right and left hepatic ducts, a *supraduodenal* segment supplying the common hepatic and upper common bile ducts, and a *retropancreatic* segment supplying the lower common bile duct. Twenty-one high-quality casts were ultimately analyzed. They described the blood supply to the supraduodenal segment as "axial," arising from named arteries related to the upper and lower ends of the duct. In their specimens, an average of eight small arteries supplied the supraduodenal duct, with the most important vessels running along the lateral borders of the duct. They called these the 3 o'clock and 9 o'clock arteries and found one or both of these to be present in all specimens. They also described several other vessels supplying the duct that arose from the retroduodenal and gastroduodenal arteries. They found that 60% of vessels reaching the supraduodenal duct ran up from these vessels, while 38% ran down from the right hepatic (25.5%), cystic (7.5%), left hepatic (3.1%), and others, including a very small percent from the common hepatic artery.

Further, they discovered arterial supply to the supraduodenal duct from a vessel not previously described; they coined this the *retroportal artery*. This vessel arises from the proximal posterior aspect of either the celiac axis or the superior mesenteric artery, with one case of joint supply and another where the vessel was essentially replaced by a replaced right hepatic artery. The vessel courses behind the portal vein and on to the back of the pancreatic head to reach the lower end of the supraduodenal duct. In about half of their specimens, the artery terminated by anastomosing with the retroduodenal artery near the lower end of the supraduodenal duct, then supplying small branches to the posterior surface of the duct. They designated this a type I pattern. A type II pattern was present in 30% of cases, where the retroportal artery passed superiorly along the back of the supraduodenal duct and joined the right hepatic artery behind the common hepatic duct. Along the way it provided branches to the pericholedochal plexus. The authors note that the connection with the right hepatic artery means that in a type I pattern this portion of the duct has some more proximal blood supply.

In their specimens, arterial supply to the hilar ducts typically arose from numerous small arteries arising from the left and right hepatic arteries that form a network on the surface of the ducts, anastomosing with the plexus around the supraduodenal duct. In some of their specimens, the 3 and 9 o'clock arteries also extended superiorly to contribute to the supply of the hilar ducts.

Iwao and Heaton revisited the retroportal artery as it relates to hepato-pancreatico-biliary and transplant surgery [25]. They noted that the retroportal artery is associated with lymphatic channels and nerves and they posited that the neural fibers associated with the vessel may have a role in modulating blood supply to the bile duct. They further suggested that surgery involving this vessel may denervate the associated splanchnic and parasympathetic nerves in the surrounding connective tissue and could also lead to ampullary dysfunction in some patients.

Cho and Lunderquist wrote about the peribiliary vascular plexus based on anatomic analysis in rabbits as well as visceral angiograms in humans [26]. After making arterial and portal casts, they sectioned the bile ducts in rabbits and found that the plexus consisted of two concentric vascular layers in the wall of the bile duct, where the inner capillary layer was arterial and the outer layer contained both arterial and portal venous vasculature, with suggestion that there was flow from the inner arterial capillary layer to the thicker outer plexus with anastomoses to portal vasculature. They also described the venous drainage of the bile duct as occurring in two ways: via lobular veins directly into the adjacent sinusoids and via interlobular veins. They also found that in animals in which the hepatic artery had been occluded, the peribiliary plexus became more prominent with an increased arterial component.

In their study, they failed to demonstrate the capillary or venous plexus in humans with normal bile ducts undergoing visceral arteriography or portal venography. In patients with occlusion of the proper hepatic artery, the authors described fine tortuous collaterals arising from the gastroduodenal artery branches, running along the common bile and hepatic ducts and anastomosing with hepatic arterial branches at the porta. They also noted similar collaterals in patients with cirrhosis.

Portal venous blood supply to the bile duct was assessed in a small study evaluating microvascular blood supply with a combination of laser Doppler flow measurement and reflectance spectrophotometry in 15 patients undergoing pancreaticoduodenectomy [27]. They found that blood flow to the common bile duct (CBD) decreased to 62% after clamping the portal vein, to 51% after clamping the hepatic artery, and to only 31% after clamping both; this led them to conclude that the contribution of the portal vein to the microvascular flow through the CBD is approximately 40% and suggest that disturbances in portal flow could contribute to the development of biliary complications after liver transplantation. One might also wonder whether patients receiving HAIP therapy who have compromised portal flow might also be at increased risk for developing CIBS for this reason. A case report in 1986 by Dikengil et al. noted HAIP FUDR-related CIBS with findings of marked portal hypertension in addition to biliary ductal dilation [21].

Radiographic Considerations and Management

Radiographic findings of HAIP CIBS have been described since early reports of this therapy. M Kemeny et al. reported that 8 of 46 (17.4%) patients in a randomized trial of HAIP with FUDR developed imaging and pathologic findings identical to those of sclerosing cholangitis associated with inflammatory bowel disease, two of whom ultimately died from their biliary disease [17]. Botet et al. described 6 of 87 (6%) patients with elevated ALK and bilirubin over 3 mg/dL with segmentally narrowed bile ducts predominantly involving the common hepatic duct and the central right and left hepatic ducts, with lesser involvement of the common bile duct and the intrahepatic ducts [28]. A common finding in almost all cases of CIBS includes involvement of the confluence of the right and left hepatic ducts.

Brown et al. reported on 30 of 282 (10.6%) patients who developed obstructive jaundice while receiving HAIP chemotherapy, 24 (overall 8.5%) of whom had obstruction related to CIBS, and who required percutaneous, transhepatic biliary drainage [29]. It was in this report that they coined the term "chemotherapy biliary sclerosis." Twenty-four of the 30 (80%) patients that required drainage and all 9 who developed a biloma had been treated with intra-arterial mitomycin C. As with other reports, they described the most common cholangiographic finding being high grade obstruction of the common hepatic duct, which extended to the confluence of the right and left hepatic ducts in 50% of cases and with frequent involvement of the more peripheral intrahepatic ducts. They further described a "striated" and "fuzzy" appearance of the stricture often with an associated flame-shaped filling defect extending inferiorly into a more normal caliber common duct (Fig. 18.1). Eight of the 30 patients had their drainage catheters converted to internal self-expanding metallic stents, with an average patency of 5.1 months. Five of the 30 (17%) patients treated had bleeding complications following biliary intervention, some of which resolved without intervention while others required embolization. In most patients with malignant bile duct obstruction who undergo percutaneous biliary intervention complicated by arterial bleeding, the injured vessel is almost always along the course of the catheter near the puncture site [30]. Interestingly, they found that abnormalities demonstrated at angiography were often along the course of the catheter but remote from the bile duct puncture site (Fig. 18.2). This may be due to the sclerosis and encasement of the portal triads described by Shea et al. based on intraoperative appearance of the bile ducts. Based on anatomic studies cited earlier, the authors hypothesized that patients whose primary blood supply to the supraduodenal duct comes from above rather than below may be more likely develop CIBS.

There is increasing evidence that HAIP therapy can prolong survival in selected patients, and this is reflected in the increasing use of HAIP across the United States and associated increase in publications [31–34]. Unfortunately, some patients receiving HAIP chemotherapy continue to develop elevated liver enzymes and CIBS [35]. Management of these patients is complicated and labor intensive, and the first step is usually to decrease or hold the dose of FUDR based on ALK and bilirubin, increasing the amount of dexamethasone in the pump, and starting oral ursodiol [36]. Some patients ultimately require intervention—to treat pruritus or normalize the bilirubin, as normal or near-normal bilirubin is often required to continue systemic treatment.

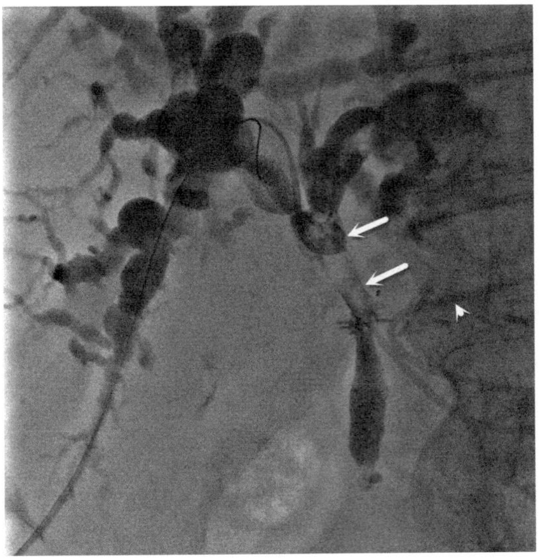

Fig. 18.1 Cholangiogram from a right-sided approach in a patient with an HAIP shows flame-shaped occlusion of the common hepatic duct (arrows) extending into the common hepatic duct with proximal biliary dilation involving the right- and left-sided ducts

In patients with persistent hyperbilirubinemia off pump therapy, we advocate waiting as long as possible to intervene in asymptomatic patients. This is especially true in patients without evidence of disease.

Evaluation of the HAIP patient with altered liver chemistries requires high-quality cross-sectional imaging, with either contrast-enhanced CT and/or contrast-enhanced MRI. Findings suggestive of CIBS include biliary ductal dilation typically involving the hilus without other explanation (e.g., tumor/perihilar nodes) and hepatic perfusion abnormalities. In one study of 60 patients treated with HAIP who did not have bile duct abnormalities attributable to tumor or adenopathy, 34 (57%) developed bile duct abnormalities detected by CT within 1 year of starting pump chemotherapy [37]. The authors found abnormalities of the common bile duct in 74%, including periductal edema, wall thickening and enhancement, and/or focal stricture, and found intrahepatic ductal dilatation in 85%. They also noted parenchymal perfusion abnormalities in 41%, all of whom also had duct abnormalities. Of the 29 patients with intrahepatic ductal dilatation, 10 had progressive clinical obstructive signs or symptoms and ultimately required endoscopic or percutaneous drainage and stenting.

Prior to undertaking any biliary intervention, high-quality CT or MRI images should be examined to assess bile duct anatomy, the level of obstruction, whether there is the suggestion of ductal isolation and the extent to which the ducts in various segments communicate with each

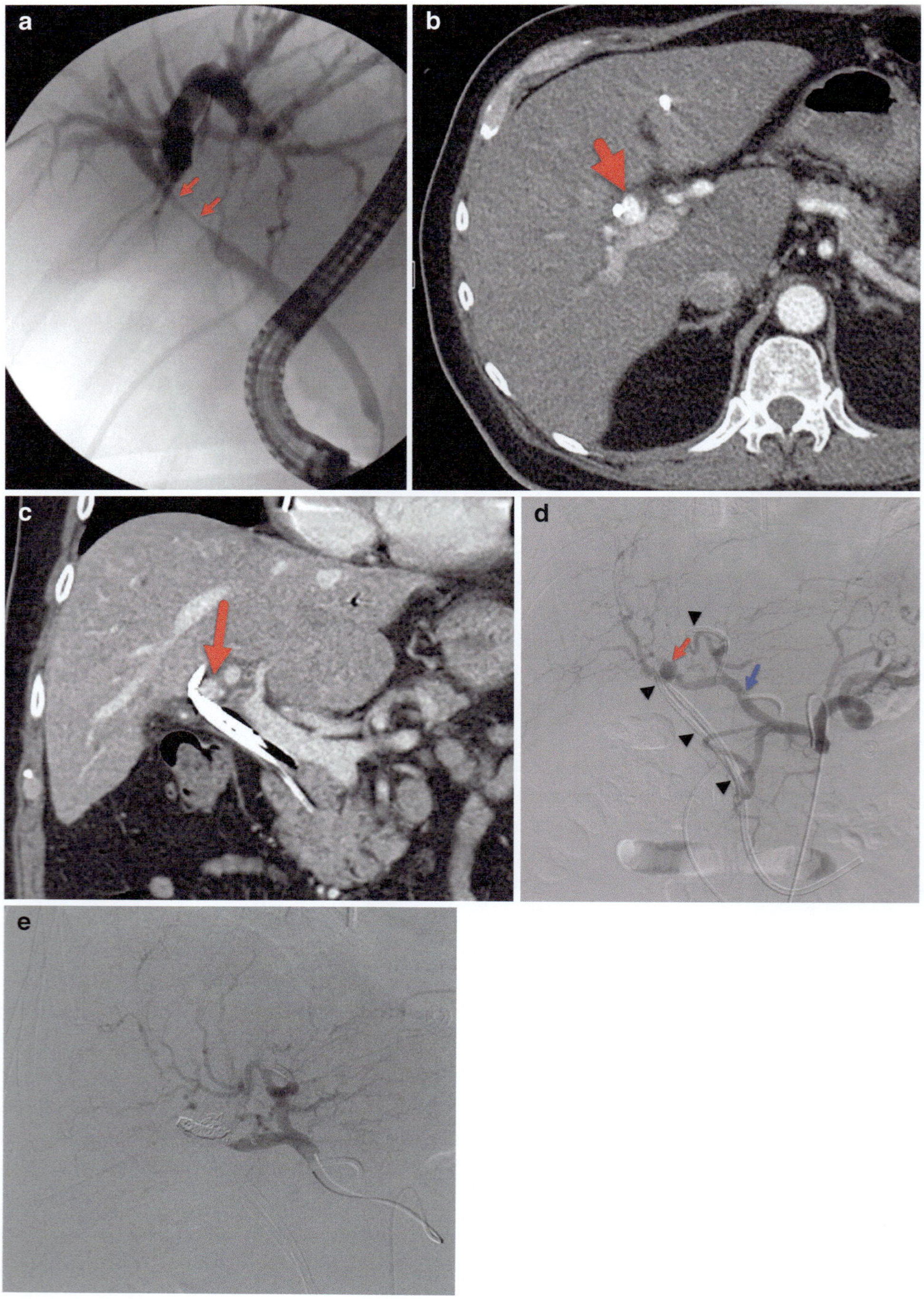

Fig. 18.2 Patient with HAIP for colon cancer liver metastases presented with elevated bilirubin precluding chemotherapy approximately 7 months after starting pump chemotherapy. (**a**) Cholangiogram at the time of endoscopic stent placement showed a short segment hilar stricture (red arrows). (**b, c**) The patient presented with melena 6 weeks after stent placement. Axial and coronal contrast-enhanced CT shows a right hepatic artery pseudoaneurysm (red arrows). (**d**) Catheter angiogram shows the pseudoaneurysm (red arrow) along the course of the indwelling endoscopic stent (black arrows). The tip of the HAIP (blue arrow) is in the expected location of the gastroduodenal artery. (**e**) Angiogram immediately after coil embolization of the right hepatic artery shows collateralization to the right liver from the left hepatic artery

other through the main lobar ducts or sectoral ducts, hepatic lobar atrophy, the location of tumors, and the patency of associated portal vein branches. In order to treat pruritus, draining even a single sector may resolve symptoms; however, in order to lower the bilirubin, the goal of intervention is to maximize the amount of functional liver drained with as few procedures and sites of access as possible [38].

Depending on the level of obstruction, biliary decompression might be performed either endoscopically or percutaneously [29, 39, 40]. We typically advocate endoscopic management for strictures involving the common hepatic duct or below without extension into the right or left main ducts, and certainly without involvement of the higher order intrahepatic ducts.

However, in patients with CIBS, the hepatic hilus is almost always involved and therefore a percutaneous approach is favored because a specific duct can be targeted and the stricture treated with either cholangioplasty, serial dilation, or stent placement above the ampulla (Figs. 18.3 and 18.4). It is our practice whenever possible to keep the stents above the ampulla to prevent reflux and enteric contamination of the bile ducts, in hopes of minimizing the risk of future episodes of cholangitis (Fig. 18.5).

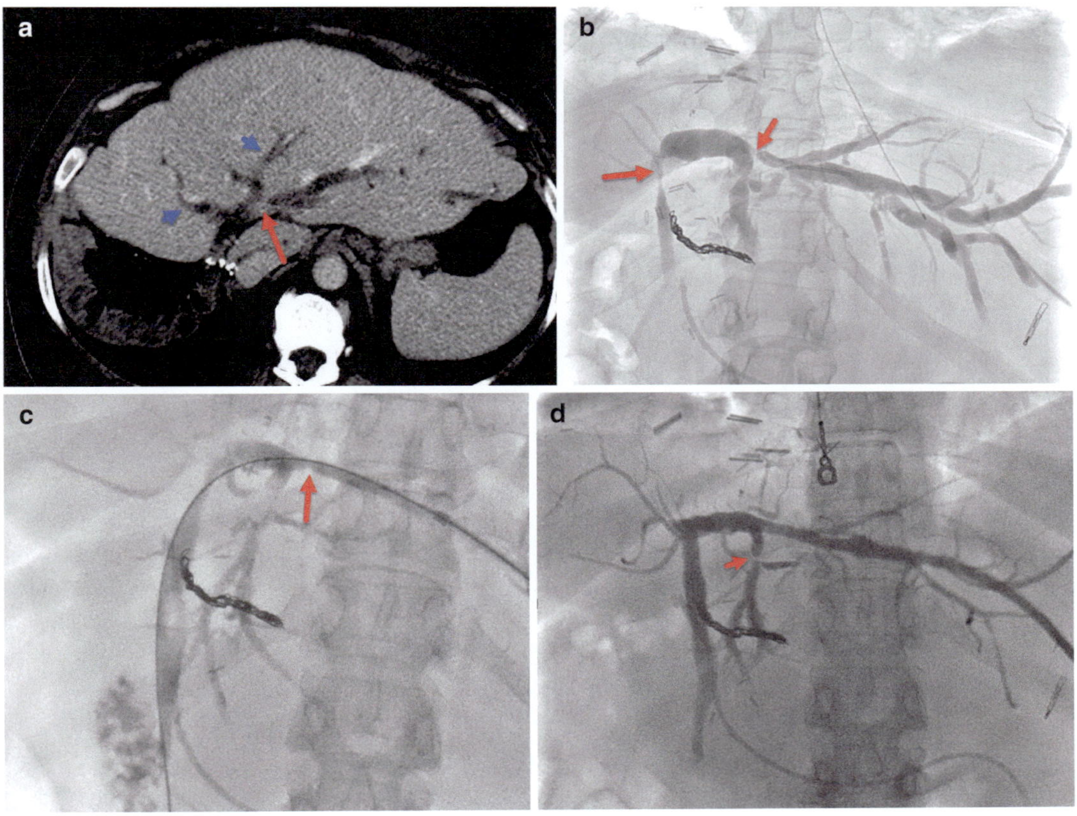

Fig. 18.3 (**a**) Contrast-enhanced CT image in a patient with an HAIP and severe pruritus showing obstruction of the central segment 2 duct (red arrow). Dilation of the segment 2 and 3 ducts (blue arrows) suggests a second level of obstruction. (**b**) Cholangiogram performed at the time of biliary drain placement confirms segmental partial occlusion of the central segment 2 duct and common hepatic duct (red arrows). (**c**) Cholangioplasty of both strictures was performed; a waist in the balloon (red arrow) was seen while dilating the segment 2 stricture. (**d**) One month after a second dilation 6 weeks later, sheath study shows near complete resolution of both the segment 2 and common hepatic duct strictures. After a capping trial of an external drain, the exteriorized catheter was removed. Stricture of the central segment 3 duct (red arrow) was noted, but pruritus had resolved and bilirubin normalized so this was not addressed

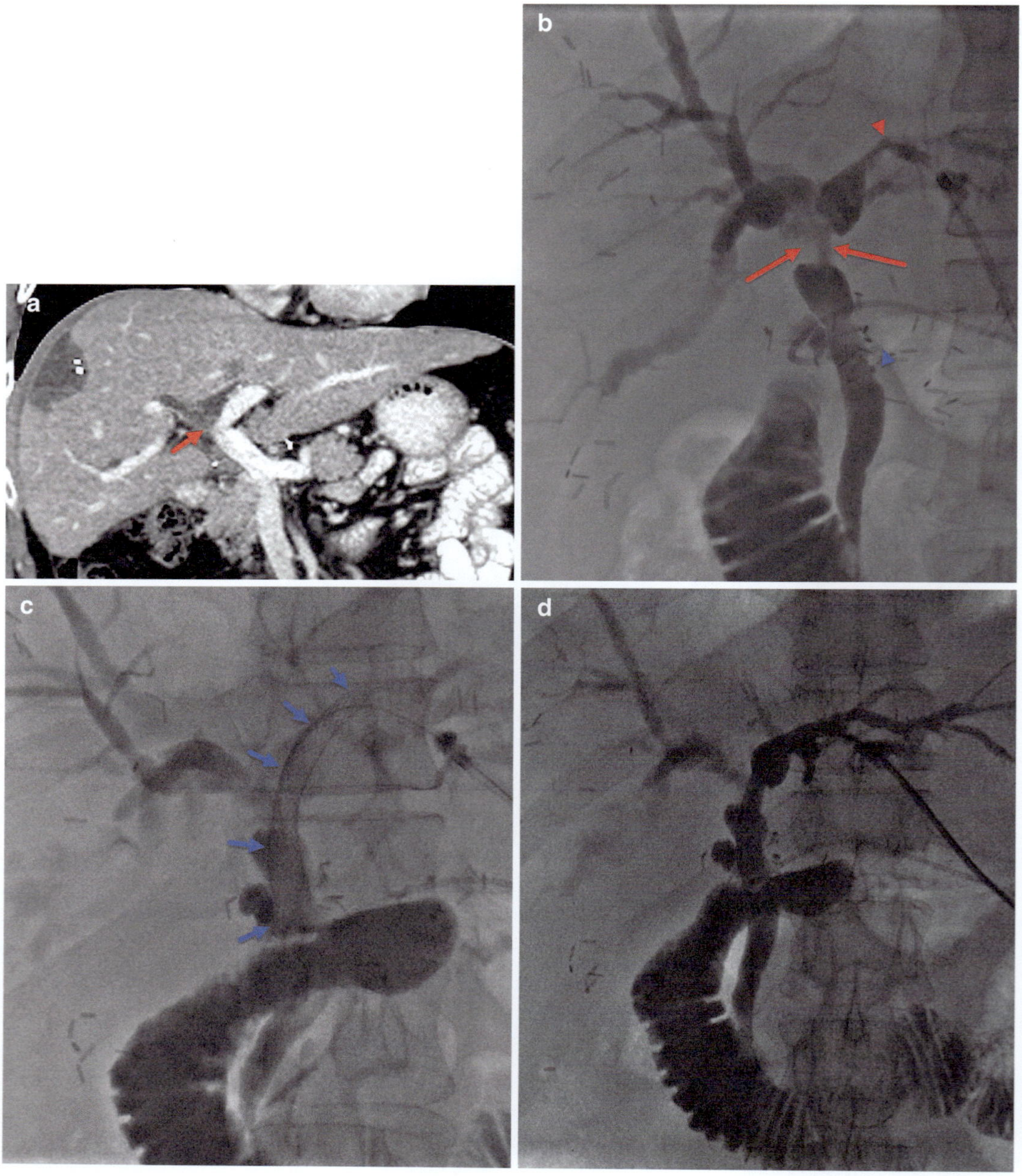

Fig. 18.4 (**a**) Contrast-enhanced CT in a patient with HAIP suggests obstruction of the biliary tree at the confluence and percutaneous cholangiogram (**b**) confirms the finding. An irregular appearing stricture of the hepatic confluence (red arrows) and a more subtle stricture of the segment 3 duct (red arrowhead) are seen. Blue arrowhead shows the tip of the HAIP catheter. (**c**) Primary placement of a self-expanding metallic stent (blue arrowheads) from the left hepatic duct terminating in the common duct above the ampulla. (**d**) Contrast injection after placement shows rapid drainage across the stent into the common bile duct. No exteriorized catheter was left in place after stent placement

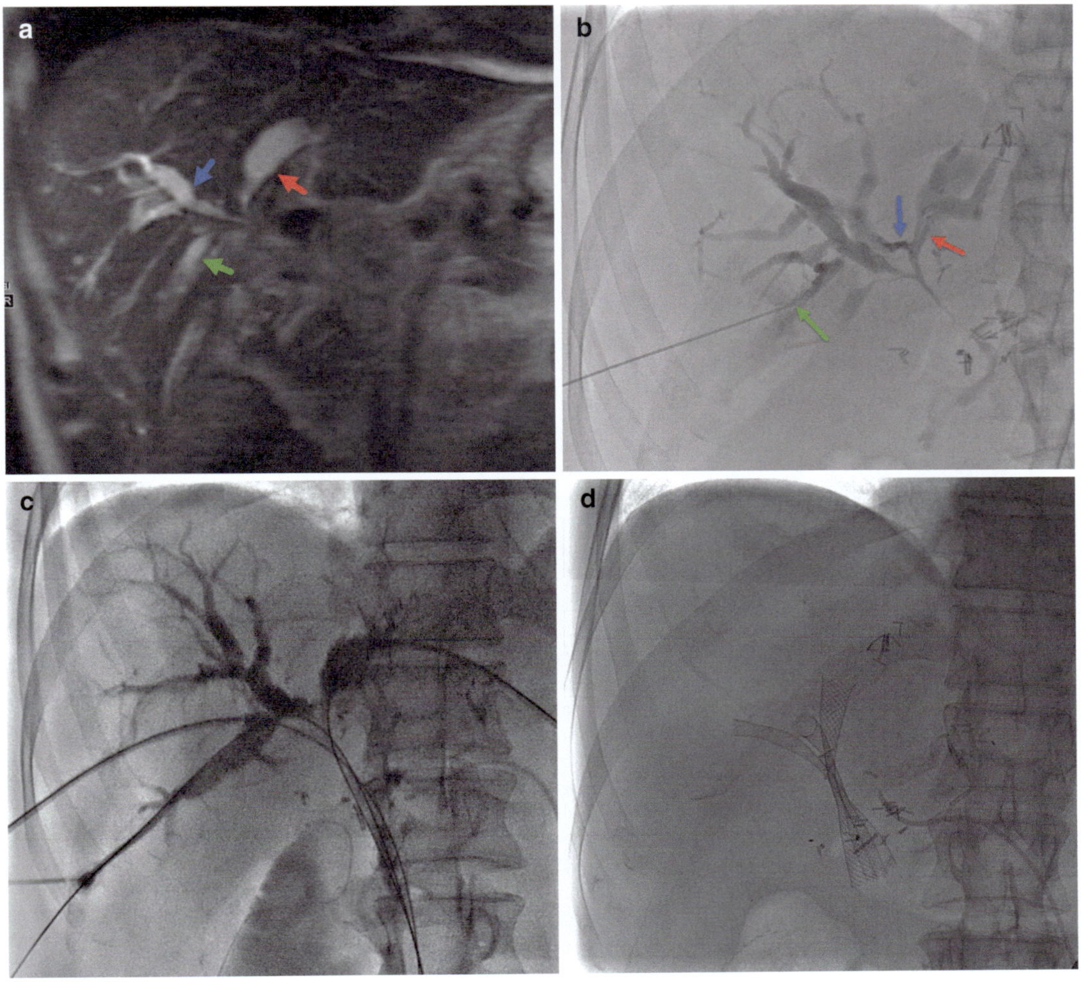

Fig. 18.5 Patient with colon cancer and HAIP. Bilirubin increased to 4.5 mg/dL precluding further treatment and patient was symptomatic with pruritus. (**a**) Single coronal image from MRCP shows dilation of multiple right- (green and blue arrows) and left-sided ducts (red arrow). (**b**) Cholangiogram from a right posterior access (green arrow) shows effective isolation of the right anterior (blue arrow) and left-sided bile ducts (red arrow). (**c**, **d**) Three stents were placed simultaneously extending to the common bile duct above the ampulla. The stents were placed suprapapillary to preserve the sphincter and minimize the risk of enteric contamination of the biliary tree. After stent placement, the bilirubin normalized to 0.6 mg/dL

Because of the risk of bleeding due to the sclerosis of the portal triads and in an effort to maintain the sterility of the biliary tree, in cases of obstruction at or above the confluence, our current practice usually involves primary placement of one or more (sometimes two, rarely three) self-expanding metal stents across the obstruction terminating above the ampulla without placement of an exteriorized catheter. If/when the patient presents with evidence of stent occlusion, depending on their clinical status and prognosis, we may choose to re-intervene either percutaneously or refer for endoscopic management.

In some patients with short segment obstruction and no evidence of disease with life expectancy measured in years, cholangioplasty and/or slow serial up-sizing of an exteriorized catheter may be appropriate. This scenario typically requires an exteriorized catheter for several months, which negatively impacts quality of life. Therefore, we recommend employing this treatment very selectively, and almost certainly in patients with good prognosis and without evidence of active disease.

References

1. Balch CM, Urist MM, McGregor ML. Continuous regional chemotherapy for metastatic colorectal cancer using a totally implantable pump. Am J Surg. 1983;145:285–90.
2. Niederhuber JE, Ensminger W, Gyves J, Thrall J, Walker S, Cozzi E. Regional chemotherapy of colorectal cancer metastastic to the liver. Cancer. 1984;53:1446–343.
3. Kemeny N, Daly J, Oderman P, Shike M, Chun H, Petroni G, et al. Hepatic artery pump infusion: toxicity and results in patients with metastatic colorectal carcinoma. J Clin Oncol. 1984;2(6):595–600.
4. Martin RCG, Edwards MJ, McMasters KM. Morbidity of adjuvant hepatic arterial infusion pump chemotherapy in the management of colorectal cancer metastatic to the liver. Am J Surg. 2004;188:714–21.
5. Kemeny N, Seiter K, Niedzwiecki D, Chapman D, Sigurdson E, Cohen A, Botet J, Oderman P, Murray P. A randomized trial of intrahepatic infusion of fluorodeoxyuridine with dexamethasone versus fluorodeoxyuridine alone in the treatment of metastatic colorectal cancer. Cancer. 1992;69(2):327–34.
6. Ensminger W, Knol J, De Remer S, Wilkinson E, Walker S, Williams D, Maybaum J. Effects of dexamethasone or celecoxib on biliary toxicity after hepatic arterial infusion of 5-fluorodeoxyuridine in a canine model. Cancer Res. 2004;64:311–5.
7. Modulation of flourouracil by leucovorin in patients with advanced colorectal cancer: evidence in terms of response rate. J Clin Oncol. 1992;10(6):896–903.
8. Kemeny N, Seiter K, Conti JA, Cohen A, Bertino JR, Sigurdson ER, Botet J, Chapman D, Mazumdar M, Budd AJ. Hepatic arterial floxuridine and leukovorin for unresectable liver metastases from colorectal carcinoma. Cancer. 1994;73:1134–42.
9. Kemeny N, Conti JA, Campana P, Huang Y, Wei JS, Botet J, Pullman S, Bertino JR. Phase II study of hepatic arterial floxuridine, leucovorin, and dexamethasone for unresectable liver metastases from colorectal carcinoma. J Clin Oncol. 1994;12(1):2288–95.
10. Davidson SB, Izzo F, Chase JL, DuBrow RA, Patt Y, Hohn DC, Curley SA. Alternating floxuridine and 5-fluorouracil hepatic arterial chemotherapy for colorectal liver metastases minimizes biliary toxicity. Am J Surg. 1996;172:244–7.
11. Sutanto-Ward E, Arisawa Y, Tremiterra S, Sigurdson ER. Regional chemotherapy for colorectal hepatic metastases: evidence for improved survival with new drug combinations. Ann Surg Oncol. 1996;3(1):36–43.
12. Kemeny N, Cohen A, Seiter K, Conti JA, Sigurdson ER, Tao Y, Niedzwiecki D, Botet J, Budd A. Randomized trial of hepatic arterial floxuridine, mitomycin and carmustine versus floxuridine alone in previously treated patients with liver metastases from colorectal cancer. J Clin Oncol. 1993;11(2):330–5.
13. Borner M, Laffer U, Ludwig C, Obrist R, Metzger U, Aeberhard P, Weber W, Castiglione M, Obrecht JP, Brunner K, Gloor F, Cavalli F, Senn HJ. Effectiveness and low toxicity of hepatic artery infusion with fluorouracil and mitomycin for metastatic colorectal cancer confined to liver. Ann Oncol. 1990;1:227–8.
14. Kemeny N, Eid A, Stockman J, Gonen M, Schwartz L, Tetzlaff E. Hepatic arterial infusion of floxuridine and dexamethasone plus high-dose mitomycin-C for patients with unresectable hepatic metastases from colorectal carcinoma. J Surg Oncol. 2005;91:7–101.
15. Cercek A, D'Angelica M, Power D, Capanu M, Gewirtz A, Patel D, Allen P, Fong Y, DeMatteo RP, Jarnagin WR, Kemeny NE. Floxuridine hepatic arterial infusion associated biliary toxicity is increased by concurrent administration of systemic bevacizumab. Ann Surg Oncol. 2014;21:479–86.
16. Ito K, Ito H, Kemeny NE, Gonen M, Allen PJ, Paty PB, Fong Y, DeMatteo RP, Blumgart LH, Jarnagin WR, D'Angelica MI. Biliary sclerosis after hepatic arterial infusion pump chemotherapy for patients with colorectal cancer liver metastasis: incidence, clinical features and risk factors. Ann Surg Oncol. 2012;19:1609–17.
17. Kemeny M, Battifora H, Blayney DW, Cecchi G, Goldberg DA, Leong LA, Margolin KA, Terz JJ. Sclerosing cholangitis after continuous hepatic artery infusion of FUDR. Ann Surg. 1985;202(2):176–81.
18. Doria MI, Shepard KV, Levin B, Riddel R. Liver pathology following hepatic arterial infusion chemotherapy. Cancer. 1986;38:855–61.
19. Shea WJ, Demas BE, Goldberg HI, Hohn DC, Ferrell LD, Kerlan RK. Sclerosing cholangitis associated with hepatic arterial FUDR chemotherapy: radiographic-histologic correlation. AJR. 1986;146:717–21.
20. Haq M, Valdes LG, Peterson DF, Gourley WK. Fibrosis of extrahepatic biliary system after continuous hepatic artery infusion of floxuridine through and implantable pump (Infusaid pump). Cancer. 1986;57:1281–3.
21. Dikengil A, Siskind BN, Morse SS, Swedlung A, Bober-Sorcinelli KE, Burrel MI. Sclerosing cholangitis from intraarterial floxuridine. Clin Radiol. 1986;8(6):690–3.
22. Hohn D, Melnick J, Stagg R, Altman D, Friedman M, Ignoffo R, Ferrell L, Lewis B. Biliary sclerosis in patients receiving hepatic arterial infusions of floxuridine. J Clin Oncol. 1985;3(1):98–102.
23. Ludwig J, Kim CH, Wiener RH, Krom RAF. Floxuridine-induced sclerosing cholangi-

tis; an ischemic cholangiopathy? Hepatology. 1989;9(2):215–8.
24. Northover MA, Terblanche J. A new look at the arterial supply of the bile duct in man and its surgical implications. Br J Surg. 1979;66:379–84.
25. Iwao Y, Heaton ND. A review of the retroportal artery in the blood supply of the biliary tree: implications for hepato-biliary and transplant surgeons. Liver Transpl. 2021;27(6):918–22.
26. Cho K, Lunderquist A. The peribiliary vascular plexus: the microvascular architecture of the bile duct in the rabbit and in clinical cases. Radiology. 1983;147:357–64.
27. Slieker J, Farid WRR, van Eijck CHJ, Lange JF, van Bommel J, Metselaar HJ, de Jonge J, Kazemier G. Significant contribution of the portal vein to blood flow through the common bile duct. Ann Surg. 2012;255(3):523–7.
28. Botet B, Watson RC, Kemeny N, Daly JM, Yeh S. Cholangitis complicating intraarterial chemotherapy in liver metastasis. Radiology. 1985;156:335–7.
29. Brown KT, Kemeny N, Berger MF, Getrajdman GI, Napp T, Fong Y, Herman S, Kurtz RC, Botet J, Blumgart LH. Obstructive jaundice in patients receiving hepatic artery infusion pump chemotherapy: etiology, treatment implications, and complications after biliary drainage. JVIR. 1997;8:229–34.
30. Perez-Johnston R, Deipolyi AR, Covey AM. Percutaneous biliary interventions. Gastroenterol Clin N Am. 2018;47(3):621–41.
31. Koerkamp BG, Sadot E, Kemeny NE, Gonen M, Leal JN, Allen PJ, Cercek A, DeMatteo RP, Kingham TP, Jarnagin WR, D'Angelica MI. Perioperative hepatic arterial infusion pump chemotherapy is associated with longer survival after resection of colorectal liver metastases: a propensity score analysis. J Clin Oncol. 2017;35(17):1938–46.
32. Kemeny NE, Chou JF, Boucher TM, Capanu M, DeMatteo RP, Jarnagin WR, Allen PJ, Fong YC, Cercek A, D'Angelica MI. Updated long-term survival for patients with metastatic colorectal cancer treated with liver resection followed by hepatic artery infusion and systemic chemotherapy. J Surg Oncol. 2016;113:477–84.
33. Srouji R, Narayan R, Boerner T, Buisman F, Seier K, Gonen M, Balachandran VP, Drebin J, Jarnagin WR, Kingham TP, Wei A, Kemeny NE. Addition of adjuvant hepatic artery infusion to systemic chemotherapy following hepatic resection of colorectal liver metastases is associated with reduced liver-related mortality. J Surg Oncol. 2020;121:1314–9.
34. Pak LM, Kemeny NE, Capanu M, Chou JF, Boucher T, Cercek A, Balachandran VP, Kingham TP, Allen PJ, De Matteo RP, Jarnagin WR, D'Angelica MI. Prospective phase II trial of combination hepatic artery infusion and systemic chemotherapy for unresectable colorectal liver metastases: long term results and curative potential. J Surg Oncol. 2018;117:634–43.
35. Muaddi H, D'Angelica MI, Wiseman JT, Dillhoff M, Latchana N, Roke R, Ko Y-J, Carpizo D, Spencer K, Fields RC, Williams G, Aucejo F, Acevedo-Moreno L-A, Billingsley KG, Walker BS, Mayo SC, Karanicolas PJ. Safety and feasibility of initiating a hepatic artery infusion pump chemotherapy program for unresectable colorectal liver metastases: a multicenter, retrospective cohort study. J Surg Oncol. 2021;123:252–60.
36. Paumgartner G, Beuers U. Ursodeoxycholic acid in cholestatic liver disease: mechanisms of action and therapeutic use revisited. Hepatology. 2002;36(3):525–31.
37. Phongkitkarun S, Kobayashi S, Varavithya V, Huang X, Curley SA, Charnsangavej C. Bile duct complications of hepatic arterial infusion chemotherapy evaluated by helical CT. Clin Radiol. 2005;60:700–9.
38. Thorton RH, Ulrich R, Hsu M, Moskowitz C, Reidy-Lagunes D, Covey AC, Brody LA, Robson PM, Sofocleous CT, Solomon SB, Getrajdman GI, Brown KY. Outcomes of patients undergoing percutaneous biliary drainage to reduce bilirubin for administration of chemotherapy. J Vasc Interv Radiol. 2012;23:89–95.
39. Siegel JH, Ramsey WH. Endoscopic biliary stent placement for bile duct stricture after hepatic artery infusion of 5-FUDR. J Clin Gastroenterol. 1986;8(6):673–6.
40. Alazami WM, McHenry L, Watkins JL, Fogel EL, Schmidt S, Sherman S, Lehman GL. Chemotherapy-induced sclerosing cholangitis: long-term response to endoscopic therapy. J Clin Gastroenterol. 2006;40(4):353–7.

19 Hepatic Failure Secondary to HAI Pump Chemotherapy

Elwin Tham, Carl Schmidt, and Anthony Scholer

Introduction

This chapter focuses on the incidence, presentation, and management of acute liver insufficiency related to hepatic arterial infusion (HAI) therapy with floxuridine (FUDR). Experiments using animal models and early human trials in the middle part of the last century established intra-arterial administration of chemotherapy as a viable treatment for malignancy. An important observation was the ability to achieve more tissue alteration and tumor regression than systemic doses of the same agents [1, 2]. In Sullivan's initial series of 21 patients with hepatic metastases treated with HAI chemotherapy, three patients died of liver failure after initiation of treatment [3]. In the current era, risk of irreversible hepatic insufficiency or death from liver failure related to HAI-delivered FUDR is rare and not reported in recent trials [4]. However, intra-arterial FUDR is associated with increases in serum hepatic enzyme and bilirubin elevations during therapy. Biliary damage, discussed in another chapter (Chap. 18), can lead to permanent liver damage.

E. Tham · C. Schmidt (✉)
Department of Surgery, West Virginia University, Morgantown, WV, USA
e-mail: carl.schmidt@hsc.wvu.edu

A. Scholer
Hackensack Meridian Medical Group, Jersey Shore University Medical Center, Neptune, NJ, USA
e-mail: Anthony.Scholer@hmhn.com

Incidence

Acute hepatic failure (AHF) has been defined as severe acute liver injury resulting in impaired synthetic liver function and encephalopathy for fewer than 26 weeks in a patient without cirrhosis or preexisting liver disease [5]. Historically, the incidence of HAI-related AHF was poorly documented, lacked a clear definition, and focused on HAI-induced mortality. As mentioned, death from hepatic failure in early studies was as high as 13–19% [3, 6, 7]. In these studies, some deaths from liver failure may have been related to liver tumor burden and other confounding factors rather than intra-arterial chemotherapy, depending on duration of treatment.

HAI with FUDR is associated with significant dose-limiting liver toxicity and manifests hepatic injury in two different ways. *Hepatocellular injury*, the focus of this chapter, typically manifests as elevated hepatic enzymes (aspartate aminotransferase [AST], alanine aminotransferase [ALT], alkaline phosphatase [ALP], and serum bilirubin). *Biliary sclerosis*, discussed in Chap. 18, results from toxic effects on the biliary sys-

M. D'Angelica, M. Lidsky (eds.), *Hepatic Arterial Infusion for Malignancy*,
https://doi.org/10.1007/978-3-031-74935-3_19

tem or ischemic changes secondary to fibrosis of the pericholangitic venous plexus, both of which can result in biliary strictures [8]. Hepatocellular injury occurs in a high proportion of patients given FUDR by HAI with reported rates of 30–70% [7]. Episodes of serum hepatic enzyme levels are usually mild to moderate in severity and resolve with temporary discontinuation of therapy, FUDR dose reduction, or both. While rarely a serious or irreversible issue, these transient elevations can cause treatment delay.

Presentation

Hepatocellular injury and AHF rarely result from complications of hepatic artery infusion pump catheter placement, specifically ischemic hepatitis secondary to catheter-induced hepatic arterial occlusion or thrombosis. Overly aggressive manipulation of the hepatic artery during pump placement can result in acute thrombosis, and intimal dissection of the gastroduodenal artery (GDA) is another possible technical complication. Rates of catheter-related complications have decreased over time from 11% to 5% or less in recent years, possibly related to evolution of catheter types and improvements in surgical technique [7]. A systematic review of over 17 studies of implantable pumps revealed thrombosis rates of 6.6% [9]. Among catheter types, percutaneous catheters were most frequently associated with hepatic artery occlusion (19%), followed by GDA catheters with an extension port (8%) and GDA catheters with implantable pumps (6%). Today, the most common method for FUDR therapy by HAI uses an implantable pump with catheter placed in the GDA. Hepatic artery thrombosis, however, rarely results in AHF.

As mentioned, the more common cause of hepatocellular injury and rarely AHF is chemical hepatitis related to the pyrimidine analogue FUDR used for HAI therapy. Patient factors increasing the risk of FUDR-related chemical hepatitis are not well defined. Interestingly, baseline hepatic function is not strongly associated with occurrence of chemical hepatitis [10–14]. FUDR may have an increased risk of chemical hepatitis over other chemotherapeutic agents including standard fluorouracil with rates as high as 34% [7]. Despite this, FUDR remains the agent of choice for HAI therapy due to its pharmacokinetic profile that results in high intratumoral drug concentrations (400 times greater than systemic administration) [15–18].

Hepatocellular injury related to HAI FUDR therapy is most often first detected by elevations in liver biochemical tests, specifically AST, ALT, ALP, bilirubin, or a combination. Most patients are asymptomatic and it is very uncommon to develop symptoms of acute hepatitis such as nausea, vomiting, anorexia, malaise, or right upper quadrant pain. Symptoms such as hepatic encephalopathy, coagulopathy, and hepatorenal syndrome are symptoms of later stage hepatic failure [5, 19]. FUDR therapy should be discontinued long before such symptoms arise.

Management

For arterial thrombosis related to catheter-related complications, an ounce of prevention is worth a pound of cure. Precise placement of the catheter tip in the GDA stump at the junction of common hepatic artery and GDA ostia is essential as protrusion of the catheter tip beyond this junction may disrupt hepatic arterial flow and cause early thrombosis. Conversely, if the catheter tip leaves too much GDA stump between catheter tip and ostia, pooling of chemotherapy may occur, leading to local arteritis, pseudoaneurysm formation, or thrombosis. Thrombolytics and/or anticoagulants can be initiated to achieve salvage rates of approximately 30% [10].

Dose reduction algorithms based on the pharmacokinetics and pharmacodynamics of FUDR are critically important for prevention of sustained hepatocellular injury and AHF [10, 11, 20]. Typical dosing of FUDR via HAI begins at 0.12 mg/kg/day of ideal body weight in combination with dexamethasone for 14 days followed by 14 days of heparin/saline solution without FUDR [21]. Hepatic enzymes and bilirubin are measured prior to each administration of FUDR and for the heparin/saline alone refills to assess for liver or biliary toxicity. When enzymes or

Table 19.1 Hepatic arterial infusion floxuridine dose reduction algorithm

Liver blood test	Values	Values	FUDR dose
AST			
Reference range	≤50 U/L	>50 U/L	
Current value	0 to <3 × ref	0 to <2 × ref	100%
	3 to <4 × ref	2 to <3 × ref	80%
	4 to <5 × ref	3 to <4 × ref	50%
	≥5 × ref	≥4 × ref	Hold
If held, restart when	<4 × ref	<3 × ref	50% of last dose
ALP			
Reference	≤90 U/L	>90 U/L	
Current value	0 to <1.5 × ref	0 to <1.2 × ref	100%
	1.5 to <2 × ref	1.2 to <1.5 × ref	80%
	≥2 × ref	≥1.5 × ref	Hold
If held, restart when	<1.5 × ref	<1.2 × ref	25% of last dose
Total bilirubin			
Reference	≤1.2 mg/dL	>1.2 mg/dL	
Current value	0 to <1.5 × ref	0 to <1.2 × ref	100%
	1.5 to <2 × ref	1.2 to <1.5 × ref	50%
	≥2 × ref	≥1.5 × ref	Hold
If held, restart when	<1.5 × ref	<1.2 × ref	25% of last dose

Adapted from [15]

bilirubin are elevated, dose-reduction or holding of therapy is required to mitigate further hepatocellular or biliary injury (Table 19.1).

References

1. Klopp CT, Alford TC, Bateman J, Berry GN, Winship T. Fractionated intra-arterial cancer; chemotherapy with methyl bis amine hydrochloride; a preliminary report. Ann Surg. 1950;132:811. https://doi.org/10.1097/00000658-195010000-00018.
2. Sullivan RD, Jones R, Schnabel TG, Mc Shorey JC. The treatment of human cancer with intra-arterial nitrogen mustard (methylbis(2-chloroethyl) amine hydrochloride). Utilizing a simplified catheter technique. Cancer. 1953;6:121. https://doi.org/10.1002/1097-0142(195301)6:1<121::AID-CNCR2820060112>3.0.CO;2-6.
3. Sullivan RD, Norcross JW, Watkins E. Chemotherapy of metastatic liver cancer by prolonged hepatic-artery infusion. N Engl J Med. 1964;270:321. https://doi.org/10.1056/nejm196402132700701.
4. Kemeny NE, Niedzwiecki D, Hollis DR, et al. Hepatic arterial infusion versus systemic therapy for hepatic metastases from colorectal cancer: a randomized trial of efficacy, quality of life, and molecular markers (CALGB 9481). J Clin Oncol. 2006;24:1395. https://doi.org/10.1200/JCO.2005.03.8166.
5. Vasques F, Cavazza A, Bernal W. Acute liver failure. Curr Opin Crit Care. 2022;28:198. https://doi.org/10.1097/MCC.0000000000000923.
6. Reed ML, Vaitkevicius VK, Al-Sarraf M, Vaughn CB, Singhakowinta A, Sexon-Porte M, Izbicki R, Baker L, Straatsma GW. The practicality of chronic hepatic artery infusion therapy of primary and metastatic hepatic malignancies: ten-year results of 124 patients in a prospective protocol. Cancer. 1981;47:402. https://doi.org/10.1002/1097-0142(19810115)47:2<402::AID-CNCR2820470231>3.0.CO;2-B.
7. Barnett KT, Malafa MP. Complications of hepatic artery infusion: a review of 4580 reported cases. Int J Gastrointest Cancer. 2001;30:147. https://doi.org/10.1385/ijgc:30:3:147.
8. Doria MI, Riddell RH, Shepard KV, Levin B. Liver pathology following hepatic arterial infusion chemotherapy: hepatic toxicity with FUDR. Cancer. 1986;58:855. https://doi.org/10.1002/1097-0142(19860815)58:4<855::AID-CNCR2820580409>3.0.CO;2-6.
9. Power DG, Kemeny NE. The role of floxuridine in metastatic liver disease. Mol Cancer Ther. 2009;8:1015. https://doi.org/10.1158/1535-7163.MCT-08-0709.
10. Doussot A, Kemeny NE, D'Angelica MI. Hepatic arterial infusional chemotherapy in the management of colorectal cancer liver metastases. Hepat Oncol. 2015;2:275. https://doi.org/10.2217/hep.15.9.
11. Muaddi H, D'Angelica M, Wiseman JT, et al. Safety and feasibility of initiating a hepatic artery infusion pump chemotherapy program for unresectable colorectal liver metastases: a multicenter, retrospective cohort study. J Surg Oncol. 2021;123:252. https://doi.org/10.1002/jso.26270.

12. Song MJ. Hepatic artery infusion chemotherapy for advanced hepatocellular carcinoma. World J Gastroenterol. 2015;21:3843. https://doi.org/10.3748/wjg.v21.i13.3843.
13. Guo W, Gao J, Zhuang W, Wu Z, Li B, Chen S. Efficacy and safety of hepatic arterial infusion chemotherapy combined with transarterial embolization for unresectable hepatocellular carcinoma: a propensity score-matching cohort study. JGH Open. 2020;4:477. https://doi.org/10.1002/jgh3.12285.
14. Baek YH, Kim KT, Lee SW, et al. Efficacy of hepatic arterial infusion chemotherapy in advanced hepatocellular carcinoma. World J Gastroenterol. 2012;18:3426. https://doi.org/10.3748/wjg.v18.i26.3426.
15. Lewis HL, Bloomston M. Hepatic artery infusional chemotherapy. Surg Clin N Am. 2016;96:341. https://doi.org/10.1016/j.suc.2015.11.002.
16. Ensminger WD, Rosowsky A, Raso V, Levin DC, Glode M, Come S, Steele G, Frei E. A clinical-pharmacological evaluation of hepatic arterial infusions of 5-fluoro-2′-deoxyuridine and 5-fluorouracil. Cancer Res. 1978;38:3784.
17. Buchwald H, Grage TB, Vassilopoulos PP, Rohde TD, Varco RL, Blackshear PJ. Intraarterial infusion chemotherapy for hepatic carcinoma using a totally implantable infusion pump. Cancer. 1980;45:866. https://doi.org/10.1002/1097-0142(19800301)45:5<866::AID-CNCR2820450507>3.0.CO;2-3.
18. Sigurdson ER, Ridge JA, Daly JM. Fluorodeoxyuridine uptake by human colorectal hepatic metastases after hepatic artery infusion. Surgery. 1986;100:285.
19. Bacchetti S, Pasqual E, Crozzolo E, Pellarin A, Cagol PP. Intra-arterial hepatic chemotherapy for unresectable colorectal liver metastases: a review of medical devices complications in 3172 patients. Med Devices. 2009;2:31. https://doi.org/10.2147/mder.s4036.
20. Dizon DS, Schwartz J, Kemeny N. Regional chemotherapy: a focus on hepatic artery infusion for colorectal cancer liver metastases. Surg Oncol Clin N Am. 2008;17:759. https://doi.org/10.1016/j.soc.2008.04.009.
21. Homsi J, Garrett CR. Hepatic arterial infusion of chemotherapy for hepatic metastases from colorectal cancer. Cancer Control. 2006;13:42. https://doi.org/10.1177/107327480601300106.

Termination of Hepatic Arterial Infusion and Pump Removal

20

Samantha M. Ruff, Kelly Koch, Jashodeep Datta, and Alex C. Kim

Introduction

Hepatic artery infusion pump (HAIP) chemotherapy is becoming increasingly utilized as part of multimodal therapy to treat patients diagnosed with colorectal cancer liver metastasis (CRLM) and intrahepatic cholangiocarcinoma. The therapy entails surgical placement of an intraperitoneal catheter into the gastroduodenal artery attached to a chemoperfusion pump in the subcutaneous space. Following placement, chemotherapy (i.e., floxuridine or FUDR) is instilled into the pump and is infused directly to the liver via hepatic arterial flow. Recent studies have demonstrated an overall complication rate of approximately 25% [1]. HAIP-specific complications include pump/pocket infection, seroma, and hematoma, GDA pseudoaneurysm, hepatic artery dissection, catheter or arterial thrombosis, catheter erosion into viscera, pump malfunction, and biliary sclerosis. Such complications may result in termination of therapy and subsequent removal of the HAIP. Additionally, HAIP removal may occur due to disease progression, completion of therapy, or patient preference. This chapter will focus on complications as drivers of HAIP chemotherapy termination as well as indications and surgical technique for pump removal.

Samantha M. Ruff and Kelly Koch are co-first author.

S. M. Ruff
Division of Surgical Oncology, University of Virginia Health Systems, Charlottesville, VA, USA
e-mail: Samantha.ruff@osumc.edu

K. Koch
Department of Surgical Oncology, Sylvester Cancer Center/University of Miami/Jackson Memorial Hospital, Miami, FL, USA

J. Datta (✉)
Department of Surgery, Sylvester Cancer Center/University of Miami/Jackson Memorial Hospital, Miami, FL, USA
e-mail: jash.datta@med.miami.edu

A. C. Kim
Division of Surgical Oncology, University of Virginia Health Systems, Charlottesville, VA, USA

Division of Surgical Oncology, University of Texas Southwestern Medical Center, Charlottesville, Dallas, USA
e-mail: Alex.kim@utsouthwestern.edu

Complication-Related Indications for Termination of Therapy and Pump Removal

A variety of pump-specific complications may result in early termination of therapy and subsequent removal of the pump, which are detailed below. For a complete review of HAI-specific complications, see Chap. 10.

Pump Pocket Complications

Subcutaneous HAIP pocket complications including seroma, hematoma, or a wound infection occur in 8–18% of patients [2, 3]. Seromas are managed expectantly and rarely require any interventions. In cases of persistent collection, needle aspiration is therapeutic and HAIP pump removal is unneces-

M. D'Angelica, M. Lidsky (eds.), *Hepatic Arterial Infusion for Malignancy*,
https://doi.org/10.1007/978-3-031-74935-3_20

sary. Aspiration can occur while accessing the pump for instillation of saline or chemotherapy. Early postoperative hematomas are a result of bleeding from deep skin perforators to the fascia and occurs in approximately 1–5% patients [4–6]. Due to concerns for wound dehiscence and secondary infectious complication, significant hematomas are managed operatively with early clot evacuation and control of the bleeding source without pump removal. Minor bruising or minimal collections of blood can be managed conservatively.

Pump pocket infection is a dreaded complication that can result in pump removal. The infection can be a result of contamination from surgery, from needle access, or as a result of foreign body contamination from wound breakdown and seeding by skin flora. In the presence of cellulitis, oral or intravenous antibiotics often resolves the underlying infection. However, severe infection, including purulent fluid or wound dehiscence, is managed in the operating room. In the operating room, the primary goal is infection control, including potential pump removal. Alternatively, the HAIP may be salvaged in two ways. The first option is to disconnect the catheter intra-abdominally and splice it to a new catheter and pump with relocation of the pump site. This allows for partial replacement of the pump rather than complete removal. Alternatively, this can be performed extraperitoneally by cutting the catheter and tunneling it to a new pump pocket site where it can be spliced to a new pump. However, this can result in an infection at the new pump pocket site as well, especially if the catheter is contaminated. A second approach, which is more likely to be a temporizing measure, is to wash out the infected pocket with antibiotic solution (or betadine), but this almost always results in pump removal weeks to months later. The success rate of these techniques is anecdotal and remains unclear. Ulceration or erosion of the pump pocket through the dermis can prelude infection and should prompt resiting of the pump pocket to avoid further complications or removal of the HAIP. The most concerning part of infectious complications is interruption of therapy [2, 7, 8].

A retrospective cohort study conducted at City of Hope examining 75 patients receiving HAIP chemotherapy reported pump removal in 3% of cases [4]. In comparison, a retrospective review of 544 patients treated at Memorial Sloan-Kettering Cancer Center (MSKCC) revealed that 14 (2.6%) patients developed a pump pocket infection. Of these 14 patients, 4 patients developed a pump pocket infection within 30 days of placement (early infection) and 10 patients more than 30 days after placement (late infection). In the early infection group, 50% of pumps were able to be salvaged and in the late infection group, 40% were salvaged [5]. Furthermore, a multicenter review of 154 patients undergoing HAIP again demonstrated a similar 4.5% rate of pump pocket infection [6]. Although pump site infection is rare, it must be treated expeditiously with antibiotics and at times in the OR.

Vascular Complications

Vascular complications occur in less than 10% of patients and include pseudoaneurysms, arterial dissection, and thrombosis [2].

Pseudoaneurysm

Pseudoaneurysms can develop from dissection of the vessel wall following local trauma during HAIP vascular catheter insertion into the gastroduodenal artery (GDA). HAIP patients are at highest risk of a hepatic artery or GDA pseudoaneurysm from migration of the catheter (seen in 5–18% of patients) and/or pooling of floxuridine that can weaken the vessel wall [2, 9].

Erosion of the catheter through the GDA occurs in less than 3–5% of patients [10]. While most are incidentally discovered on restaging scans, in rare instances, patients can present with life-threatening emergency secondary to the ensuing GDA pseudoaneurysm. In this setting, intervention entails either coil embolization or placement of a covered metal stent in the common hepatic artery crossing the origin of the GDA, both of which render the HAIP nonfunctional [2]. Compared to the GDA, hepatic artery pseudoaneurysms are less common and are secondary to hepatic artery dissection and injury at the time of catheter placement [11–14]. Following vascular intervention, HAIP removal is considered, ideally, when a break in systemic therapy is appropriate.

Thrombosis

Another vascular complication is thrombosis of the hepatic artery that renders the HAIP nonfunctional, at which time pump removal may be considered. In the MSKCC series of 544 patients, arterial thrombosis was the most frequent complication. In total, 33 patients (6% of the study population) experienced arterial thrombosis with 13 patients developing an arterial thrombosis within 30 days of having the pump placed (31% of pumps were salvaged) and 20 experiencing the complication more than 30 days after placement (30% of pumps were salvaged). On average, thrombosis occurred 16 months after pump placement and mostly developed in the common hepatic artery [5]. Early thrombosis is usually related to catheter malposition (e.g., catheter tips terminates in the hepatic artery) [15]. The protrusion of the catheter tip into the hepatic artery from the GDA causes impedance of blood flow, increased turbulence, and ultimately thrombosis. Late thrombosis occurs secondary to placement of the catheter tip away from the GDA takeoff from the hepatic artery, which can result in stagnant flow of chemotherapy in the GDA, followed by sclerosis of the artery and subsequent thrombosis and propagation into the hepatic artery [14].

Pump and Catheter Malposition

There are several complications that are specific to having an indwelling foreign body. Migration or dislodgement of the catheter has been found in 5–18% of patients [2]. As discussed throughout this chapter, catheter migration can lead to GDA pseudoaneurysm or erosion into the nearby structures (like the duodenum) [2, 4, 16–19]. Following discontinuation of the Codman3000 HAIP, a few centers utilized the Medtronic SynchroMed™ II pump, often under FDA compassionate use approval. This pump requires splicing or linking of a native catheter to the Intera® vascular catheter prior to insertion. Anecdotally, there were isolated reports of catheter separation at the site of linkage, requiring an operative revision of the catheter and/or removal of the HAIP.

Erosion of the HAIP catheter into the duodenum has been previously reported. In these scenarios, catheter erosions were discovered via upper endoscopy incidentally or during workup for abdominal pain, gastrointestinal bleeding, and/or concern for bowel perforation [2]. This can result in pump removal secondary to infectious complications.

The HAIP can also become detached from the fascia and flip. This usually requires operative repair but can result in poor flow rates or injury to the catheter. If this cannot be salvaged, it may require removal of the pump. Occasionally, pump flow rates can change independent of a catheter obstruction and require either replacement of the pump (and splicing to the old catheter) or removal.

Extrahepatic Perfusion of Chemotherapy

One final pump-related complication that may necessitate removal is extrahepatic perfusion that cannot be corrected. Extrahepatic perfusion is often due to incomplete dissection of small periportal vessels that originate higher up on the hepatic arteries and carry blood away from the liver to other organs (e.g., posterior–superior pancreaticoduodenal artery off of the right hepatic artery). This can lead to downstream complications such as gastric or duodenal ulcers and pancreatitis. Vessels causing extrahepatic perfusion are commonly treated angiographically, but occasionally require surgery [20, 21], In the MSKCC study, 16 patients had extrahepatic perfusion (9 less than 30 days after placement with 100% salvaged, 7 more than

30 days after placement with 57% salvaged) [5]. Often the HAIP pump can be salvaged through interventional radiology procedures to embolize these vessels. If extrahepatic perfusion cannot be salvaged, termination of HAIP therapy is recommended, and then the pump may be removed to decrease the risk of further complications.

Biliary Complications

Biliary toxicity is the direct result of HAIP therapy and remains the most challenging complication (see Chap. 18 for complete review of chemotherapy-induced biliary sclerosis, CIBS). The hepatic artery is the dominant blood supply to the biliary tree. Due to the delivery of FUDR through the hepatic arterial system, the biliary tree is at risk of increased toxicity. Chemotherapy-induced injury to the bile ducts and subsequent inflammation lead to biliary strictures and sclerosis in approximately 2–8% of patients [2]. Due to the frequency of the complication, the addition of transarterial dexamethasone with FUDR is now standard, though the risk is not completely mitigated [22]. Interestingly, it is most commonly observed in adjuvant HAIP therapy following liver resection for CRLM [2]. Biliary injury or inflammation is suspected in the setting of persistently elevated liver function tests in asymptomatic patients. In severe cases, diagnostic imaging may demonstrate common bile duct or hepatic duct strictures with intrahepatic biliary ductal dilation [2, 23]. Severe cases usually require termination of HAIP therapy including HAIP removal and in some instances biliary stenting to decompress the biliary tree. In rare cases, patients may progress to hepatic failure despite immediate cessation of HAIP therapy [2].

In a multicenter retrospective study examining 154 HAIP patients, biliary sclerosis was observed in 8.4% [6]. Moreover, a study comparing patients who received systemic therapy and HAIP versus systemic therapy alone demonstrated a 6.7% rate of biliary sclerosis in HAIP patients and it was the cause of death in four patients [24]. The toxicity is increased with addition of other chemotherapy via HAIP including mitomycin C (MMC). A phase II study examining high-dose MMC (15 mg/m^2) in conjunction with FUDR demonstrated higher response rates at the expense of increased biliary complications including liver bilomas (7.9%), hyperbilirubinemia (22%), and biliary sclerosis (9.5%) [25]. As a result, delivery of concurrent HAIP chemotherapy with FUDR and MMC is not recommended.

Moreover, bevacizumab was identified as a significant risk factor for biliary complications. A review of 203 patients with HAIP from prospective studies found an association between the use of bevacizumab (VEGF inhibitor) in combination with HAIP chemotherapy and biliary toxicity. It is hypothesized that VEGF inhibitors may alter the normal hepatic vasculature and increase the permeability of vessels. The result is a greater influx of chemotherapy into the bile ducts resulting in significant cellular damage and inflammation. Secondary to the antiangiogenic effects of VEGF inhibitors, the healing process can also be impaired. Together, all these factors likely contribute to biliary strictures [23]. As such, the consensus recommendation is against concomitant bevacizumab therapy in HAIP patients due to significantly increased risk of biliary sclerosis and stricture.

Disease-Related Indications for Termination of HAI and Pump Removal

Disease Progression/Ineffectiveness of Therapy

Although hepatic artery infusion (HAI) is highly efficacious in well-selected patients, eliciting response rates of 24–81% for CRLM [26, 27] and 27–59% in patients with intrahepatic cholangiocarcinoma [28], a significant proportion of patients selected for HAIP chemotherapy will experience disease progression or treatment resistance. Some providers may continue HAI in the setting of extrahepatic progression, especially if the hepatic disease burden remains under control with HAIP chemotherapy but is thought to have the greatest impact on prognosis. However, hepatic progression suggests failure of HAI and the provider may terminate therapy, or at least transition to alternative strategies (increasing intensity of systemic therapy), while considering the risks of leaving the pump in place (complications noted in the first half of the chapter) versus the benefit of future clinical trial enrollment.

Completion of Therapy

Defining "completion of therapy" can be difficult. For patients with unresectable disease, much like systemic chemotherapy, hepatic artery infusion chemotherapy typically continues until progression (above), intolerance or unacceptable toxicity, conversion to resection, and/or complete response. Even in patients who convert to resection or are treated with adjuvant HAI, the pump is often left in place and maintained for future use if the patient experiences hepatic recurrence. If the pump is not actively delivering chemotherapy, it can be maintained with glycerin (Codman3000 or Intera3000) or heparinized saline (Medtronic SynchroMed™) to keep the pump functional for future therapy, akin to flushing a subcutaneous intravenous chemotherapy port. If no further HAIP chemotherapy will be delivered, such as in the scenario of biliary sclerosis, the pump may be removed. Moreover, the HAIP can also be removed at the time of liver transplantation (see Chap. 21), a treatment strategy for unresectable CRLM and intrahepatic cholangiocarcinoma that is becoming more frequent.

In patients deemed free of cancer, especially after many years, discussion regarding pump removal may take place. These conversations should be conducted with the patient following a multidisciplinary discussion, weighing the risk of long-term pump-related complications (e.g., infection or erosion) with hepatic recurrence. In the adjuvant setting, hepatic recurrences become very uncommon after 3 years and this is around the time to consider pump removal.

Patient Request

Although uncommon, patients also request pump removal for various reasons. A common scenario is a patient who is traveling great distances to the pump center for pump maintenance with low likelihood of using their pump in the future. Alternatively, some patients request pump removal due to pain related to abutment of the costal margin or anterior superior iliac spine, aesthetic concerns, or impairment in quality of life or daily intended activities.

Technical Considerations of HAIP Removal

In most instances of removal, it is only necessary to remove the pump itself. This is most often performed under MAC or general anesthesia. The pump pocket is surgically incised, entering the capsule to extract the device. The catheter is then ligated with a silk (or other nonabsorbable) suture with the end tacked to or placed beneath the anterior fascia to prevent catheter migration through the pocket incision. Once the pump is removed, the capsule is excised to facilitate healing and minimize the risk of seroma, with attention to leave the anterior rectus sheath intact. The capsule can also simply be fulgurated with cautery. If excision is done for infection, further debridement of the pocket may be necessary. The closure of the pump pocket is at the discretion of the surgeon.

In rare instances (e.g., persistent bacteremia or duodenal erosion), removal of the catheter may also be necessary. The catheter can be extracted from the GDA, typically after preemptive coverage of the GDA orifice with a covered stent.

Conclusion

HAIP removal is a straightforward procedure, often done as an outpatient, yet the decision to remove the pump is much more nuanced. While some complications are clear indications for termination of therapy and pump removal, such as biliary sclerosis, rescue from other complications, such as infection, can prolong the viability of the device and extend therapy. The surgeon, oncologist, and multidisciplinary team should assess both patient and disease-specific factors for each individual patient, as termination of HAIP chemotherapy and pump removal should be considered permanent. Only in rare circumstances can a new HAIP be implanted to resume therapy in the future.

References

1. Bacchetti S, Pasqual E, Crozzolo E, Pellarin A, Cagol PP. Intra-arterial hepatic chemotherapy for unresectable colorectal liver metastases: a review of medical devices complications in 3172 patients. Med Devices (Auckl). 2009;2:31–40.
2. Sharib JM, Creasy JM, Wildman-Tobriner B, Kim C, Uronis H, Hsu SD, et al. Hepatic artery infusion pumps: a surgical toolkit for intraoperative decision-making and management of hepatic artery infusion-specific complications. Ann Surg. 2022;276(6):943–56.
3. Brajcich BC, Bentrem DJ, Yang AD, Cohen ME, Ellis RJ, Mahalingam D, et al. Short-term risk of performing concurrent procedures with hepatic artery infusion pump placement. Ann Surg Oncol. 2020;27(13):5098–106.
4. Roybal JJ, Feliberti EC, Rouse L, Wagman LD. Pump removal in infected patients with hepatic chemotherapy pumps: when is it necessary? Am Surg. 2006;72(10):880–4.
5. Allen PJ, Nissan A, Picon AI, Kemeny N, Dudrick P, Ben-Porat L, et al. Technical complications and durability of hepatic artery infusion pumps for unresectable colorectal liver metastases: an institutional experience of 544 consecutive cases. J Am Coll Surg. 2005;201(1):57–65.
6. Muaddi H, D'Angelica M, Wiseman JT, Dillhoff M, Latchana N, Roke R, et al. Safety and feasibility of initiating a hepatic artery infusion pump chemotherapy program for unresectable colorectal liver metastases: a multicenter, retrospective cohort study. J Surg Oncol. 2021;123(1):252–60.
7. Creasy JM, Napier KJ, Reed SA, Zani S Jr, Wong TZ, Kim CY, et al. Implementation of a hepatic artery infusion program: initial patient selection and perioperative outcomes of concurrent hepatic artery infusion and systemic chemotherapy for colorectal liver metastases. Ann Surg Oncol. 2020;27(13):5086–95.
8. Chakedis J, Beal EW, Sun S, Galo J, Chafitz A, Davidson G, et al. Implementation and early outcomes for a surgeon-directed hepatic arterial infusion pump program for colorectal liver metastases. J Surg Oncol. 2018;118(7):1065–73.
9. Buisman FE, Grünhagen DJ, Homs MYV, Grootscholten C, Filipe WF, Kemeny NE, et al. Adjuvant hepatic arterial infusion pump chemotherapy after resection of colorectal liver metastases: results of a safety and feasibility study in The Netherlands. Ann Surg Oncol. 2019;26(13):4599–607.
10. Turley MC, Moore C, Creasy JM, Sharib J, Lan B, Thacker JKM, et al. Combined primary resection with hepatic artery infusion pump implantation is safe for unresectable colorectal liver metastases. J Gastrointest Surg. 2022;26(4):764–71.
11. Kemeny N, Huang Y, Cohen AM, Shi W, Conti JA, Brennan MF, et al. Hepatic arterial infusion of chemotherapy after resection of hepatic metastases from colorectal cancer. N Engl J Med. 1999;341(27):2039–48.
12. Liu LX, Zhang WH, Jiang HC, Zhu AL, Wu LF, Qi SY, et al. Arterial chemotherapy of 5-fluorouracil and mitomycin C in the treatment of liver metastases of colorectal cancer. World J Gastroenterol. 2002;8(4):663–7.
13. Samaras P, Pfammatter T, Pestalozzi BC. Hemorrhage associated with hepatic artery pseudoaneurysms after regional chemotherapy with floxuridine: case report. Int Semin Surg Oncol. 2008;5:17.
14. Strnad BS, Ludwig DR, Gilcrease-Garcia B, Fraum TJ, Shetty AS, Doyle MBM, et al. Contemporary imaging of the surgically placed hepatic arterial infusion chemotherapy pump. AJR Am J Roentgenol. 2021;217(3):633–43.
15. Leal JN, Kingham TP. Hepatic artery infusion chemotherapy for liver malignancy. Surg Oncol Clin N Am. 2015;24(1):121–48.
16. Cherqui D, Garden OJ, Bismuth H. Duodenal erosion complicating an implanted hepatic arterial access device. Br J Surg. 1988;75(6):556.
17. Pozniak MA, Babel SG, Trump DL. Complications of hepatic arterial infusion chemotherapy. Radiographics. 1991;11(1):67–79.
18. Maeshiro T, Miyamoto S, Umekita N, Fukutome A, Yamada F, Awane Y. Two cases of catheter tip dislocation to the duodenal bulb: a rare complication of hepatic arterial infusion chemotherapy. Gan To Kagaku Ryoho. 1995;22(11):1687–9.
19. Ha NB, Wang CW, El-Nachef N. An unusual mechanical cause of upper gastrointestinal hemorrhage. Gastroenterology. 2021;160(6):e1–4.
20. Talbot ML, Clark JR, Clingan PC, Morris DL. Gastroduodenal ulceration following hepatic arterial chemotherapy: the role of methylene blue endoscopy in the investigation of pain. HPB (Oxford). 2002;4(1):29–34.
21. Doria MI Jr, Doria LK, Faintuch J, Levin B. Gastric mucosal injury after hepatic arterial infusion chemotherapy with floxuridine. A clinical and pathologic study. Cancer. 1994;73(8):2042–7.

22. Kemeny N, Seiter K, Niedzwiecki D, Chapman D, Sigurdson E, Cohen A, et al. A randomized trial of intrahepatic infusion of fluorodeoxyuridine with dexamethasone versus fluorodeoxyuridine alone in the treatment of metastatic colorectal cancer. Cancer. 1992;69(2):327–34.
23. Cercek A, D'Angelica M, Power D, Capanu M, Gewirtz A, Patel D, et al. Floxuridine hepatic arterial infusion associated biliary toxicity is increased by concurrent administration of systemic bevacizumab. Ann Surg Oncol. 2014;21(2):479–86.
24. Srouji R, Narayan R, Boerner T, Buisman F, Seier K, Gonen M, et al. Addition of adjuvant hepatic artery infusion to systemic chemotherapy following resection of colorectal liver metastases is associated with reduced liver-related mortality. J Surg Oncol. 2020;121(8):1314–9.
25. Kemeny N, Eid A, Stockman J, Gonen M, Schwartz L, Tetzlaff E, et al. Hepatic arterial infusion of floxuridine and dexamethasone plus high-dose mitomycin C for patients with unresectable hepatic metastases from colorectal carcinoma. J Surg Oncol. 2005;91(2):97–101.
26. Karanicolas PJ, Metrakos P, Chan K, Asmis T, Chen E, Kingham TP, et al. Hepatic arterial infusion pump chemotherapy in the management of colorectal liver metastases: expert consensus statement. Curr Oncol. 2014;21(1):e129–36.
27. Chapelle N, Matysiak-Budnik T, Douane F, Metairie S, Rougier P, Touchefeu Y. Hepatic arterial infusion in the management of colorectal cancer liver metastasis: current and future perspectives. Dig Liver Dis. 2018;50(3):220–5.
28. Holster JJ, El Hassnaoui M, Franssen S, IJzermans JNM, de Jonge J, Mostert B, et al. Hepatic arterial infusion pump chemotherapy for unresectable intrahepatic cholangiocarcinoma: a systematic review and meta-analysis. Ann Surg Oncol. 2022;29(9):5528–38.

Transplant After HAI

21

Alejandro Pita, Federico Aucejo, and William C. Chapman

Introduction

In recent decades, liver-directed therapy via intra-arterial chemotherapy has become a well-established modality in the treatment of unresectable colorectal metastasis confined to the liver [1]. While the largest experience demonstrating improvement in overall survival has mostly originated from Memorial Sloan Kettering Cancer Center, recent multicenter studies have been aimed to corroborate these results. Hepatic artery infusion therapy has also been successfully utilized to downstage patients from unresectable to resectable disease, and it has shown encouraging results in the management of unresectable intrahepatic cholangiocarcinoma [1, 2]. Despite its proven benefits, a small portion of patients treated via hepatic artery infusion pump (HAIP) can develop complex complications such as biliary sclerosis (see Chaps. 18 and 19). If severe biliary sclerosis has occurred, liver transplantation would present a good option for the management of hepatic failure, simultaneously providing oncologic treatment. Similarly, patients having favorable response to HAIP therapy resulting in limited yet still unresectable disease can also potentially benefit from liver transplantation as a definitive intervention for residual disease. However, liver transplantation following treatment with intra-arterial chemotherapy can be technically challenging as a result of adhesion formation from repeated surgical manipulation and inflammatory reaction, most notably at the liver hilum. In this chapter, we will describe our experience with liver transplantation after treatment with hepatic artery infusion pump, including the indications, technical considerations, and overall outcomes.

Indications for Liver Transplantation

The administration of intra-arterial chemotherapy through surgically placed devices can be associated with both acute and long-term adverse effects. When these are not promptly diagnosed and adequately treated, these complications can have ominous consequences and potentially be an indication for liver transplantation as the only available treatment option. A critical example is the dose-dependent damaging effect that intra-arterial chemotherapy can have on the biliary tree. In the long-term, biliary sclerosis remains a

A. Pita (✉) · F. Aucejo
Department of General Surgery, Digestive Disease and Surgery Institute, Cleveland Clinic, Cleveland, OH, USA
e-mail: pitaa@ccf.org; AUCEJOF@ccf.org

W. C. Chapman
Section of Abdominal Organ Transplant, Department of Surgery, Washington University School of Medicine, Washington University, St Louis, MO, USA
e-mail: chapmanw@wustl.edu

M. D'Angelica, M. Lidsky (eds.), *Hepatic Arterial Infusion for Malignancy*,
https://doi.org/10.1007/978-3-031-74935-3_21

well-described complication of HAIP therapy, occurring in 5.5–8.4% of cases [3, 4]. In the early stages, mild symptoms can be managed with biliary stent placement, which can provide adequate symptomatic relief. When extensive biliary sclerosis develops, patients are at risk of recurrent cholangitis (Fig. 21.1), which may require the placement of percutaneous transhepatic biliary drains. Dose adjustments and concurrent intra-arterial steroid administration can be aimed at minimizing the risk of biliary complications; however, significant decreases in the amount or frequency of drug delivered can potentially compromise its effect on tumor control. The occurrence of biliary sclerosis can not only have a detrimental effect on the quality of life of these patients, but it can also have fatal consequences. As a result, these patients may require liver transplantation as a salvage treatment. Even in patients with limited residual intrahepatic disease, transplantation can be a viable treatment option for both the biliary complication and the metastatic disease. Unfortunately, the paucity of available organs remains an important limitation to the widespread utilization of liver transplantation as a potentially curative intervention in these cases. Living donor liver transplantation can be an excellent alternative option, since patients would not have to spend longer than necessary waiting for an organ to become available, and it would not impact the deceased donor pool.

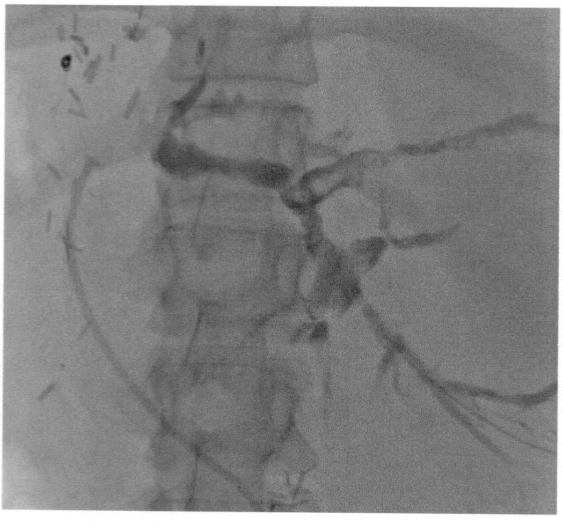

Fig. 21.1 Cholangiogram demonstrating alternating strictures and dilated segments secondary to HAIP therapy, with complete obstruction of the central left bile duct; status post right hepatectomy

Systemic chemotherapy regimens used for the treatment of disseminated colorectal metastases, often given in combination with HAIP therapy, have demonstrated hepatotoxic effects ranging from mild to severe. Mechanisms of hepatotoxicity include development of nonalcoholic fatty liver disease or steatohepatitis (NAFLD/NASH), sinusoidal obstruction syndrome, and potential progression to cirrhosis, although the exact mechanisms remain poorly understood [5]. When more advanced stages of fibrosis develop, patients can present with complications typically associated with cirrhosis, including portal hypertension with development of varices, splenomegaly, thrombocytopenia, and other complications of advanced liver disease, as it was the case for a patient undergoing deceased donor liver transplantation at a North American institution (Table 21.1, Patient #3). Liver transplantation can be offered in this setting, granted there is persistent lack of malignant disease progression during the process of transplant evaluation and while the patient remains on the waiting list.

HAIP therapy, in combination with systemic chemotherapy, has demonstrated utility in downstaging metastatic disease via conversion from unresectable to resectable disease [6]. However, some patients may demonstrate a good treatment response without complete conversion to resection. In the absence of either conversion to resection or complete radiologic response, patients who experience decreased yet persistently unresectable metastatic burden with good disease control after a period of surveillance can still be offered liver transplantation as a treatment modality. It is in these patients with limited yet persistent unresectable disease that liver transplantation can be considered. Transplantation protocols in these cases mirror those being developed for patients who show adequate response to systemic chemotherapy without receiving HAIP therapy. In general, in order to be eligible for transplantation, patients must have histologically confirmed unresectable liver metastasis, with adenocarcinoma of the colon or rectum resected with adequate margins at least 1 year prior to the planned date of liver transplant. Local recurrence on colo-

Table 21.1 Summary of findings in patients who underwent HAIP therapy followed by liver transplantation at two US institutions

Pt no.	Previous resection/therapies	Pre-LT PET findings	Indication for LT	Donor type and estimated blood loss	Grafts required for vascular reconstruction	Intraoperative complications	Viable tumor on explant	Recurrence
1	Two-stage hepatectomy including PV embolization; systemic chemotherapy	No residual disease	Biliary sclerosis/secondary sclerosing cholangitis requiring PTHC catheter drainage	LDLT EBL: 0.5 L	No	No	No	No (3 years post LT)
2	HAI used for downstaging, followed by partial right hepatectomy and multiple ablations; systemic chemotherapy	Periaortic lymph node with SUV 7.9. No additional evidence of metastatic disease	RFA leading to biloma and bleeding from HA, requiring embolization resulting in HAT, biliary necrosis requiring PTHC, portal vein thrombosis with development of portal hypertension	DBD-OLT EBL: 56 L	Cadaveric iliac vein graft from recipient SMV to donor main PV; aortic conduit with iliac artery graft from recipient right common iliac artery	Intraoperative death (right heart failure due to massive RA clot prior to implantation; hemodynamic collapse following reperfusion)	No. periaortic LN biopsy negative for malignancy.	NA
3	Left hepatectomy, MWA, external beam radiation; systemic chemotherapy	Hypermetabolic focus with SUV 8.3 in hepatic dome. No additional evidence of metastatic disease	Cirrhosis with portal HTN secondary to chemotherapy-induced hepatotoxicity. Persistent metastatic disease confined to the liver	DBD-OLT EBL: 25 L	Recipient splenic artery anastomosed end-to-end to donor celiac artery (no graft required)	No	Yes	Resection of one pulmonary metastasis 1 year after transplant. No further recurrence 3 years post LT
4	Laparoscopic ablation (x3), followed by open partial right hepatectomy; systemic chemotherapy	Non-FDG avid hypodense mass consistent with treated lesion	Chronic portal vein thrombosis with cavernous transformation, resulting in bleeding esophageal varices	LDLT EBL: 5.4 L	Cadaveric iliac vein graft from recipient coronary vein shunt	No	No	No (2 years post LT)

(continued)

Table 21.1 (continued)

Pt no.	Previous resection/ therapies	Pre-LT PET findings	Indication for LT	Donor type and estimated blood loss	Grafts required for vascular reconstruction	Intraoperative complications	Viable tumor on explant	Recurrence
5	Systemic chemotherapy	N/A	Acute decompensation; cholangiopathy	DBD-OLT EBL: 2 L	No	No	No	Yes (1.6 years RFS)
6	Partial hepatectomy (segment 4), Y90, immunotherapy	N/A	Cholangiopathy	DBD-OLT EBL: 2 L	No	Diaphragmatic injury due to adhesions—Needed diaphragmatic repair and right chest tube placement	No	No (1.4 years post LT)
7	Right hepatectomy, systemic chemotherapy, and immunotherapy	Multiple FDG-avid lesions throughout remnant left hemiliver	Persistent unresectable disease	DBD-OLT EBL: 7.9 L	No	No	Yes (3 viable lesions)	Yes (10 months RFS)
8	Left hepatectomy	N/A	Cholangiopathy	DBD-OLT EBL: 5.8 L	No	No	No	No (5 years post LT)
9	Left lateral sectionectomy	N/A	Cholangiopathy	DCD-OLT EBL: 1.5 L	No	No	No	No (4 years post LT)
10	Left lateral sectionectomy, immunotherapy for recurrence	No residual disease	Cholangiopathy	DBD-OLT EBL: 0.5 L	No	No	No	No (2 years post LT)
11	HAIP therapy alone	N/A	Persistent unresectable disease	DCD-OLT EBL: 0.25 L	No	Difficult dissection due to HAIP pump effect noted	No	No (5 months post LT)

LDLT living donor liver transplant, *DBD-OLT* orthotopic liver transplantation from a deceased from brain death donor, *DCD* deceased from circulatory death, *RFS* recurrence-free survival noscopy or pelvic imaging, or evidence of extrahepatic metastatic disease in the 12 months preceding liver transplantation would be considered a contraindication to transplantation. Tumor markers are also often included as part of the eligibility criteria, with a preferred level of carcinoembryonic antigen (CEA) of less than 80–100 ng/dL at the time of liver transplantation. Similarly, molecular and pathological factors might be taken into consideration as they can be associated with unfavorable outcomes, as is the case of BRAF V600E mutant tumors. Of note, RAS mutations have not been significantly associated with worse outcomes. Additionally, patients should receive at least 3–6 months of chemotherapy with no increase in the size or number of lesions. In order to assess the biological tumor behavior of the liver metastases, the International Hepato-Pancreato-Biliary Association (IHPBA) consensus guidelines recommend against liver transplantation if the metabolic tumor volume exceeds 70 cm^3 or total lesion glycolysis is greater than 260 g on pretransplant ^{18}F-FDG PET/CT [7]. Lastly, a good ECOG performance status (0–1) is required, with no significant weight loss or physical deconditioning in the months preceding transplantation. It should be clear that the role of transplantation for colorectal liver metastases is in its infancy and guidelines are in evolution.

As the field of transplant oncology continues to expand, centers have also established protocols for the treatment of intrahepatic cholangiocarcinoma through liver transplantation. Further, as the role of HAIP therapy in the treatment of intrahepatic cholangiocarcinoma continues to be defined, there is a possibility that liver transplantation will play a role in the management of complications associated with this treatment modality in future years.

Intraoperative Considerations

Liver transplantation in patients who have undergone HAIP placement can be extremely challenging due to the technical difficulty associated with the procedure. These patients have usually undergone multiple abdominal surgeries, including hepatic resections and HAIP placement; therefore, extensive adhesions are common (Fig. 21.2). The presence of portal hypertension can significantly contribute to intraoperative blood loss, as portosystemic collaterals that are disrupted during the dissection can bleed extensively. More importantly, the delivery of intra-arterial chemotherapy agents generally results in a significant inflammatory reaction within the hepatic hilum, making the dissection of the hilar structures challenging. In these cases, the sur-

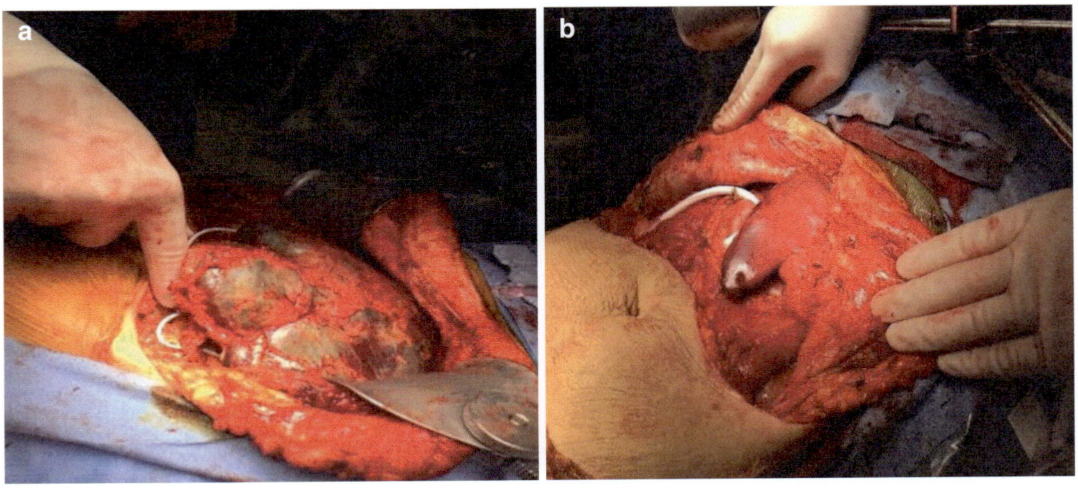

Fig. 21.2 Intraoperative findings during living donor liver transplantation following HAIP therapy. (**a**) Extensive adhesions, hilar inflammation, and scarring of the native liver. (**b**) Completion of left lobe graft liver transplant

geon might have to employ alternative techniques such as mass clamping of the hilum in order to expedite the hepatectomy, followed by dissection of the individual hilar structures after the hepatectomy has been completed. In three out of four patients undergoing transplantation in one of the centers, the mass clamping technique was utilized (Table 21.1, Patients 2–4), emphasizing the level of technical difficulty seen in these cases.

A well-described complication of HAIP placement is hepatic arterial thrombosis, which occurs in 1–2% of HAIP therapy cases [3]. Acute postoperative hepatic arterial pseudoaneurysms following HAIP placement that require percutaneous interventional radiologic procedures such as embolization, placement of covered stents, or reoperations can also result in the development of thrombosis. As a result, at the time of liver transplantation, the use of arterial grafts may be required for vascular reconstruction. Several techniques must be at the surgeon's disposal for arterial reconstruction, including placement of a supraceliac, infrarenal, or common iliac artery grafts, or the use of alternative inflow such as the splenic artery (Table 21.1, Patients 2 and 3).

Similarly, venous reconstruction might be required at the time of liver transplantation. While chronic portal vein thrombosis is not directly associated with HAIP therapy, it can occur in the setting of cirrhosis resulting from chemotherapy-induced hepatotoxicity, and it can add to the overall complexity of the transplant operation. Alternative portal flow inflow may be required in the cases where thrombectomy is not feasible, such as placement of a cadaveric iliac vein graft onto the SMV, large shunt, or renoportal interposition graft in the presence of a large splenorenal shunt (Table 21.1, Patients 2 and 4). As such, adequate preoperative planning is crucial to ensure the availability of alternative vessels in cases where reconstruction might be required. In the case of deceased donor liver transplantations, cadaveric arterial grafts should be accessible as they would be retrieved at the time of the procurement. For living donors, on the other hand, the availability of sufficient preserved cadaveric vessels must be ensured, as reconstruction might be required for both inflow and outflow of the graft.

In the specific case of chronic hepatic artery thrombosis, arterial collateralization from perihepatic structures (diaphragm, stomach, duodenum, and retroperitoneum) can be extensive. These collateral vessels tend to be diffuse and can also result in extensive bleeding throughout the procedure.

When evaluating the type of biliary reconstruction, intraoperative assessment of the distal common bile duct (CBD) by the surgeon should determine the feasibility of duct-to-duct reconstruction or if hepaticojejunostomy will be needed.

Due to the degree of difficulty associated with these cases, they should generally be performed at a time when experienced surgeons are readily available for assistance, and they should be reserved for large-volume centers with high level of expertise.

Postoperative Follow-Up

Liver transplantation for colorectal metastases in highly selected patients has been shown to have good survival outcomes, comparable to patients who undergo liver transplantation for other indications [7]. Currently, survival data on patients who were treated with HAIP therapy and subsequent liver transplantation are not available in the literature. In the combined experience of two US centers, seven out of ten patients who had HAIP therapy and successfully underwent liver transplantation have remained free of recurrent disease, although follow-up is limited. One of the three patients that experienced recurrence underwent posttransplantation pulmonary metastasectomy and is currently disease-free (Table 21.1, Patient 3). Considering the original extent of disease in these patients and the interventions required during the course of treatment, these results are promising. Future studies will be critical to reveal the long-term outcomes in these cases.

An important point of consideration is the correlation between the pretransplant imaging with

PET/CT and the pathology examination of the explanted organs (Table 21.1). Two out of six patients with available pretransplant PET/CT images had evidence of active intrahepatic disease based on imaging, and the same findings were confirmed on explant pathology. The PET/CT findings for the other patients correlated with the absence of viable intrahepatic malignancy on final pathology. These findings are encouraging, as they support the utility of HAIP therapy in achieving effective results in the management of metastatic liver disease.

Monitoring for complications following liver transplantation should follow routine posttransplantation protocols, with the addition of serial imaging and tumor maker checks for the long-term surveillance for recurrence of malignant disease. Some studies have shown decrease oncogenicity with the use of mTOR inhibitors for prolonged immunosuppression following liver transplantation. As a result, the immunosuppression protocol within the IHPBA consensus guidelines recommends conversion from calcineurin inhibition to mTOR inhibitor in the 4–6 weeks following liver transplantation [7].

Conclusion

The delivery of intra-arterial chemotherapy through surgically inserted devices have gained traction in recent years in the management of unresectable hepatic colorectal metastases, with encouraging results. Unfortunately, complications related to the use of HAIP therapy such as biliary sclerosis and hepatotoxicity can be severe, resulting in significant morbidity. When complications arise, or when patients with live-confined metastatic disease derive long-standing disease control yet remain unresectable, liver transplantation may be considered as a definitive and potentially curative option in adequate responders to regional and systemic therapy, with satisfactory overall outcomes.

References

1. Thiels CA, D'Angelica MI. Hepatic artery infusion pumps. J Surg Oncol. 2020;122(1):70–7. https://doi.org/10.1002/jso.25913. Epub 2020 Mar 25.
2. Cercek A, Boerner T, Tan BR, et al. Assessment of hepatic arterial infusion of floxuridine in combination with systemic gemcitabine and oxaliplatin in patients with unresectable intrahepatic cholangiocarcinoma: a phase 2 clinical trial. JAMA Oncol. 2020;6(1):60–7. https://doi.org/10.1001/jamaoncol.2019.3718.
3. Muaddi H, D'Angelica M, Wiseman JT, et al. Safety and feasibility of initiating a hepatic artery infusion pump chemotherapy program for unresectable colorectal liver metastases: a multicenter, retrospective cohort study. J Surg Oncol. 2021;123(1):252–60. https://doi.org/10.1002/jso.26270. Epub 2020 Oct 23.
4. Ito K, Ito H, Kemeny NE, et al. Biliary sclerosis after hepatic arterial infusion pump chemotherapy for patients with colorectal cancer liver metastasis: incidence, clinical features, and risk factors. Ann Surg Oncol. 2012;19(5):1609–17. https://doi.org/10.1245/s10434-011-2102-8. Epub 2011 Oct 12.
5. McWhirter D, Kitteringham N, Jones RP, et al. Chemotherapy induced hepatotoxicity in metastatic colorectal cancer: a review of mechanisms and outcomes. Crit Rev Oncol Hematol. 2013;88(2):404–15. https://doi.org/10.1016/j.critrevonc.2013.05.011. Epub 2013 Jun 17.
6. Kemeny NE, Melendez FD, Capanu M, et al. Conversion to resectability using hepatic artery infusion plus systemic chemotherapy for the treatment of unresectable liver metastases from colorectal carcinoma. J Clin Oncol. 2009;27(21):3465–71.
7. Bonney GK, Chew CA, Lodge P, et al. Liver transplantation for non-resectable colorectal liver metastases: the International Hepato-Pancreato-Biliary Association consensus guidelines. Lancet Gastroenterol Hepatol. 2021;6(11):933–46. https://doi.org/10.1016/S2468-1253(21)00219-3. Epub 2021 Sep 8. Erratum in: Lancet Gastroenterol Hepatol. 2021 Nov;6(11):e7.

Part VI

Starting a New Hepatic Arterial Infusion Program

22 Starting a New HAI Program: Building a Team

Andrew Crocker, Jason Castellanos, and Lee Ocuin

Team Recruitment

More so than most cancer treatments, implementation and delivery of hepatic arterial infusion pump (HAIP) chemotherapy requires intensive multidisciplinary collaboration. At every stage of programmatic development, a team-based approach with invested clinician leaders and well-educated support staff is necessary. For this reason, creating a multidisciplinary care team is one of the earliest steps in the process of developing a new HAIP program. The shared workflow, clinical decision-making, and consensus formed by members of the HAIP team is essential to success in the planning, patient selection, drug delivery, and follow-up for patients receiving HAIP therapy.

Physician team members should include surgical oncologists or transplant surgeons with expertise in related surgical fields (hepatopancreatobiliary, colorectal), medical oncology, radiology (diagnostic and interventional), and nuclear medicine. Exact team roles will vary by institution and practice location. Identification of team leaders and defining roles ensures clarity and continuity throughout the preoperative, intraoperative, and postoperative clinical course of these complex patients. In a survey completed in conjunction with the HAI Consortium Research Network (HCRN) assessing factors for establishing a successful HAI program, surgical and medical oncologists were ranked as the most crucial members of the multidisciplinary team [1]. Ultimately, the role of team lead is usually best assumed by the team member who is most invested in the development and success of the new program. Most frequently, this will be a surgical or medical oncologist [1–3]. Ideally, leadership is shared as it will maximize buy-in and allocation of resources between specialties, as the surgical, medical, and oncologic needs of the patient will evolve throughout a patient's treatment course.

Prior experience with HAIP therapy at outside institutions is an important but not absolute necessity for team leaders at any level. However, for those starting new programs who do not have direct experience with HAIP program implementation, site visits to more experienced centers are an important step prior to program activation and should be considered mandatory (see Chap. 26) [3–5]. In the survey by Cavnar and colleagues, site visits were felt to be "indispensable for

A. Crocker
St. Elizabeth's Medical Center, Boston, MA, USA
e-mail: andrew.crocker@steward.org

J. Castellanos
Department of Surgical Oncology, Fox Chase Cancer Center, Philadelphia, PA, USA
e-mail: Jason.Castellanos@fccc.edu

L. Ocuin (✉)
Division of Surgical Oncology, Lehigh Valley Topper Cancer Institute, Allentown, PA, USA

M. D'Angelica, M. Lidsky (eds.), *Hepatic Arterial Infusion for Malignancy*,
https://doi.org/10.1007/978-3-031-74935-3_22

knowledge, team building, and future questions" [1]. Notably, the majority of surgeons polled in this survey traveled off-site for training with respective medical oncology and clinic staff team members as part of their educational preparation prior to roll out. We strongly recommend a site visit with a multidisciplinary team to a high volume HAIP program to ensure team leaders have cohesive understanding of the clinical and logistical challenges with HAIP therapy planning, delivery, and use.

Support Staff

The inclusion and training of support staff is necessary for a successful HAIP team. Ideally, team members at all levels of care will maintain involvement throughout preparation, rollout, and troubleshooting for developing HAIP programs. Therefore, a conscientious and targeted approach toward recruitment of ancillary staff is important to facilitate this continuity of education and care. Departmental staff to include when building an HAIP team will vary by institution. Important team members can be divided into broad categories: pharmacy and infusion, operating room staff, and diagnostic and interventional radiology staff, including nuclear medicine. HAIP program team leaders should identify a lead pharmacist to assist with obtaining and maintaining an adequate floxuridine (FUDR) (or other agent) supply, as well as mixing chemotherapy for the HAIP and intervening refills, and ensuring proper storage of therapeutic agents. Protocols should be established and put in place to streamline this workflow including order sets for outpatient infusion and inpatient fills. The pharmacist is also tasked with ensuring appropriate FUDR and concurrent systemic therapy dosing based on established protocols. Infusion nurses should be trained on pump access and refill protocols. Nursing leadership and staff on the patient wards should also be engaged, trained, and educated on the management of these complex patients, including proper pump access and refill protocols as this may be required over the duration of a patient's treatment course. Most hospitals have general or service line-specific nurse coordinators and leads in the operating room (OR), and they are essential to ensuring proper equipment (e.g., HAIP and tapered catheters) is in adequate supply and available. Additionally, an OR team including a circulating nurse and scrub technician should be trained on the intraoperative pump priming and filling protocol. Both leading up to pump implantation and in the operating room, a device representative should be present to assist with education of staff and troubleshooting of pump-specific concerns. Utilizing representative expertise will help on several fronts: both with planning and actual pump insertion.

All patients are required to undergo a nuclear medicine pump flow scan (Tc-99-MAA pump study), whether on an inpatient or outpatient basis, and nuclear medicine leadership should be engaged on these protocols, which are similar to those used for planning for Y90 radioembolization [3, 6]. In the initial phase of program activation, a core member of the HAIP team should be prepared to perform the pump access and bolus of Tc-99-MAA. Lastly, interventional radiology should be engaged in the program as their expertise is important in the management of cases of extrahepatic perfusion identified on pump studies, preoperative or postoperative embolization of difficult to access accessory or replaced arteries, and rescue from complications such as GDA pseudoaneurysm.

Team Culture and Outreach

Prior to developing and implementing a successful HAIP program, a realistic understanding of peer experience and opinions toward HAIP therapy as a clinically valuable modality is essential. Put bluntly, if any members of the multidisciplinary team do not subscribe to the general viability and efficacy of HAIP therapy, it will be challenging to generate the necessary patient volume to gain adequate team experience and/or provide optimal patient care. This is especially true of team leaders in surgical or medical oncology who actively drive patient treatment decisions. While fostering open discourse and sharing of literature that supports HAIP therapy use can improve this situation, it is important to understand the opinions and clinical treatment patterns of your peers when deciding to undertake the development of an HAIP program. Similarly, nonaffiliated and community connections are essential for patient referral and sustained patient volume. Gauging clinical opinions toward HAIP chemotherapy and fostering outreach among community oncology faculty, regional private practices as well as smaller or community-based healthcare systems will increase the likelihood of smooth rollout and long-term survival of an HAIP program.

Conclusion

HAIP chemotherapy represents an important therapeutic tool in the management of well-selected patients with liver metastatic colorectal cancer and unresectable intrahepatic cholangiocarcinoma. Team planning and recruitment represents a crucial challenge in the development of a new HAIP program. Clearly defined team roles, team member experience, and overall team impression of the role of HAIP therapy, all will contribute toward program success. Ultimately, a collaborative and multidisciplinary team-based approach incorporating physician and support staff expertise at all levels will be most important in the development and implementation of a new HAIP program.

References

1. Cavnar M, Ghalambor T, Lidsky ME, et al. Considerations and barriers to starting a new HAI pump program: an international survey of the HAI Consortium Research Network. HPB. 2022;24(12):2104–11. https://doi.org/10.1016/j.hpb.2022.08.008.
2. Karanicolas PJ, Metrakos P, Chan K, et al. Hepatic arterial infusion pump chemotherapy in the management of colorectal liver metastases: expert consensus statement. Curr Oncol. 2014;21(1):e129–36. https://doi.org/10.3747/co.21.1577.
3. Creasy JM, Napier KJ, Reed SA, et al. Implementation of a hepatic artery infusion program: initial patient selection and perioperative outcomes of concurrent hepatic artery infusion and systemic chemotherapy for colorectal liver metastases. Ann Surg Oncol. 2020;27(13):5086–95. https://doi.org/10.1245/s10434-020-08972-y.
4. Muaddi H, D'Angelica M, Wiseman JT, et al. Safety and feasibility of initiating a hepatic artery infusion pump chemotherapy program for unresectable colorectal liver metastases: a multicenter, retrospective cohort study. J Surg Oncol. 2021;123(1):252–60. https://doi.org/10.1002/jso.26270.
5. Buisman FE, Grünhagen DJ, Homs MYV, et al. Adjuvant hepatic arterial infusion pump chemotherapy after resection of colorectal liver metastases: results of a safety and feasibility study in The Netherlands. Ann Surg Oncol. 2019;26(13):4599–607. https://doi.org/10.1245/s10434-019-07973-w.
6. D'Angelica MI, Correa-Gallego C, Paty PB, et al. Phase II trial of hepatic artery infusional and systemic chemotherapy for patients with unresectable hepatic metastases from colorectal cancer: conversion to resection and long-term outcomes. Ann Surg. 2015;261(2):353–60. https://doi.org/10.1097/SLA.0000000000000614.

Device and Drug Procurement

23

Thomas J. Chirichella III, Kelly J. Lafaro, and Jane S. Han

Hospital Support

Success begets success, so a strong start with adequate materials is important to building and maintaining momentum. Appealing to the business side of hospital administrators is important in garnering financial support of a hepatic arterial infusion (HAI) pump program. Representatives from a multidisciplinary team (including surgery, medical oncology, pharmacy, nuclear medicine, interventional radiology, and outpatient infusion center), as discussed in the previous chapter (Chap. 22), should contribute their unique perspectives. A carefully prepared and presented business plan includes the following:

1. Basic background information regarding HAI and systemic chemotherapy
2. Literature on how HAI can be used as neoadjuvant and adjuvant therapy for resected colorectal liver metastases
3. Literature on how HAI can provide durable disease control and, in some patients, convert unresectable colorectal metastases to resectable status
4. Literature on how HAI is used for unresectable intrahepatic cholangiocarcinoma
5. Synopsis of HAI outcomes and applicability to the local population
6. Anticipated patient accrual rate

Anticipated accrual should be backed by concrete evidence, such as the number of patients in one's current practice or referral base that would have been potential candidates for HAI. It is highly recommended to target a goal accrual rate of one to two patients per month for the first year, with 5% growth per year. This helps justify long-term commitment in the eyes of a hospital administrator who needs to support overhead cost, acquisition, and physician and hospital reimbursements.

Consider the effect of nonmaterial factors on cost and hospital reimbursement as well. The current CPT codes are as follows: 36260 for insertion of an implantable arterial pump, 36261 for revision of an implantable arterial pump, and 36262 for removal of implantable arterial pump. Furthermore, infusion center CPTs are as follows: 96425 for chemotherapy treatment more

T. J. Chirichella III (✉)
Department of Surgery, Mercy Health St. Elizabeth Youngstown Hospital, Youngstown, OH, USA
e-mail: tjchirichella@mercy.com

K. J. Lafaro
Department of Surgery, Johns Hopkins University School of Medicine, Baltimore, MD, USA
e-mail: klafaro1@jhmi.edu

J. S. Han
Department of Surgery, NYU Langone Hospital Brooklyn, Brooklyn, NY, USA
e-mail: janehan@alum.mit.edu

M. D'Angelica, M. Lidsky (eds.), *Hepatic Arterial Infusion for Malignancy*,
https://doi.org/10.1007/978-3-031-74935-3_23

than 8 hours and 96522 for refill and maintenance. Additional codes will apply to select patients, including 47562 (laparoscopic cholecystectomy), 47600 (open cholecystectomy), 38747 (portal lymphadenectomy), 47120 (partial hepatectomy), 47370 (ablation), 44207 (segmental colectomy), 45116 (proctectomy), and 44346 (creation of ostomy). Codes may vary for open versus laparoscopic/robotic approach.

Performance of a concurrent liver resection and/or ablation with the method of HAI pump placement (open versus robotic) may influence operative time and patients' hospital length of stay. If pump implantation is performed by a minimally invasive (e.g., robotic) approach, the CPT is considered an unlisted laparoscopic procedure (47379); however, the surgeon and coders will need to add the equivalent CPT code for an open case [1–4].

Nuclear flow testing must be readily accessible postoperatively, as it will be needed to confirm hepatic-only perfusion without nontarget extrahepatic perfusion from the pump. Nuclear medicine will need to acquire technetium-99 (Tc-99) isotope to inject the pump and confirm placement. Interventional radiology services may also be needed to exclude any extrahepatic perfusion. Finally, follow-up computed tomography (CT) scans should be obtained at 2–3-month intervals to assess response to therapy and restage the patients [5, 6].

Once the business plan is completed, it is essential to enlist the support of the section chief and/or Chair of Surgery prior to delivering the plan to the division/department administrator and ultimately to the hospital's supply chain market advisor.

Acquisition and Supply Chain

Currently, there is only one hepatic artery infusion therapy pump approved by the Food and Drug Administration (FDA)—the Intera 3000, manufactured by Intera Oncology (Wellesley, MA, USA). The hospital's supply chain market advisor will need to request a quote from the manufacturer for the pump and its accessories. The required materials specific to different departments (surgery, nuclear medicine, interventional radiology, and infusion center) will be required by the pump manufacturer: the hepatic artery infusion pump, silicone tapered catheter(s), special bolus needles (1–3/8″ and 2″) along with refill kit(s) and non-coring refill needles must be acquired.

Once a quote is obtained, hospital purchasing will review and clarify any questions or concerns with the pump manufacturer. It is advisable to ask the hospital staff for any requirements around supplier registration, credentialing, or any other deliverables that need to be completed prior to pump approval. The operating room (OR) staff then submits the quote to a value analysis committee or equivalent to begin the approval process.

Documentation is provided around reimbursement coding, pump specifications, and FDA approvals that will be requested from the pump manufacturer. A purchasing agreement/contract is drafted and sent to the pump manufacturer for review and negotiation—this process takes the longest amount of time. The hospital system and pump manufacturer lawyers will undergo several rounds of negotiations before an agreement is fully executed. Once approval is granted and signed by hospital administration, the agreement/contract is fully executed, and supplier registration is complete.

The supply chain marketing advisor must place the HAI pump order in advance of the first implantation surgery. As stated earlier in the business plan, the first order for the surgery department should include a pump, a backup pump, and two tapered catheters (rarely used but advisable to keep on the shelf as backup). Prior to the first implantation, nuclear medicine should also order a box of special bolus needles (in the event the extra needle that comes with the pump is misplaced or contaminated), the outpatient infusion center must order refill kits, and the pharmacy needs to obtain sufficient chemotherapy (floxuridine—FUDR) for the extent of the patient's expected treatment course (anticipate one vile of FUDR per month for 6 months). It should also be noted that one vile of FUDR is 500 mg and can be used for multiple patients, but has a shelf life of only 24 h after suspending the drug. This means patients should be scheduled on the same day in the treatment center, when possible, to maximize drug utilization and minimize waste. Once the orders are approved and supplies delivered, the surgeon can schedule the operation and notify the pump manufacturer. This allows the manufacturer to perform an in-service for all staff involved (OR staff, nuclear medicine, and chemotherapy infusion nurses), which will be discussed in an upcoming chapter (Chap. 25). The pump manufacturer will also send a clinical support expert to the new center for on-site support during the first and subsequent cases until the team is proficient and self-sufficient.

The time this process takes depends on the hospital and the different committees that must approve. Involving the division chief and administrator early on is helpful for navigating the nuances of a particular hospital's procedures and for connecting with proper contacts that will facilitate the creation of a HAI pump program. The support from the chief and administrator may also become key to overcoming unexpected barriers that can arise at any point along the approval process.

Drug Procurement

Currently, floxuridine (FUDR®) is the only approved chemotherapy for HAI pump use in the United States. While it is a very old chemotherapeutic agent, it is not on every hospital's formulary. The head of pharmacy at the hospital's infusion center will know whether FUDR is on formulary and can help complete a formulary request if it is not. Most formulary requests are online applications that require to following information:

- Generic/brand name
- Manufacturer
- Dosage forms
- Cost
- Indication
- Alternative medications that can be used
- Predicted number of patients that will be treated per month
- Justification for placement on formulary—citing literature

Large institutions may have an Oncology Specialty Panel that meets to approve a potential formulary request before it is forwarded to the hospital-wide formulary committee. Once FUDR is approved, the pharmacy buyer will contact the manufacturer to create an account. The manufacturer will send the pharmacy buyer documentation as well as a credit application to complete. Once these are returned and processed, the manufacturer will create an account for the hospital and provide the pharmacy buyer with the order form used to purchase the FUDR. It is important that this process be completed prior to scheduling the first HAI pump placement.

Depending on how the pharmacy, infusion center, and medical oncologists wish to proceed, the pharmacist may need to create a "chemotherapy treatment plan" in the electronic medical record. This plan will need to include FUDR dosing as well as heparin/saline and dexamethasone dosing. Glycerin dosing should also be included in this build. See Chap. 11 for full details on HAI drugs.

Conclusion

Starting a HAI pump program differs for each hospital or hospital system, so the business plan should be appropriately tailored. However, the basic tenants remain regardless of the environment. It is imperative to have a team of people involved in the planning and organizing from the beginning, often with a surgeon as the lead, and inclusive of representatives from medical oncology, pharmacy, nuclear medicine, interventional radiology, and the infusion center. It is critical to have all aspects of the program approved and to have the pumps, supplies, and infusion drug physically in the hospital prior to scheduling the first surgery.

References

1. Centers for Medicare and Medicaid Services, CPT/HCPCS codes. www.cms.gov/medicare/regulations-guidance/physician-self-referral/list-cpt/hcpcs-codes.
2. Thiels CA, D'Angelica MI. Hepatic artery infusion pumps. J Surg Oncol. 2020;122(1):70–7. https://doi.org/10.1002/jso.25913. Epub 2020 Mar 25. PMID: 32215927; PMCID: PMC9014308.
3. Qadan M, D'Angelica MI, Kemeny NE, Cercek A, Kingham TP. Robotic hepatic arterial infusion pump placement. HPB (Oxford). 2017;19(5):429–35. https://doi.org/10.1016/j.hpb.2016.12.015. Epub 2017 Jan 26. PMID: 28132735; PMCID: PMC5633044.
4. Buisman FE, Homs MYV, Grünhagen DJ, et al. Adjuvant hepatic arterial infusion pump chemotherapy and resection versus resection alone in patients with low-risk resectable colorectal liver metastases—the multicenter randomized controlled PUMP trial. BMC Cancer. 2019;19:327. https://doi.org/10.1186/s12885-019-5515-6.
5. Napier KJ, Lidsky ME, James OG, Wildman-Tobriner B. Hepatic arterial infusion pumps: what the radiologist needs to know. Radiographics. 2021;41(3):895–908.
6. Bailey JJ, Dewaraja Y, Hubers D, Srinivasa RN, Frey KA. Biodistribution of 99mTc-MAA on SPECT/CT performed for 90Y radioembolization therapy planning: a pictorial review. Clin Transl Imaging. 2017;5(5):473–85. https://doi.org/10.1007/s40336-017-0245-8. Epub 2017 Sep 11. Erratum in: Clin Transl Imaging. 22 March 2018; https://doi.org/10.1007/s40336-018-0273-z. PMID: 29423383; PMCID: PMC5798624.

Regulatory and Safety Issues Surrounding Hepatic Arterial Infusion Devices: The Past, Present, and Future

24

Charles J. Schneider, Benjamin A. Bleiberg, Hannah G. McDonald, and Michael J. Cavnar

Early Hepatic Arterial Infusion Devices With and Without Regulatory Oversight

Implantable drug delivery systems are surgically placed devices that provide a mechanism for administering drugs in therapeutic concentrations to a specific target tissue. By focusing a pathology-altering treatment on the affected organ or disease-site, these devices should ideally provide local disease-control while limiting toxicity from often deescalated systemic therapy. All the while, the properly devised device and medication it delivers should not preclude the ability to concurrently administer intravenous and/or non-intravenous treatments, although dosage or schedule limitations may be necessary depending on the expected cumulative toxicity to the treated organ from the combination of localized and nonlocalized therapies.

To understand relatively recent regulatory issues surrounding hepatic artery infusion (HAI) devices, we must first understand the history of hepatic artery infusion and the evolution of pump infusion systems. The first modern implantable drug-reservoir delivery system was tested in Folkman and Long's studies of antiarrhythmic drug delivery in canine models of heart block with a silicone rubber reservoir coupled with a semipermeable membrane in close proximity to the ventricular myocardium [1]. This specific application had limited success and a concerning safety profile, and as such was not advanced to human trials. However, studies in canine models demonstrated the practicality of directed drug delivery systems, leading to expansion of these approaches to the realm of human medicine and cancer treatment, with liver-directed chemotherapy delivered through the hepatic artery developing as a specific research and treatment focus during this timeframe.

Dr. Bierman was credited with the first administration of generalized arterial chemotherapy in which he accessed the aorta percutaneously through the brachial artery for delivery of nitrogen mustard in 1950 [2]. Meanwhile, understanding of the physiologic mechanism supporting HAI therapy was evolving, based on experiments performed in a rabbit model. These showed that the primary blood supply of liver metastases is the hepatic artery, in contrast to normal liver tissue, which is supplied predominantly by the portal vein [3]. By the early 1960s, percutaneous and transabdominal approaches had been developed

C. J. Schneider · B. A. Bleiberg
Department of Medicine, University of Pennsylvania Pearlman College of Medicine, Philadelphia, PA, USA
e-mail: Charles.Schneider@pennmedicine.upenn.edu; Benjamin.Bleiberg@pennmedicine.upenn.edu

H. G. McDonald · M. J. Cavnar (✉)
Department of Surgery, University of Kentucky College of Medicine, Lexington, KY, USA
e-mail: hannah.mcdonald@uky.edu; michael.cavnar@uky.edu

M. D'Angelica, M. Lidsky (eds.), *Hepatic Arterial Infusion for Malignancy*,
https://doi.org/10.1007/978-3-031-74935-3_24

for administration of HAI therapy [4]. In 1963, external spring-driven pumps were designed for experimental use of HAI therapy. These 340-g devices were secured by a harness and utilized a hand wound mechanism similar to a mechanical watch, delivering the drug from a 25-mL reservoir via polyvinyl tubing. The drug was delivered on an 8-h schedule, and allowed for prolonged arterial infusion for up to 7 days. However, these devices were prone to malfunction and user error, and were vulnerable to disruption with activity [5].

In 1977, the first human underwent administration of regional intra-arterial infusion of chemotherapy for colorectal metastases to the liver through a fully implantable infusion pump utilizing the Shiley Infusaid pump system, produced by a subsidiary of Pfizer [6]. A key distinction of implantable pumps as compared to their external spring activated predecessors was a reliance on vapor pressure from evaporating fluorocarbons in the pump bellow to generate the force needed to provide a steady infusion rate. The first published report providing long-term follow-up of liver-directed chemotherapy utilized a trans-brachial approach to cannulate the hepatic artery, with an infraclavicular refillable drug reservoir. This two-patient case series demonstrated no technical mishaps or device malfunction at 7–10 weeks of follow-up for either patient [7]. Subsequent studies demonstrated the practicality and reliability of implantable, percutaneous refillable infusion pumps for the durable delivery of HAI therapy. An early study of five patients with Infusaid systems treated up to 29 weeks noted no pump malfunction, with adverse events during the study period exclusively associated with FUDR toxicity. [8]

By 1981, trials of implanted drug delivery systems for hepatic artery infusional (HAI) delivery of chemotherapy soon followed utilizing direct access of the hepatic artery, which became standard of care in the following years. As in the Cohen two-patient case report, other early HAI trials involved patients with unresectable colorectal cancer liver metastases and utilized the same Infusaid pump (Shiley) system [9–11]. The Infusaid model 100 device became commercially available in March 1982 to administer 5-fluorodeoxyuridine (FUDR) and obtained FDA approval that year for hepatic artery and IV antibiotic administration. Although the initial Infusaid model 100 was suitable for direct hepatic artery catheterization and implantation, it was ultimately upgraded (Infusaid model 400) with an improved catheter flushing system, allowing for more reliable administration of liver-directed FUDR. These Infusaid pump models were characterized by the innovative use of a gas–liquid propellant system harnessing body temperature rather than a battery to create a driving pressure source, reducing a potential cause of pump failure, decreasing maintenance, and reducing risks of alterations in the rate of drug delivery, which persisted in subsequent infusion pumps [12]. The new and improved Infusaid model 400 pump (Fig. 24.1) was approved by the FDA in 1992 for both the administration of FUDR for hepatic metastases, as well as for site-specific heparin administration in recurrent venous thromboembolic disease. In March 1996, a second manufacturer, Arrow International, gained FDA approval for their internalized Arrow 3000 HAI pump system. The Arrow pump system, while mechanistically similar to the Infusaid pump, was not widely adopted and the company closed in 2002 [13].

At that time, the largest trial included 20 patients who underwent implantation with the Infusaid pump, and identified only six relatively minor device safety issues including three catheter migrations requiring repositioning in two patients, and three broken catheters requiring catheter replacement over a course of 3210 patient days. During the study treatment period, there were no documented catheter occlusions or pump malfunctions [9]. A follow-up trial of 22 patients with liver-only metastatic colorectal cancer (mCRC) treated with FUDR administered through an Infusaid pump alternating every 2 weeks with a saline solution system demonstrated a >50% reduction in the size of metastatic

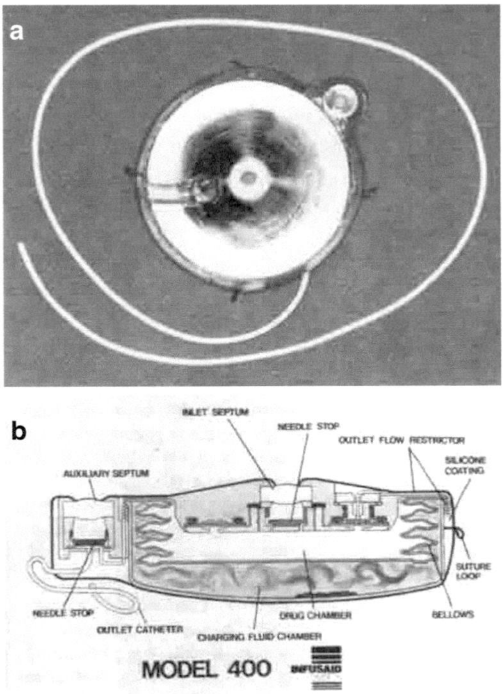

Fig. 24.1 (**a**) Infusaid Model 400 pump and attached infusion catheter. (**b**) Schematic of internal components of Infusaid 400 pump including drug chamber and charging fluid chamber which drives flow by expanding with body heat. (Used with permission, Baker, S.R., Wheeler, R.H., Ensminger, W.D., Niederhuber, J.E., 1981. Intraarterial infusion chemotherapy for head and neck cancer using a totally implantable infusion pump. Head & Neck Surgery 1981 Nov-Dec;4(2):118–24)

lesions in 22% of patients and <50% reduction in an additional 18% of patients. This combined cohort of "pump responders" had a mean survival of 13.6 months as compared to the 11.1 months for the 59% of patients who did not have a >50% reduction in liver metastatic disease burden. Implantation complications included three patients developing seromas, and two requiring pump removal for refractory pump pocket infections. One patient experienced catheter thrombosis requiring reinsertion of a new pump, one had chemotherapy extravasation into the abdominal cavity, and one required a repeat laparotomy due to catheter dislodgement. Although this trial did not demonstrate a significant survival benefit, it did demonstrate the reliability of the Infusaid pump system to deliver drug effectively with a tolerable safety profile, and with local disease-regression noted in 41% of patients as described above [14].

Despite this efficacy, case reports emerging in 1981 highlighted associations of these early pump systems with several adverse events related to patient-specific alterations or variations in gastroduodenal artery perfusion, leading to extrahepatic administration of chemotherapy and gastric or duodenal ulcer formation. For instance, isolated cases of duodenal atony resulting from this extrahepatic infusion of FUDR into the duodenum were described, and reportedly reversed with subcutaneous administration of urecholine [15, 16]. In another study of 40 patients with Infusaid pump-delivered FUDR, the symptom of abdominal pain was related to gastroduodenal ulcerations in 19 patients, and erosion of the infusion catheter into the duodenum in two patients [17]. Larger studies monitoring safety by Ramming et al. demonstrated no issues with pump malfunction or catheter clotting in a 2-year follow-up of 55 patients, but did identify a troubling number of gastric ulcers (24%), duodenal ulcers (7%), small bowel obstructions (2%), transaminitis (24%), sclerosing cholangitis (2%), and duodenal atony requiring gastroenterostomy (2%). Despite these complications, 88% of patients had a >50% reduction in pretreatment carcinoembryonic antigen (CEA) level, and the median survival from time of diagnosis of hepatic metastases and the time of pump implantation was 19.2 months and 10.1 months, respectively [18].

A similar case series of 55 patients treated with FUDR using the Infusaid pump was notable for the development of elevated liver enzymes not associated with disease progression in 96% of patients, biliary toxicity in 56% of patients, biliary sclerosis documented radiographically in 29% of patients, and acalculous cholecystitis in 9.1% of patients. In this study, no patients experienced gastroduodenal ulceration, which they attributed to improvements in hepatic arterial cannulation procedures decreasing rates of gut malperfusion and subsequent ischemia [19]. More aggressive vessel ligation minimizing extrahepatic delivery of hepatic-directed therapies also gained favor and was associated with decreased off-target organ injury. Further studies noted that the rates of technical complications associated with pump implantation and cannulation declined with surgeon experience, from 37% in surgeons who had completed <10 procedures to 7% for surgeons who had completed >10 procedures [20].

Despite these associations with adverse events, the FDA-approved Infusaid model 400 pump system was widely utilized over the following years including in the randomized controlled trial by Kemeny et al. [21], comparing adjuvant HAI with systemic chemotherapy vs. systemic chemotherapy alone for colon cancer patients after resection of liver metastases. A review of published complications from 1950 to 2001 reflecting combined safety data from 101 studies accounting for 4580 patients noted a mortality rate of 1% with 22% of patients experiencing GI symptoms, 19% suffering from chemical hepatitis, and 8% demonstrating bone marrow toxicity. Regarding the catheter itself, the most common complications appreciated were hepatic artery occlusion (6%), catheter thrombosis (5%), and catheter displacement (7%) [22]. These persistent safety issues despite decades of experience paved the way for the development of new devices with improved safety profiles and eventual discontinuation of the Infusaid pump, which fell out of favor with clinicians largely due to the high complication rates listed here.

The Codman 3000 Pump: Earning Sole FDA Approved Due to Improved Safety

Over time, the dominant HAI delivery device became the Codman 3000 pump (Fig. 24.2), which was FDA approved in 1996 and manufactured by Cerenovus, a subsidiary of Johnson & Johnson. While this pump utilized a gas–liquid propellant system similar to prior pump systems, it differed from prior models structurally with a raised, more easily accessible septum, and a safety valve-equipped bolus pathway [23]. The primacy of this pump was cemented following the pump's utilization in the 2009 phase I trial by Kemeny et al., demonstrating impressive efficacy of HAI in patients with unresectable liver metastases and ultimately becoming the only FDA-approved device for HAI therapy delivery. A multisite follow-up of 154 patients who underwent Codman 3000 pump placement between 2003 and 2017 demonstrated that 14% of patients developed acute pump-related complications including infection (4.5%), hematoma (1.3%), and catheter occlusion or dislodgement (1.9%). A total of 11% of patients developed a "late" pump-related complications during long-term follow-up, most notably biliary sclerosis that was seen in 8.4% of patients [24]. A 2009 Cochrane review of 1277 patients from 10 randomized clinical trials of HAIP for unresectable colorectal liver metastasis demonstrated significantly higher response rates for HAI therapy compared to systemic chemotherapy (43% vs. 18% with a pooled risk ratio of response of 2.26), but without significant improvements in overall survival (15.9 vs. 12.4 months). Long-term HAI pump complications in this cohort included duodenal ulcers (0.6%), delayed pump site infection (1.3%), and pump migration (0.6%) [24]. Overall, in comparison with the Infusaid pump, the Codman pump offered a safer delivery system with a much lower incidence of serious complications and toxicity, along with generally improved efficacy.

Given the apparent superiority of the Codman pump in effectiveness and safety, the Codman 3000 pump emerged as the only FDA-approved device for delivery of intrahepatic chemotherapy infusion, from June 1, 2014, to its discontinuation on April 1, 2018. The package insert noted the following potential risks associated with the device: catheter thrombosis, bolus path

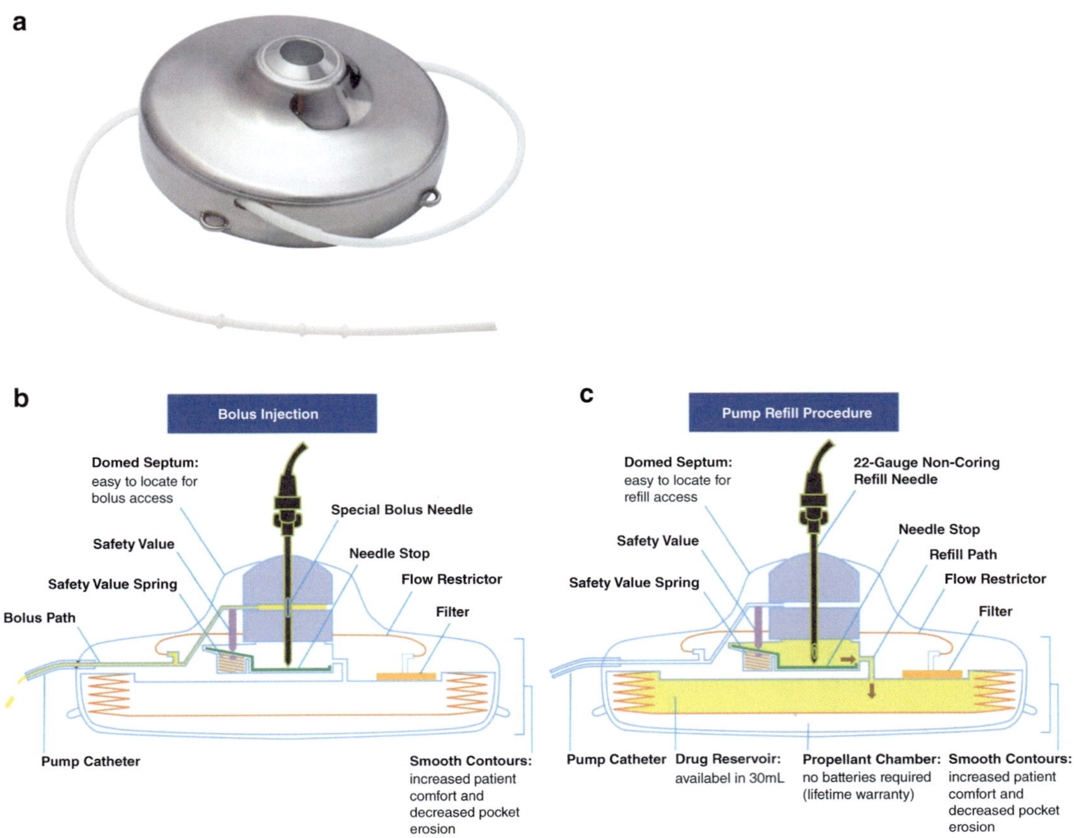

Fig. 24.2 The Intera 3000 and Codman 3000 hepatic artery infusion pump. (**a**) The Intera 3000 pump is identical to the previous Codman 3000 pump, featuring pump/reservoir pre-attached to the silicone vascular catheter fitted with beads for intravascular securement. Bolus injection and pump refill are accomplished via the same access diaphragm on the pump's raised septum but accomplished with different needles. For bolus injection (**b**), a needle with a side hole allows direct infusion into the catheter, while a needle with its hole situated at the end fills the 30 mL drug reservoir shown in yellow (**c**). Surrounding the expandable drug reservoir bellows is a propellant chamber containing Freon, which expands with body heat, driving the drug through a flow restrictor accomplishing a 1.2–1.3 mL per day flow rate. ()

occlusion, vessel thrombosis, pump dislodgement, seroma, recurrent hematoma, infection, extravasation, catheter shear, dislodgement, leakage, and migration. A 2014 FDA commentary on implantable infusion pumps details approvals for the Codman 3000 HAI pump as well as an array of non-liver-directed pump systems. Examples of these include the Medtronic Synchromed pump (approved in 1991) and the Prometra II pump (approved in 2012) designed for intrathecal administration of agents such as baclofen and morphine for chronic pain and spasticity [12]. This commentary established a consensus agreement with a 2013 NCI summary statement describing the medical necessity of implantable hepatic infusion pumps for patients with primary liver cancer and metastatic colorectal cancer.

Codman 3000 Pump Discontinuation: An "Orphan" Device Crisis Leading to International Uproar

On April 1, 2018, Cerenovus ceased production of the pump and provided a letter notifying physicians of this decision 3 days later, citing "raw material supply constraints within the manufacturing process" as the main determinant leading to discontinuation. On further queries from physicians and the media, the company noted low sales with an estimated 300 pumps sold to institutions in the United States annually as well as challenges identifying suppliers of highly specialized essential materials like the titanium rods utilized within the pump, making further production unsustainable [25]. In response, physicians cited promising phase I and II randomized controlled trials, expressing optimism for the increased utilization of HAI pumps in patients with hepatic colorectal metastases as well as ethical concerns regarding the abrupt discontinuation of the sole FDA-approved device without a comparable alternative in development. Physicians involved directly in HAI therapy programs at major academic centers noted that while the decision of a publicly traded medical device company to concentrate limited resources to potentially more widely applicable (and profitable) avenues was defensible from a business perspective, the lack of coordination with physicians and regulators to explore and identify alternatives prior to discontinuation could be considered unethical [26]. In abruptly discontinuing an essential product without advanced warning to physicians and patients, the company could be seen as violating the medical ethics principle of improper termination of a patient relationship and disregarding the impact of pump discontinuation on patients.

Despite efforts from physicians and patient advocacy groups including many patients who had personally benefitted from pump implantation and HAI, the Codman pump's production was halted as scheduled in 2018 and the remaining stockpiles of the device were exhausted later that year. Physicians appealed to medical device companies and healthcare industry regulators that to avoid future similar situations, device manufacturers should reaffirm their commitment to maintaining supplies of narrow indication devices. Additionally, a plea was made for minimum time requirements between device discontinuation and product cessation, potentially with oversight from an independent ethical group or FDA subcommittee. Lastly, physician groups requested consideration of economic incentives not just for narrow indication device research but also for maintenance [26]. Clinicians were called upon to reinforce the body of evidence supporting these devices more effectively with ongoing comparative effectiveness trials against newer therapies to ensure their continued production [26].

Medtronic Pump with Codman 3000 Catheter "Solution": An Off-Label "Hybrid" Device Pleading for Regulatory Oversight

At the time of the Codman pump's discontinuation, physicians had identified a pump from Medtronic medical devices, the Medtronic Synchromed II, approved for intrathecal medication infusion, as the most similar product available in the market. A previous generation of this pump had hepatic intra-arterial administration of FUDR listed as an indication, but it never achieved a substantial market share due to dominance of the Codman pump. Thus, when the Synchromed II (Fig. 24.3) was released, an FDA indication for this new Medtronic device was not pursued. As such, this pump notably lacked the style of the extended, beaded arterial catheter associated with the Codman pump (Fig. 24.2) as it was not intended for intra-arterial placement and usage. Of interest and particularly applicable to the Codman pump

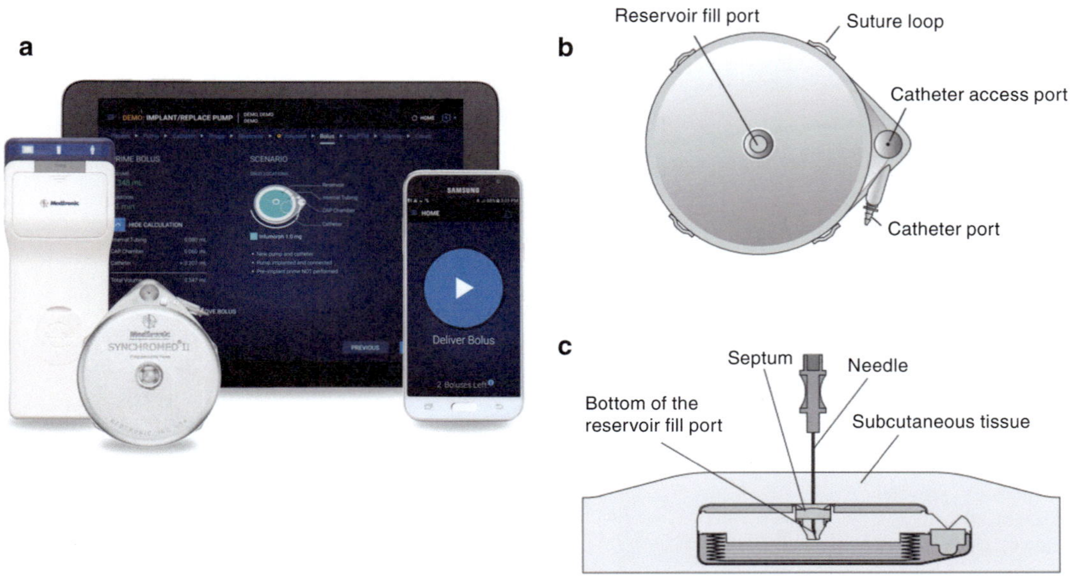

Fig. 24.3 The Medtronic Synchromed II pump. (**a**) The Synchromed II pump is a Bluetooth enabled device with a programmable rate using a Samsung tablet or smartphone. (**b**) The pump has a port for reservoir refill in the center and a catheter access side port for direct infusion. Inadvertent bolus during a refill procedure is prevented by the larger caliber of the refill needle. (**c**) Side view of the pump showing the reservoir during access for refill. (© Medtronic 2020. All rights reserved. Used with permission from Medtronic)

discontinuation dilemma is that during the course of a previous clinical trial using the Codman pump at Memorial Sloan Kettering Cancer Center, a production shortage made this pump unavailable for a period of time. Out of necessity, in order to avoid a prolonged hold on the trial, the physicians leading that trial decided to employ an off-label combination of the Medtronic Synchromed II pump with the Codman vascular catheter, the latter of which was available as a stand-alone product. After discontinuation of the Codman 3000 pump in 2018, as several centers began to consider reintroducing this off-label combination, Medtronic issued a statement advising physicians to "use their best clinical judgment when evaluating the use of any commercially available pump outside its labeling" [25]. This led to the current off-label use of the Medtronic pump retrofitted with a Codman arterial catheter (further referred to as MCHP; Fig. 24.4) for HAI chemotherapy administration.

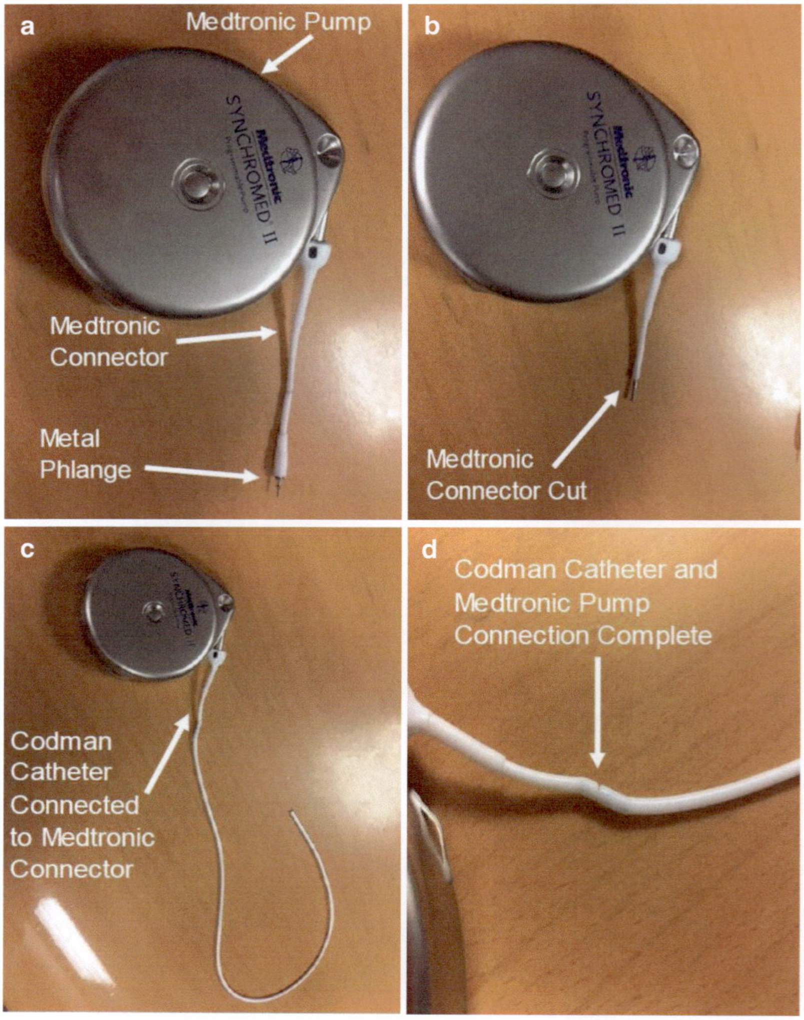

Fig. 24.4 The hybrid Medtronic Synchromed II pump/Codman vascular catheter. (**a**) The Synchromed II pump is connected to the Medtronic Sutureless connector. The Sutureless connector has been cut in half and the Codman metal splice connector inserted (**b**), then connected to the stand-alone Codman vascular catheter (**c**) and (**d**). After connection, silk ties are placed on either side of the connector to prevent disconnection (not shown). (Personal pictures used with permission from Dr. Nancy Kemeny)

Off-Label Usage of Medical Treatments and Devices: General Considerations and Risk

Off-label use occurs when physicians identify an opportunity to use a medication or device approved for an indication differing from the indication being treated in order to address an unmet patient need [27]. Off-label use is characterized by use outside of the summary of product characteristics (SmPC) laid out by the market authorization holders (MAH) or regulatory authorities. This principle is distinct from unauthorized or unlicensed usage, which constitutes use in a country in which market authorization has not been granted [28]. The FDA recognizes that physicians must use best clinical practice and medical decision-making to act in the interest of the patient they are treating. Especially in situations where there is no approved or efficacious alternative, a physician may use legally available devices or drugs on a case-by-case basis, using best medical knowledge and judgment.

Off-label use is often necessary for underrepresented indications or populations such as children, elderly, pregnant, or breastfeeding women. The practice is widespread in rare diseases, oncology, pediatrics, and psychiatry, all of which represent understudied or underfunded populations. This also applies to patients with unstudied comorbid conditions. The most common types of off-label use include modification of dosage, administration route, pharmaceutical form, application for different indication, or unstudied age group or patient characteristic. Studies show approximately 50% of cancer therapy is off-label, especially with increasing prevalence of targeted therapies used to augment standard-of-care regimens [28]. Another example of this is evident in self-expanding endoprostheses in vascular surgery, which have more off-label usage than on-label [29].

There are little published safety and efficacy data for off-label use and it can be difficult to track these data, which may lead to unpredictable outcomes. For example, safety monitoring is achieved through a combination of spontaneous reports, observational studies, registries, and clinical trials. Furthermore, manufacturers are prohibited from advertising or promoting off-label use, therefore communication of this is generally done via discussion with colleagues and presentation of case reports/series. With this complex and unpredictable pattern of information dissemination, there is risk of incomplete information such as instances where regulatory agencies may have previously declined approval for a specific indication, but it is still being applied [27]. In the case of an adverse event, the physician may be held legally responsible. A dramatic example of this led to the passage of the 1962 Kefauver-Harris Drug Amendments, signed into law by President John F. Kennedy in response to the tragedy of phocomelia and other birth defects seen in babies born to women who used off-label thalidomide for treatment of morning sickness in Europe, Australia, and Canada. This act led to close monitoring in all stages of safety and efficacy testing [30].

While there is now regulation to limit and monitor off-label use to optimize safety, there are also substantial barriers to achieving market approval for expanded use, including long development times, high costs, and lack of incentives for exploring expanded indications. Incentives do exist, however, including through the office of Orphan Drug Development (FDA), which offers market exclusivity, research and development grants, tax credits, waiver of regulatory fees, and expedited approval for marketing [28].

There have been several pivotal movements within the regulatory sector of the FDA over the past several decades. The Safe Medical Devices Act (SMDA) of 1990 provided the framework for the post-market surveillance and device tracking. This allowed for closer monitoring of adverse events and off-label use and led to the Medical Device Reporting (MDR) regulation in 1996. The MDR serves as an outlet for reporting serious adverse events (SAEs) involving devices. The SMDA requires reporting of on- and off-label device-related deaths, serious injuries, and general annual reports to both the FDA and the manufacturer [31]. However, SAEs from off-label usage are likely far underreported.

Off-Label Usage of Medical Devices: Specific Mechanisms for Meeting Regulatory Compliance

There are three main pathways for expanded access of approved devices, including emergency use, compassionate use, and investigational device exemption (IDE) (Table 24.1).

Emergency use is applicable for patients with life-threatening conditions who require immediate treatment and for which no acceptable alternative exists. FDA approval is not required as the indication for emergency use is an application in which the patient's clinical condition precludes time to allow for existing protocols to obtain FDA approval. This can apply to a device being studied in a clinical trial or for which an IDE is in process, but this is not a requirement. In order to obtain approval for emergency use, specific patient protection measures must be met. These include the patient (or legal representative) providing consent, institutional clearance in accordance with local policies, concurrence of the IRB chairperson, an independent assessment by an uninvolved physician, and authorization from the

Table 24.1 Mechanisms of regulatory compliance for off-label usage of medical devices

Use application	FDA review prior to use	Prespecified monitoring schedule	Indication	Applied to	Patient protection measures required	FDA indication expansion
Emergency use	No	No	Immediately life-threatening use without suitable alternative	Individuals and small groups	Patient consent, IRB chair approval, independent physician assessment, manufacturer authorization	No
Compassionate use	Yes	Yes	Essential treatment without acceptable approved alternative	Individuals and small groups	Patient consent, IRB chair approval, independent physician assessment, manufacturer authorization	No
Investigational device exemption	Yes	Yes	Essential treatment without acceptable approved alternative	Larger groups, typically within a clinical trial	Full clinical trial protocol with IRB approval, trial informed consent, institutional regulatory oversight of trial	Possible

device manufacturer. Physicians seeking emergency use authorization must document the nature of the patient's emergency situation to the FDA and are recommended to obtain local ethical board review prior to device utilization.

Compassionate use best applies to life-threatening or serious conditions without a comparable or satisfactory alternative therapy to diagnose, monitor, or treat the disease/condition. This is best applied to an individual or small group of patients. FDA approval is required (unlike with emergency use) in addition to the same patient protection measures and follow-up reporting including patient outcomes as with emergency use. This FDA review requires the submission of a prespecified device monitoring schedule to detect potential device adverse events. Additionally, the Center for Devices and Radiological Health (CDRH) requires notification of device placement within 5 days for non-FDA-approved devices not on clinical trials. In general, emergency use and compassionate use authorizations are used for a small number of patients and would not be expected to lead to expansion of FDA indication.

IDEs similarly apply to patients with life-threatening or serious conditions without a comparable or satisfactory alternative therapy; however, this is used on a larger scale, typically within the setting of a clinical trial, and these are usually done with the intent of expansion of indication. As such, IDEs require a substantial amount of work to prepare, with submission of a full IRB-approved clinical trial protocol to the FDA along with the application. The process to expansion of indication after initial FDA approval is lengthy and complex, which is summarized in Fig. 24.5. After initial market approval (following successful phase I, II, and III clinical trials), a clinician or member of industry may identify an unmet need requiring expanded indication use for an approved existing technology. After institutional regulatory processes are completed, including IRB approval of a clinical trial protocol, and, if applicable, additional NCI-mandated approvals, an investigator must complete an investigational device exemption (IDE) application with the FDA. Within 30 days of submission, the application will be approved, approved with revisions, or disapproved. Once approval is granted, there are important IDE requirements for the approved clinical trial. The device must be properly labeled, bearing the statement: "CAUTION—Investigational Device. Limited

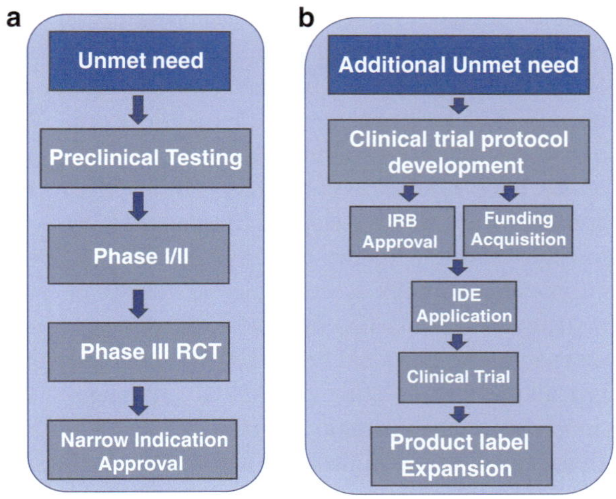

Fig. 24.5 Schematic showing the (**a**) initial process of FDA device approval for a narrow indication and (**b**) subsequent process for product label expansion for broader indications

by Federal (or United States) law to investigational use." The device may only be distributed to qualified investigators. There are standardized requirements for the informed consent process, specifically related to disclosure of the investigational status of the expanded use of the device. Subject monitoring and protocol compliance are mandated, and regular reporting of safety and efficacy data to both IRB and FDA officials is required.

In the case of the institutional safety trials using the MCHP (see below), the process for writing and obtaining IRB approval of a full clinical trial protocol, obtaining funding, and preparing the application and obtaining IDE approval ranged from 1 to 2 years. Sometimes the length of time, amount of effort, and expense required to complete this process is prohibitive. In some cases, due to these barriers, investigators do not seek expanded indication for devices and drugs, and the number of off-label uses for a specific device may surpass the number of on-label uses. An example of this is the Gore® Viabahn® endoprosthesis, which has been approved for use in the superficial femoral and distal iliac arteries as well as with arteriovenous grafts [32]. The actual use reported in the literature expands to use in popliteal and axillary arteries, for TIPS, and even in-stent stenosis, to name a few [29, 33–36].

Expanded Access to HAI Using the Medtronic Pump–Codman Catheter "Hybrid" Device: Compassionate Use, Emergency Use, and FDA-Mandated Safety Trials Under IDE at Two Academic Centers

As a result of the abrupt discontinuation of the Codman 3000 pump, clinicians were thrust into a situation where the only system available to a population of patients in dire need of potentially lifesaving liver-directed chemotherapy was a "hybrid" HAI delivery system that had very little usage history and lacked regulatory approval. We present here detailed examples of how our programs continued to provide this crucial therapy to patients using these three expanded access pathways.

In an effort stay within the FDA-regulated avenues and continue with off-label administration of HAI therapy, some institutions, including the Hospital of the University of Pennsylvania, addressed the crisis initially by applying on an individual "case-by-case" basis for single-patient emergency and compassionate use expanded access of the non-FDA-approved Medtronic HAI pump–Codman catheter hybrid (MCHP). This was a cumbersome process, with individual applications required for each patient requiring separate submission, review, and approval on a per patient basis. A total of 22 patients at the Hospital of the University of Pennsylvania underwent HAI under an emergency ($N = 15$) or compassionate ($N = 7$) use authorization by the FDA of the hybrid device combination. On average, approximately 10 days elapsed from application to approval of emergency or compassionate use. Ultimately, the FDA deemed that the volume of patients undergoing this process at the site was untenable and mandated that in order to continue implanting and utilizing the MCHP investigational device, the institution would be required to create and initiate a clinical trial to formally study feasibility, safety, and patient outcomes.

Thus, a phase I trial was initiated at the Hospital of the University of Pennsylvania in July 2021 to establish the safety of the non-FDA-approved combined Medtronic II Synchromed pump and Codman catheter hybrid device. Likewise, at the University of Kentucky, a similar phase I trial was initiated under an FDA IDE in May 2020. Design of these trials was influenced by discussions with peers at institutions already using the hybrid device combination off-label (in the absence of one of these standard FDA mechanisms for off-label use), who cited rare device combination-related issues. Thus, the trials were opened to formally prove the safety of the combination.

As of the date of this writing, 34 patients were registered on the Hospital of the University of Pennsylvania FDA-mandated device-safety trial and continue to be followed for device-related complications. Six patients had their pumps removed with two related to pump failures: specifically, a pump catheter thrombosis that prevented drug delivery in one, and a pump found to be disconnected from its catheter discovered inadvertently during a non-pump-related laparotomy. The remaining four pump removals were related to the following issues: persistent fungemia related to HAI pump seeding, FUDR-related biliary stricture, removal for patient preference, and removal during ventral hernia repair. One of the patients experienced a post-pump removal complication in the form of a bleed from the pump site and pocket hematoma that may have been related to increased bleeding risk from systemic administration of trifluidine and tipiracil (Lonsurf).

At the University of Kentucky, 21 patients underwent implantation of the hybrid device combination under an IRB-approved Phase I safety and feasibility clinical trial with an IDE. There were no device component disconnects; however, one patient (4.8%) suffered erosion of the catheter into the Roux limb of a Roux-en-Y gastric bypass, related to an underlying Axios™ stent in place for endoscopic access to the excluded gastric remnant for repeated endoscopic retrograde pancreatocholangiography (ERCP) and stent placement for the patient's malignant biliary obstruction from intrahepatic cholangiocarcinoma. This was felt to be due to the position of the catheter itself, and not due to the hybrid device. Another patient (4.8%) had a device dosing error due to misprogramming of the device via the tablet and more rapid drug infusion than intended; however, this did not result in patient harm. One pump (4.8%) was removed for infection many months after completion of treatment while on surveillance. One patient (4.8%) died of rapid progression of disease after pump implantation and never received HAI therapy, while all of the others received a median of 4 cycles of treatment. One patient (4.8%) died of COVID-19 infection on study (in the peak of the pandemic; unvaccinated). Another patient (4.8%) withdrew from the study after several months of HAI and underwent a liver transplantation at another institution on a clinical trial. As with the Hospital of the University of Pennsylvania trial and consistent with previously published studies, patients in both cohorts experienced low rates of biliary sclerosis, sclerosing cholangitis, but elevated liver enzymes resulting in dose reductions were common, though considered unrelated to off-label use of the hybrid pump.

The Codman Pump "Reborn" and Renamed: The Intera HAI Delivery System

In response to the absence of an FDA-approved device for HAI therapy, investors including former patients who had received liver-directed chemotherapy worked alongside company founders Dr. Johnathan Reis and Dr. David Dove to reestablish production of the Codman pump, renamed and remarketed as the Intera 3000 pump (Fig. 24.2). The manufacture reestablishment process took 3 years to ensure the device would meet specifications of the previously FDA-approved pump and could demonstrate equivalency. Premarket approval was granted on 4/13/2021, but due to the COVID-19 pandemic, on-site premarket inspection of the Intera 3000 manufacturing site was delayed, preventing distribution of the device. However, following the advocacy of members of the HAI Consortium Research Network urging the prioritization of review, the manufacturing site inspection was the first conducted by the FDA upon resumption of inspections. The FDA approval of the new manufacturing location was received on 6/22/2021 and the device became available for patient use in short order with the first Intera 3000 pump implanted at Duke University in August 2021.

A 2025 review of HAI patients treated at a new and expanding center that included use of the FDA-approved Intera pump system reported postoperative HAI-specific complications occurring in 23% of patients, including 11% related to the pump pocket (infection, hematoma, seroma, pump migration/erosion), 3% related to the catheter 4% with vascular complications (dissection, pseudoaneurysm), and 6% with biliary sclerosis. Only 3 (3%) of patients in this series experienced a pump malfunction, all of which were salvaged with pump replacement. This review noted that most patients with complications do not require pump extraction and with early identification of the problem, most are able to continue HAI [37].

The Intera 3000 hepatic artery infusion pump has demonstrated a favorable safety profile since its initial approval in April 2021. However, on July 10, 2022, in the wake of several reports to the FDA's adverse event reporting program documenting pumps delivering infusional solutions including chemotherapy at flow rates higher than expected, a recall was announced. The recall affected devices distributed between August 12, 2021 and May 17, 2022, comprising a total of 50 devices. Three incidents were associated with the recall without reports of patient safety events including injury or death. Physicians were advised to monitor flow rate and liver toxicity per standard protocols and increase frequency of patient follow-up to sooner than every 2 weeks with plans to consider pump replacement if alterations in flow rate significantly impacted delivery of the infusate [38].

Conclusions

Significant progress has been made during four decades of hepatic artery infusion pumps for intrahepatic delivery of chemotherapy: from external devices to implantable; from battery-powered to self-sustaining; from high complication rates to relative safety and low toxicity when inserted and used properly; and from "orphan" use to an evolving, more universal applicability that will hopefully provide life-prolonging treatment to a growing population of patients with colorectal cancer liver metastases and potentially other cancers. We have navigated successfully through the regulatory rapids of the Medtronic pump–Codman catheter hybrid to emerge in the still waters of FDA reapproval of the Codman pump, reborn as the Intera 3000. However, more challenges may lie ahead. In the last several years, with the formation of the HAI Consortium Research Network (HCRN), a group of over 70 HAI institutions in the United States and around the world, organized and coordinated leadership has emerged, with the goal of collaboration for research and outcomes tracking, mentorship of new programs to facilitate safe dissemination of HAI, and development of collaborative group clinical trials. Applying the lessons and challenges of the early era of HAI, these leaders will help guide the HAI community into the next era. In particular, it will be critical to assure that safe, reliable, and effective regulatory-body-approved HAI devices remain on the healthcare market for the growing patient-in-need population.

References

1. Folkman J, Long DM. The use of silicone rubber as a carrier for prolonged drug therapy. J Surg Res. 1964;4:139–42. https://doi.org/10.1016/S0022-4804(64)80040-8.
2. Bierman HR, Byron RL Jr, Miller ER, Shimkin MB. Effects of intra-arterial administration of nitrogen mustard. Am J Med. 1950;8:535. https://doi.org/10.1016/0002-9343(50)90263-4.
3. Breedis C, Young G. The blood supply of neoplasms in the liver. Am J Pathol. 1954;30:969–77.
4. Sullivan RD, Norcross JW, Watkins E Jr. Chemotherapy of metastatic liver cancer by prolonged hepatic-artery infusion. N Engl J Med. 1964;270:321–7. https://doi.org/10.1056/nejm196402132700701.
5. Watkins E Jr. Chronometric infusor—an apparatus for protracted ambulatory infusion therapy. N Engl J Med. 1963;269:850–1. https://doi.org/10.1056/nejm196310172691607.
6. Johnston J, Reich S, Bailey A, Sluetz J. Shiley Infusaid pump technology. Ann N Y Acad Sci. 1988;531:57–65. https://doi.org/10.1111/j.1749-6632.1988.tb31812.x.
7. Cohen AM, et al. Transbrachial hepatic arterial chemotherapy using an implanted infusion pump. Dis Colon Rectum. 1980;23:223–7. https://doi.org/10.1007/bf02587086.
8. Buchwald H, et al. Intraarterial infusion chemotherapy for hepatic carcinoma using a totally implantable infusion pump. Cancer. 1980;45:866–9. https://doi.org/10.1002/1097-0142(19800301)45:5<866::AID-CNCR2820450507>3.0.CO;2-3.
9. Cohen AM, et al. Treatment of hepatic metastases by transaxillary hepatic artery chemotherapy using an implanted drug pump. Cancer. 1983;51:2013–9. https://doi.org/10.1002/1097-0142(19830601)51:11<2013::aid-cncr2820511109>3.0.co;2-#.
10. Ensminger W, Niederhuber J, Dakhil S, Thrall J, Wheeler R. Totally implanted drug delivery system for hepatic arterial chemotherapy. Cancer Treat Rep. 1981;65:393–400.
11. Barone RM, et al. Intra-arterial chemotherapy using an implantable infusion pump and liver irradiation for the treatment of hepatic metastases. Cancer. 1982;50:850–62. https://doi.org/10.1002/1097-0142(19820901)50:5<850::AID-CNCR2820500508>3.0.CO;2-2.
12. Fayzullin A, Bakulina A, Mikaelyan K, Shekhter A, Guller A. Implantable drug delivery systems and foreign body reaction: traversing the current clinical landscape. Bioengineering. 2021;8:205. https://doi.org/10.3390/bioengineering8120205.
13. Allen PJ, et al. Technical complications and durability of hepatic artery infusion pumps for unresectable colorectal liver metastases: an institutional experience of 544 consecutive cases. J Am Coll Surg. 2005;201:57–65. https://doi.org/10.1016/j.jamcollsurg.2005.03.019.
14. Rustin RB, Vogt DP, Bukowski RM, Shepard KV. Hepatic artery infusion chemotherapy for colorectal liver metastases. Cleve Clin J Med. 1990;57:692–6. https://doi.org/10.3949/ccjm.57.8.692.
15. Hall DA, Clouse ME, Gramm HF. Gastroduodenal ulceration after hepatic arterial infusion chemotherapy. Am J Roentgenol. 1981;136:1216–8. https://doi.org/10.2214/ajr.136.6.1216.
16. Silberman AW, et al. A complication of the Infusaid pump: duodenal atony reversed by urecholine. J Surg Oncol. 1987;36:210–4. https://doi.org/10.1002/jso.2930360312.
17. Shike M, Gillin JS, Kemeny N, Daly JM, Kurtz RC. Severe gastroduodenal ulcerations complicating hepatic artery infusion chemotherapy for metastatic colon cancer. Am J Gastroenterol. 1986;81:176–9.
18. Ramming KP, O'Toole K. The use of the implantable chemoinfusion pump in the treatment of hepatic metastases of colorectal cancer. Arch Surg. 1986;121:1440–4. https://doi.org/10.1001/archsurg.1986.01400120090015.
19. Hohn DC, et al. Toxicities and complications of implanted pump hepatic arterial and intravenous floxuridine infusion. Cancer. 1986;57:465–70. https://doi.org/10.1002/1097-0142(19860201)57:3<465::aid-cncr2820570311>3.0.co;2-s.
20. Campbell KA, et al. Regional chemotherapy devices: effect of experience and anatomy on complications. J Clin Oncol. 1993;11:822–6. https://doi.org/10.1200/jco.1993.11.5.822.
21. Kemeny N, Huang Y, Cohen AM, Shi W, Conti JA, Brennan MF, Bertino JR, Turnbull AD, Sullivan D, Stockman J, Blumgart LH, Fong Y. Hepatic arterial infusion of chemotherapy after resection of hepatic metastases from colorectal cancer. N Engl J Med. 1999;341(27):2039–48. https://doi.org/10.1056/NEJM199912303412702. PMID: 10615075.
22. Barnett KT, Malafa MP. Complications of hepatic artery infusion : a review of 4580 reported cases. Int J Gastrointest Cancer. 2001;30:147–60. https://doi.org/10.1385/ijgc:30:3:147.
23. Ethans KD, Schryvers OI, Nance PW, Casey AR. Intrathecal drug therapy using the Codman Model 3000 Constant Flow Implantable Infusion Pumps: experience with 17 cases. Spinal Cord. 2005;43:214–8. https://doi.org/10.1038/sj.sc.3101684.
24. Muaddi H, et al. Safety and feasibility of initiating a hepatic artery infusion pump chemotherapy program for unresectable colorectal liver metastases: a

multicenter, retrospective cohort study. J Surg Oncol. 2021;123:252–60. https://doi.org/10.1002/jso.26270.
25. Grady D, Kaplan S. A lifesaving pump for cancer patients is being phased out. The New York Times. 2018.
26. Ellis RJ, Angelos P, Jarnagin WR, Kemeny NE, Merkow RP. Abrupt discontinuation of the Codman hepatic artery infusion pump: considerations in the era of precision medicine. J Am Coll Surg. 2019;229:217–9. https://doi.org/10.1016/j.jamcollsurg.2019.03.002.
27. Russell ME, Friedman MI, Mascioli SR, Stolz LE. Off-label use: an industry perspective on expanding use beyond approved indications. J Interv Cardiol. 2006;19:432–8. https://doi.org/10.1111/j.1540-8183.2006.00185.x.
28. Rusz C-M, et al. Off-label medication: from a simple concept to complex practical aspects. Int J Environ Res Public Health. 2021;18:10447. https://doi.org/10.3390/ijerph181910447.
29. Ni Q, et al. Viabahn stent graft for the endovascular treatment of occlusive lesions in the femoropopliteal artery: a retrospective cohort study with 4-year follow-up. Ann Vasc Surg. 2020;66:573–9. https://doi.org/10.1016/j.avsg.2019.11.018.
30. Paine M. Therapeutic disasters that hastened safety testing of new drugs. Clin Pharmacol Ther. 2017;101:430–4. https://doi.org/10.1002/cpt.613.
31. Administration, F. U. F. D (2018). Medical Device Reporting Regulation History. https://www.fda.gov/medicaldevices/mandatory-reporting-requirements-manufacturers-importers-and-device-user-facilities/medical-devicereporting-regulation-history.
32. FDA (2014). Instructions for use for Gore Viabahn Endoprosthesis with Heparin Bioactive Surface. https://www.accessdata.fda.gov/cdrh_docs/pdf4/P040037S060c.pdf.
33. Arase H, et al. Viabahn stent graft in the treatment of traumatic axillary artery pseudoaneurysm. Cardiovasc Interv Ther. 2022;37:580–2. https://doi.org/10.1007/s12928-021-00806-2.
34. Patel SR, et al. A systematic review and meta-analysis of endovascular popliteal aneurysm repair using the Hemobahn/Viabahn stent-graft. J Endovasc Ther. 2015;22:330–7. https://doi.org/10.1177/1526602815579252.
35. Liu J, et al. A new choice of stent for transjugular intrahepatic portosystemic shunt creation: Viabahn ePTFE covered stent/bare metal stent combination. J Interv Med. 2021;4:32–8. https://doi.org/10.1016/j.jimed.2020.10.003.
36. Al Shammeri O, Bitar F, Ghitelman J, Soukas PA. Viabahn for femoropopliteal in-stent restenosis. Ann Saudi Med. 2012;32:572–82. https://doi.org/10.5144/0256-4947.2012.575.
37. Liu A, et al. Ann Surg Oncol. 2025;32(2):1033–1042. PMID: 39565488
38. Medwatch F. Intera Oncology recalls Intera 3000 hepatic artery infusion pump due to faster than expected flow rates that may impact infusion delivery. FDA. 2022.

25 Starting a New HAI Pump Program: How to Train a New HAI Team

Sepideh Gholami, Deborah Small, and Maria Diab

The initiation of a new hepatic arterial infusion pump (HAIP) program is an exciting endeavor that can be very rewarding when done well using a systematic approach. As clinical research and patient health literacy and advocacy expand, there has been a growing interest in HAIP treatment. With that growing interest, there is an increasing need to expand our ability to offer this treatment modality to a larger patient population, since historically only a few centers in the country offered this highly specialized treatment. When setting up a new HAIP program, it is crucial to ensure the availability of the required infrastructure to support the delivery of such a specialized cancer treatment; in particular, the assembly of a fully trained multidisciplinary team of healthcare providers including medical oncology, surgical oncology, diagnostic and interventional radiology, gastroenterology, pharmacy, nursing, and social work. In the early stages of program implementation, it is recommended that a champion from each specialty is selected to help train additional team members as the program expands. This includes trainees on all involved teams who will take part in caring for these patients. Furthermore, given the rapid expansion of HAIP programs in recent years, new programs must identify engaged mentors to help guide patient selection and troubleshoot both clinical and programmatic issues one will face while building a new program. Therefore, it is advised to send team members for training at an experienced HAIP center, not only for the hands-on experience but also for the additional opportunity to establish a relationship with potential mentors for the future. This chapter focuses on the training of the HAIP team members at the local institution. For details on specific in-service training at an experienced center (e.g., site visit), refer to Chap. 26 for further details.

Supplementary Information The online version contains supplementary material available at https://doi.org/10.1007/978-3-031-74935-3_25.

S. Gholami (✉)
Division of Surgical Oncology, Northwell Health Cancer Institute, Northwell Health, New Hyde Park, NY, USA
e-mail: sgholami@northwell.edu

D. Small
Department of Nursing, University of California Davis, Sacramento, CA, USA

M. Diab
Division of Hematology and Medical Oncology, Department of Internal Medicine, Henry Ford Health, Detroit, MI, USA
e-mail: mdiab2@hfhs.org

Training the Surgical Team

Programs are instituted and led by surgeons with advanced training in either surgical oncology, hepatobiliary surgery, or transplant surgery,

M. D'Angelica, M. Lidsky (eds.), *Hepatic Arterial Infusion for Malignancy*,
https://doi.org/10.1007/978-3-031-74935-3_25

in conjunction with a medical oncology champion. Historically, HAIP surgeons have completed fellowship training at one of the founding HAIP programs or were trained by a colleague who trained at these centers. Despite most having fellowship-level training in HAIP implantation, it remains advisable that new teams participate in a site visit at a high-volume HAI center. In a recently published survey, among surgeons starting a new HAIP program, over half performed a site visit at MSKCC as a refresher prior to program initiation, despite prior HAIP experience. However, given the rapid expansion of HAIP programs in the last decade [1], more surgeons are learning HAIP outside of this traditional pathway. For surgeons with an HAIP-experienced partner, it is important to double-scrub cases with them to gain experience in the technical nuances of HAIP implantation. For those who do not have this opportunity, in-person observation of HAIP implantation is key. It is our opinion that attempting to build an HAIP program without direct mentorship from an experienced HAIP surgeon and medical oncologist carries a significant risk of program failure. Likewise, it is important to engage residents and fellows in the care of HAIP patients, both in the clinical setting and the operating room, as some may build their own HAIP programs in the future.

Surgical trainees and advanced practice providers also play a key role in the perioperative management of HAIP patients. It is advised that the surgeon champion meet with rotating house staff to provide education on HAI conceptually, technical considerations, commonly encountered HAI-specific complications and their workup and management, as well as general HAI-specific perioperative care. In doing so, the inpatient surgical team can help optimize perioperative outcomes, including being the first to identify early signs of impending complications. An additional resource that may be of benefit is a recently published HAI toolkit that reviews intraoperative considerations and the workup and management of many HAI-specific complications [2].

Training the Medical Oncology Team and Pharmacist

The medical oncologist is the primary team member responsible for the delivery of locoregional and systemic chemotherapy, as well as management of toxicity. For medical oncologists (physicians and advanced practice providers) who are new to HAI, but also for providers with prior experience, it is advised that they participate in a site visit at a high-volume center, as described above and in Chap. 26, where they learn about HAI chemotherapy dosing and general HAIP management.

The oncologist will need to ensure seamless communication with the pharmacy team, as floxuridine (FUDR) and systemic dosing must be carefully managed and synchronized. While some pharmacists may participate in the team site visit, another common practice is to connect a pharmacist champion at a new HAI center with the pharmacist at an established center. Given the complexity of FUDR dosing, especially in conjunction with systemic chemotherapy, it is prudent for the medical oncologist to review all dosing with a pharmacist who is regularly involved in HAIP therapy. The pharmacist will need to keep track of adequate FUDR supply and assure appropriate formulation with dexamethasone, which should be included with all FUDR treatments. For maintenance fills with glycerin, programs should be aware that sterile glycerin is only available from specialty compounding pharmacies and requires special acquisition. Pharmacy orders are required not only for basic aspects such as dosing of agents (FUDR, heparin, etc.) but also for dose adjustment algorithms in settings when adverse events occur and/or laboratory results dictate dose reductions or dose holds. It is helpful if order sets for future visits can include required laboratory values and, preferably, clinic and infusion visit requests to make for a smoother scheduling process and avoid delays. Special attention should be paid to scheduling and coordination of visits for patients who will be receiving HAIP FUDR as well as systemic chemotherapy (FOLFOX, FOLFIRI, etc.).

At the beginning of program building, it is advised to group HAIP patients on selected days to allow for ease of scheduling and workflow at the infusion center. This can also prevent unnecessary waste of FUDR, since multiple patients can often be treated from a single vial depending on the dose they are receiving.

Nursing and Operating Room Staff Training

It is important to include nursing staff (both in the operating room and at the infusion centers where most of the pumps are refilled) in a comprehensive training program. At most institutions, pump refills are performed by a trained chemotherapy infusion nurse. Therefore, it is key to find a dedicated nursing champion for the program. This champion will need to understand all aspects of care for HAIP patients ranging from appropriate patient selection and education to the pump refill procedure and potential complications. If possible, it is recommended that the nurse champion participate in the HAI team site visit to shadow a nurse at a well-established program. If a site visit is not possible, finding a way for the nurse champion to connect with a mentor at an established center virtually (for training and troubleshooting) is invaluable. The pump manufacturers also have educators and representatives who provide valuable in-service training on the implantation and the refill procedure for nursing staff. A breach in sterile technique must be avoided as this can lead to pump pocket infection and subsequent pump loss. Nurses need to be made aware of the possibility of inaccessible reservoirs due to reservoir rotation or flipping. In this case, the surgeon should be available to assist in troubleshooting difficult access. In the rare event of challenging pump access, interventional radiology can facilitate access under fluoroscopic guidance. As the program grows, the treatment room nursing champion will be responsible for training additional nurses to access and refill pumps, which mitigates scheduling dilemmas in the absence of trained staff. It is advised that training of new nurses in the treatment room follows a protocolized process inclusive of observation, hands-on assistance with pump access, and proctoring until proficiency is achieved.

Operating room nurses and technicians also require training in the nuances of HAIP implantation. To streamline the setup for the HAIP implantation procedure, the operating surgeon must establish a "pick list." This includes typical retractors for a laparotomy and instruments necessary for portal dissection, vessel loops, gentle bulldog clamps, and a vein pick. In the case of a minimally invasive, robotic-assisted placement, appropriate instrumentation must be ensured. It is recommended that the pump company representative is present to provide technical support for early cases to ensure that necessary disposables (refill and bolus needles) are available and the HAIP is flushed and primed with the correct heparin doses at the time of the implantation. The operating room pharmacy needs to be prepared with an appropriate orderset to provide necessary drugs including heparinized saline (high and low dose), papaverine for possible dilation of the gastroduodenal artery, methylene blue for extrahepatic perfusion testing, and antibiotic solution for irrigation of the surgical pump pocket depending on individual surgeon practice. The surgical scrub and operating room circulator nurse will need to be trained about the conduct of pump implantation including pump priming.

Special Training for Nuclear Medicine, Diagnostic (DR) and Interventional Radiology (IR), and Gastroenterology (GI)

Prior to the initial pump refill, it is required to obtain a SPECT/CT after injection of Tc-MAA solution to assess for extrahepatic perfusion (see Chap. 9). Most nuclear medicine radiologists have some experience with liver perfusion scans performed before Y90 radioembolization, which can be leveraged to develop a protocol for HAIP perfusion studies. It is critical to educate radiologists on the most common sites of extrahepatic perfusion, specifically the stomach, duodenum, and pancreas.

Diagnostic radiologists (DR) also play a key role in the preoperative and postoperative assessment of HAI patients. Preoperatively, evaluation of the extent of disease, specifically the presence of extrahepatic disease and/or hepatic disease burden, as well as assessment of hepatic arterial anatomy, is crucial. The DR team must also become familiar with both normal and abnormal radiographic findings in patients with implanted pumps, including catheter position and the development of vascular and biliary changes that may be indicative of impending or active complications [3].

The IR staff needs to be trained and comfortable with pump access, specifically for obese patients with difficult to palpate pumps, as well as to perform pump angiograms when pump flow rate is found to be concerningly low. Additionally, advanced IR expertise is required to rescue patients from HAI-specific complications, including embolization of vessels to address extrahepatic perfusion and other possible life-threatening complications, such as bleeding from a ruptured pseudoaneurysm.

Lastly, GI needs to be made aware of potential gastrointestinal ulceration or catheter erosion, which can present with persistent abdominal pain, especially during FUDR treatment. Given the possibility of biliary sclerosis, the GI and IR teams need to be equipped to deal with such a complication, which is further detailed in Chap. 18.

Multidisciplinary Patient Selection

When training the new HAIP team, it is of utmost importance to include patient selection, which is multifaceted. First, the extent of disease should be defined. Liver-only disease is preferable, though patients with liver-dominant disease and limited extrahepatic involvement may be considered. Second, the patient's age, support system, and anticipated future compliance should be reviewed. Transportation challenges are potential barriers to pump care, and social work may be of assistance in such situations. Third, a review of each patient's hepatic arterial anatomy is required for preoperative planning. Fourth, while most patients received concurrent systemic therapy with HAI, nuanced decisions to omit such therapy may be made after weighing potential toxicities with goals of treatment. It is critical to discuss patient candidacy in the multidisciplinary setting of a tumor board, for example, to ensure consensus from all involved teams.

Patient Education

Training the HAI team to educate patients is an important component of patient selection, informed consent, and patient compliance. Team members should become proficient in discussing HAI-specific considerations with patients. These specific factors should be considered when educating patients intended to receive HAI, and this education is likely to be reiterated during their pre- and postsurgical visits in different capacities. First, demonstrating what the pump looks like and displaying an actual pump or model to show how it is accessed is extremely helpful to patients. Simplifying complex anatomical descriptions by the surgeon may also improve the patient's conception of HAIP. Industry partners who manufacture the pump also provide educational media, which can be a great resource for patient education. Important limitations to some lifestyle practices that might potentially modify the flow rate of the pump are important to review with patients and their support systems. Those lifestyle practices include travel to high elevations, flying in unpressurized aircraft, scuba diving, and practices that involve exposure to prolonged elevated temperatures (such as the use of hot tubs, saunas, or heating pads). Most patients treated with HAI will also receive concurrent systemic chemotherapy, often inclusive of infusional 5-fluorouracil (5-FU). Here, it is important to differentiate the two "pumps" and the differences in scheduling between the two. A comprehensive review of current medications is important, as well as explaining the reasoning behind avoiding some medications in the setting of HAIP, such as antiangiogenesis agents. If the patient is not already on them, H2 blockers or, more commonly, proton pump inhibitors should be initiated. The rationale behind this is that the hypothesized excretion of FUDR into the bile is in itself ulcerogenic, leading to inflammation or ulceration in up to 50% of patients. Lastly, limiting alcohol consumption and hepatic-metabolized drugs such as acetaminophen is advised. For more information on patient education, see Chap. 28.

Continued Education and Quality Control

Once your staff has been trained, it is critical to work in a collaborative manner and engage the staff in the review of outcomes and the quality of the care provided. Any trends outside the expected complication rates [2, 4–6] should raise concerns and be looked at as an opportunity to improve outcomes. A successful program also requires that the team leader stays engaged with all stakeholders of the team. This involves sharing new data from patients treated in the form of direct communication and presentations to encourage and engage new team members to grow one's program. Also, it is recommended that new programs review policy, procedures, and workflow to address any shortcomings and improve outcomes with an in-depth quality control review method. Taking part as active members in HAIP working groups, most notably, the HAI Consortium Research Network (HCRN) not only provides a convenient platform for knowledge sharing but also serves as a venue to brainstorm about new clinical research ideas and clinical trial participation.

Conclusions

As we witness a growing demand for HAIP therapy, it is important for centers embarking on establishing their new program to be systematic in their approach. This starts by identifying champions from the multiple different specialties involved to serve as ambassadors who will acquire the appropriate skillset and work within their institution to ensure the readiness of all the elements required for the success of such program. Training should be tailored to the practices that each team member will be responsible for. Crucial aspects, such as patient selection, are best conducted in a multidisciplinary fashion to ensure the fulfillment of prerequisites for HAI. Maintaining a relationship with mentors at high volume centers is important not only from a mentorship/troubleshooting standpoint but also to serve as grounds for future collaborations, including designing and conducting clinical trials in this area of unmet need.

References

1. Cavnar M, Ghalambor T, Lidsky ME, et al. Considerations and barriers to starting a new HAI pump program: an international survey of the HAI Consortium Research Network. HPB. 2022;24(12):2104–11. https://doi.org/10.1016/j.hpb.2022.08.008.
2. Sharib JM, Creasy JM, Wildman-Tobriner B, et al. Hepatic artery infusion pumps: a surgical toolkit for intraoperative decision-making and management of hepatic artery infusion-specific complications. Ann Surg. 2022;276(6):943–56. https://doi.org/10.1097/sla.0000000000005434.
3. Napier KJ, Lidsky ME, James OG, et al. Hepatic arterial infusion pumps: what the radiologist needs to know. Radiographics. 2021;41:895–908.
4. Allen PJ, Nissan A, Picon AI, et al. Technical complications and durability of hepatic artery infusion pumps for unresectable colorectal liver metastases: an institutional experience of 544 consecutive cases. J Am Coll Surg. 2005;201(1):57–65. https://doi.org/10.1016/j.jamcollsurg.2005.03.019.
5. Creasy JM, Napier KJ, Reed SA, et al. Implementation of a hepatic artery infusion program: initial patient selection and perioperative outcomes of concurrent hepatic artery infusion and systemic chemotherapy for colorectal liver metastases. Ann Surg Oncol. 2020;27(13):5086–95. https://doi.org/10.1245/s10434-020-08972-y.
6. Muaddi H, D'Angelica M, Wiseman JT, et al. Safety and feasibility of initiating a hepatic artery infusion pump chemotherapy program for unresectable colorectal liver metastases: a multicenter, retrospective cohort study. J Surg Oncol. 2021;123(1):252–60.

26 Hepatic Arterial Infusion Team Site Visit

Carleton Scott Ellis, Lisa Vlastelica, Hope E. Uronis, Michael Lidsky, and Reema Anil Patel

Introduction

Hepatic arterial infusion (HAI) team members must be well-versed in the data surrounding hepatic arterial infusion (HAI) and the benefits it can provide to patients diagnosed with colorectal cancer with liver metastases or intrahepatic cholangiocarcinoma. However, starting a HAI program can be a daunting task. A site visit should be considered mandatory to bring the team in contact with a seasoned team. It allows for multi-institutional collaboration but also each member can learn from their HAI expert counterpart, as well as gain exposure to key aspects of HAI that are outside their typical scope (e.g., surgeon learns about chemotherapy dosing). This face-to-face one-on-one time will be invaluable for team members to network and understand logistics of the process as it is related to their department/expertise. There are many team members whose buy-in into the program is imperative, equipment that needs to be attained, and questions to be answered. In this chapter, we will outline key points of consideration from the perspective of a surgical oncologist, medical oncologist, and pharmacist.

Pre-site Visit

Prior to launching a clinical hepatic artery infusion pump program, it is prudent to recruit invested and collaborative experts to assemble your team (see Chap. 22) and educate all team members about HAI, which should include a review of the literature and patient selection criterion broadly used (see Chap. 25) [1, 2]. Once the team is in place, it should be considered mandatory to travel to an established HAI program for a site visit. In our experience, having launched a successful new HAI program, the ideal time for the site visit is just before HAI program activation and treatment of the first patient. This establishes deadline for putting draft protocols in print format for official review, enables all members of the team together to get to know each other and enhance collaboration, and provides a chance to review the plans with a functioning program to

C. S. Ellis
University of Kentucky College of Pharmacy, Lexington, KY, USA
e-mail: carleton.ellis@uky.edu

L. Vlastelica
Duke Cancer Institute, Durham, NC, USA

H. E. Uronis
Division of Medical Oncology, Department of Medicine, Duke Health, Durham, NC, USA
e-mail: hope.uronis@duke.edu

M. Lidsky
Department of Surgery, Duke University, Durham, NC, USA
e-mail: Michael.lidsky@duke.edu

R. A. Patel (✉)
Medical Oncology, Markey Cancer Center, University of Kentucky, Lexington, KY, USA
e-mail: reema.patel@uky.edu

M. D'Angelica, M. Lidsky (eds.), *Hepatic Arterial Infusion for Malignancy*,
https://doi.org/10.1007/978-3-031-74935-3_26

identify potential pitfalls and details that may have been overlooked, as well as troubleshoot potential hurdles or challenges.

Choosing Your Site

Prior to the last decade, most site visits for new HAI programs were conducted at Memorial Sloan Kettering Cancer Center (MSKCC) in New York City, the institution that has pioneered and optimized HAI over the past five decades. While a site visit to MSKCC is an opportunity to learn from the original founders and developers of the therapy, the option now exists to organize a site visit to a newer and thriving program. Newer but established programs allow one to not only understand the challenges of initiating a new clinic program but also collaborate with sites close to your own center and allows your team to establish touch points for their individual roles. It is recommended that the host site has at least 2–3 years of experience and treats at least 20 patients per year, such that the team is well beyond their learning curve inherent to starting any new clinical program. The high-volume component is also important so that the site visit lends itself to observing and discussing the management of multiple HAI patients in the oncology clinic, ideally including new patients being considered for HAI as well as patients on active treatment.

Who to Bring to Your Site Visit

An HAI team has many experts from various specialties, including representatives from surgery, medical oncology, pharmacy, nursing (treatment room), operating room staff, diagnostic and interventional radiology, gastroenterology, and nuclear medicine. It is imperative to consider all stakeholders of the program, including prior expertise, so that you may identify individuals who should participate in the site visit. We suggest starting with the following providers: surgical oncologist, medical oncologist, pharmacist, infusion nurse, advanced practice provider, and/or operating room nurses or managers. Providing the host site with a list of providers and their roles in the team will allow the host institution to pair up each team member with their corresponding counterparts for one-on-one experiential teaching. This will also encourage networking and effective communication about individual responsibilities, workflow logistics, electronic health record challenges, and troubleshooting institutional differences. Emphasis should be on team building and communication, trouble shooting, and collaboration.

How to Prepare for a Site Visit

Preparing for a site visit requires a substantial amount of coordination between the two institutions, as well as between multiple departments within each institution. Depending on the size of the group that you plan to bring and the amount of time that you plan to spend there, it is advisable to start planning months in advance with an eye toward favorable weather, lack of holidays, competing conferences or national commitments, and flexibility around the moving parts that are required when considering complex patient care. It is recommended to plan for a 2–3-day visit: Day 1 for clinic observation, Day 2 for operating room observation, and Day 3 for meeting with other members of the team that may not have been present on previous days. A few examples include nuclear medicine personnel, who protocols and reads pump perfusion studies, and interventional radiology and gastroenterology personnel, who help in managing HAI-specific complications.

It is beneficial also to have your planned protocol outlined with intention to have incomplete portions completed during the visit. Even things such as travel arrangements for a team of this size, funding, time off from the department, and potential CME opportunities should be considered prior to the day of the site visit. It is also prudent to inquire about requirements from the host institution, such as required paperwork and approvals, or even tuberculosis testing requirements.

Additionally, the site visit should be timed around a combination of adequate HAI pump patient clinic volume and operative cases. Ideally, the visiting team will have the opportunity to observe at least two HAI pump implantations, which allows for unexpected findings in the operating room that may result in an aborted case (e.g., unexpected finding of peritoneal disease). In terms of clinic volume, it is beneficial to observe the evaluation and management of at least five patients, including those being considered for HAI, those receiving treatment either for unresectable disease or adjuvant therapy, and patients in the maintenance phase of their care who are receiving glycerin via the pump..

What to Learn During the Site Visit

The following table includes the minimum specialist representation and key learning objectives that should be incorporated into the site visit. Note that advanced practice providers in surgery and medical oncology are key members of any new team and should also participate in the site visit.

Team member	Learning objectives
Surgery (surgical oncology, HPB surgery, transplant surgery) [3]	• Technical aspects of HAI pump implantation, including management of aberrant anatomy • Patient selection • Identification and management of HAI-specific complications • Basics of FUDR and systemic chemotherapy dosing algorithms
Medical oncology (including APP)	• Basics and nuances of FUDR dosing algorithms and modification schema • Concurrent systemic chemotherapy dosing algorithms • Management of FUDR toxicity • Patient selection
Pharmacy	• FUDR and systemic chemotherapy dosing algorithms • EMR order set optimization
Nursing (infusion)	• HAI pump access and refill procedure—Including routine fill, glycerin fill, and post-glycerin procedures
OR staff	• Conduct of HAI pump implantation • HAI pump priming procedure

We have covered some of the logistics of a site visit but what each team member needs to understand and gain from a site visit may differ from the suggestions above based on prior expertise. Below, we have specifically asked for the opinions of a medical oncologist (MO), surgical oncologist (SO), and HAI pharmacist (PharmD) to help understand how they think about ways to operationalize an HAI program at their institution.

What Are the Key Factors to Understand About HAI?

MO: The most important thing to learn from the perspective of an oncologist is the dosing of FUDR for HAI along with management of complications. During our site visit, it was imperative to practice calculating the dose on the patients we saw with the experts. It allowed for learning in real time along with feedback. Also developing your own method to track patient's labs and FUDR dosing can help you identify patterns for them. Often the oncologist is the main point of contact once HAI therapy begins and thus it is also important to learn when surgery may need to intervene on complications (pump pocket infection) versus managing the complication in oncology clinic (hyperbilirubinemia). I would also highly recommend keeping open lines of communication with the experts from the site visit. It is helpful to discuss dosing, complications, and management as you learn the process for your patients.

SO: HAI, though seemingly straightforward, is actually highly complex. A successful HAI program requires significant buy-in and support from a highly collaborative team comprised of experts across many disciplines. Patient selection is the key, and maintaining an open dialogue with the medical oncologist to facilitate choosing the patients most likely to achieve favorable results from this therapy cannot be overlooked. Not every patient will derive benefit from HAI, and it is often unpredictable who will derive great benefit versus those who derive little to no benefit. The surgeon is equally important as the medical oncologist in optimizing patient selection, and therefore it is essential that the surgeon learns from the experts at the site visit about how they select patients, how selection has evolved with experience, and which specific patient populations should not to be considered for HAI. It must also be stated that the surgeon's role in the management of HAI patients does not end after the pump is successfully implanted or when the patient initiates therapy; rather, the surgeon should remain engaged in the patient's care and ongoing evaluation throughout the entirety of their HAI journey. While the surgeon will learn the technical maneuvers for pump implantation and management of HAI-specific complications during the site visit, it is not possible to learn about all operative nuances/hurdles and aspects of management during what is a brief visit. Thus, the surgeon should maintain open lines of communication with the host surgeon who can serve as a mentor and provide real-time guidance for future patients as the new program launches and unforeseen complexities arise.

PharmD: There are two primary roles that a pharmacist can play in an HAI program—clinical and operational. For a clinical pharmacist, the most important thing to learn about HAI is the dosing schema. Dosing of FUDR is more complicated than most other chemotherapy drugs and requires knowledge of the pumps being implanted at your institution and the algorithms for dosing FUDR based on a patient's weight and lab values. It is important to have multiple checks in place so that a patient is dosed correctly. For an operational pharmacist, the most important thing to learn about HAI is how to maintain a consistent inventory of the drugs needed for an HAI program and the compounding and administration process for HAI drugs.

What Needs to Be in Place Prior to Starting an HAI Program? [4]

MO: The collaboration with your pharmacy team will be the most important asset to have in place at your institution. They will assist in management and procurement of the therapies involved in HAI. Involving your pharmacist early on, as well as participating in a site visit, allows them to ensure the program will flow smoothly from all angles in the medical oncology clinics. Having prior discussions about workflow and building order sets for these complex therapies is a collaborative effort between you and your pharmacy team.

SO: The first requirement is recruitment and training of a collaborative multidisciplinary team. Typically, a medical oncologist champion is required; this person is not only invested in the development of the new clinical program and committed to its success but also serves as the coleader of the entire team. In parallel, it is important to secure institutional support (hospital system, department, division) to acquire the device, relevant drugs, and equipment, as well as to establish clinical and pharmaceutical protocols. These steps are all required before the site visit.

PharmD: Most importantly, a pharmacist must be able to procure the medications required for an HAI program—specifically FUDR and glycerin. The only indication for FUDR is for use in a hepatic arterial infusion pump, so most institutions will not have this medication on formulary unless they have an HAI program. The pharmacy department can take responsibility for shepherding FUDR through the pharmacy & therapeutics (P&T) committee process and ultimately ensuring an adequate and stable supply of FUDR. Glycerin is not a requirement for a functional HAI program as alternatives exist for maintaining pump catheter patency (i.e., heparin or fondaparinux), but for the best patient experience it is ideal to have a mechanism to either procure or compound sterile glycerin for use in HAI pumps, which reduces the amount of clinic visits necessary when a patient is not actively on therapy in their HAI pump.

What Are Some Questions and Potential Barriers to Starting an HAI Program? [4]

MO:

1. Do we have an oncologist(s) and advanced practitioner support with full-time equivalent (FTE) to devote time to this complex therapy?

2. Do we have the appropriate support from nursing, infusion, and pharmacy who understand the goals and complications of HAI?
3. Do we have clear expectations and a training protocol for each oncology team member? How can HAI manufacturers help us in training?
4. Do we have support to build and maintain HAI order sets?
5. Do we have all the supportive medications and processes in place?
6. Do we have contingency processes in place in case a patient has problems with their pump such as it is running too fast and/or running dry?
7. Is our surgical oncology team available to coordinate care for patients?
8. Do we have interventional radiology and gastroenterology teams with the skills needed to rescue patients from FUDR toxicity (biliary sclerosis)?

SO:

1. Does medical oncology support the start of a new HAI team? This is often the most important consideration, because a new program will not be successful without support and investment from medical oncology.
2. Is there a medical oncologist who will be the champion from that specialty?
3. Are other specialties going to oppose the HAI program because it competes with other therapies (e.g., radioembolization)?
4. What patient population will be prioritized? Unresectable? Adjuvant?
5. Is there infrastructure in place to manage HAI patients, including rescuing them from complications?
6. Will insurance pay for the device and therapy?
7. How long will it take from conceptualization to implementation of a new HAI program?
8. How many patients should we/can we treat per month? Per year?
9. Do we have an interventional radiology team with the skills needed to rescue patients from pump complications (e.g., extrahepatic perfusion, pseudoaneurysms, arterial dissection, catheter thrombosis, biliary sclerosis)?

PharmD:

1. Do we have a process in place to ensure adequate supply of FUDR and glycerin?
   (a) Can my institution compound high-risk products, or if not, do we have a relationship with a 503(b) pharmacy or manufacturer that can compound the product for us?
2. Do we have a clinical pharmacist FTE who can work with surgical oncology and medical oncology to appropriately dose and monitor FUDR?
3. Do we have support to build and maintain HAI order sets?
4. Have patient-specific factors for safe receipt of HAI been considered, such as patients who live at high altitude or have heparin allergies?
5. Do we have an infusion area with capacity to house patients with an HAI pump and nurses trained in accessing these pumps?
6. Do we have contingency processes in place in case a patient has problems with their pump such as it is running too fast and/or running dry?
7. Are there educational materials for patients that detail logistics of being treated with HAI and expectations?

These are all examples of questions that need to be discussed before starting a HAI program, and the involvement of all the stakeholders in obtaining reassurance and answers to their unique concerns and questions is vital to successfully addressing them.

What Advice Would You Give to Someone Starting a New HAI Program?

MO: Use your resources! As soon as discussions begin about bringing an HAI program to your institution, start with a literature search. It is imperative to have some working knowledge about HAI, history, criticisms, and successes to make the program flow at your institution. Only you will understand how your current oncology system functions, and after learning about HAI, you can develop an understanding on how to incorporate HAI into that system. Your immediate counterparts will be surgery, nursing, and pharmacy; thus, it is important to involve them early so they can help with institutional system navigation. Along with the systematic hurdles, understanding and identifying the patients who will benefit the most from HAI therapy is imperative. Having multidisciplinary conferences about each patient allows every team member to weigh in on the risk and benefits from their viewpoint. The need for oral H_2 blockade (or proton pump inhibition) during therapy to avoid complicating gastritis or ulcers that may occur is an imperative but easy intervention to forget. Our goal is to provide personalized cancer care for each unique patient, and this truly involves all team members critically analyzing each case.

SO: Take your time and build a team of truly invested experts who will dedicate themselves to the success of the new program. A successful HAI program cannot rest on the shoulders of a single provider; it really does take a village. In fact, the success of a new HAI program is measured by sustainability, not volume. Therefore, optimize patient selection and prioritize patient outcomes, including morbidity and oncologic outcomes, which will pave the way for volume later. To achieve the best outcomes, collaboration and communication between all providers and HAI team members is critical. To augment your team at a local level, it is advised that you remain in close contact with mentors from peer institutions, especially where the site visit was conducted, to help navigate the inevitable unforeseen obstacles or nuanced decisions that must be overcome when evaluating and treating a highly complex patient population.

PharmD: Use your resources! Every institution starting an HAI program has to overcome different hurdles and in doing so learn valuable lessons. If you are experiencing issues in starting a program, you are not the only pharmacy department or institution that has had those issues. The HAI consortium is filled with institutions that are happy to help and answer questions you may have when starting a new program.

Conclusion

Hepatic arterial infusion is a highly nuanced and complex therapy that requires a large, collaborative, multidisciplinary team. Regardless of prior experience, a new HAI team should travel to an established, high-volume HAI center for a site visit where they can learn about patient selection, pump implantation, HAI and systemic chemotherapy dosing and modifications, pump access and refill procedures, HAI-specific complications, and general HAI patient management. Such an experience should be considered mandatory, and this chapter details how to plan for the site visit, who to bring, and learning objectives. Armed with this information, we wish you a great HAI Site Visit!

References

1. Creasy JM, Napier KJ, Reed SA, et al. Implementation of a hepatic artery infusion program: initial patient selection and perioperative outcomes of concurrent hepatic artery infusion and systemic chemotherapy for colorectal liver metastases. Ann Surg Oncol. 2020;27:5086. https://doi.org/10.1245/s10434-020-08972-y.
2. McDonald HG, Patel RA, Ellis CS, et al. Starting a successful hepatic artery infusion pump program: a practical guide. Surgery. 2023;174(1):101–5. https://doi.org/10.1016/j.surg.2023.03.026.
3. Sharib JM, Creasy JM, Wildman-Tobriner B, et al. Hepatic artery infusion pumps: a surgical toolkit for intraoperative decision-making and management of hepatic artery infusion-specific complications. Ann Surg. 2022;276(6):943–56. https://doi.org/10.1097/SLA.0000000000005434.
4. Cavnar M, Ghalambor T, Lidsky ME, et al. Considerations and barriers to starting a new HAI pump program: an international survey of the HAI Consortium Research Network. HPB (Oxford). 2022;24(12):2104–11. https://doi.org/10.1016/j.hpb.2022.08.008.

27 Establishing and Sustaining a New Hepatic Arterial Infusion Program: Early Program and Patient Selection Considerations

Lauren M. Janczewski, Kristoffer Lassen, and Ryan P. Merkow

Considerations Prior to Establishing a Program

Prior to establishing a new hepatic artery infusion (HAI) program, there are several key considerations that providers need to review, starting with assessing an institution's suitability to build and sustain a successful program. Not all institutions are appropriate for development of an HAI program. Determining suitability at an institution involves careful evaluation, including ensuring that there is adequate case volume, ability to perform the procedure safely, manage potential complications including expertise in interventional radiology and gastroenterology, and medical oncology engagement in order to deliver HAI chemotherapy safely [1]. Institutional suitability largely relies on the training and availability of providers, but also depends on previously established infrastructure [2]. Of note, European centers will need to prepare for a dedicated process of floxuridine (FUDR) import from the United States (US) as the drug is not approved for sale in the European Union (EU). New HAI programs should already have a framework in place and be well equipped to handle the complexity of patients receiving HAI chemotherapy with a mechanism for close monitoring.

Program suitability also relies on assembling a multidisciplinary team of providers both dedicated and knowledgeable with HAI delivery. Early and extensive buy-in from all stakeholders is crucial to build a new program, including surgical oncologists experienced in complex hepatobiliary surgery, medical oncologists and an infusion team, diagnostic radiologists with nuclear medicine technicians, interventional radiologists (IR), interventional gastroenterologists (iGI), both floor and operating room nursing staff, and pharmacists (Table 27.1) [2, 3]. Surgical oncologists not only need specific training in HAI pump insertion and postoperative management but should also be comfortable with complex hepatic resections for conversion to resectable disease following HAI chemotherapy [4, 5]. Medical oncologists in collaboration with pharmacists and an infusion team should be specialized in HAI delivery including management of follow-up and dosing protocols with timely dose reductions or termination as needed [2].

L. M. Janczewski
Department of Surgery, Northwestern University Feinberg School of Medicine, Chicago, IL, USA
e-mail: lauren.janczewski1@nm.org

K. Lassen
Department of HPB-Surgery, Oslo University Hospital at Rikshospitalet, Oslo, Norway

Department of Clinical Medicine, UiT The Arctic University of Norway, Tromsø, Norway
e-mail: krlass@ous-hf.no

R. P. Merkow (✉)
Division of Surgical Oncology, Department of Surgery, University of Chicago, Chicago, IL, USA
e-mail: rpmerkow@uchicago.edu

M. D'Angelica, M. Lidsky (eds.), *Hepatic Arterial Infusion for Malignancy*,
https://doi.org/10.1007/978-3-031-74935-3_27

Table 27.1 Necessary stakeholders and their role in establishing a new HAI program

Stakeholder	Role description
Surgical oncology	• Received training in HAI pump placement • Knowledgeable and equipped to handle postoperative complications • Experienced in complex hepatobiliary cases including extended hepatic resections and ablation • Experienced in colorectal resection (may partner with colorectal surgeons) • Participates in multidisciplinary tumor board
Medical oncology	• Received training in HAI chemotherapy management and dosing protocols • Knowledgeable of potential HAI-specific complications • Initiates close and continued follow-up for patients receiving HAI chemotherapy • Participates in multidisciplinary tumor board
Pharmacy	• Knowledgeable of potential HAI chemotoxicities • Received training in HAI dosing protocols • Closely follows patient labs while receiving HAI chemotherapy and monitors for HAI-specific complications, i.e., biliary sclerosis • Maintains adequate supply of pump chemotherapy
Oncology infusion nursing leaders	• Knowledgeable in HAI dosing protocols and HAI pump access • Prepared to provide education on HAI pump access to ancillary infusion staff
Nuclear medicine	• Experienced diagnostic radiologists in interpreting nuclear medicine studies • Knowledgeable of potential HAI-specific complications such as extrahepatic, incomplete, or non-perfusion • Nuclear medicine technicians trained in facilitating HAI-pump studies
Interventional radiology	• Knowledgeable of potential HAI-specific complications • Equipped to handle catheter-related, vascular, or infectious complications requiring potential catheter thrombolysis, coil embolization for hemorrhage, arterial stenting, or percutaneous drainage of the biliary tree and abscesses • Trained in ablation techniques for liver tumors
Interventional gastroenterology	• Knowledgeable of potential HAI-specific complications, i.e., biliary sclerosis • Equipped to handle sequelae of sclerosing cholangitis with urgent biliary stent placement
Inpatient nursing leaders	• Received training in postoperative and HAI-specific complications • Prepared to provide education on caring for postoperative patients following HAI pump placement to ancillary nursing staff
Operating room nursing leaders	• Received training in necessary operative equipment • Knowledgeable of intraoperative protocols during HAI pump placement
Industry	• Provide in-service training for the above stakeholders in pump priming, access, refilling, and troubleshooting • Provide clinical support in the OR for pump implantation
Supply chain	• Maintains device inventory

Additionally, the radiology department at an HAI program must have the capabilities to perform and interpret nuclear medicine studies, which is necessary to exclude extrahepatic, incomplete, or non-perfusion for all patients after HAI pump insertion [6, 7]. Availability of IR and iGI physicians who are well equipped to manage potential postoperative complications such as catheter-related or vascular complications requiring embolization, or biliary complications requiring stent placement, is also critical [8–10]. Lastly, floor nurses should be educated on postoperative patient management and operating room staff should have general knowledge of necessary operative equipment and intraoperative protocols [2]. Institutions interested in establishing a new HAI program will not succeed without the availability and engagement of all multidisciplinary team members who are educated on HAI chemotherapy management and prepared to both identify and treat potential complications.

Before moving forward with establishing a new HAI program, it is important to develop a clear guide for initial patient selection as well as goals for both patient outcomes and the program overall, preferably as part of a research protocol. Additionally, key providers should organize a site visit to an established HAI program to learn from those with first-hand experience and identify areas for improvement in their current infrastructure. The team traveling to a high-volume HAI center should include at least surgery, medical oncology, and nursing representatives [1, 2]. Moreover, providers should receive extensive training by the hepatic pump representatives to ensure the basic foundational education is accomplished, and prior to proceeding with treatment of the initial group of patients, providers should also discuss long-term program goals. Stakeholder buy-in, engagement, and commitment is essential to success as issues will inevitably arise as the program develops [1, 2]. Lastly, all patients selected for HAI chemotherapy should be discussed, at least initially, at a multidisciplinary tumor board meeting once a program is established. This includes discussion of the indication for pump placement for each patient, which should be understood and agreed upon by all involved providers. Review of patients being considered for HAI at a multidisciplinary tumor board is fundamental to improving the expertise and collective knowledge of patient selection, complication management, and outcomes among the team of providers.

Considerations for Building a Successful Program

The objective for new HAI programs is not just to establish a program but to ensure program growth and sustainability as well as to achieve successful patient outcomes. The primary consideration for building a successful program is safety. For many years, most HAI pumps were placed at only a few high-volume, very specialized centers; however, as more providers gain interest in offering HAI as a potential therapy, there has been growing interest in establishing HAI programs [11].

When assessing safety, providers at HAI programs must consider post-pump management. Two time frames when measuring the associated risk of HAI include the initial postoperative period with complications related to pump placement as well as HAI-specific complications following the delivery of trans-arterial chemotherapy. Rates of non-pump-related postoperative complications most commonly range from 15% to 20% including intraabdominal abscess, surgical site infection, and bile leak, although these are inconsistently reported [5, 12–14]. Additionally, rates of pump or HAI-specific complications such as biliary sclerosis, arterial thrombosis, catheter dislodgement, and extrahepatic perfusion, which can cause pancreatitis, duodenal ulcers, or hemorrhage, range from 10% to 20%, leading to significant patient morbidity [3, 4, 8, 15–17]. Specifically, close attention and avoidance of the development of biliary sclerosis as a result of HAI chemotherapy is critical for new HAI programs. If biliary obstruction does occur, swift recognition and management is essential to prevent and treat cholangitis [8, 18]. It is important to ensure that the incidence of both postoperative and HAI-specific complications is within these general ranges to minimize the associated risks with HAI delivery.

In addition to ensuring safety, another main component to developing a successful HAI program is feasibility. When institutional infrastructure and HAI protocols are finalized by the multidisciplinary team, program feasibility should be assessed by monitoring the delivery of HAI chemotherapy to the early patient cohort [1]. This includes keeping track of the percentage of patients who receive HAI chemotherapy and the time to HAI chemotherapy initiation after pump placement [2]. Following pump insertion, the percentage of patients who receive HAI chemotherapy reported by established HAI programs is typically greater than 95% and the time to HAI initiation is most frequently between 2 and 4 weeks, depending on whether the patient underwent a concomitant hepatic resection [3, 12, 19]. New HAI programs should place a strong emphasis on close follow-up after HAI pump insertion during the postoperative phase and delivery of chemotherapy for their initial patient cohort. This will minimize the incidence and morbidity of potential complications and ensure all patients receive HAI chemotherapy within an appropriate timeline, increasing the likelihood for successful outcomes.

As programs begin treating patients with HAI chemotherapy, communication through both individual and team meetings is important to evaluate the initial safety and efficacy so that programs can adapt based on their preliminary outcomes. Following the first case, including both pump insertion and delivery of HAI chemotherapy, new programs should organize a team meeting with the opportunity for all providers to debrief [2]. It is essential not to skip this step and continue frequent multidisciplinary team meetings as new programs start treating patients with HAI chemotherapy. Lack of communication while building a new program can lead to provider miscommunication and inability to effectively address problems that will inevitably arise. This will significantly risk program failure over time. Of note, this should not be limited to only the surgical and medical oncologists on the team [1]. It is important to ensure that everyone's voice including nursing, pharmacy, nuclear medicine, gastroenterology, operating room staff, and interventional radiology is heard. All concerns should be taken seriously and immediately addressed to optimize successful patient outcomes. The importance of nonphysician engagement and buy-in should not be underestimated as this is critical to ensure best treatment practices for this difficult-to-treat subset of patients. Similarly, having a collaborative relationship with other physician members, such as IR, is equally important as the treatment of hepatic metastases should be viewed as a partnership, not competition.

Early Patient Selection

Criteria for early patient selection at newly established HAI programs should start with a narrow scope of practice that is agreed upon by all providers to facilitate early treatment success. Following multidisciplinary evaluation, all providers should have a clear understanding of the pattern and extent of disease and goals of therapy prior to proceeding with HAI pump insertion. It has been generally recommended that early patient selection should primarily focus on patients with unresectable hepatic metastases from colorectal cancer and locally unresectable liver-confined intrahepatic cholangiocarcinoma. The optimal patient has had stable to responsive disease after first- or second-line chemotherapy, or has become intolerant to cytotoxic therapy [3, 20, 21]. Such stringent selection ensures a new program can safely implant pumps, get patients through the perioperative period, and safely and effectively deliver HAI chemotherapy without jeopardizing other effective lines of therapy. As HAI programs continue to develop and evolve overtime, adjuvant HAI in patients with completely resectable colorectal liver metastases (CRLM) can be considered; however, HAI-related complications in this potentially curable group of patients is particularly devastating and therefore should be avoided in new programs [22–27]. Patient selection within the initial cohort should largely consist of patients with liver-only metastases as well [3, 11, 21, 22], unless a dedicated protocol has been agreed upon. Transitioning to treat patients with extrahepatic metastatic disease (i.e., resectable lung metastases) can be carefully evaluated in formal protocols as HAI programs gain experience but should not be the primary focus for new programs to ensure early treatment success.

In addition to the pattern and extent of disease, new programs should pay close attention to the underlying disease biology when selecting patients for HAI chemotherapy. Particular consideration should be given to tumor mutation status. We recommend excluding colorectal cancer patients with BRAF mutations due to their elevated risk of extrahepatic metastatic disease and overall poor prognosis [28]. Although this is a relatively small subset of patients (<10% of advanced colorectal cancers), BRAF-mutated colorectal cancer is an identified negative prognostic biomarker with limited response to traditional systemic chemotherapy as well as increased risk for recurrence and extrahepatic metastatic disease [28, 29]. Excluding patients with BRAF mutations within the early patient cohort is an important consideration, again, to increase successful patient outcomes. A multidisciplinary assessment of the underlying disease response to systemic chemotherapy is also warranted when selecting patients for HAI chemotherapy at new programs [1]. If not part of a formalized protocol with complete follow-up, early patient selection should exclude patients with progressing hepatic metastases and focus on disease that has reached a point of stability in response to systemic chemotherapy [21].

In summary, emphasis on patient selection for new HAI programs is an imperative aspect to ensure the success of a new HAI program. Early patient selection at new HAI centers should concentrate on patients with liver-only metastatic colorectal cancer and intrahepatic cholangiocarcinoma with favorable biology. After demonstrating acceptable outcomes within the early patient cohort, HAI programs may then consider broadening their selection criteria and expand their patient population; however, this should be done with extensive and deliberate multidisciplinary discussion after substantial gained experience at the program level or as part of a prospective trial.

Surgical Planning and Technical Aspects

HAI chemotherapy cannot be delivered without insertion of the pump; thus, some of the most important aspects of treating this complex group of patients are the technical components of the operation, ensuring that the pump functions appropriately prior to proceeding with HAI chemotherapy [15, 17]. This can be optimized by identifying patients with favorable preoperative characteristics and verifying the necessary materials, supplies, and equipment for pump placement are available prior to proceeding with the operation.

The preoperative evaluation should place particular emphasis on a thorough surgical history and review of necessary imaging prior to HAI pump insertion. Patients with extensive surgical history, specifically open abdominal surgeries with dissection of or near the porta hepatis, should be avoided initially as this increases the operative difficulty and potential for complications [17]. All patients should undergo a dedicated abdominal computed tomography angiography (CTA) preoperatively. This is done not only to evaluate the presence of potential extrahepatic metastases but also to delineate the gastroduodenal artery (GDA) and hepatic vasculature for verification of a suitable target vessel for the pump catheter insertion [4, 6, 15]. Variant hepatic artery anatomy is common, and new programs should identify patients with favorable anatomy, that allows for GDA canulation to minimize the initial technical complexity and minimize pump complications. While a dominant replaced left hepatic artery may be sacrificed in most cases, it may prove a challenge if the patient responds well to HAI treatment and is considered for a right hemi-hepatectomy at a later stage. Additionally, new programs may consider implanting pumps in patients who have an unsuitable GDA. In these scenarios, conduits or non-GDA targets are used, but this may increase the risk of a nonusable pump and/or major morbidity.

Following preoperative evaluation, a clear surgical plan should be prepared prior to proceeding with HAI pump insertion. Although HAI pumps can be placed via both an open and robotic approach, it is recommended that pump insertion at new programs be done initially through an open approach, with the potential to transition to a robotic practice as operative experience is gained with demonstrated success [30, 31]. Additionally, a plan for management of the primary tumor for CRLM should be developed as well. Concomitant colectomy with HAI pump placement in patients with CRLM has been shown to be safe and poses minimal increased risk of postoperative complications, including infection; however, management of the primary tumor for CRLM should be planned on an individualized basis and warrants multidisciplinary discussion prior to proceeding [13, 14].

The degree of liver disease should also be carefully assessed both preoperatively and intraoperatively, and a plan developed for addressing the hepatic tumor burden. For patients with unresectable disease undergoing HAI pump placement alone, a pathway for potential conversion prior to pump placement should be established for future resection [20, 21, 32, 33]. For example, an initial operation could consist of clearing the left hepatic lobe of all disease, HAI pump placement, and colorectal primary resection, with a plan for future staged right hepatectomy following HAI chemotherapy. Although patients may not convert to resectability along their treatment course, the goal for conversion in patients with unresectable metastases is important to define prior to moving forward. For patients with CRLM, the specific plan may change based on intraoperative ultrasound, and the surgeon should be prepared to adapt the preoperative plan as needed.

Program Evolution

As new HAI programs exhibit growth with gained experience, broadening the patient selection criteria can be considered based on the level of comfort within each specific institution. As mentioned previously, once surgeons have sufficient experience and have demonstrated success with HAI placement via an open approach, expanding the surgical practice to include robotic HAI pump insertion for surgeons with an already established robotic skillset is possible [30, 31]. However, this should only be done after the learning curve for placing HAI pumps has been achieved through an open abdominal approach. Although there is no published literature on a clearly defined learning curve, the work of Allen et al. demonstrated decreased complication rates for surgeons who had placed more than 25 pumps [4].

Another area for HAI practice expansion includes developing a protocol for HAI patient selection in the setting of extrahepatic disease [2]. The appropriateness of each patient for HAI chemotherapy should be thoroughly discussed on an individualized basis, and basic criteria should be developed to guide patient selection within this population. When transitioning to include patients with extrahepatic metastatic disease, a thorough understanding of the tumor biology with evaluation of the pattern and extent of extrahepatic disease burden is crucial. Overall, patients should have low volume extrahepatic disease with a well-defined plan to address these lesions [34–36]. For example, a starting point for HAI programs seeking to expand their practice could consider patients with a single pulmonary metastasis in the setting of CRLM that is deemed readily resectable by a thoracic surgeon. Patients with extrahepatic metastatic disease with more aggressive biology (e.g., portal nodes, peritoneal disease) are generally not candidates for HAI chemotherapy [34].

After HAI programs have demonstrated success in managing patients with unresectable disease, programs can consider transitioning their practice to include delivery of adjuvant HAI chemotherapy. Programs should have extensive multidisciplinary discussions to develop a clear outline for patients that are appropriate for adjuvant HAI and a prospective protocol is preferable as there will be no assessable tumor to monitor [23, 25]. Although the use of adjuvant HAI is less common due to concerns regarding toxicity (in particular biliary toxicity), in this potentially curable group of patients, its safety and survival implications have been described [5, 19, 24]. Much of this initial experience and current literature regarding adjuvant HAI comes from Memorial Sloan Kettering Cancer Center (MSKCC), where the majority of research and development of HAI chemotherapy originated [26, 27, 37]. In particular, when comparing patients with unresectable and resectable CRLM, researchers at MSKCC found the median overall survival for patients who received adjuvant HAI was 67 months compared to 44 months for those who only underwent resection, despite the HAI group having more advanced disease [26]. Similar results have been demonstrated at additional HAI institutions as well, confirming the safety and feasibility of adjuvant HAI when patients are appropriately selected [19, 23–25]. The number of resectable liver metastases considered for adjuvant HAI may vary at the institutional level as there is no specific number of liver metastases deemed necessary for adjuvant HAI in the literature; however, an agreed upon protocol must be developed by the multidisciplinary team prior to moving forward. In a similar fashion to beginning an HAI program, expanding an HAI program must be done by carefully evaluating safety and feasibility as the program evolves.

Conclusion

With gaining interest in providing HAI chemotherapy as a potential treatment modality for this difficult-to-treat subset of patients, centers need to consider program suitability and institutional infrastructure prior to establishing a new HAI program. Early patient selection, stakeholder buy-in, and successful initial outcomes are critical to ensure long-term program sustainability. Although HAI chemotherapy was previously restricted to select highly specialized center, establishing new HAI programs is both safe and feasible when considering these specific factors in their initial development. To ensure the growth of our common knowledge base, new efforts should preferably be within prospective protocols with adequate follow-up.

References

1. Cavnar M, et al. Considerations and barriers to starting a new HAI pump program: an international survey of the HAI Consortium Research Network. HPB (Oxford). 2022;24:S100.
2. Karanicolas PJ, et al. Hepatic arterial infusion pump chemotherapy in the management of colorectal liver metastases: expert consensus statement. Curr Oncol. 2014;21(1):e129–36.
3. Creasy JM, et al. Implementation of a hepatic artery infusion program: initial patient selection and perioperative outcomes of concurrent hepatic artery infusion and systemic chemotherapy for colorectal liver metastases. Ann Surg Oncol. 2020;27(13):5086–95.
4. Allen PJ, et al. Technical complications and durability of hepatic artery infusion pumps for unresectable colorectal liver metastases: an institutional experience of 544 consecutive cases. J Am Coll Surg. 2005;201(1):57–65.
5. Chakedis J, et al. Implementation and early outcomes for a surgeon-directed hepatic arterial infusion pump program for colorectal liver metastases. J Surg Oncol. 2018;118(7):1065–73.
6. Napier KJ, et al. Hepatic arterial infusion pumps: what the radiologist needs to know. Radiographics. 2021;41(3):895–908.
7. Perez DR, et al. Angiographic identification of extrahepatic perfusion after hepatic arterial pump placement: implications for surgical prevention. HPB (Oxford). 2014;16(8):744–8.
8. Ito K, et al. Biliary sclerosis after hepatic arterial infusion pump chemotherapy for patients with colorectal cancer liver metastasis: incidence, clinical features, and risk factors. Ann Surg Oncol. 2012;19(5):1609–17.
9. Sofocleous CT, et al. Arterial embolization for salvage of hepatic artery infusion pumps. J Vasc Interv Radiol. 2006;17(5):801–6.
10. Bloom AI, et al. Transcatheter embolization for the treatment of misperfusion after hepatic artery chemoinfusion pump implantation. Ann Surg Oncol. 1999;6(4):350–8.
11. Ko YJ, Karanicolas PJ. Hepatic arterial infusion pump chemotherapy for colorectal liver metastases: an old technology in a new era. Curr Oncol. 2014;21(1):e116–21.
12. Muaddi H, et al. Safety and feasibility of initiating a hepatic artery infusion pump chemotherapy program for unresectable colorectal liver metastases: a multicenter, retrospective cohort study. J Surg Oncol. 2021;123(1):252–60.
13. Brajcich BC, et al. Short-term risk of performing concurrent procedures with hepatic artery infusion pump placement. Ann Surg Oncol. 2020;27(13):5098–106.
14. Turley MC, et al. Combined primary resection with hepatic artery infusion pump implantation is safe for unresectable colorectal liver metastases. J Gastrointest Surg. 2022;26(4):764–71.
15. Curley SA, et al. Technical considerations and complications associated with the placement of 180 implantable hepatic arterial infusion devices. Surgery. 1993;114(5):928–35.
16. Kemeny NE, et al. Hepatic arterial infusion versus systemic therapy for hepatic metastases from colorectal cancer: a randomized trial of efficacy, quality of life, and molecular markers (CALGB 9481). J Clin Oncol. 2006;24(9):1395–403.
17. Sharib JM, et al. Hepatic artery infusion pumps: a surgical toolkit for intraoperative decision-making and management of hepatic artery infusion-specific complications. Ann Surg. 2022;276(6):943–56.
18. Kemeny MM, et al. Sclerosing cholangitis after continuous hepatic artery infusion of FUDR. Ann Surg. 1985;202(2):176–81.
19. Walker BS, et al. Hepatic arterial infusion pump chemotherapy combined with systemic therapy for patients with advanced colorectal liver metastases: outcomes in a newly established program. J Surg Oncol. 2022;126(3):513–22.
20. Pak LM, et al. Prospective phase II trial of combination hepatic artery infusion and systemic chemotherapy for unresectable colorectal liver metastases: long term results and curative potential. J Surg Oncol. 2018;117(4):634–43.
21. Datta J, et al. Role of hepatic artery infusion chemotherapy in treatment of initially unresectable colorectal liver metastases: a review. JAMA Surg. 2019;154(8):768–76.
22. Alberts SR, et al. Alternating systemic and hepatic artery infusion therapy for resected liver metastases from colorectal cancer: a North Central Cancer Treatment Group (NCCTG)/National Surgical Adjuvant Breast and Bowel Project (NSABP) phase

II intergroup trial, N9945/CI-66. J Clin Oncol. 2010;28(5):853–8.
23. Buisman FE, et al. Adjuvant hepatic arterial infusion pump chemotherapy after resection of colorectal liver metastases: results of a safety and feasibility study in The Netherlands. Ann Surg Oncol. 2019;26(13):4599–607.
24. Lorenz M, et al. Randomized trial of surgery versus surgery followed by adjuvant hepatic arterial infusion with 5-fluorouracil and folinic acid for liver metastases of colorectal cancer. German Cooperative on Liver Metastases (Arbeitsgruppe Lebermetastasen). Ann Surg. 1998;228(6):756–62.
25. Mitry E, et al. Adjuvant chemotherapy after potentially curative resection of metastases from colorectal cancer: a pooled analysis of two randomized trials. J Clin Oncol. 2008;26(30):4906–11.
26. Groot Koerkamp B, et al. Perioperative hepatic arterial infusion pump chemotherapy is associated with longer survival after resection of colorectal liver metastases: a propensity score analysis. J Clin Oncol. 2017;35(17):1938–44.
27. Kemeny NE, et al. Updated long-term survival for patients with metastatic colorectal cancer treated with liver resection followed by hepatic arterial infusion and systemic chemotherapy. J Surg Oncol. 2016;113(5):477–84.
28. Ciombor KK, et al. BRAF-mutated advanced colorectal cancer: a rapidly changing therapeutic landscape. J Clin Oncol. 2022;40(24):2706–15.
29. Grassi E, et al. Current therapeutic strategies in BRAF-mutant metastatic colorectal cancer. Front Oncol. 2021;11:601722.
30. Dhir M, et al. Robotic-assisted placement of an hepatic artery infusion pump and catheter for regional chemotherapy of the liver. Ann Surg Oncol. 2016;23(Suppl 5):755–6.
31. Qadan M, et al. Robotic hepatic arterial infusion pump placement. HPB (Oxford). 2017;19(5):429–35.
32. Levi FA, et al. Conversion to resection of liver metastases from colorectal cancer with hepatic artery infusion of combined chemotherapy and systemic cetuximab in multicenter trial OPTILIV. Ann Oncol. 2016;27(2):267–74.
33. D'Angelica MI, et al. Phase II trial of hepatic artery infusional and systemic chemotherapy for patients with unresectable hepatic metastases from colorectal cancer: conversion to resection and long-term outcomes. Ann Surg. 2015;261(2):353–60.
34. Ammori JB, et al. Hepatic artery infusional chemotherapy in patients with unresectable colorectal liver metastases and extrahepatic disease. J Surg Oncol. 2012;106(8):953–8.
35. Pawlik TM, Schulick RD, Choti MA. Expanding criteria for resectability of colorectal liver metastases. Oncologist. 2008;13(1):51–64.
36. Carpizo DR, et al. Liver resection for metastatic colorectal cancer in patients with concurrent extrahepatic disease: results in 127 patients treated at a single center. Ann Surg Oncol. 2009;16(8):2138–46.
37. Kemeny N, et al. Hepatic arterial infusion of chemotherapy after resection of hepatic metastases from colorectal cancer. N Engl J Med. 1999;341(27):2039–48.

Patient Education for Hepatic Arterial Infusion

28

Sree B. Chalasani, Ann E. Stevens, and Cornelius A. Thiels

Introduction

Patient education is a key component of providing high-quality care and is essential from an ethical standpoint. It is even a fundamental patient right in many countries [1]. It is also essential for the safe delivery of therapies and improved outcomes [2]. In the setting of advanced or metastatic cancer, patient education is critically important given the risk of progression or recurrence, and physicians need to account for the quality-of-life implications of the therapies and patients' overall goals.

Patient education should be a core component of all hepatic artery infusion (HAI) pump programs as there are unique aspects of HAI therapy that must be clearly conveyed to patients before and during their treatment journey. In this chapter we, will review the components of a robust patient education program, including surgical, medical oncology, and nursing education. We will also discuss the development of patient education materials. Lastly, we will emphasize the unique aspects of HAI education, as an incomplete understanding of the logistics associated with pump fills and the physical limitations associated with having a pump can lead to life-threatening consequences for patients if they are not properly educated.

S. B. Chalasani (✉)
Memorial Sloan Kettering Cancer Center, New York, NY, USA
e-mail: Chalasas@mskcc.org

A. E. Stevens · C. A. Thiels
Mayo Clinic, Rochester, MN, USA
e-mail: Stevens.Ann@mayo.edu; Thiels.Cornelius@mayo.edu

Developing a HAI Patient Education Program

General Patient Education

Patient education for HAI requires a multidisciplinary approach that includes surgeons, medical oncologists, nurses, pharmacists, and patient education specialists. Patient education for HAI is not a single event, but an ongoing process. It should begin at the first clinic consultation and continue throughout the duration of the patient's pump therapy, until the pump has been removed. Patient education for HAI must include everything from mechanism and scientific data to support pump placement, details of pump placement surgery and recovery, explanation of the pump fill process, education on chemotherapy side effects, the potential oncologic risks and benefits, and pump maintenance and/or removal process. This education must be done simultaneously with routine oncologic education, especially since pump therapy is often delivered concurrently with other cancer therapies. Therefore, patient education cannot be delivered in a single appointment or via a single educational document and instead should delivered in a comprehensive

M. D'Angelica, M. Lidsky (eds.), *Hepatic Arterial Infusion for Malignancy*,
https://doi.org/10.1007/978-3-031-74935-3_28

manner by a team of nurses and physicians, ideally combined with traditional patient education materials when possible.

Patient Education When Evaluating a Patient for Pump Placement

Prior to proceeding with HAI pump placement and chemotherapy, it is essential that patients receive thorough education on the rationale for pump placement and the potential risks, benefits, and alternatives to HAI therapy. In addition, unlike many other therapies, patients must have a thorough understanding of the intensiveness of pump treatments, the potential financial and logistical implications, and the physical limitations, as these can impact their candidacy for HAI therapy. It is important that patients meet with both a surgeon and medical oncologist familiar with HAI pump placement and chemotherapy prior to proceeding with pump placement.

Patients should be educated on the rationale for pump placement as well as the data to support HAI in the setting of their individual cancer diagnosis. Although the level of detail physicians provide on the mechanism of action and data to support pump chemotherapy may vary by health literacy and patient wishes, all patients should be offered this information. The following information on the mechanism of action of HAI therapy may be beneficial to discuss with patients: the anatomic principle that liver metastases are primarily perfused by the hepatic artery [3]; the selected chemotherapeutic agents for HAI have a high extraction by the liver followed by rapid clearance; and the result that higher concentrations of chemotherapy can be administered locally to the liver while minimizing systemic side effects [4].

Types of HAI Pumps

The specific type of pump placed depends on institutional preference and what pump is approved for HAI therapy, which can vary by country. There are currently two implanted pumps being used to deliver HAI chemotherapy in the United States.

Patient Considerations When Receiving the Intera 3000 HAI Pump (Previously Known as the Codman pump)

The Intera 3000 HAI pump is manufactured by Intera Oncology (Wellesley, MA, USA). The pump flow rate is constant, and the exact flow rate is specified by the company in the product packaging. The Intera 3000 pump is MRI conditional and patients with this implanted device can be safely scanned with MRI so long as the machine meets the conditions specified by the company. Patients should be educated to notify their physicians that they have a HAI pump as exceeding the listed MRI parameters could result in increased drug delivery and/or excessive force or torque leading to patient injury. An example of the Intera 3000 HAI pump is shown in Fig. 28.1 and should be shown to patients prior to surgery.

Patient Considerations on Medtronic SynchroMed II Pump

This pump *is not FDA approved* for HAI therapy but may be used off-label. The Medtronic SynchroMed II pumps have distinct nuances that are important for patients to be aware of. Medtronic pumps are programmed at a set flow rate that can be adjusted using a Clinician Medtronic Programmer (a tablet that connects to the pump via Bluetooth). It is important for patients to understand that this pump is battery

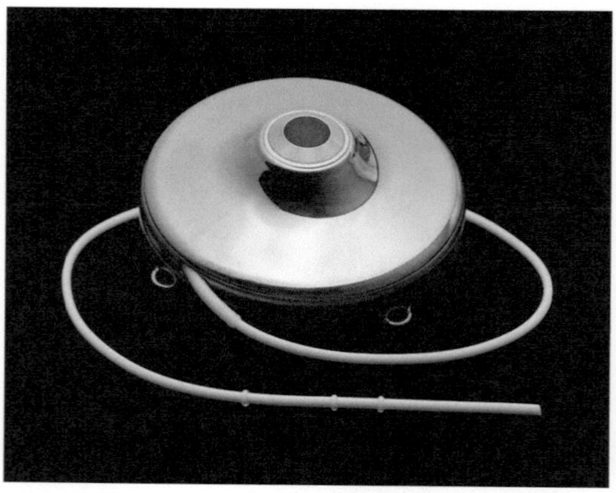

Fig. 28.1 Example of the Intera 3000 HAI pump. (Copyright Intera Oncology, permission provided)

operated and the life expectancy of the pump is estimated at 7 years. These pumps are also MRI compatible; however, the patient should inform their physician about the pump prior to undergoing an MRI. The device temporarily shuts off in the presence of the magnet; therefore, the pump should be interrogated by the Clinician Medtronic Programmer within 24 h of completion of the imaging study. The Clinician Medtronic Programmer can interact with other devices such as cochlear implants, deep brain stimulators, defibrillators, and pacemakers, and these devices should be kept away from the programmer. If the pump malfunctions or dries up, the pump can create an audible alert, which warns patients to seek urgent medical evaluation.

Logistics of Pump Therapy

Numerous logistical factors must be considered before patients proceed with HAI pump placement. One of the most important concepts for patients to understand is the time commitment and frequency of appointments during HAI treatment. Once the pump is placed, the first pump fill is required within 2 weeks of the last pump fill (date of pump priming in OR). Depending on institutional protocols, this first pump fill can be performed during the hospital admission or shortly after discharge. Patients then begin 2-week cycles of pump fills for the duration of their treatment. It is critically important for patients to understand that pump fill appointments cannot be missed or delayed more than a few days without risking irreversible pump failure as fluid in the pump is necessary to maintain patency.

To prevent noncompliance, it is imperative to explain to patients why their HAI pump must be refilled every 2 weeks while they are on treatment. Patients need to understand that without sufficient circulating solution, the HAI pump catheter can clot and become nonfunctional. It is also important for patients to understand that if a HAI pump becomes nonfunctional, it typically cannot be replaced.

A typical course of HAI treatment lasts approximately 4–6 months, although occasionally can last longer. Patients need to be able to reliably travel to the medical center for every pump fill appointment and they must be aware that these refills typically cannot be completed at centers that do not specialize in HAI pump therapy. Potential barriers to travel, including weather and travel delays, should be anticipated in advance and mitigation strategies discussed with the patient. Although patient eligibility should not be limited by social, logistical, or financial factors, it is important to address any barriers prior to pump placement, particularly in patients who are traveling to receive this therapy. Preoperative consultation with social work may be beneficial given the significant time and resource commitment needed to receive HAI therapy and the potential physical limitations (see below) when the pump is in place.

While some HAI centers will collaborate with local oncologists or surgeons for saline fills and/or systemic chemotherapy, it is important for patients to understand that most centers require them to transfer all of their oncologic care to the center that surgically places their HAI pump and administers HAI chemotherapy. It is also important for patients to understand that they will typically continue to receive systemic chemotherapy during HAI treatment, and most centers require that patients receive their systemic chemotherapy at the HAI center. Patients should be informed that most providers are not familiar with managing HAI pumps, chemotherapy, or complications, and therefore they need to routinely return to the HAI center for close monitoring of liver function, titration of medications, and to manage any complications.

Activity Guidelines and Restrictions

Patients must be counseled on activity restrictions prior to committing to HAI pump placement as it can impact their ability to work or engage in social and recreational activities that may be important to them. Most of the restrictions are related to avoiding changes in pressure, elevation, and body temperature, which can impact the pump infusion flow rate. This may result in excessive delivery of pump chemotherapy and unintended toxicity and/or rapid evacuation of drug reservoir contents, which can result in pump failure. Patients should be counseled to observe the following suggested guidelines (Box 28.1) or be referred to the individual pump manufacture guidelines [5]. It is important to note that these are based on manufacturer guidance and experience of the authors and are not necessarily evidence based. Some of these restrictions only apply while receiving HAI chemotherapy or in the setting of liver dysfunction (e.g., alcohol and acetaminophen avoidance). Lastly, these restrictions should be emphasized prior to proceeding with pump placement and reemphasized before and during HAI therapy. The patient should also be made aware that patients often can feel the pump and even less vigorous physical activity can result in pain or discomfort.

Box 28.1 Suggested Patient Activity Restrictions

Do not participate in rough physical activity such as contact sports. This may cause a hit or blow to the pump site and can damage the pump. Less intensive physical activity may also result in discomfort
Do not go deep sea or scuba diving. The increased pressure experienced during these activities will affect the flow rate of the pump
Do not fly in small, private planes that are not pressurized. Traveling by commercial airplanes that are pressurized is safe
Changes in elevation can impact the flow rate of the pump. Always consult the physician managing your pump prior to engaging in an activity with the potential for changes in elevation
Do not place heating pads, hot water bottles, or electric blankets over the pump site
Do not use hot tubs or saunas and avoid prolonged direct sun exposure. An increase in local pump site temperature or an elevated body temperature will cause the pump to flow faster
Do not take any medications that contain acetaminophen without consulting your physician
Avoid alcohol while receiving HAI chemotherapy

Patient Education from Surgical Perspective

This section will cover the important aspects of patient education related to surgery. Although many surgeons who place HAI pumps will remain involved in the patient's care throughout their journey, this section will focus on patient education related to the surgical consultation, preoperative consent, surgery, and recovery. Patient education at these time points, however, should seamlessly include medical oncology (chemotherapy) and nursing education as discussed below.

Informed Consent and Complications

Surgeons have an ethical and legal obligation to engage in an informed consent process with patients considering HAI pump placement. While most hospitals have a consent form that requires a signature, the language found in these consent forms cover only a small fraction of the informed consent process. Therefore, a thorough informed consent is an important aspect of the patient education process. It is important to confirm adequate mental capacity of the patient and then discuss all the standard components of informed consent with the patient, which should include the disease diagnosis, proposed procedure, procedure-related risks, long-term HAI-specific risks, likelihood of success of the procedure and HAI therapy, and alternative treatment options [6]. However, unique to HAI pump placement, patients should also be clearly informed that the device will be implanted and remain in their body.

As with any surgical procedure, it is important to discuss with patients the expected recovery process and potential complications. The individual risks of pump placement, including complications related to the device, pump pocket, catheter, artery, malperfusion, biliary tree, and non-function, are discussed in other sections of this book. However, unique to other surgeries, it is important to discuss the risk and implications of extrahepatic perfusion and pump failure with the patient. It is also important to emphasize (before and after surgery) any unique complications that patients should watch for. For example, a surgical site hematoma or infection in the setting of an implanted device may require urgent attention and treatment. A fever should also be reported as it can increase the flow rate of the pump and may warrant moving up the next pump refill appointment. Therefore, in addition to the routine signs and symptoms to watch for, patients should be informed about the unique pump site and systemic symptoms to watch for, all of which should prompt notification of the HAI treatment team as soon as concerning signs or symptoms are encountered.

Combined Procedures

HAI pump placement is often performed concurrently with additional procedures. Patients should be informed that they will undergo cholecystectomy at the time of pump placement if they have not already had a cholecystectomy in the past. Lastly, it is important to discuss with the patient any combined surgeries, including liver resections or ablations and/or colorectal resections. Each of these combined procedures has unique patient education implications that are outside the scope of the chapter. However, it is important to discuss with patients how each of these combined procedures may increase the morbidity and/or recovery process after HAI pump placement. For example, major liver resections may delay the initiation of pump therapy slightly and although there is no definitive evidence to support an increased infection risk when HAI pump placement is combined with colorectal procedures, surgeons may choose to discuss this risk with patients at their discretion.

Postoperative Follow-Up

Each institution and surgeon typically have a slightly different postoperative follow-up regimen. However, it is important that patients understand that in the first few weeks after their pump placement, they may have numerous follow-up appointments. These appointments may include surgical follow-up, consultation with medical oncology, the first pump fill, and a nuclear medicine study depending on the institutional protocol. Patients should also be informed that they will be given an identification card around the time of surgery (most commonly mailed to the patient). Patients should be counseled to carry this identification card with them for use in emergency departments, airports, or other security areas (Fig. 28.2). Lastly, patients should be educated to inform healthcare providers about their pump as this can impact their ability to receive MRIs depending on the type of pump and type of MRI machine.

Nuclear Medicine Study

Institutions must utilize postoperative nuclear medicine scans to check the perfusion of the pump after surgery and before patients start HAI therapy. This procedure is typically done either during the hospital admission or shortly after discharge. If done after discharge, then it is important to inform patients of this required procedure prior to pump implantation as it may impact their travel arrangements. Patients should also be educated on the rationale for this procedure and that it is used to verify the absence of extrahepatic perfusion. If there is perfusion outside of the liver, this must be addressed before chemotherapy can be administered through the HAI pump and thus additional tests or procedures may be needed. This procedure can be uncomfortable and take up to 2 h; therefore, patient education prior to this procedure to discuss expectations is beneficial. This education should include the appropriate use of pain medications or topical anesthetics prior to the procedure as indicated.

Pump Maintenance After Therapy and the Process of Removing a Pump

After patients complete their course of HAI chemotherapy, it is important to discuss with them the logistics and options for pump maintenance or removal. This conversation should occur

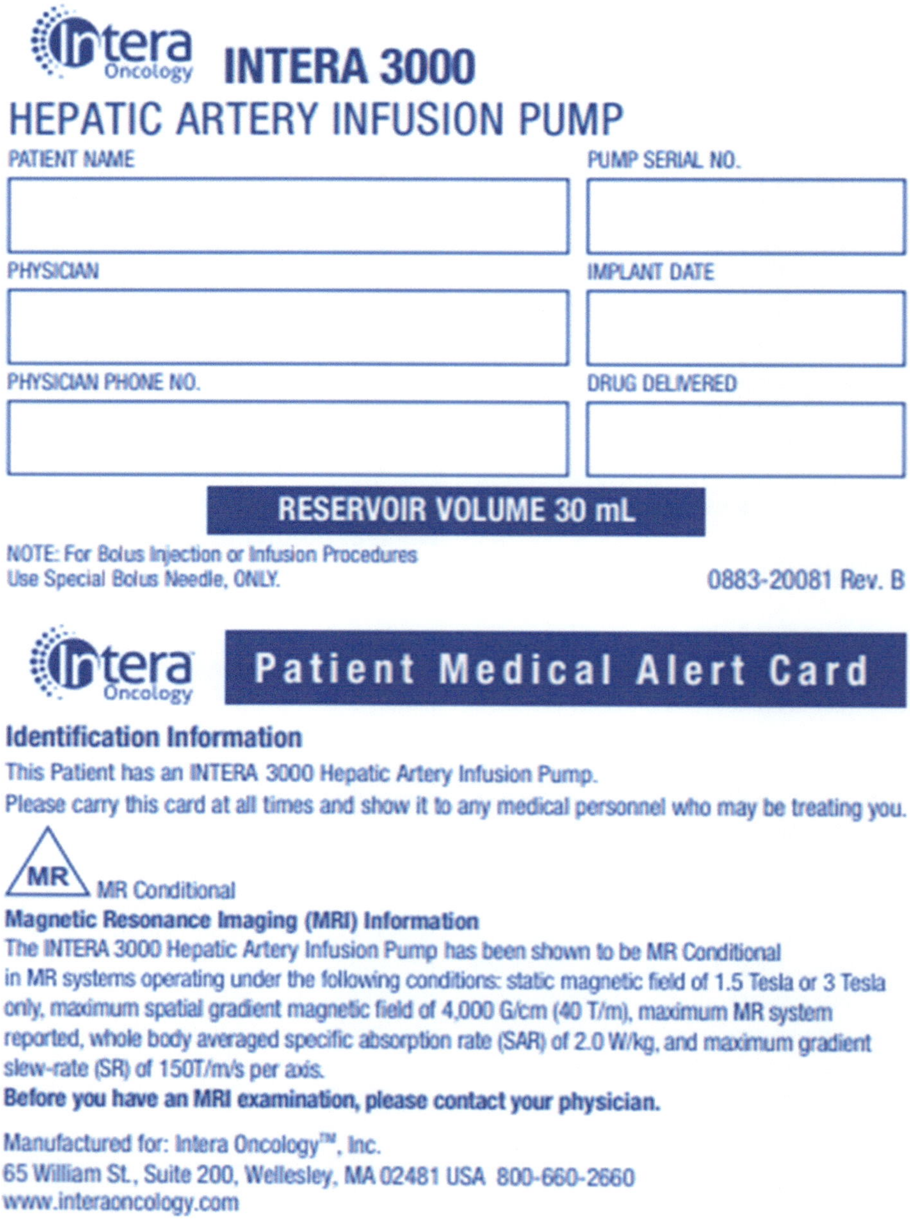

Intera Oncology INTERA 3000

HEPATIC ARTERY INFUSION PUMP

PATIENT NAME

PUMP SERIAL NO.

PHYSICIAN

IMPLANT DATE

PHYSICIAN PHONE NO.

DRUG DELIVERED

RESERVOIR VOLUME 30 mL

NOTE: For Bolus Injection or Infusion Procedures
Use Special Bolus Needle, ONLY.

0883-20081 Rev. B

Intera Oncology Patient Medical Alert Card

Identification Information

This Patient has an INTERA 3000 Hepatic Artery Infusion Pump.
Please carry this card at all times and show it to any medical personnel who may be treating you.

MR

MR Conditional

Magnetic Resonance Imaging (MRI) Information

The INTERA 3000 Hepatic Artery Infusion Pump has been shown to be MR Conditional in MR systems operating under the following conditions: static magnetic field of 1.5 Tesla or 3 Tesla only, maximum spatial gradient magnetic field of 4,000 G/cm (40 T/m), maximum MR system reported, whole body averaged specific absorption rate (SAR) of 2.0 W/kg, and maximum gradient slew-rate (SR) of 150T/m/s per axis.

Before you have an MRI examination, please contact your physician.

Manufactured for: Intera Oncology™, Inc.
65 William St., Suite 200, Wellesley, MA 02481 USA 800-660-2660
www.interaoncology.com

Fig. 28.2 Example of patient medical alert card. (Copyright Intera Oncology, permission provided)

before the pump is placed and again after they complete HAI therapy. It is important to emphasize that although HAI treatments typically last only 4–6 months, many patients will continue to keep the pump in place for much longer (up to 2–5 years or longer). It is important to explain to patients that pumps do not have to be removed unless there is a complication. Patients again need to understand that once a pump is removed, they very rarely can be replaced.

Patients should be educated on the option of transitioning to glycerin solution fills, which allow them to prolong the interval between pump fills. Although the pump is filled every 2 weeks while on active HAI therapy, patients can transition to pump fills every 6–8 weeks once they are in maintenance mode. This allows patients to keep their HAI pump patent for potential future use while decreasing return visit frequency. It is also important to inform patients in advance that the pump removal does require an outpatient surgical procedure. Lastly, it is crucial that patients understand that when a pump is removed, the catheter (tubing) is typically left in the abdomen. Some patients might find this unsettling and therefore it is essential to explain this to the patient prior to pump placement.

Patient Education from Medical Oncology Perspective

This section will cover important aspects of patient education related to pump fill appointments, HAI chemotherapy, concurrent systemic chemotherapy, side effects, and other medications used during HAI treatment. A typical course of HAI treatment can last up to 4–6 months; however, it can vary from patient to patient depending on the indication. Patients should be informed that not all patients are able to receive all the planned doses of HAI treatments and that the dose is often reduced during the therapy. During the first consultation, it is important not only to review the overall outline of therapy but also to educate patients that their therapy can change based on operative findings and clinical course. Patients' expectations should be managed throughout their treatment and any change in the planned treatment course should be discussed with patients in a timely manner. The next steps should be planned after an informed discussion with patients where all the options are reviewed.

Process of Pump Fills and Follow-Up Appointments

During appointments, patients will have labs drawn, meet with a member of their medical oncology team, and undergo a refill of their HAI pump. Liver function testing is an important aspect of HAI treatment as the chemotherapy dose may need adjusting based on patient's liver function tests. Patients will need imaging periodically throughout their treatment to assess tumor response to HAI treatment.

Filling the pump itself typically takes 15–20 min; however, the duration of these appointments can vary from less than an hour to a full day depending on additional testing and appointments. Outside of normally scheduled appointment dates, patients also need to be prepared to come to the medical center on short notice if complications arise. Pump site seromas can be a problem after surgery and might have to be aspirated prior to or at the time of pump access. The pump can flip and necessitate repositioning. This procedure is performed by the surgeon in the operating room under general anesthesia. Patients should be advised to be on the lookout for pump pocket infection which can present as fevers, pain or redness around the pump site, or drainage from the pump pocket incision, and can occur at any interval of time after pump placement and/or pump refills. They should reach out to their physician immediately if these signs or symptoms are observed. It is also important to educate patients on the process of having the pump filled. Particularly, during the first few fill appointments, it is important that the oncologist or nurse who fills the pump explains the procedure to the patient. An example of how the pump is accessed is shown in Fig. 28.3 and is also reviewed in the video atlas.

HAI Chemotherapy and Side Effects

The most widely used chemotherapy agent for HAI treatment is floxuridine (FUDR). The most severe complications of FUDR include biliary sclerosis, which can result in liver failure if not addressed promptly, as well as stomach or duodenal ulceration as a result of malperfusion. Patients should be educated on the warning signs that should prompt them to reach out to their oncologist immediately. Symptoms of biliary sclerosis include pruritis and jaundice, while those of upper gastrointestinal ulcers include severe acid reflux symptoms, upper abdominal pain, and melena. All these symptoms may indicate FUDR toxicity and should be considered

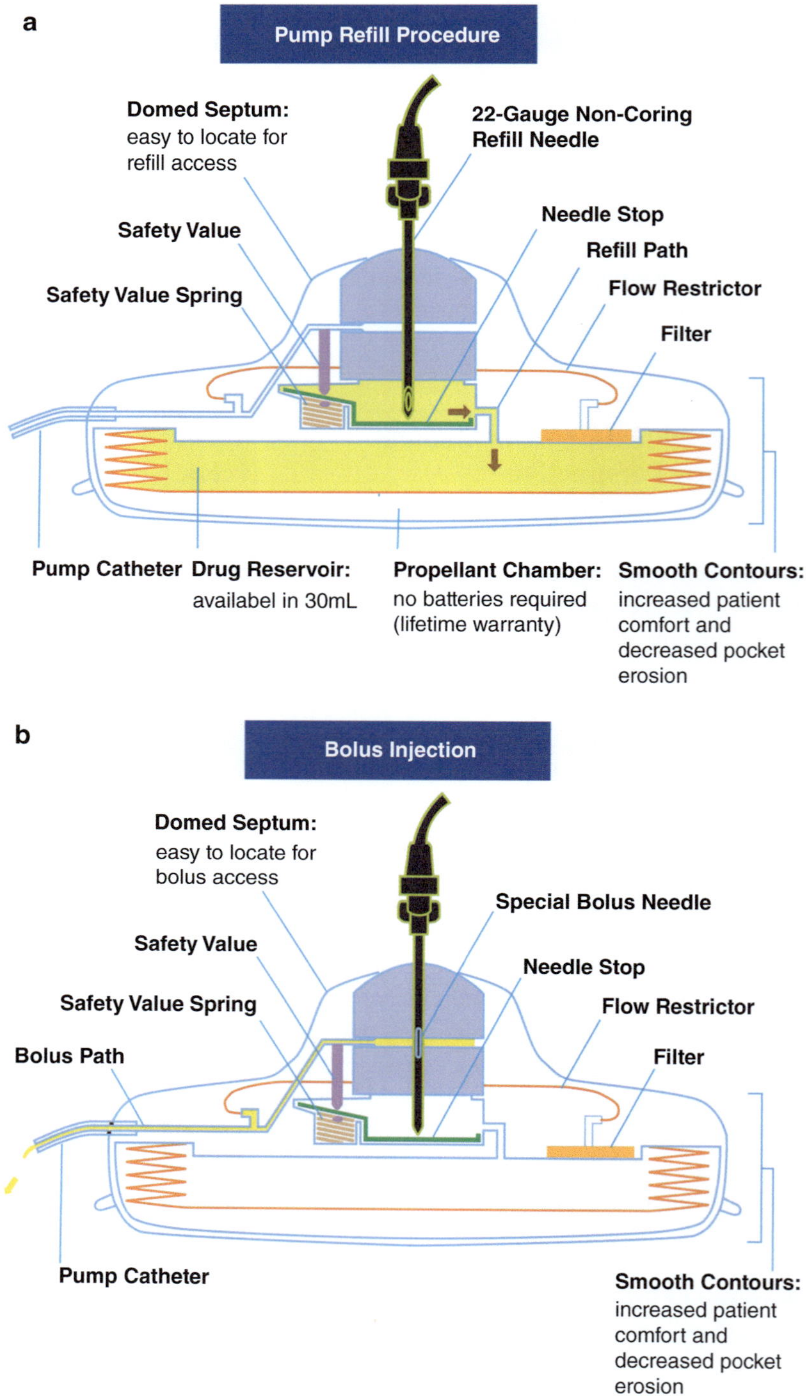

Fig. 28.3 Education figure for how pump is filled during refills (**a**) and when bolus injection is needed (**b**). (Copyright Intera Oncology, permission provided)

as red flags. These symptoms or an asymptomatic elevation of liver function tests may require the FUDR to be emptied out of the pump as soon as possible.

Mitomycin is another chemotherapy agent used in HAI treatment, particularly in FUDR-refractory patients with liver-only disease progression [7]. Given that mitomycin is a vesicant, patients need to be aware that a pump flow scan must be repeated to ensure the pump is functioning appropriately before administering the first dose. Mitomycin is given as an infusion using the special bolus needle to access the Intera pump; while it can be administered through the Medtronic pump, special considerations must be taken, such as needle access under fluoroscopy to ensure mitomycin is not injected inadvertently into the pocket. Patients should be informed about the possibility of low platelet counts as a result.

To decrease the risk of stomach ulceration, patients are always prescribed a proton pump inhibitor (PPI) when they begin HAI chemotherapy, if not already included in their routine medical management. Patients should be advised not to stop this medication unless directed by their medical oncologist. Ensure compliance with the PPI at every visit.

Dexamethasone

Patients should be educated on the use of dexamethasone or other steroids in their HAI pump. Administration of dexamethasone along with FUDR is shown to decrease the risk of biliary complications and improve response rates [8]. For patients with diabetes and prediabetes, an endocrinologist or primary care physician may need to be involved to coordinate the patient's medications as patients may require a different diabetic regimen when they have steroids in their pump. Other long-term side effects of dexamethasone must be reviewed with patients. This is especially important for patients who may warrant long-term steroid administration in the pump for bile duct inflammation.

Concurrent Systemic Chemotherapy

Patients should be educated that their systemic chemotherapy dose is adjusted to allow for the addition of HAI pump chemotherapy. A more in-depth discussion of individual chemotherapy regimens is beyond the scope of this chapter (see Chap. 12). An important note, however, for patients to understand is that any bevacizumab regimen is contraindicated with HAI chemotherapy given the increase in biliary toxicity [9]. Patients needs to be aware of this information in the rare event they receive their systemic chemotherapy locally.

All patients should be educated on the general side effects of systemic chemotherapy. These include, but are not limited to nausea, vomiting, diarrhea, constipation, low blood counts, lower immunity and resultant increased risk for infection, the possibility of requiring blood transfusion, an increase in bleeding risk, allergic reactions, loss of taste, loss of appetite, mouth sores, fatigue, infertility, dry skin, sun sensitivity, nail and hair changes, and hair loss. Everyone of child-bearing age should be referred for fertility counselling as needed. With the increasing incidence of young onset colorectal cancers, this is particularly important to keep in mind. Patients also need education on the distinct adverse effects of systemic chemotherapy regimens frequently used with HAI chemotherapy. Common side effects include:

5-Fluorouracil: vasospasm resulting in heart attack and DPD deficiency resulting in life-threatening complications (rare possibility, but patients should be counselled). Avoid supplements with folate.

Oxaliplatin: short- and long-term peripheral neuropathy and cold intolerance.

Irinotecan: diarrhea requiring antimotility agents, UGT1A deficiency resulting in life-threatening complications (rare).

Panitumumab: maculopapular acneiform rash that is severe.

Gemcitabine: flu-like symptoms.

Glycerin

Once the HAI chemotherapy is complete, Intera pumps can be maintained with glycerin. Given its high viscosity, glycerin slows the pump infusion rate and must be filled every 6–8 weeks.

Developing Patient Education Materials [5]

Although direct (face-to-face or virtual) patient education between patients and their physicians and nurses is the foundation of a successful HAI program, additional written-based patient education materials can be highly beneficial. Clinic consultation can often be stressful for patients and their families, and they may not remember all the details discussed or be able to relay this information to caregivers who are not present for the appointment. Therefore, printed patient education materials can be beneficial to provide in addition to verbal education.

In addition, studies have shown many cancer patients access their information through websites. Although institution-specific, non-branded, patient education materials are ideal [10], the manufacturers of the pump devices also have patient education available for patients [11]. Additional video-based education can also be beneficial. As discussed below, it is important that patient education materials are written at a reading level suitable for all patients. An example of Mayo Clinic's approach to written patient education is provided in Box 28.2. The manufactures of the pump may also provide patient education documents that should be made available to patients [11].

Box 28.2 Summary of the Sections of the Mayo Clinic HAI Patient Education Booklet

For your careful consideration	This disclaimer section summarizes some of the essential logistical implications of pump placement and therapy (including the need for refills every 2 weeks) so that this is not overlooked later in the material
Introduction	This section provides an overview for patients including a very general description of when HAI is used
What is a pump?	This section includes an illustration and description of the pump and its size and weight to help patients understand what will be implanted in their body
How does the chemotherapy get delivered?	This section explains how the pump is used to deliver chemotherapy
What is the process for having this treatment?	This section explains the pump surgery and recovery
What happens after the pump is implanted?	This section explains what will feel like to have the pump in place. A very general overview of potential complications is also provided
When does chemotherapy from the pump begin?	This section describes the logistics of filling the pump and receiving treatments
What happens during the refill appointments?	This section describes what to expect at a refill appointment
What are the activity guidelines and restrictions?	This section summarizes important activity restrictions
What happens after you no longer receive chemotherapy from the pump?	This section summarizes what happened after pump chemotherapy is finished
Can the pump be removed?	This discusses pump removal
When should you contact your health care provider?	Information on things to watch for and when to contact your healthcare provider

An ideal patient education program tailors to the needs of all patients in a patient-specific manor. For some patients, this may include the use of smart phone and digital patient education tools, which have found to be beneficial in general surgery patients [12]. Educational videos and patient support groups are also an ideal resource for some patients and should be made available if possible. Some manufacturers of the HAI pumps also provide "How HAI Therapy Works" videos, which can be helpful for patients to understand

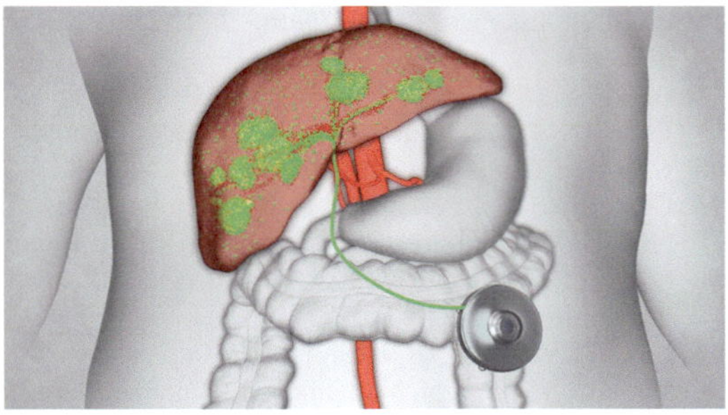

Fig. 28.4 3D rendering demonstration of how a hepatic artery infusion pump delivers chemotherapy to patients. (Copyright Intera Oncology, permission provided)

the HAI placement and treatments [11]. An example of a 3D animation that can be used for patient education is shown in Fig. 28.4.

Important Considerations When Developing Patient Education

It is important to consider the patient's cognitive resources when educating patients. However, this can be particularly challenging with a treatment as intensive and complex as HAI. Therefore, it is essential to understand the patient's baseline cognitive resources and provide patient education tailored to each patient needs [10]. In general, when developing written patient education material, it is important to consider that the average adult in the United States reads five grade levels lower than their highest educational level that they obtained [13, 14]. Furthermore, according to the National Adult Literacy Survey, close to half of the adult population in the United States is either functionally or marginally illiterate (reading at level below the eighth grade) [15]. Therefore, the American Medical Association (AMA) recommends that medical information be provided at a sixth-grade level or lower [16–20]. In addition to traditional barriers including language, education, and health literacy, it is also important to note that cancer patients may have additional cognitive decline as a result of the cancer treatments [21].

Conclusion

Robust patient education is a core component of any HAI pump program and it takes a multidisciplinary approach to be successful. This education should occur throughout a patient's treatment journey, from the first consultation to when their HAI pump is removed, and it should be tailored to the individual patient's learning needs. As discussed in this chapter, there are many unique aspects of HAI therapy to include in patient education as well as methods to deliver this information. These unique aspects include the risks, benefits, and complications of HAI as well as the logistical implications, activity restrictions, side effects of HAI, and long-term implications of pump placement. With proper patient education, all patients can be engaged and active participants in their HAI care and many complications can be avoided.

Acknowledgments None.

References

1. Government of South Australia, SA Health. South Australian Health Commission. Your rights and responsibilities: a charter for consumers of the South Australian public health system. 2008; p. 7–8. Accessed 9 Oct 2023.
2. Martínez-Miranda P, Casuso-Holgado MJ, Jesús Jiménez-Rejano J. Effect of patient education on quality-of-life, pain and fatigue in breast cancer survivors: a systematic review and meta-analysis. Clin Rehabil. 2021;35(12):1722–42.
3. Breedis C, Young G. The blood supply of neoplasms in the liver. Am J Pathol. 1954;30(5):969–77.
4. Ensminger WD, Rosowsky A, Raso V, Levin DC, Glode M, Come S, et al. A clinical-pharmacological evaluation of hepatic arterial infusions of 5-fluoro-2′-deoxyuridine and 5-fluorouracil. Cancer Res. 1978;38(11 Pt 1):3784–92.
5. InteraOncology, Intera 3000 hepatic artery infusion (HAI) pump patient education brochure. Accessed 9 Oct 2023.
6. Bagnall NM, Pucher PH, Johnston MJ, Arora S, Athanasiou T, Faiz O, et al. Informing the process of consent for surgery: identification of key constructs and quality factors. J Surg Res. 2017;209:86–92.

7. Schneider A, Kemeny N, Chapman D, Niedzwiecki D, Oderman P. Intrahepatic mitomycin C as a salvage treatment for patients with hepatic metastases from colorectal carcinoma. Cancer. 1989;64(11):2203–6.
8. Kemeny N, Seiter K, Niedzwiecki D, Chapman D, Sigurdson E, Cohen A, et al. A randomized trial of intrahepatic infusion of fluorodeoxyuridine with dexamethasone versus fluorodeoxyuridine alone in the treatment of metastatic colorectal cancer. Cancer. 1992;69(2):327–34.
9. D'Angelica MI, Correa-Gallego C, Paty PB, Cercek A, Gewirtz AN, Chou JF, et al. Phase II trial of hepatic artery infusional and systemic chemotherapy for patients with unresectable hepatic metastases from colorectal cancer: conversion to resection and long-term outcomes. Ann Surg. 2015;261(2):353–60.
10. Vaartio-Rajalin H, Huumonen T, Iire L, Jekunen A, Leino-Kilpi H, Minn H, et al. Patient education process in oncologic context: what, why, and by whom? Nurs Res. 2015;64(5):381–90.
11. Intera Oncology. Hepatic artery infusion therapy. 2023. https://interaoncology.com/. Accessed 9 Oct 2023.
12. Morte K, Marenco C, Lammers D, Bingham J, Sohn V, Eckert M. Utilization of mobile application improves perioperative education and patient satisfaction in general surgery patients. Am J Surg. 2021;221(4):788–92.
13. Cutilli CC, Bennett IM. Understanding the health literacy of America: results of the National Assessment of Adult Literacy. Orthop Nurs. 2009;28(1):27–32; quiz 3–4.
14. Berkman ND, Dewalt DA, Pignone MP, Sheridan SL, Lohr KN, Lux L, et al. Literacy and health outcomes. Evid Rep Technol Assess (Summ). 2004;87:1–8.
15. Centers for Disease Control and Prevention. Statistics NCfH. Hospital utilization (in non-Federal short-stay hospitals). https://www.cdc.gov/nchs/fastats/hospital.htm. Accessed 3 May 2017.
16. U.S. Department of Health and Human Services. National Library of Medicine. MedlinePlus. https://medlineplus.gov/index.html. Accessed 21 Oct 2013.
17. Weiss BD, Schwartzberg JG, Davis TC, Parker RM, Sokol PE, Williams MV. Health literacy and patient safety: help patients understand—manual for clinicians. Chicago: American Medical Association Foundation and American Medical Association; 2007.
18. Weiss BD, Coyne C. Communicating with patients who cannot read. N Engl J Med. 1997;337(4):272–4.
19. Cotugna N, Vickery CE, Carpenter-Haefele KM. Evaluation of literacy level of patient education pages in health-related journals. J Community Health. 2005;30(3):213–9.
20. Doak LG, Doak CC, Meade CD. Strategies to improve cancer education materials. Oncol Nurs Forum. 1996;23(8):1305–12.
21. Pendergrass JC, Targum SD, Harrison JE. Cognitive impairment associated with cancer: a brief review. Innov Clin Neurosci. 2018;15(1–2):36–44.

Starting a New HAIP Program: International Perspective

29

F. E. Buisman, I. Dominguez-Rosado, P. J. Karanicolas, and K. F. D. Kuhlmann

Hepatic arterial infusion pump (HAIP) chemotherapy has been mostly a single institution therapy for many decades. It has gained international interest over the past decade, leading to multiple international initiatives. Some of these initiatives have been successful, while others have failed [1]. Setting up a HAIP program is complex and requires significant training, infrastructure, perseverance, and dedication of a multidisciplinary team. HAIP chemotherapy is now available in multiple centers in the USA beyond Memorial Sloan Kettering Cancer Center (MSKCC); however, experience outside the USA is currently limited to a few centers. This chapter will discuss the issues unique to the international context in establishing a new HAIP program.

The Historic Perspective

HAIP was developed in the 1970s–1980s at the University of Michigan, the Lahey Clinic, and MSKCC where the therapy has since been optimized, and has since then been adopted in only a small number of centers. The main target population for HAIP chemotherapy is patients with colorectal liver metastases (CRLM) and intrahepatic cholangiocarcinoma (ICC). Multiple reasons hampered widespread international adoption of HAIP. First, concerns have been raised that efficacy results reported from a tertiary high volume center were not generalizable to other low volume centers. HAIP chemotherapy is not feasible in a setting of low volume due to the risk of inexperience and consequently higher failure rates. Furthermore, initial randomized controlled trials on HAIP for resectable colorectal liver metastases (CRLM) were published in an era where new and effective systemic regimens such as oxaliplatin and irinotecan for colorectal cancer patients were discovered [2, 3]. Both agents are effective for unresectable metastatic colorectal cancer administration but demonstrated little or no survival benefit in the perioperative setting for CRLM [2–6]. Intravenous drug administration is simple compared to pump implantation and sub-

F. E. Buisman
Department of Surgical Oncology, Erasmus University Medical Center, Rotterdam, the Netherlands
e-mail: f.buisman@erasmusmc.nl

I. Dominguez-Rosado
Department of Surgery, Instituto Nacional de Ciencias Medicas y Nutricion Salvador Zubiran, Mexico City, Mexico

P. J. Karanicolas
Department of Hepatobiliary, Pancreatic, and GI Surgical Oncology, The Edmond Odette Cancer Centre @ Sunnybrook Health Sciences Centre, Toronto, ON, Canada
e-mail: Paul.Karanicolas@sunnybrook.ca

K. F. D. Kuhlmann (✉)
Department of Surgical Oncology, The Netherlands Cancer Institute, Amsterdam, the Netherlands
e-mail: k.kuhlmann@nki.nl

M. D'Angelica, M. Lidsky (eds.), *Hepatic Arterial Infusion for Malignancy*,
https://doi.org/10.1007/978-3-031-74935-3_29

sequent combined treatment with HAIP and systemic therapy, which requires new technical skills and close collaboration within dedicated multidisciplinary teams. In the early years of HAIP chemotherapy, the reports on complications of HAIP chemotherapy such as arterial thrombosis, liver toxicity, biliary sclerosis, and pump-related technical complications might have discouraged physicians [7, 8]. However, these concerns have been proven false as multiple studies demonstrated that HAIP chemotherapy is safe, and technical complication rates are low [9–12]. Finally, many logistical hurdles have to be taken to start a HAIP program, such as availability and distribution of floxuridine (FUDR) and implantable infusion pumps.

Requirements and Challenges of a New HAIP Program

Developing a new HAIP program is challenging but will be successful if the essential hurdles can be overtaken. Many of these hurdles are identical for each center, independent of the country or state.

Mandatory Materials and Regulatory Considerations

Infusion Pumps

The subcutaneous pump is a key component of intra-arterial chemotherapy, because FUDR has a half-life of only 10 min [13]. In the USA, the Codman 3000 pump had been used for many years. The advantage of this pump is that it is simple and easy to use. It is a non-programmable pump, with a fixed infusion that is controlled by pressurized Freon gas. In 2018, the production of the Codman 3000 pump was abruptly discontinued. Raw material shortage was mentioned to be the reason of discontinuation [14]. Economic considerations may also have been part of the decision to discontinue the production of the Codman pump. Solid scientific evidence supporting the indication for HAIP is limited, and only a few hundred patients are treated with this pump in the USA annually. Shortly after, Johnson & Johnson and Intera Oncology™ entered into an agreement for the sale of the Drug Delivery (FUDR) and Codman* Model 3000 Series Pumps and accessories. Intera Oncology has since been the supplier of FUDR and infusion pumps and the Codman 3000 pump was renamed the Intera 3000 HAI pump.

Because of temporary interruption of pump supply, the Medtronic SynchroMed II infusion pump was temporarily used in the USA and is still used in other countries such as Canada. This is a technically much more complex infusion pump, it is programmable, and more difficult to refill, causing a higher potential risk for technical failure of the therapy.

Centers in the European Union were not able to use the Codman 3000 pump as Freon gas is not allowed due to European Union environmental regulations. In these centers, the Tricumed IP2000V non-programmable infusion pump from Germany is used. This pump was initially developed for intrathecal treatment of patients with chronic pain and spasticity and is currently permitted for use in HAIP-related clinical trials. This pump has similar specifications as the Codman 3000. The main difference is that butane rather than Freon pressurizes the reservoir, resulting in FUDR propulsion. Codman/Intera 3000 and Tricumed IP2000V infusion pumps and accessories have never been registered in Mexico and South America as well.

Floxuridine

Floxuridine (FUDR) is the preferred drug for HAIP chemotherapy and was registered in the USA in 1971. It is not registered outside the USA. In some countries, it can only be used in registered clinical trials, while in other countries, floxuridine is allowed for compassionate use requiring a special government import permit. Alternatives for HAIP chemotherapy such as oxaliplatin and 5-FU are less effective and more toxic and do not have the same regional delivery advantage [15–17].

Over the last decades, FUDR has only been distributed by Hikma Pharmaceuticals. Intera Oncology more recently spun off a sister company called Cerona Therapeutics (Wellesley, MA), which now supplies FUDR, still manufactured by Hikma. FUDR is a relatively low-priced anti-cancer drug compared to current modern systemic chemotherapies. This has probably resulted in the absence of incentive to apply for registration and authorization. Due to the limited use of FUDR and potential growth in the future, manufacturing should be increased to avoid issues with availability. International Collaboration of HAI centers and pharmaceutical partners such as Intera Oncology are important to generate the evidence needed for registration and authorization and is essential for broad implementation and accessibility in the future.

Toward Safety and Feasibility

According to the NCCN guidelines, HAIP chemotherapy is a recommended alternative treatment option, restricted to centers with the experience to allow safe and feasible administration of HAIP chemotherapy. In the European Union, HAIP chemotherapy is not recommended as a treatment option, however. Several feasibility studies have been performed to ensure safe introduction of HAIP programs outside the MSKCC [1, 8–10, 12, 15, 18]. A recent Dutch phase II safety feasibility study included 20 patients in two centers that were treated with adjuvant HAIP chemotherapy after resection of CRLM [10]. Safety was determined by the 90-day HAIP-related postoperative complications from the day of pump placement (Clavien-Dindo classification, grade III or higher) and feasibility by the successful administration of the first cycle of HAIP chemotherapy. HAIP chemotherapy was considered safe and feasible, since only two patients developed HAIP-related postoperative complications that could be resolved with reoperation to replace the pump or to reposition a flipped pump. After a median of 43 days (IQR 29–52) following surgery, all patients received the first dose of HAIP chemotherapy, which was completed uneventfully in all patients. Performing a pilot study that focuses on safety and feasibility is an essential phase in the development of a HAIP program as it ensures that potential pitfalls and hurdles can be addressed.

Starting a pump program in a non-high income country (HIC) is a challenging but not impossible task. It is indispensable to have a medical and surgical oncologist fully trained on HAIP and in close contact with other more experienced centers, in order to troubleshoot problems that might occur.

For example, from 2020 to 2022, eight cases were performed at one of the author's (ID) institutions in Mexico City (three unresectable ICC, three unresectable CRLM, and two as adjuvant CRLM therapy) with technical success, using the combination of the Medtronic pump and the Braun catheter devices. One 90-day mortality occurred due to COVID-19 pneumonia, with no pump-related complications. Particularly during the early learning curve of implementation, case selection by a multidisciplinary team is extremely important.

The safety and feasibility of initiating a HAIP program for patients with unresectable CRLMs were also retrospectively analyzed in 154 patients at six North American centers. Major complications occurred in 7 (4.6%) patients during their hospitalization and 13 (8.4%) patients developed biliary sclerosis during follow-up. A total of 148 patients (96.1%) received at least one-dose of HAIP chemotherapy with a median of 5 (4–7) cycles [11]. A single-center study from Duke University Medical center showed safety and feasibility of introducing a HAIP program in 21 patients between 2018 and 2020.

Rigorous training of a multidisciplinary team, comprising of surgeons, medical oncologists, interventional radiologists, nuclear physician pharmacist, and nurse practitioners/physician assistants is of utmost importance for safe HAIP treatment. Special attention should be paid to the proctoring of the team members, which should be executed by organizing workshops for the multidisciplinary teams at MSKCC and proctor visits of experienced HAIP providers. In situations where local surgeons lack experience in pump placement, we recommended performing pump implantations during the pilot phase together with a visiting surgeon from an expert center. The learning curve for pump placement has not yet been investigated. In the Dutch PUMP Study

(NTR7493), pump placement procedures were extended from two to eight centers and it was agreed upon to proctor the first five procedures [10]. The step from open pump placement procedure to robot-assisted pump placement will result in a new learning curve [19].

Effective pump placement is obviously very important and can only be achieved with specialized training and experience. For safe HAIP after pump placement, the complete treatment team needs in-depth knowledge about complications and side effects, postoperative radiological pump assessment, indications for dose adjustments of FUDR or systemic treatment, intervention methods, and surgical decision-making. HAIP protocols from experienced centers should be adopted, introduced, and adapted to the local situation. A collaboration with an experienced HAIP center is particularly essential as it facilitates expert opinions in case of difficult decisions, for example, in cases of various vascular anatomy anomalies, dose adjustments in between HAIP cycles, and local treatment strategies after HAIP.

Toward Definitive Implementation

Clinical trials will help to gather evidence that supports national and international guidelines. However, many publications demonstrate that HAIP chemotherapy is associated with improved survival in both patients with CRLM (unresectable and resectable) and intrahepatic cholangiocarcinoma (ICC) (unresectable) [2, 20–23]. With this evidence, it is surprising that this treatment is not widely implemented and introduced in existing guidelines. The national guidelines in Europe have not adopted HAIP chemotherapy as a treatment option for both CRLM and ICC. Insurance companies do not reimburse HAIP chemotherapy in most countries where FUDR is not registered, making it difficult to start a new HAIP program. With the increasing popularity of HAIP chemotherapy, several initiatives have been undertaken to further investigate the role of HAIP chemotherapy. Efforts of starting a local HAIP program have largely been a result of international (research) fellows from the MSKCC who received training in HAIP at MSKCC and were inspired to develop a new HAIP program in their own center.

New clinical trials may refine the number of indications, improve patient selection and cost-efficiency, and could lead to broader implementation and reimbursement of HAIP. In The Netherlands, four clinical trials (PUMP I–III and PUMP IT) were initiated for patient with CRLM and ICC (NL7277, NL8234, NL9294, NCT04552093). The research group from Oslo (Norway) has developed two randomized controlled trials (EXCALIBUR I–II) on patients with CRLM (NCT04898504). In the USA, new trials are actively enrolling (NCT05863195).

HAI Consortium Research Network

The MSKCC efforts to gather evidence and guiding others in their efforts have resulted in an international network, the HAI Consortium Research Network (HCRN), which is a collaboration of over 70 international HAIP centers and was founded in 2020. The network has been working on growing evidence for HAIP chemotherapy by developing (inter) national trials, developing a prospective HAIP database, formulating a consensus statement, and collectively discussing potential future opportunities that may be more successful if preformed within the international consortium rather than locally. A large prospectively maintained database will allow for the development of rigorous models that focus on optimizing patient selection for HAIP chemotherapy. Also locally developed models may be validated within the HCRN dataset.

Conclusions

Safe introduction and implementation of a HAIP program outside the USA is challenging. Multiple logistical and regulatory hurdles have to be overcome, and a well-trained large multidisciplinary team as well as close collaboration with an experienced HAIP center is essential. Proctoring of the team is advisable and pilot studies that focus on safety and feasibility ensure that hurdles in the beginning of a new HAIP program will be recognized and avoided in the future. An important problem that needs to be addressed is the registration and authorization of the infusion pump and FUDR.

For broad international acceptance, implementation, and reimbursement of HAIP, the development of randomized trials for the different indications is mandatory. International collaboration offers new opportunities, including the development of a large, international, multicenter HAIP database. This database, currently underway, will facilitate the study of HAIP-specific topics and offers hope that this therapy will soon become more widely available.

References

1. Lorenz M, Müller HH, Schramm H, Gassel HJ. Randomized trial of surgery vs. surgery followed by adjuvant hepatic arterial infusion with 5-fluorouracil and folinic acid for liver metastases of colorectal cancer. German Cooperative on Liver Metastases (Arbeitsgruppe Lebermetastasen). Ann Surg. 1998;228:756–62.
2. Kemeny N, Huang Y, Cohen AM, Shi W, Conti JA, Brennan MF, et al. Hepatic arterial infusion of chemotherapy after resection of hepatic metastases from colorectal cancer. N Engl J Med. 1999;341(27):2039–48.
3. Kemeny NE, Gonen M. Hepatic arterial infusion after liver resection. N Engl J Med. 2005;352(7):734–5.
4. Nordlinger B, Sorbye H, Glimelius B, Poston GJ, Schlag PM, Rougier P, et al. Perioperative chemotherapy with FOLFOX4 and surgery versus surgery alone for resectable liver metastases from colorectal cancer (EORTC Intergroup trial 40983): a randomised controlled trial. Lancet. 2008;371(9617):1007–16.
5. Nordlinger B, Sorbye H, Glimelius B, Poston GJ, Schlag PM, Rougier P, et al. Perioperative FOLFOX4 chemotherapy and surgery versus surgery alone for resectable liver metastases from colorectal cancer (EORTC 40983): long-term results of a randomised, controlled, phase 3 trial. Lancet Oncol. 2013;14(12):1208–15.
6. Ychou M, Hohenberger W, Thezenas S, Navarro M, Maurel J, Bokemeyer C, et al. A randomized phase III study comparing adjuvant 5-fluorouracil/folinic acid with FOLFIRI in patients following complete resection of liver metastases from colorectal cancer. Ann Oncol. 2009;20(12):1964–70.
7. Ammori JB, Kemeny NE. Regional hepatic chemotherapies in treatment of colorectal cancer metastases to the liver. Semin Oncol. 2010;37(2):139–48.
8. Allen PJ, Nissan A, Picon AI, Kemeny N, Dudrick P, Ben-Porat L, et al. Technical complications and durability of hepatic artery infusion pumps for unresectable colorectal liver metastases: an institutional experience of 544 consecutive cases. J Am Coll Surg. 2005;201(1):57–65.
9. Allen PJ, Nissan A, Picon AI, Kemeny N. Technical complications and durability of hepatic artery infusion pumps for unresectable colorectal liver metastases: an institutional experience of 544 consecutive cases. J Am Coll Surg. 2005;201(1):57–65.
10. Buisman FE, Grünhagen DJ, Homs MYV, Grootscholten C, Filipe WF, Kemeny NE, et al. Adjuvant hepatic arterial infusion pump chemotherapy after resection of colorectal liver metastases: results of a safety and feasibility study in The Netherlands. Ann Surg Oncol. 2019;26(13):4599–607.
11. Muaddi H, D'Angelica M, Wiseman JT, Dillhoff M, Latchana N, Roke R, et al. Safety and feasibility of initiating a hepatic artery infusion pump chemotherapy program for unresectable colorectal liver metastases: a multicenter, retrospective cohort study. J Surg Oncol. 2021;123(1):252–60.
12. Chakedis J, Beal EW, Sun S, Galo J, Chafitz A, Davidson G, et al. Implementation and early outcomes for a surgeon-directed hepatic arterial infusion pump program for colorectal liver metastases. J Surg Oncol. 2018;118(7):1065–73.
13. Ensminger WD, Gyves JW. Clinical pharmacology of hepatic arterial chemotherapy. Semin Oncol. 1983;10(2):176–82.
14. Ellis RJ, Angelos P, Jarnagin WR, Kemeny NE, Merkow RP. Abrupt discontinuation of the Codman hepatic artery infusion pump: considerations in the era of precision medicine. J Am Coll Surg. 2019;229(2):217–9.
15. Lorenz M, Muller HH, Schramm H, Gassel HJ, Rau HG, Ridwelski K, et al. Randomized trial of surgery versus surgery followed by adjuvant hepatic arterial infusion with 5-fluorouracil and folinic acid for liver metastases of colorectal cancer. German Cooperative on Liver Metastases (Arbeitsgruppe Lebermetastasen). Ann Surg. 1998;228(6):756–62.
16. Guthoff I, Lotspeich E, Fester C, Wallin I, Schatz M, Ehrsson H, et al. Hepatic artery infusion using oxaliplatin in combination with 5-fluorouracil, folinic acid and mitomycin C: oxaliplatin pharmacokinetics and feasibility. Anticancer Res. 2003;23(6D):5203–8.
17. Dzodic R, Gomez-Abuin G, Rougier P, Bonnay M, Ardouin P, Gouyette A, et al. Pharmacokinetic advantage of intra-arterial hepatic oxaliplatin administration: comparative results with cisplatin using a rabbit VX2 tumor model. Anti-Cancer Drugs. 2004;15(6):647–50.
18. Gassel HJ, Müller HH, Mattes P, Stieger R, Schramm H, Lorenz M. Intra-arterial (5-FU/FA and FUDR) versus systemic chemotherapy (5-FU/FA) of nonresectable colorectal liver metastases. Langenbecks Arch Chir Suppl Kongressbd. 1998;115:1458–60.

19. Qadan M, D'Angelica MI, Kemeny NE, Cercek A, Kingham TP. Robotic hepatic arterial infusion pump placement. HPB. 2017;19(5):429–35.
20. Kemeny NE, Chou JF, Boucher TM, Capanu M, DeMatteo RP, Jarnagin WR, et al. Updated long-term survival for patients with metastatic colorectal cancer treated with liver resection followed by hepatic arterial infusion and systemic chemotherapy. J Surg Oncol. 2016;113:477.
21. Kemeny NE, Jarnagin WR, Capanu M, Fong Y, Gewirtz AN, Dematteo RP, et al. Randomized phase II trial of adjuvant hepatic arterial infusion and systemic chemotherapy with or without bevacizumab in patients with resected hepatic metastases from colorectal cancer. J Clin Oncol. 2011;29(7):884–9.
22. Kemeny NE, Melendez FD, Capanu M, Paty PB, Fong Y, Schwartz LH, et al. Conversion to resectability using hepatic artery infusion plus systemic chemotherapy for the treatment of unresectable liver metastases from colorectal carcinoma. J Clin Oncol. 2009;27(21):3465–71.
23. Kemeny MM, Adak S, Gray B, Macdonald JS, Smith T, Lipsitz S, et al. Combined-modality treatment for resectable metastatic colorectal carcinoma to the liver: surgical resection of hepatic metastases in combination with continuous infusion of chemotherapy—an intergroup study. J Clin Oncol. 2002;20(6):1499–505.

Part VII

The Future of Hepatic Arterial Infusion

Device Development: The Future

30

Benjamin D. Ferguson and Hari Nathan

The devices used to deliver hepatic arterial infusion (HAI) chemotherapy have existed essentially in their current form for several decades without substantial evolution. While several different devices have been used at various points in the history of HAI therapy, the technology used to deliver HAI therapy has not fundamentally changed over the past 30 years. This chapter will review the history of HAI pump technology and some opportunities for future development.

HAI pumps are implantable reservoirs that are filled with a drug, allowing extended delivery of chemotherapy into the hepatic artery at a continuous rate through an attached outflow catheter that is surgically inserted into an appropriate artery. Modern pumps that are now used for the delivery of HAI chemotherapy have their roots in devices initially developed in the 1940s and brought to clinical use in the 1970s and 1980s [1], primarily for intrathecal drug delivery for pain management. Early pump designs underwent subsequent iterations, allowing for slight differences in performance and clinical applications. In particular, programmable pumps with battery-driven roller motors, such as the Medtronic SynchroMed II, were eventually developed to more closely tailor the delivery of drugs in certain clinical settings [2], although these features have not been widely applied in HAI therapy.

Non-programmable constant-rate pumps, such as the discontinued Codman 3000 (Johnson & Johnson) and currently available Intera 3000 (Intera Oncology, Wellesley, MA, USA) have generally been preferred for their simplicity and reliability. The Intera 3000 is currently the most common HAI pump in use. Non-programmable pumps employ a propellant liquid/gas mixture that can be pressurized by filling the pump reservoir. Subsequent re-expansion of the propellant due to body heat drives pump flow (Fig. 30.1). In the United States, Freon™ is used as a propellant, while a variant pump popular primarily in Europe, manufactured by Tricumed, instead uses *n*-butane due to European Union regulations against the use of Freon™ [3, 4]. The battery-driven Medtronic SynchroMed II programmable pump came into off-label use for HAI chemotherapy delivery in 2018 as an alternative device following discontinuation of production of Codman 3000 pumps by Johnson & Johnson [5]. Intera Oncology reintroduced this pump with essentially the same design under the name Intera 3000 HAI pump in 2021, so an FDA-approved device for this indication is once again available.

While HAI pumps are generally reliable and time-tested devices, they are not without limitations that present opportunities for improvement. One inherent property of all HAI pumps is the frequency with which reservoir refills are needed,

B. D. Ferguson · H. Nathan (✉)
Department of Surgery, University of Michigan, Ann Arbor, MI, USA
e-mail: benferg@med.umich.edu; drnathan@umich.edu

M. D'Angelica, M. Lidsky (eds.), *Hepatic Arterial Infusion for Malignancy*,
https://doi.org/10.1007/978-3-031-74935-3_30

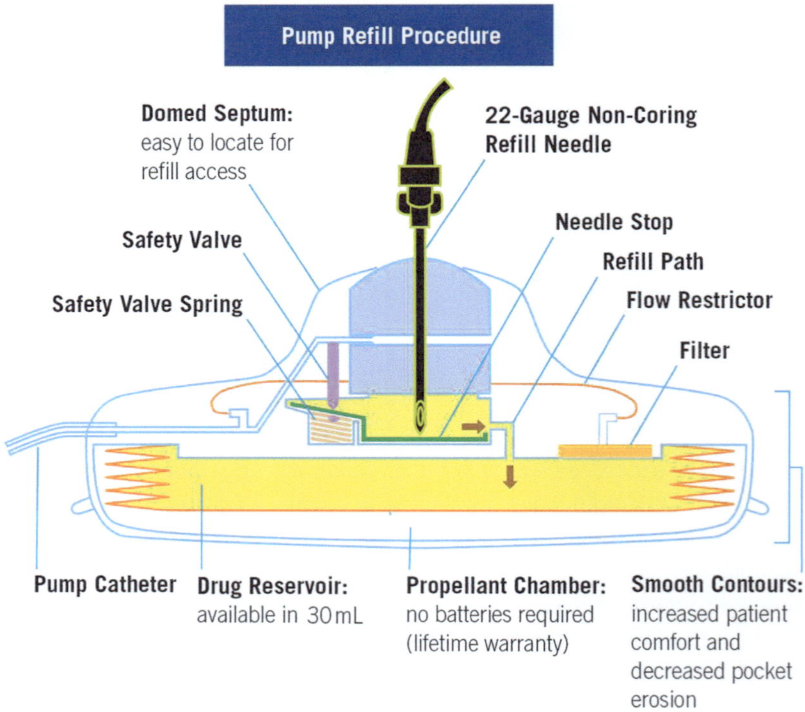

Fig. 30.1 Schematic of the Intera 3000 pump during refill. (Image Copyright 2022 Intera Oncology. All rights reserved. Used with the permission of Intera Oncology)

typically every 2 weeks while receiving HAI chemotherapy, to continue functioning and deliver chemotherapy. This is a natural limitation based on the size of the pump reservoir, which must be sufficiently small to allow for subcutaneous implantation, and the rate of drug delivery, which must be sufficiently rapid to allow for meaningful target organ concentration. Pumps with larger reservoirs have also been available, but the other reason for this interval has been that HAI chemotherapy is typically delivered over 2 weeks, followed by 2 weeks of heparinized saline infusion (often with dexamethasone), requiring the pump to be emptied and refilled every 2 weeks. In theory, a pump that could automatically switch from chemotherapy to heparinized saline could allow for refill visits every 4 weeks, which would particularly benefit patients who travel long distances for HAI chemotherapy.

Novel ways to alter the continuous flow rate of programmable pumps could be an area of future investigation to vary the infusion rate over time to improve efficacy, reduce toxicity, or both. Such modifications should be formally studied in clinical trials to confirm safety and efficacy. For patients not actively receiving HAI chemotherapy, extended refill intervals can be achieved by filling Intera 3000 pumps with glycerin, which allows for an interval of 6–8 weeks between refills. For propellant-driven pumps, flow can be affected by environmental conditions such as body temperature, external temperature, and changes in barometric pressures that occur during certain activities like scuba diving and air travel or simply moving across various elevations. Future pump developments may focus on addressing this limitation to optimize patient convenience. Additional pump developments may focus on using alternative pressure-generating agents other than Freon™ or *n*-butane, which may mitigate some differences in flow rates based on environmental perturbations.

While not inherent to the pump itself, there may exist further opportunities to optimize drug concentrations. Though drug bioavailability and metabolism in the liver have been studied extensively over the past several decades [6], optimal drug concentrations for oncologic efficacy are still poorly understood, especially since HAI chemotherapy is now used in combination with modern systemic chemotherapy regimens and with certain targeted therapies. The original work defining dosing protocols were carried out in an era when HAI chemotherapy was commonly used as a single modality or in combination with more limited chemotherapy regimens (e.g., infusional 5-FU alone). Lower concentrations than those established in early HAI studies may achieve adequate response in the era of multimodality therapy, potentially with less risk of toxicity. Additionally, HAI delivery of drugs other than FUDR has been explored to a limited extent [7, 8], and other work has aimed to establish HAI chemotherapy regimens under a personalized medicine approach [9, 10]. Further investigations into optimal drug combinations and doses are still needed.

Patients with liver tumors frequently undergo magnetic resonance (MR) imaging to monitor response and assess resectability. Currently available HAI pumps are rated as MR conditional, meaning that certain precautions are required to avoid overheating during the scan (which can transiently increase the flow rate of the Intera 3000 pump due to heating) and confirm appropriate pump function afterward (because of motor stalls in the Medtronic SynchroMed II pump caused by the magnetic field). While extensive experience has shown MR imaging to be generally safe with implanted HAI pumps [11], the development of devices with unrestricted MR compatibility is another potential area for innovation. Currently available pumps also cause significant artifacts in MR and, to a less troublesome degree, CT images. Placing the pump on the left side of the abdomen can ameliorate the impact on liver imaging, but the use of materials that do not cause this problem may be another area for innovation.

As stated above, the currently utilized HAI pumps are reliable, though developing a device that takes advantage of the programable options could prove beneficial. Such innovation could result in a "smart pump" that can provide real-time data pertaining to the programable flow rate (e.g., significant deviations from programmed flow rate could trigger an alert to the patient and/or provider), actual volume remaining in the reservoir (rather than just expected volume remaining), time to required refill, and notifications warning the patient or provider when low reservoir volume is reached. Despite these opportunities, to the authors' knowledge, no significant HAI pump innovations are currently in development. Major innovations in the near future of HAI chemotherapy are likely to focus on tailored therapies, nuances of drug combinations and dosing, and expanded disease indications for HAI therapy, rather than changes to pump technology itself. Many of these considerations are discussed elsewhere in this volume and are worthy of substantial excitement for the future of HAI therapy, while the time-tested HAI pumps now in use will likely continue to be used for the foreseeable future.

References

1. Anteby R, Kemeny NE, Kingham TP, D'Angelica MI, Wei AC, Balachandran VP, et al. Getting chemotherapy directly to the liver: the historical evolution of hepatic artery chemotherapy. J Am Coll Surg. 2021;232(3):332–8.
2. Jones R. 41—Spinal cord stimulation and implanted intrathecal drug infusion. In: Lennard TA, Walkowski S, Singla AK, Vivian DG, editors. Pain procedures in clinical practice. 3rd ed. Saint Louis: Hanley & Belfus; 2011. p. 483–506.
3. Kemeny N, Fata F. Hepatic-arterial chemotherapy. Lancet Oncol. 2001;2(7):418–28.
4. Chappel E. Chapter 7—Implantable drug delivery devices. In: Chappel E, editor. Drug delivery devices and therapeutic systems. Academic Press; 2021. p. 129–56.
5. Ellis RJ, Angelos P, Jarnagin WR, Kemeny NE, Merkow RP. Abrupt discontinuation of the Codman hepatic artery infusion pump: considerations in the era of precision medicine. J Am Coll Surg. 2019;229(2):217–9.
6. Sigurdson ER, Ridge JA, Kemeny N, Daly JM. Tumor and liver drug uptake following hepatic artery and portal vein infusion. J Clin Oncol. 1987;5(11):1836–40.
7. Boilève A, De Cuyper A, Larive A, Mahjoubi L, Najdawi M, Tazdait M, et al. Hepatic arterial infusion of oxaliplatin plus systemic chemotherapy and targeted therapy for unresectable colorectal liver metastases. Eur J Cancer. 2020;138:89–98.
8. Pernot S, Pellerin O, Mineur L, Monterymard C, Smith D, Lapuyade B, et al. Phase III randomized trial comparing systemic versus intra-arterial oxaliplatin, combined with LV5FU2 +/− irinotecan and a targeted therapy, in the first-line treatment of metastatic colorectal cancer restricted to the liver (OSCAR): PRODIGE 49. Dig Liver Dis. 2022;54(3):324–30.

9. Lévi F, Karaboué A, Etienne-Grimaldi MC, Paintaud G, Focan C, Innominato P, et al. Pharmacokinetics of irinotecan, oxaliplatin and 5-fluorouracil during hepatic artery chronomodulated infusion: a translational European OPTILIV study. Clin Pharmacokinet. 2017;56(2):165–77.
10. Hill RJW, Innominato PF, Lévi F, Ballesta A. Optimizing circadian drug infusion schedules towards personalized cancer chronotherapy. PLoS Comput Biol. 2020;16(1):e1007218.
11. De Andres J, Villanueva V, Palmisani S, Cerda-Olmedo G, Lopez-Alarcon MD, Monsalve V, et al. The safety of magnetic resonance imaging in patients with programmable implanted intrathecal drug delivery systems: a 3-year prospective study. Anesth Analg. 2011;112(5):1124–9.

31 Novel Agents and Drug Development

Issac R. Schwantes, Paul Wong, Ajay V. Maker, and Skye C. Mayo

Overview of HAI Chemotherapy

Key to understanding hepatic arterial infusion (HAI) is the role it plays in the treatment of patients with liver malignancies. Specifically, the most common clinical indications are for patients with unresectable colorectal cancer liver metastases (uCRLM), advanced hepatocellular carcinoma (HCC), or unresectable intrahepatic cholangiocarcinoma (uICC). HAI is also utilized as an adjuvant therapy for resectable CRLM. Rarely, patients with malignancies such as pancreatic adenocarcinoma, neuroendocrine liver metastases, or metastatic melanoma have been considered for liver-directed therapy with HAI. Regardless of pathology, malignancies that would be considered candidates for HAI are most often at an advanced stage in which HAI therapy is given in combination with systemic therapy. Patients with liver metastases, particularly uCRLM, have the greatest potential to be converted from an unresectable to resectable status [1].

The success of HAI therapy is predicated on differential blood supply between normal hepatocytes and liver metastases. Liver metastases derive nearly all their blood supply from the hepatic arterial circulation, whereas hepatocytes derive their blood supply predominantly from the portal vein, and to a lesser extent, the hepatic artery [2]. The same is true for primary hepatic malignancies. In addition, the use of drugs with a high first-pass metabolism, such as floxuridine, can result in high hepatic and low systemic concentrations, thereby minimizing systemic toxicity. Sigurdsson et al. provided the first demonstration of increased floxuridine concentration in tumor cells following arterial infusion compared to portal vein infusion [3]. Floxuridine has the highest first-pass extraction of any agents studied, being concentrated up to 400-fold compared to serum concentrations (Table 31.1). High hepatic clearance rates are also optimal for arterial delivery, as the hepatic artery blood flow can be upward of 1.5 L/min, and agents with low clearance rates would be at risk for recirculation into the systemic circulation [4]. Floxuridine shows a very high clearance (>95%) compared to 5-fluorouracil (5-FU), and with its other pharma-

I. R. Schwantes · S. C. Mayo (✉)
Division of Surgical Oncology, Oregon Health and Science University, Knight Cancer Institute, Portland, OR, USA
e-mail: schwante@ohsu.edu; mayos@ohsu.edu

P. Wong
Division of Surgical Oncology, University of California-San Francisco, San Francisco, CA, USA
e-mail: pwong@ucsf.edu

A. V. Maker (✉)
Division of Surgical Oncology, University of California-San Francisco, San Francisco, CA, USA

UCSF Helen Diller Family Comprehensive Cancer Center, University of California San Francisco, San Francisco, CA, USA
e-mail: ajay.maker@ucsf.edu

M. D'Angelica, M. Lidsky (eds.), *Hepatic Arterial Infusion for Malignancy*,
https://doi.org/10.1007/978-3-031-74935-3_31

Table 31.1 Pharmacokinetics of various agents studied in hepatic arterial infusion

Drug	Half-life (min)	Hepatic arterial exposure
5-Fluoro-2-deoxyuridine (floxuridine)	10	100–400-fold
Fluorouracil	10	5–10-fold
Mitomycin C	10	6–8-fold
Dichloromethotrexate	–	6–8-fold
Bis-chloroethyl-nitrosourea	5	6–7-fold
Cisplatin	20–30	4–7-fold
Doxorubicin	60	2-fold

Adapted from Ensminger, WD, Gyves JW: Clinical pharmacology of hepatic arterial chemotherapy. *Semin Oncol* 10:176–182, 1983

cokinetic properties, it is an excellent drug for arterial delivery and remains the dominant drug delivered via HAI [5]. However, HAI delivery of floxuridine is associated with biliary toxicity, leading to biliary sclerosis in a not insignificant number of patients. This has historically been, and remains, a potential limiting factor for the implementation of HAI therapy programs [6].

Current Cytotoxic Clinical Investigations

A query of the U.S. National Library of Medicine sponsored clinical trials website (clinicaltrials.gov) in November 2022 revealed 115 unique clinical trials evaluating HAI. Thirty-nine involve the use of HAI pump therapy. There is a paucity of level 1 data using the HAI pump therapy, and none in the setting of modern chemotherapy agents that have become the mainstay of current regimens for patients with advanced liver malignancies. Given the established role of HAI FUDR in multiple early phase I/II trials, the overwhelming majority of trials focus on the use of floxuridine with FOLFOX or FOLFIRI, with few providing data regarding novel agent delivery. Herein, all studies performed since 2010 are summarized with a focus on new agents and immunotherapies. After analysis of each trial, pertinent details and associated results are summarized in Table 31.2.

Table 31.2 Recent clinical trials involving novel agents or major advancements hepatic arterial infusion since 2010

Disease	Intervention	Outcome	Phase	Approach	Publication
Advanced hepatocellular carcinoma	HAI interferon B with HAI 5-FU in advanced HCC previously unresponsive to HAIC 5-FU/ cisplatin	60% of patients responded to therapy with decreasing tumor markers. Median overall survival was 108 days, with 1-year overall survival of 10%	Pilot	Repeated percutaneous catheterization port	Shakado et al. (2014) [29]
Advanced liver cancer	HAI nab-paclitaxel	HAI of nab-paclitaxel up to 300 mg/m^2 over 4 h was well tolerated	1	Percutaneous	Siqing et al. (2016) [30]
Colorectal cancer or pancreatic cancer liver metastasis	HAI of anti-CEA CAR-T cells	HAI of anti-CEA CAR-T was not associated with any serious adverse events above grade 3 and there were no on-target/ off-tumor. Complete metabolic response within liver sustained for 13 months	1	Percutaneous	Katz et al. (2020) [17]
Advanced hepatocellular carcinoma	HAI FOLFOX and HAI NK cells	HAI of escalating doses of NK cells following HAI FOLFOX did not cause adverse events or toxicity	1	Percutaneous	Bae et al. (2022) [31]
Colorectal cancer liver metastasis	HAI NV1020 HSV oncolytic virus	Initial post-viral infusion increases in tumor size (69% of patients) or in standardized uptake value (SUV) (80%) that qualified as progressive disease. Subsequent decreases seen in tumor size (64% of patients) or SUV (83%) that classified as partial response or stable disease	1	Percutaneous	Sze et al. (2012) [18]
Unresectable colorectal cancer liver metastasis	HAI of decitabine	HAI administration of decitabine can be safely conducted; proposed dose level of 20 mg/m^2/day on 5 consecutive days every 4 weeks	1	Percutaneous arterial catheter port	Jansen et al. (2019) [32]
Alcoholic cirrhosis	HAI of stem cells CD34+ and MSC (mesenchymal stem cells)	HAI infusion of autologous hematopoietic and mesenchymal stem cells was safe, and no postoperative complications observed	1	Percutaneous	Sharma et al. (2022) [19]
Alcoholic cirrhosis	HAI of autologous bone marrow-derived endothelial progenitor cells (EPCs) in EtOH cirrhosis	HAI infusion of autologous bone marrow-derived EPCs was not associated with any severe adverse events, and significant improvement in MELD score was seen	1	Percutaneous	D'Avola et al. (2017) [20]

(continued)

Table 31.2 (continued)

Disease	Intervention	Outcome	Phase	Approach	Publication
Unresectable HCC	HAI Theraspheres (Y90) in HCC patients with PV thrombosis	Yttrium-90 therapy appears to be a safe and viable therapy. Long-term health-related quality of life was preserved following Y90 radioembolization	2	Percutaneous	Kokabi et al. (2015) [33] Xing et al. (2018) [34]
Unresectable HCC with portal vein thrombosis	HAI FOLFOX + Sorafenib	Combination treatment was clinically tolerable, and 65% of patients reached 3-month progression-free survival	2	Percutaneous	He et al. (2018) [35]
Unresectable HCC with portal vein thrombosis	HAI FOLFOX + sorafenib vs. sorafenib alone	Median OS: 16.3 months with sorafenib plus HAIC and 6.5 months with sorafenib alone ($P < 0.001$)	2	Percutaneous arterial catheter port	Zheng et al. (2022) [10]
Unresectable colorectal cancer liver metastasis	HAI floxuridine + systemic FOLFIRI	Overall response rates were 76%, with four complete responses. 23 patients (47%) achieved conversion to resection at a median of 6 months from treatment initiation	2	HAI pump	D'Angelica et al. (2015) [1]
Resectable colorectal cancer liver metastasis	HAI floxuridine + systemic FOLFIRI with panitumumab vs. without panitumumab	3-year recurrence-free survival: 57% with Pmab and 42% without Pmab 3-year OS: 97% with Pmab and 91% without Pmab	2	HAI pump	Kemeny et al. (2021) [36]
Alcoholic cirrhosis	HAI of stem cells in EtOH cirrhosis	HAI of MSCs was associated with histological improvements (Laennec fibrosis system) in six patients (54.5%). Improvements in child-Pugh score seen in ten patients (90.9%) and significant decreases observed in levels of transforming growth factor-β1, type 1 collagen, and α-smooth muscle actin	2	Percutaneous	Jang et al. (2014) [21]
Unresectable colorectal cancer liver metastasis	HAI of irinotecan beads with systemic FOLFOX	9-month PFS: 53.6% Objective response rate (RECIST 1.1): 73.2% Secondary R0 surgery rate: 33% Median OS: 37.4 months	2	Percutaneous	Pernot et al. (2020) [37]
Unresectable colorectal cancer liver metastasis	HAI FOLFIRI+ systemic cetuximab	29.7% of treatment arm underwent R0/R1 resection	2	Percutaneous arterial catheter port	Levi et al. (2016) [7]
Unresectable colorectal cancer liver metastasis	HAI raltitrexed/ oxaliplatin (TOMOX) vs. HAI FOLFOX	PFS: 5.8 months for FOLFOX arm and 4.6 months for TOMOX arm Median OS: 17.6 months for FOLFOX arm and 13.1 months for TOMOX arm	2	Percutaneous	Feng et al. (2022) [38]
Unresectable intrahepatic cholangiocarcinoma	HAI floxuridine + systemic SOC gemcitabine/ oxaliplatin	Median overall survival was 25.0 months, median 1 year OS was 89.5%	2	HAI pump	Cercek et al. (2020) [9]

(continued)

Table 31.2 (continued)

Disease	Intervention	Outcome	Phase	Approach	Publication
Resectable colorectal cancer liver metastasis	HAI floxuridine with alternating systemic capecitabine/ oxaliplatin	2-year survival rate: 88%	2	HAI pump	Alberts et al. (2010) [39]
Unresectable HCC	HAI FOLFOX vs. TACE in unresectable HCC	Median OS: 23.1 months in HAI group vs. 16.1 months in TACE group	3	Repeated percutaneous catheterization	Li et al. (2022) [13]
Advanced HCC	Sorafenib plus HAI FOLFOX vs. sorafenib alone	Median OS was similar in the sorafenib plus HAIC and sorafenib monotherapy groups (11.8 vs. 11.5 months)	3	Percutaneous arterial catheter port	Kudo et al. (2018) [12] Ueshima et al. (2015) (Phase ½) [40]
Advanced HCC or unresectable HCC	HAI FOLFOX vs. standard of care with sorafenib	Median OS: 13.9 months for HAI FOLFOX and 8.2 months for sorafenib	3	Percutaneous arterial catheter port	Lyu et al. (2022) [11]
Unresectable HCC with portal vein invasion	HAI FOLFOX + systemic sorafenib vs. sorafenib alone	Median OS: 13.37 months in HAIC + sorafenib group and 7.13 months in sorafenib alone group	3	Percutaneous	He et al. (2019) [41]
Unresectable metastatic melanoma	HAI of melphalan vs. best alternative therapy (BAC)	Overall PFS: 5.4 months for HAI melphalan and 1.6 months for BAC ($P < 0.0001$) Median OS not significantly different (HAI melphalan 10.6 vs. BAC 10.0 months)	3	Percutaneous	Boone et al. (2018) [42]
Metastatic ocular melanoma	HAI fotemustine vs. systemic fotemustine	Trial terminated due to futility at overall survival analysis at 171 patients	3	Percutaneous	Leyvraz et al. (2014) [43]
Resectable colorectal cancer liver metastasis	HAI floxuridine, oxaliplatin, mitomycin C preoperatively vs. surgery alone	5-year DFS rate: 77% in HAI treatment arm and 65% in control arm ($P = 0.001$) 5-year liver metastasis rate: 7% in HAI treatment and 16% in control ($P < 0.001$) 5-year OS rate: 84% HAI arm and 76% control arm ($P = 0.005$)	3	Percutaneous arterial catheter port	Zhu et al. (2021) [44]

Cytotoxic Therapy: Notable Phase II/III Clinical Trials

The OPTILIV trial was a non-randomized multicenter phase II trial evaluating the impact of HAI irinotecan, oxaliplatin, and 5-FU delivered via a percutaneously implanted HAI access port in combination with intravenously delivered cetuximab in patients with uCRLM that were KRAS wild-type [7]. The primary outcome, conversion to complete resection (R0/R1), was obtained in 30% of the study population. During this study, phase I pharmacokinetic data was obtained for FOLFIRI and reported elsewhere [8].

Cercek et al. evaluated HAI FUDR with systemic gemcitabine and oxaliplatin in patients with unresectable intrahepatic cholangiocarcinoma (uICC) in a phase II single arm trial involving two centers. The addition of HAI FUDR resulted in median overall survival of 25.0 months (compared to 11.7 months with systemic treatment alone in historical controls) with an associated 1-year overall survival of 89.5% [9].

The results of adding HAI therapy to systemic sorafenib for patients with advanced hepatocellular carcinoma have been mixed. A 2022 phase II clinical trial demonstrated an increased median OS of 16.3 months with sorafenib plus HAI-delivered FOLFOX compared to 6.5 months with sorafenib alone ($P < 0.001$) [10]. Similar findings were seen in the FOHAIC-1 trial, which compared HAI FOLFOX to single-agent sorafenib and showed a median OS of 13.9 months vs. 8.2 months ($P < 0.001$) [11]. However, the earlier multicenter SILUS phase III clinical trial revealed no difference in median overall survival between HAI FOLFOX and sorafenib versus sorafenib alone [12].

Recently, a phase III multicenter randomized controlled trial for patients with unresectable hepatocellular carcinoma investigated HAI delivery of FOLFOX (FOLFOX Bolus, followed by fluorouracil infusion for 24 h) compared to trans-arterial chemoembolization (TACE) with epirubicin, lobaplatin, and lipiodol and polyvinyl alcohol particles. There was an increased overall survival in patients treated with HAI FOLFOX compared to TACE (23.1 months vs. 16.1 months, $P < 0.001$). Additionally, the HAI group experienced a lower incidence of adverse events (30% vs. 19%, $P = 0.03$) and longer progression-free survival (PFS, 9.6 months vs. 5.4 months, $P < 0.001$) [13].

HAI-Delivered Biologic Therapies

The discovery of novel biological therapies, including immune checkpoint inhibitors, has prompted the further exploration of these agents through HAI delivery. For patients with microsatellite stable disease, there has been little research to date reporting on the potential of HAI delivery of immune checkpoint inhibitors, such as antibodies to PD1/PDL-1, for both primary HCC and liver metastases. This may be due to the hypothesized limited efficacy of this therapy in the pro-metastatic and immunosuppressive environment of the liver, making it difficult to impact durable antitumor immune responses [14, 15]. Liver metastases, in particular, are regarded as major contributors to immunotherapy resistance and have been shown to contribute to fewer amounts of antigen-specific CD8+ T-cells in the tumor microenvironment [16]. However, localized delivery of these biological agents has been proposed to optimize their efficacy in the liver.

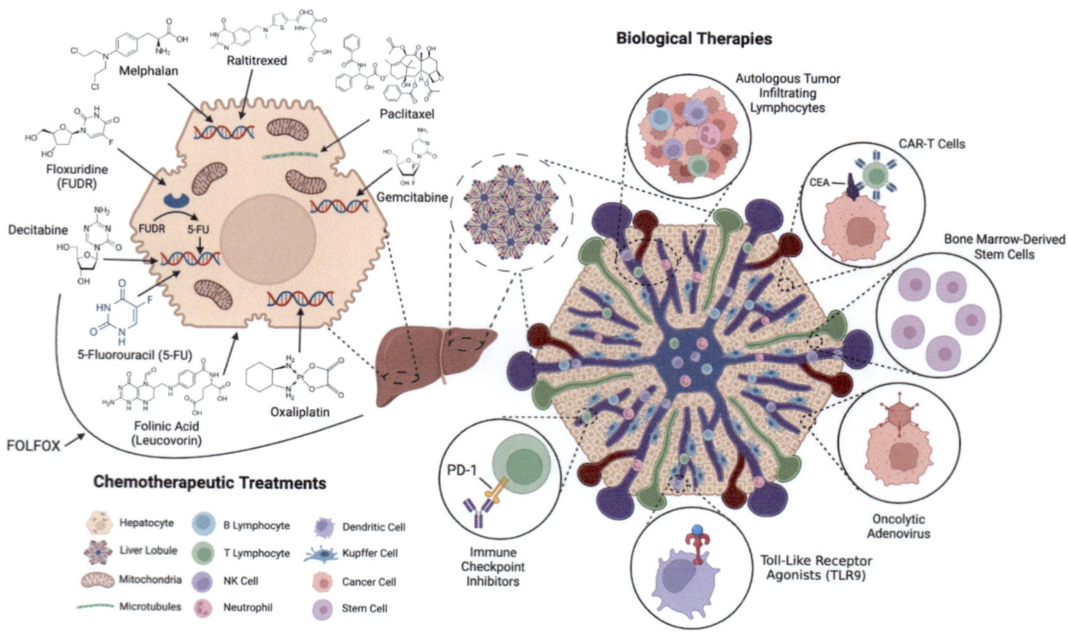

Fig. 31.1 Chemotherapeutic and biological agents explored in hepatic artery infusion clinical trials

Figure 31.1 illustrates chemotherapeutic and biological agents that have been investigated through HAI delivery in clinical trials.

HAI Biologic Therapy: Notable Clinical Trial Findings

Currently, only a few published clinical trials have explored the delivery of biological therapies through the hepatic artery, with treatments ranging from oncolytic viruses to chimeric antigen receptor (CAR) T-cells. While these studies have piloted the delivery of biologics through the hepatic artery, only percutaneous approaches have been featured without utilization of a HAI pump.

A phase Ib trial evaluated the safety and efficacy of CAR T-cells targeting carcinoembryonic antigen (CEA) in a single patient with pancreatic adenocarcinoma metastatic to the liver, treated via hepatic arterial infusion (HAI) using pressure-enabled drug delivery (PEDD) technology. Three doses of anti-CEA CAR T-cells were delivered regionally, while interleukin-2 (IL-2) was administered intravenously to enhance CAR T-cell activity. Previous studies from this group demonstrated that PEDD significantly improves CAR T-cell delivery to CEA-positive liver metastases, increasing delivery efficiency by over five-fold compared to standard microcatheters. Importantly, HAI of anti-CEA CAR T-cells was not associated with any serious adverse events (SAEs) greater than grade 3, and no on-target/off-tumor SAEs were observed. Serum tumor markers decreased during treatment in this single subject.

Delivery of oncolytic virotherapy through the hepatic artery was investigated in a phase I/II trial by Sze et al. [18]. The oncolytic herpes virus NV1020 was delivered in combination with systemic therapy in patients with previously treated colorectal liver metastases. The trial of 22 patients included quantitative FDG-PET and CT responses that were analyzed and compared to clinical outcomes. Following initial viral infusion, 69% of patients demonstrated increases in tumor size and 80% showed increases in standardized uptake value (SUV) on FDG-PET meeting criteria to be classified as progressive disease. However, in those patients who experienced initial increases in tumor size, 64% went on to have objective clinical responses and 83% experienced decreases in SUV to be reclassified as partial response or stable disease.

In the context of alcoholic cirrhosis, there have been several trials studying the delivery of autologous bone marrow-derived progenitor and stem cells through the hepatic artery. Sharma et al. conducted a phase I trial in which autologous hematopoietic and mesenchymal stem cells were infused through the hepatic artery [19]. No adverse effects or post-procedural complications were noted, highlighting that HAI of stem cells can be safely performed for patients with decompensated liver cirrhosis. Similarly, a phase I/II trial by D'Avola et al. evaluated the safety and efficacy of autologous bone marrow-derived endothelial progenitor cells (EPCs) in patients with decompensated liver cirrhosis [20]. Following bone marrow harvest for ex vivo differentiation of EPC, a single administration of EPCs was given, and no adverse events related to the treatment were observed. Patients did experience significant improvement in baseline MELD score by an average of 6 points in the first 90 days after treatment. The antifibrotic effects of administering bone marrow-derived cells through the hepatic artery was reported in a phase II trial of patients with alcoholic cirrhosis by Jang et al. [21]. Patients were treated with mesenchymal stem cells with the rationale that these cells possess the ability to differentiate into hepatocytes and produce antifibrotic effects. Results from the trial showed that six (54.5%) patients demonstrated histological improvement according to the Laennec fibrosis system. Additionally, improvements in Child-Pugh score were seen in ten patients (90.9%), and statistically significant decreases in transforming growth factor-$\beta 1$, type 1 collagen, and α-smooth muscle actin were observed.

Future Trials of HAI-Delivered Biologic Therapy

There are multiple ongoing clinical trials investigating the delivery of biological therapies through the hepatic artery for which published results are eagerly anticipated. This includes early phase clinical trials leveraging PEDD technology to study the pressure-enabled HAI delivery of a TLR 9 agonist (SD-101) [22] with systemic administration of checkpoint inhibitors for primary liver tumors (NCT05220722) and metastatic uveal melanoma (NCT04935229). Furthermore, two phase I trials are investigating the safety and feasibility of HAI delivery of modified lymphocytes. One trial features the administration of engineered T cells with a human antibody domain against the anti-HLA-A02/AFP complex, which is widely expressed in HCC (NCT03888859). The second trial is exploring the HAI delivery of autologous tumor infiltrating lymphocytes followed by subcutaneous injection of IL-2 for patients with metastatic melanoma (NCT04812470).

Oncolytic virotherapy is another avenue of treatments that is being pursued in ongoing HAI clinical trials. There is currently a phase I trial assessing the safety and highest tolerable dose for the rRp450 herpes simplex virus when infused into the hepatic artery for liver metastases and primary liver tumors (NCT01071941). Similarly, a phase I/IIa trial is evaluating the safety of HAI administrations of AdVince, which is an oncolytic adenovirus that has been engineered to treat metastatic neuroendocrine tumors (NCT02749331) [23].

There are ongoing trials assessing the HAI delivery of immune checkpoint inhibitors including anti-PD-1 antibodies in a phase II trial for patients with unresectable HCC (NCT04814030) and HAI-delivered PD-1/PD-L1 inhibitors via microcatheter versus standard peripheral vein infusion in a Phase III trial for patients with advanced HCC (BCLC Stage C) (NCT03949231).

Potential for PRRT

Initially developed in 1997, peptide receptor radioligand therapy (PRRT) utilizes a somatostatin receptor analog to bind somatostatin receptors and deliver radioligands to metastatic neuroendocrine tumors. Treatment of neuroendocrine tumors with PRRT has shown to produce profound clinical responses and be well tolerated [24]. Given that neuroendocrine cancers commonly metastasize to the liver, there has been interest in the HAI delivery of PRRT to patients with extensive liver metastatic disease. More recently, pilot studies have shown that intra-arterial delivery of Yttrium-90 labeled tetraazacyclododecane-tetraacetic acid modified Tyr3-octreotide ([90Y-DOTA]-TOC) induces significant radiographic responses and has high-first-pass effect in the liver [25]. A confirmatory pilot study failed to replicate the original data and was terminated early due to poor treatment response [26]. Given the stark contrast in the results of the studies, further studies are needed to determine safety and efficacy of utilization of PRRT via HAI.

Future Directions in Drug Development

Most current studies on HAI focus on historical regimens using floxuridine or other fluorouracil derivatives. Recent research focused on combining HAI with intravenously delivered agents, primarily biologics, rather than developing novel HAI-specific agents or optimizing existing therapeutics.With the advent of targeted immunotherapy and personalized medicine, a significant number of agents will continue to be explored in early phase clinical trial investigations, which may leave less incentive or ability to thoroughly investigate traditional existing cytotoxic agents such as oxaliplatin and irinotecan. Reformulating these or other existing cytotoxic agents could offer potential benefits, such as reducing toxicity and increasing their residence time in target tissues. Toxicity trials using floxuridine have replicated hepatic injury consistent with biliary sclerosis in various animal models, yet the underlying mechanism remains unknown despite nearly 40 years of clinical use [27, 28]. The reported rates of biliary sclerosis highlight an urgent need to elucidate the mechanism driving this toxicity. Modifications to the floxuridine molecule could potentially reduce the risk of biliary sclerosis while preserving its high first-pass metabolism and antimetabolite efficacy. Furthermore, there are hundreds of cytotoxic and antimetabolite therapies currently used for other malignancies that would be good candidates for early-phase trials to evaluate the pharmacokinetics of intra-arterial infusion for liver-directed therapy.

Though there exist major challenges for HAI drug development, there is great potential in the local delivery of concentrated agents directly to liver cancer that supports broadening the repertoire of agents for available for delivery by HAI. The role of regional delivery of novel immunotherapeutics holds particular appeal.

References

1. D'Angelica MI, Correa-Gallego C, Paty PB, et al. Phase II trial of hepatic artery infusional and systemic chemotherapy for patients with unresectable hepatic metastases from colorectal cancer: conversion to resection and long-term outcomes. Ann Surg. 2015;261(2):353–60. https://doi.org/10.1097/SLA.0000000000000614.
2. Breedis C, Young G. The blood supply of neoplasms in the liver. Am J Pathol. 1954;30(5):969–77. https://www.ncbi.nlm.nih.gov/pubmed/13197542.
3. Sigurdson ER, Ridge JA, Kemeny N, Daly JM. Tumor and liver drug uptake following hepatic artery and portal vein infusion. J Clin Oncol. 1987;5(11):1836–40. https://doi.org/10.1200/JCO.1987.5.11.1836.
4. Collins JM. Pharmacologic rationale for hepatic arterial therapy. Recent Results Cancer Res. 1986;100:140–7. https://doi.org/10.1007/978-3-642-82635-1_18.
5. Ensminger WD, Rosowsky A, Raso V, et al. A clinical-pharmacological evaluation of hepatic arterial infusions of 5-fluoro-2′-deoxyuridine and 5-fluorouracil. Cancer Res. 1978;38(11 Pt 1):3784–92. https://www.ncbi.nlm.nih.gov/pubmed/151583.
6. Hohn DC, Stagg RJ, Friedman MA, et al. A randomized trial of continuous intravenous versus hepatic intraarterial floxuridine in patients with colorectal cancer metastatic to the liver: the Northern California Oncology Group trial. J Clin Oncol. 1989;7(11):1646–54. https://doi.org/10.1200/JCO.1989.7.11.1646.
7. Levi FA, Boige V, Hebbar M, et al. Conversion to resection of liver metastases from colorectal cancer with hepatic artery infusion of combined chemotherapy and systemic cetuximab in multicenter trial OPTILIV. Ann Oncol. 2016;27(2):267–74. https://doi.org/10.1093/annonc/mdv548.
8. Levi F, Karaboue A, Etienne-Grimaldi MC, et al. Pharmacokinetics of irinotecan, oxaliplatin and 5-fluorouracil during hepatic artery chronomodulated infusion: a translational European OPTILIV study. Clin Pharmacokinet. 2017;56(2):165–77. https://doi.org/10.1007/s40262-016-0431-2.
9. Cercek A, Boerner T, Tan BR, et al. Assessment of hepatic arterial infusion of floxuridine in combination with systemic gemcitabine and oxaliplatin in patients with unresectable intrahepatic cholangiocarcinoma: a phase 2 clinical trial. JAMA Oncol. 2020;6(1):60–7. https://doi.org/10.1001/jamaoncol.2019.3718.
10. Zheng K, Zhu X, Fu S, et al. Sorafenib plus hepatic arterial infusion chemotherapy versus sorafenib for hepatocellular carcinoma with major portal vein tumor thrombosis: a randomized trial. Radiology. 2022;303(2):455–64. https://doi.org/10.1148/radiol.211545.
11. Lyu N, Wang X, Li JB, et al. Arterial chemotherapy of oxaliplatin plus fluorouracil versus sorafenib in advanced hepatocellular carcinoma: a biomolecular exploratory, randomized, phase III trial (FOHAIC-1). J Clin Oncol. 2022;40(5):468–80. https://doi.org/10.1200/JCO.21.01963.
12. Kudo M, Ueshima K, Yokosuka O, et al. Sorafenib plus low-dose cisplatin and fluorouracil hepatic arterial infusion chemotherapy versus sorafenib alone in patients with advanced hepatocellular carcinoma (SILIUS): a randomised, open label, phase 3 trial. Lancet Gastroenterol Hepatol. 2018;3(6):424–32. https://doi.org/10.1016/S2468-1253(18)30078-5.
13. Li QJ, He MK, Chen HW, et al. Hepatic arterial infusion of oxaliplatin, fluorouracil, and leucovorin versus transarterial chemoembolization for large hepatocellular carcinoma: a randomized phase III trial. J Clin Oncol. 2022;40(2):150–60. https://doi.org/10.1200/JCO.21.00608.
14. Lee JC, Green MD, Huppert LA, Chow C, Pierce RH, Daud AI. The liver-immunity nexus and cancer immunotherapy. Clin Cancer Res. 2022;28(1):5–12. https://doi.org/10.1158/1078-0432.CCR-21-1193.
15. Liu Z, Liu X, Liang J, et al. Immunotherapy for hepatocellular carcinoma: current status and future prospects. Front Immunol. 2021;12:765101. https://doi.org/10.3389/fimmu.2021.765101.
16. Yu J, Green MD, Li S, et al. Liver metastasis restrains immunotherapy efficacy via macrophage-mediated T cell elimination. Nat Med. 2021;27(1):152–64. https://doi.org/10.1038/s41591-020-1131-x.

17. Katz SC, Moody AE, Guha P, et al. HITM-SURE: hepatic immunotherapy for metastases phase Ib anti-CEA CAR-T study utilizing pressure enabled drug delivery. J Immunother Cancer. 2020;8(2):e001097. https://doi.org/10.1136/jitc-2020-001097.
18. Sze DY, Iagaru AH, Gambhir SS, De Haan HA, Reid TR. Response to intra-arterial oncolytic virotherapy with the herpes virus NV1020 evaluated by [18F]fluorodeoxyglucose positron emission tomography and computed tomography. Hum Gene Ther. 2012;23(1):91–7. https://doi.org/10.1089/hum.2011.141.
19. Sharma M, Pondugala PK, Jaggaihgari S, et al. Safety assessment of autologous stem cell combination therapy in patients with decompensated liver cirrhosis: a pilot study. J Clin Exp Hepatol. 2022;12(1):80–8. https://doi.org/10.1016/j.jceh.2021.03.010.
20. D'Avola D, Fernandez-Ruiz V, Carmona-Torre F, et al. Phase 1-2 pilot clinical trial in patients with decompensated liver cirrhosis treated with bone marrow-derived endothelial progenitor cells. Transl Res. 2017;188:80–91.e2. https://doi.org/10.1016/j.trsl.2016.02.009.
21. Jang YO, Kim YJ, Baik SK, et al. Histological improvement following administration of autologous bone marrow-derived mesenchymal stem cells for alcoholic cirrhosis: a pilot study. Liver Int. 2014;34(1):33–41. https://doi.org/10.1111/liv.12218.
22. Krieg AM. Toll-like receptor 9 (TLR9) agonists in the treatment of cancer. Oncogene. 2008;27(2):161–7. https://doi.org/10.1038/sj.onc.1210911.
23. Yu D, Leja-Jarblad J, Loskog A, et al. Preclinical evaluation of AdVince, an oncolytic adenovirus adapted for treatment of liver metastases from neuroendocrine cancer. Neuroendocrinology. 2017;105(1):54–66. https://doi.org/10.1159/000448430.
24. Imhof A, Brunner P, Marincek N, et al. Response, survival, and long-term toxicity after therapy with the radiolabeled somatostatin analogue [90Y-DOTA]-TOC in metastasized neuroendocrine cancers. J Clin Oncol. 2011;29(17):2416–23. https://doi.org/10.1200/JCO.2010.33.7873.
25. Kratochwil C, Lopez-Benitez R, Mier W, et al. Hepatic arterial infusion enhances DOTATOC radiopeptide therapy in patients with neuroendocrine liver metastases. Endocr Relat Cancer. 2011;18(5):595–602. https://doi.org/10.1530/ERC-11-0144.
26. Lawhn-Heath C, Fidelman N, Chee B, et al. Intraarterial peptide receptor radionuclide therapy using (90)Y-DOTATOC for hepatic metastases of neuroendocrine tumors. J Nucl Med. 2021;62(2):221–7. https://doi.org/10.2967/jnumed.119.241273.
27. Andrews JC, Knol J, Wollner I, et al. Floxuridine-associated sclerosing cholangitis. A dog model. Invest Radiol. 1989;24(1):47–51. https://doi.org/10.1097/00004424-198901000-00011.
28. Zeng ZS, Zhang ZF, Sigurdson ER. Toxicity study of hepatic artery infusion chemotherapy with massive dose FUDR in rats. Surg Oncol. 1995;4(3):147–55. https://doi.org/10.1016/s0960-7404(10)80019-2.
29. Shakado S, Iwata K, Tsuchiya N, et al. Pilot study of hepatic arterial infusion chemotherapy with interferon-beta and 5-fluorouracil: a new chemotherapy for patients with advanced hepatocellular carcinoma. Hepatogastroenterology. 2014;61(131):557–62. https://www.ncbi.nlm.nih.gov/pubmed/26176035.
30. Siqing F, Culotta KS, Falchook GS, et al. Pharmacokinetic evaluation of nanoparticle albumin-bound paclitaxel delivered via hepatic arterial infusion in patients with predominantly hepatic metastases. Cancer Chemother Pharmacol. 2016;77(2):357–64. https://doi.org/10.1007/s00280-015-2946-x.
31. Bae WK, Lee BC, Kim HJ, et al. A phase I study of locoregional high-dose autologous natural killer cell therapy with hepatic arterial infusion chemotherapy in patients with locally advanced hepatocellular carcinoma. Front Immunol. 2022;13:879452. https://doi.org/10.3389/fimmu.2022.879452.
32. Jansen YJL, Verset G, Schats K, et al. Phase I clinical trial of decitabine (5-aza-2′-deoxycytidine) administered by hepatic arterial infusion in patients with unresectable liver-predominant metastases. ESMO Open. 2019;4(2):e000464. https://doi.org/10.1136/esmoopen-2018-000464.
33. Kokabi N, Camacho JC, Xing M, et al. Open-label prospective study of the safety and efficacy of glass-based yttrium 90 radioembolization for infiltrative hepatocellular carcinoma with portal vein thrombosis. Cancer. 2015;121(13):2164–74. https://doi.org/10.1002/cncr.29275.
34. Xing M, Kokabi N, Camacho JC, Kim HS. Prospective longitudinal quality of life and survival outcomes in patients with advanced infiltrative hepatocellular carcinoma and portal vein thrombosis treated with Yttrium-90 radioembolization. BMC Cancer. 2018;18(1):75. https://doi.org/10.1186/s12885-017-3921-1.
35. He MK, Zou RH, Li QJ, et al. Phase II study of sorafenib combined with concurrent hepatic arterial infusion of oxaliplatin, 5-fluorouracil and leucovorin for unresectable hepatocellular carcinoma with major portal vein thrombosis. Cardiovasc Intervent Radiol. 2018;41(5):734–43. https://doi.org/10.1007/s00270-017-1874-z.
36. Kemeny NE, Chou JF, Capanu M, et al. A randomized phase II trial of adjuvant hepatic arterial infusion and systemic therapy with or without panitumumab after hepatic resection of KRAS wild-type colorectal cancer. Ann Surg. 2021;274(2):248–54. https://doi.org/10.1097/SLA.0000000000004923.
37. Pernot S, Pellerin O, Artru P, et al. Intra-arterial hepatic beads loaded with irinotecan (DEBIRI) with mFOLFOX6 in unresectable liver metastases from colorectal cancer: a phase 2 study. Br J Cancer. 2020;123(4):518–24. https://doi.org/10.1038/s41416-020-0917-4.
38. Feng AW, Guo JH, Gao S, et al. A randomized phase II trial of hepatic arterial infusion of oxaliplatin plus raltitrexed versus oxaliplatin plus 5-fluorouracil for unresectable colorectal cancer liver metastases. Front

Oncol. 2022;12:913017. https://doi.org/10.3389/fonc.2022.913017.

39. Alberts SR, Roh MS, Mahoney MR, et al. Alternating systemic and hepatic artery infusion therapy for resected liver metastases from colorectal cancer: a North Central Cancer Treatment Group (NCCTG)/National Surgical Adjuvant Breast and Bowel Project (NSABP) phase II intergroup trial, N9945/CI-66. J Clin Oncol. 2010;28(5):853–8. https://doi.org/10.1200/JCO.2009.24.6728.
40. Ueshima K, Kudo M, Tanaka M, et al. Phase I/II study of sorafenib in combination with hepatic arterial infusion chemotherapy using low-dose cisplatin and 5-fluorouracil. Liver Cancer. 2015;4(4):263–73. https://doi.org/10.1159/000367751.
41. He M, Li Q, Zou R, et al. Sorafenib plus hepatic arterial infusion of oxaliplatin, fluorouracil, and leucovorin vs sorafenib alone for hepatocellular carcinoma with portal vein invasion: a randomized clinical trial. JAMA Oncol. 2019;5(7):953–60. https://doi.org/10.1001/jamaoncol.2019.0250.
42. Boone BA, Perkins S, Bandi R, et al. Hepatic artery infusion of melphalan in patients with liver metastases from ocular melanoma. J Surg Oncol. 2018;117(5):940–6. https://doi.org/10.1002/jso.24984.
43. Leyvraz S, Piperno-Neumann S, Suciu S, et al. Hepatic intra-arterial versus intravenous fotemustine in patients with liver metastases from uveal melanoma (EORTC 18021): a multicentric randomized trial. Ann Oncol. 2014;25(3):742–6. https://doi.org/10.1093/annonc/mdt585.
44. Zhu D, Xia J, Gu Y, et al. Preoperative hepatic and regional arterial chemotherapy in patients who underwent curative colorectal cancer resection: a prospective, multi-center, randomized controlled trial. Ann Surg. 2021;273(6):1066–75. https://doi.org/10.1097/SLA.0000000000004558.

32 Totally Percutaneous Hepatic Arterial Infusion Chemotherapy

Daniel P. Nussbaum
and Chandrasekhar Padmanabhan

In the United States, hepatic arterial infusion (HAI) chemotherapy is predominantly administered via a surgically implanted catheter connected to a subcutaneous reservoir pump system; however, percutaneous catheter placement—with or without attachment to a subcutaneous port—represents an alternative delivery strategy that is widely used in Europe and Asia. The origins of HAI chemotherapy, in fact, directly parallel early advances in visceral arteriography, and the first reports of HAI chemotherapy relied on these inchoate techniques. Using approaches first reported by Bierman [1] and Byron [2] in the mid-twentieth century to cannulate the visceral arteries via peripheral access with a Cournand catheter, the first large series of HAI chemotherapy was reported by Clarkson and colleagues at Memorial Hospital in New York in 1962 [3]. In this study of 28 patients with primary liver cancers or hepatic metastases of various origin, arterial access was obtained (and left in situ throughout treatment) via cutdown over the left brachial artery, which was ligated distally, and patients were administered drugs still widely employed for HAI today, including 5-fluorouricil (5-FU) and floxuridine (FUDR). Similar approaches for patients with diverse primary and metastatic liver tumors were reported over the next several years [4, 5].

The first randomized controlled trial of HAI chemotherapy was performed at the University of Minnesota and reported in 1975, testing 5-FU versus mitomycin C (MMC) delivered totally percutaneously via femoral artery access using the Fenwald closed pressure system [6]. This 25-patient trial demonstrated an improvement in response rate (83% vs. 46%) and survival (median 12 vs. 9.5 months) associated with HAI 5-FU. That same year, a retrospective series of patients treated predominantly with totally percutaneous HAI 5-FU (411 of 419 patients) demonstrated a clinical improvement rate of 55%, based on objective physical examination findings and laboratory changes. Most patients had metastases from a variety of gastrointestinal primaries, and patients with clinical improvement demonstrated improved overall survival relative to patients without improvement (11.6 vs. 7.3 months, $p < 0.001$). In these early series, variant hepatic arterial anatomy was only identified at the time of planned treatment and, if addressed, required interventions such as separate cannulation of the right and left hepatic arteries. Likewise, extrahepatic perfusion was accepted as a necessary consequence of certain arterial orientations (e.g.,

D. P. Nussbaum (✉)
Department of Surgery, Duke University, Durham, NC, USA
e-mail: daniel.nussbaum@duke.edu

C. Padmanabhan
Department of Surgery, Vanderbilt University, Nashville, TN, USA
e-mail: Sekhar.padmanabhan@vumc.org

M. D'Angelica, M. Lidsky (eds.), *Hepatic Arterial Infusion for Malignancy*,
https://doi.org/10.1007/978-3-031-74935-3_32

takeoff of the right gastric artery from the right or left hepatic artery), and the technical constraints of the early experience with HAI chemotherapy resulted in high rates of complications such as gastrointestinal ulceration [3, 5]. Catheter-related morbidity such as dislodgement, arterial thrombosis, limb ischemia, and infection were also common [3–5].

Over the ensuing four decades, advances in interventional techniques have resulted in decreased morbidity associated with percutaneous access and visceral arteriography. Improvements in the ability to selectively exclude (e.g., via embolization) aberrant or accessory hepatic arteries permits whole-liver treatment with lower rates of extrahepatic perfusion. Today, totally percutaneous HAI chemotherapy can be administered as either a single treatment or serially, the latter via separate percutaneous access at each treatment visit, obviating the need for prolonged catheterization. The vast majority of the published experience with totally percutaneous HAI chemotherapy has been in patients with hepatocellular carcinoma, including several randomized controlled trials. There has also been a relatively robust experience in patients with colorectal cancer, including as neoadjuvant treatment prior to resection of the primary tumor to prevent hepatic metastasis, as well as to treat known hepatic metastases, typically in the unresectable setting. Finally, scattered reports of totally percutaneous HAI chemotherapy have been published among patients with various other primary and metastatic liver tumors, including biliary tract cancers, pancreatic cancer, breast cancer, melanoma, gastric cancer, and neuroendocrine tumors. The more mature experiences with hepatocellular carcinoma and colorectal cancer will be separately discussed, and then data in other tumor types will be summarized. Notably, this chapter will not focus on HAI chemotherapy requiring vascular isolation (e.g., hepatic perfusion), HAI chemotherapy associated with chemo- or radioembolization, or drug-eluting bead therapy, all of which are beyond the scope of this chapter.

Hepatocellular Carcinoma

One of the first descriptions of HAI chemotherapy for hepatocellular carcinoma (HCC) was in the 1970 report by Geddes and Falkson in which the authors noted an improved mean survival with intra-arterial infusion of methotrexate in five patients with histologically confirmed HCC [7]. This was followed by a report by Cady and Oberfield on the use of intra-arterial FUDR in patients with HCC in 1974 [8]. Much of the early experience with percutaneous HAI for HCC has been reported in the form of small, retrospective series, or early phase I clinical trials studying novel combinations of chemotherapeutic agents for safety and efficacy [9–21]. In the last two decades, most of the clinical investigation has occurred in East Asia where the overwhelming majority of patients have HCC secondary to chronic viral hepatitis. This brings into the question the generalizability of these studies to Western populations where HCC predominantly occurs in patients with fatty liver disease. Nevertheless, HAI has been studied both as a perioperative/periprocedural strategy with liver resection/ablation and as definitive therapy in patients with locally advanced/unresectable and even metastatic disease.

Perioperative/Periprocedural HAI Chemotherapy

One phase II randomized controlled trial has addressed the role of periprocedural HAI chemotherapy in patients with early-stage HCC [22]. Seventy patients were enrolled in this study with the following inclusion criteria: (1) pathologically confirmed or imaging-proven HCC, (2) tumor size $\leq$3 cm, (3) three or more tumors, (4) no extrahepatic disease, (5) no prior treatment, (6) Child-Pugh score $\leq$9, (7) Eastern Cooperative Oncology Group (ECOG) performance status of 0–1. Patients were randomized to angiography alone followed by radiofrequency ablation (RFA) 1 week later or hepatic arterial infusion of cisplatin (65 mg/m^2) over 30 min followed by RFA 1 week later. In both cases, angiography was performed using the Seldinger technique, though access site was not specified. Post RFA CT scan was performed in all cases and if RFA was incomplete, repeat RFA was performed. Patients were serially imaged every 3 months for at least 3 years. The overwhelming majority of patients in each group had excellent performance status (ECOG 0) and preserved liver function (Childs-Pugh A). Median alpha fetoprotein (AFP) was 41 ng/mL (range: 1.8–665 ng/mL) in the HAI group and 32.1 ng/mL (range: 1.6–502.3 ng/mL) in the non-HAI group. Median tumor size was 14.5 mm (range: 6–28 mm) in the HAI group and 14.5 mm (range: 6–28 mm) in the non-HAI group. The primary endpoint of the study was recurrence-free survival (RFS) with a median follow-up period of 55.3 months (range: 13.1–85.1 months).

Recurrence was observed in 41/70 patients (58.6%). The cumulative 1- and 3-year RFS rates were 82.9% and 54.3% in the HAI chemotherapy group versus 74.3% and 34.3% in the non-HAI chemotherapy group though this difference was not statistically significant (HR: 0.597, 95% CI: 0.320–1.091, $p = 0.094$). Subgroup analysis suggested patients with Childs A cirrhosis, and specifically a score of 5, may benefit from HAI chemotherapy prior to RFA, but these subgroups were not prespecified. Though local tumor progression rates were similar in each arm, distant recurrence was significantly improved with HAI chemotherapy with 37.1% distant recurrence in the HAI chemotherapy arm and 54.3% in the non-HAI chemotherapy arm (HR 0.468, 95% CI: 0.235–0.896, $p = 0.022$). One- and 3-year distant RFS were 91.4% and 65.7% in the HAI chemotherapy arm and 80% and 40% in the non-HAI chemotherapy arm. Adverse events were seen only in the HAI chemotherapy arm: one patient had grade 2 cholecystitis and another had grade 2 hyperkalemia.

There were several limitations to this study in terms of overall generalizability. First, nearly all the patients in this study had viral hepatitis-induced cirrhosis and subsequent HCC development. Second, not all patients were adequately treated for hepatitis C prior to treatment initiation. In addition, all patients in this study were Japanese. Nevertheless, it appears that periprocedural HAI chemotherapy with cisplatin reduced distant recurrence rates in patients undergoing RFA for early-stage HCC.

The above clinical trial was preceded by a single-center, retrospective study that tested hepatic arterial infusion of epirubicin (mean dose: 28.2 mg, range: 10–40 mg), mitomycin (mean dose: 6.2 mg, range: 4–10 mg), and lipiodol (mean dose: 2.1 mL, range: 1–3 mL) prior to radiofrequency ablation (RFA) in patients with solitary HCC and compared intrahepatic distant recurrence to patients treated with RFA alone [23]. Mean tumor size was 2.06 cm in the HAI group and 1.97 cm in the RFA-alone group. Mean AFP (ng/mL) was 111.2 in the HAI group and 120.7 in the RFA-alone group. Baseline characteristics were otherwise similar in both groups with most patients having viral hepatitis. Post-RFA intrahepatic distant recurrence-free survival at 1, 2, and 3 years were 90.8%, 74.8%, and 70% in the HAI group and 74%, 50.8%, and 34.9% in the RFA-alone group ($p < 0.001$). Local tumor progression rates were similar in each group. Cumulative 1-, 3-, and 5-year overall survival was 96%, 83.7%, and 71.1% in the HAI group and 96%, 79.6%, and 51% in the RFA-alone group ($p = 0.048$). This study was limited by its retrospective nature as well as the fact that patients with incomplete RFA were subsequently excluded from the study, thereby rendering the true denominator in each group unknown. In addition, this combination of chemotherapy is not standard for patients with HCC. Nevertheless, the results suggest that HAI chemotherapy prior to ablation of solitary HCC leads to improved recurrence-free and overall survival.

Three retrospective studies have tested the role of adjuvant HAI chemotherapy after curative-intent liver resection in patients with HCC [24–26]. The first was a study of 85 patients with previously untreated HCC and a Childs Score of A–B with no evidence of portal vein thrombosis or distant metastatic disease. In this cohort, 42 of 85 patients underwent two treatments of adjuvant HAI chemotherapy. HAI chemotherapy consisted of percutaneous catheterization of the common or proper hepatic artery followed by 2-h infusion of oxaliplatin (85 mg/m^2), 5-h infusion of 5-FU (1000 mg/m^2), and >1-h infusion of mitomycin C (6 mg/m^2). Treatment was initiated 3 weeks after liver resection and given as two sessions, 4 weeks apart. Baseline characteristics were similar in each group with mean tumor size of 6.2 cm in the HAI chemotherapy group and 5.7 cm in the non-HAI chemotherapy group. Mean AFP was 562.4 ng/mL in the HAI chemotherapy group and 547.5 ng/mL in the non-HAI chemotherapy group. Again, most patients in each group had viral hepatitis-associated liver disease with preserved liver function. Intrahepatic RFS (HR: 0.56, 95% CI: 0.32–0.97, $p = 0.03$), disease-free survival (DFS) (HR: 0.59, 95% CI: 0.36–0.97, $p = 0.03$), and OS (HR: 0.58, 95% CI: 0.35–0.96, $p = 0.03$) were all significantly higher in the HAI chemotherapy group.

The second study reported on 221 patients with resected T2–T4 HCC. Sixty-one patients received adjuvant cisplatin (10 mg/m^2), 5-FU (150 mg/m^2), leucovorin (15 mg/m^2), and epirubicin (15 mg/m^2) delivered via a completely percutaneous approach (access via the left subclavian artery) within 3 months after resection [25]. HAI chemotherapy was administered in patients deemed to have high-risk disease as determined by later tumor stage and microvascular invasion. Patients receiving adjuvant HAI chemotherapy were planned for three courses. Fifty-one of 61 patients completed at least two courses. Baseline clinical characteristics were similar in both groups except for a higher percentage of larger tumors and later stage tumors in the HAI chemotherapy group. A higher percentage of patients in the HAI chemotherapy group received anatomic liver resections and a higher percentage of patients in the HAI chemotherapy group had final resection margins >1 cm. Neither OS nor DFS were different between groups (56.4 months vs. 56.9 months and 50.6 months vs. 54.5 months, respectively). In patients with microvascular invasion, HAI chemotherapy was associated with improved OS (69.7 months vs. 54.6 months, $p = 0.036$) but not improved DFS (58.6 months vs. 56.3 months). In patients with tumors >5 cm, HAI chemotherapy was also associated with improved OS (69.7 months vs. 47.3 months, $p = 0.006$). As in the previously discussed studies, most patients had viral hepatitis and were male bringing the generalizability of this study in question.

The third study reported on 122 patients with T3 or T4 HCC including 89 patients with portal vein invasion [26]. Thirty-seven patients were treated with resection followed by adjuvant HAI chemotherapy and 85 were treated with resection alone. HAI chemotherapy comprised of a single injection of cisplatin (65 mg/m^2) at least 4 weeks after hepatectomy. There was no statistically significant difference on OS or RFS in this study; however, the authors noted that 2-year recurrence rates after hepatectomy were 31% in the HAI chemotherapy group vs. 43% in the surgery-alone group.

As can be seen by the studies above (Table 32.1), the role for adjuvant or periprocedural HAI chemotherapy for HCC remains unclear. Current data suggest there may be a role for HAI chemotherapy in patients with early-stage HCC undergoing percutaneous ablation as well as patients with large tumors and/or microvascular invasion on final pathology. Whether or not these results are applicable to Western patients with fatty liver disease is yet to be determined. Phase III randomized clinical trials are needed to confirm these findings.

HAI Chemotherapy for Locally Advanced/Metastatic Disease

Three phase III trials have been conducted in China that have studied the role of percutaneous HAI chemotherapy in patients with locally advanced or metastatic HCC (Table 32.2). The first of these was the recently published FOHAIC-1 study that randomized treatment naïve patients to percutaneous HAI chemotherapy consisting of oxaliplatin (130 mg/m^2), 5-FU (400 mg/m^2 bolus followed by 24-h infusion of 2400 mg/m^2), and leucovorin (200 mg/m^2) vs. sorafenib monotherapy (400 mg orally twice daily) [27]. Importantly, 83% of patients in this study had macrovascular invasion with or without

Table 32.1 Perioperative/periprocedural HAI chemotherapy for HCC

Study site(s)	Patient population	Study design	Treatment group(s)	Outcomes
Japan, 7 centers	Treatment naïve HCC 3 or more tumors ≤3 cm ECOG: 0–1 Childs-Pugh ≤9	Phase II, randomized, single-blinded ($n = 71$)	• Experimental arm: RFA + HAI cisplatin (65 mg/m^2) • Control arm: RFA alone	**1-year RFS** 82.9% (HAI) 74.3% (no HAI) **3-year RFS** 54.3% (HAI) 34.3% (no HAI) **HR:** 0.597 **95% CI**: 0.32–1.09 $p = 0.094$
Japan, single center	Treatment naïve HCC Solitary lesion treated with complete RFA	Retrospective cohort ($n = 182$)	• RFA + HAI (epirubicin, mitomycin, and lipiodol) • RFA alone	**1-year intrahepatic distant RFS** 90.8% (HAI) 74% (no HAI) **2-year intrahepatic distant RFS** 74.8% (HAI) 50.8% (no HAI) **3-year intrahepatic distant RFS** 70% (HAI) 34.9% (no HAI)
China, single center	Resected HCC	Retrospective cohort ($n = 85$)	• Hepatectomy + adjuvant HAI oxaliplatin (85 mg/m^2), 5-FU (1000 mg/m^2), and mitomycin C (6 mg/m^2) Hepatectomy alone	**5-year intrahepatic RFS** 45% (HAI) 32.6% (no HAI) **HR**: 0.56 **95% CI**: 0.32–0.97 $p = 0.03$ **5-year OS** 35.7% (HAI) 20.9% (no HAI) **HR**: 0.58 **95% CI**: 0.35–0.96 $p = 0.03$
Taiwan, single center	Resected T2–T4 HCC	Retrospective cohort ($n = 221$)	• Hepatectomy + adjuvant HAI cisplatin (10 mg/m^2), 5-FU (150 mg/m^2), leucovorin (15 mg/m^2), and epirubicin (15 mg/m^2) • Hepatectomy alone	**Median OS** 56.4 months (HAI) 56.9 months (no HAI) p = NS **Median DFS** 50.6 months (HAI) 54.5 months (no HAI) p = NS
Japan, single center	Resected T3–T4 HCC Portal vein invasion included	Retrospective cohort ($n = 122$)	• Hepatectomy + HAI cisplatin (65 mg/m^2) • Hepatectomy alone	No significant difference in OS or RFS

low volume oligometastatic extrahepatic disease and >85% of patients in each arm had hepatitis B. HAI was performed with sequential femoral artery puncture and catheterization. Median OS was 13.9 months in the HAI chemotherapy arm and 8.2 months in the sorafenib arm (HR 0.41, $p < 0.001$). Median PFS was 7.8 months in the HAI chemotherapy arm and 4.3 months in the sorafenib arm (HR 0.45, $p < 0.001$). Major response evaluation criteria in solid tumors (RECIST) response was noted in 31.5% of patients in the HAI chemotherapy arm vs. 1.5% in the sorafenib arm ($p < 0.001$). Sixteen patients (12%) in the HAI chemotherapy arm had significant downstaging of their tumor and 15 of those patients underwent curative locoregional treatments. Seven of the 16 down-staged patients were alive with no evidence of disease at a median fol-

Table 32.2 Phase III randomized controlled trials in patients with locally advanced/metastatic HCC

Study site(s)	Patient population	Treatment group(s)	Outcomes
Sun-Yat-sen University Cancer Center, China	Treatment naïve HCC Macrovascular invasion and/or oligometastatic extrahepatic disease allowed	• Experimental arm: HAI oxaliplatin (130 mg/m^2), 5-FU (400 mg/m^2 bolus followed by 24-h infusion of 2400 mg/m^2), and leucovorin (200 mg/m^2), $n = 130$ • Control arm: Sorafenib (400 mg twice daily), $n = 132$	**Median OS** 13.9 months (HAI) 8.2 months (sorafenib) HR: 0.41, $p < 0.001$ **Median RFS** 7.8 months (HAI) 4.3 months (sorafenib) HR: 0.45, $p < 0.001$ **Major RECIST response** 31.5% (HAI) 1.5% (sorafenib) $p < 0.001$
Multicenter, China	Unresectable, liver limited, treatment naïve HCC BCLC A-B	• Experimental arm: HAI oxaliplatin (130 mg/m^2), 5-FU (400 mg/m^2 bolus followed by 2400 mg/m^2 infusion), leucovorin (400 mg/m^2), $n = 159$ • Control arm: TACE (50 mg epirubicin, 50 mg lobaplatin, and lipiodol), $n = 156$	**Median OS** 23.1 months (HAI) 16.1 months (TACE) $p < 0.001$ **Median PFS** 9.6 months (HAI) 5.4 months (TACE) $p < 0.001$ **Major RECIST response** 46% (HAI) 18% (TACE) $p < 0.001$ **Complete clinical response** 13% (HAI) 3% (TACE) $p < 0.001$
Multicenter, China	Treatment naïve HCC with portal vein invasion	• Experimental arm: HAI oxaliplatin (85 mg/m^2), 5-FU (400 mg/m^2 bolus followed by 2400 mg/m^2), leucovorin (400 mg/m^2) + sorafenib (400 mg twice daily), $n = 125$ • Control arm: Sorafenib (400 mg twice daily), $n = 122$	**Median OS** 13.4 months (HAI) 7.1 months (no HAI) $p < 0.001$ **Median PFS** 7 months (HAI) 2.6 months (no HAI) $p < 0.001$ **Major RECIST response** 40.8% (HAI) 2.5% (no HAI) $p < 0.001$ **Complete clinical response** 11.2% (HAI) 0% (no HAI) $p < 0.001$

low-up time of 17 months. Of the 132 patients in the HAI chemotherapy arm, only two patients were unable to receive HAI chemotherapy due technical considerations; no main feeding artery could be found at angiography. Catheter-related adverse events were observed in six patients (5%).

A second phase III trial compared percutaneous HAI chemotherapy (similar dosing of FOLFOX in the previous study) with transarterial chemoembolization (50 mg epirubicin, 50 mg lobaplatin, lipiodol) for patients with Barcelona Liver Clinic (BCLC) stage A–B, unresectable tumors, ≥7 cm in size [28]. Patients were treatment naïve and had excellent performance status (ECOG: 0–1). Macrovascular invasion and extrahepatic metastases were strict exclusion criteria.

HAI was performed with sequential femoral arterial puncture and catheterization. Patients in the HAI chemotherapy arm had a median OS of 23.1 months compared to 16.1 months in the chemoembolization arm ($p < 0.001$). Median PFS was 9.6 months in the HAI chemotherapy arm and 5.4 months in the chemoembolization arm ($p < 0.001$). Major RECIST response was noted in 46% of patients in the HAI chemotherapy arm vs. 18% of patients in the chemoembolization arm ($p < 0.001$). Complete response rate was seen in 13% of patients in the HAI chemotherapy arm vs. 3% in the chemoembolization arm ($p < 0.001$). Of note, most patients had hepatitis B (88% in the HAI chemotherapy arm and 90% in the chemoembolization arm) and the PFS benefit associated with HAI chemotherapy was not evident in patients without hepatitis B. Vascular complications associated with the indwelling catheter were noted in 12 patients in the HAI chemotherapy arm, all of which were salvaged with repeat angiography.

The third phase III trial compared sorafenib plus percutaneous HAI chemotherapy (SoraHAI) with FOLFOX to sorafenib alone in patients with HCC and portal vein invasion [29]. Patients in this study were limited to Childs A cirrhotics with good performance status (ECOG: 0–2) and no prior treatment. Patients were stratified by grade of portal vein invasion (Vp1–2, Vp3, and Vp4). HAI chemotherapy was performed with sequential femoral artery puncture and catheterization. The chemotherapy regimen used in the HAI chemotherapy arm was as follows: oxaliplatin (85 mg/m^2), leucovorin (400 mg/m^2), 5-FU (400 mg/m^2 bolus followed by 2400 mg/m^2 infusion over 46 h). Patients in both arms received sorafenib (400 mg orally twice daily). Approximately 80% of the patients in each arm had hepatitis B. Patients in the SoraHAI arm had a median OS of 13.4 months compared to 7.1 months in the sorafenib arm ($p < 0.001$). When stratified by grade of portal vein invasion, median OS was improved in the SoraHAIC arm (Vp1–2: 18.2 months vs. 10.9 months, $p = 0.002$; Vp3: 13.5 months vs. 6.3 months, $p < 0.001$; Vp4: 9.5 months vs. 4.4 months, $p < 0.001$). Patients in the SoraHAI arm had a median PFS of 7 months vs. 2.6 months in the sorafenib arm ($p < 0.001$). Major RECIST response rate was 40.8% in the SoraHAI arm compared to 2.5% in the sorafenib arm ($p < 0.001$). Fourteen out of 125 patients in the SoraHAI arm achieved a complete clinical response. Ten out of 125 patients experienced vascular complications associated with the indwelling catheter. All were salvaged with repeat angiography.

In summary, HAI chemotherapy has a clear role in patients with locally advanced/unresectable HCC and in patients with limited extrahepatic disease. However, the data above should be interpreted with caution. As mentioned, all three of these phase III trials were performed in China where the primary cause of HCC is chronic hepatitis B infection. On subgroup analysis, one study suggested that patients without hepatitis B infection did not benefit from HAI chemotherapy. This puts into question the generalizability of this treatment modality to patients in Western countries where hepatitis C and fatty liver disease are more commonly associated with the development of HCC.

Colorectal Cancer and Colorectal Cancer Liver Metastases

Percutaneous HAI chemotherapy has predominantly been tested in patients with advanced (typically unresectable) colorectal cancer liver metastases, although no randomized trials have been performed in this population. The majority of modern retrospective and nonrandomized prospective studies have utilized a strategy of recurrent access [30–35], typically via the femoral artery, where arterial access and hepatic artery catheterization is performed and subsequently removed after each treatment; however, single-treatment HAI chemotherapy has also been reported in conjunction with systemic therapy [36]. Diverse regimens have been tested, making it difficult to make comparisons across studies or with historical control populations, but the existing literature can largely be stratified based on whether patients were treatment-naïve or previously received systemic therapy, as these groups represent distinct populations with respect to anticipated treatment response and longer-term outcomes.

Three prospective, nonrandomized trials (Table 32.3) have tested totally percutaneous HAI chemotherapy in patients with treatment-naïve colorectal cancer liver metastases (not excluding adjuvant chemotherapy after primary tumor resection) [30, 31, 36]. A phase II study of 38 patients in the United States (University of Nebraska) tested single-dose HAI FUDR (60 mg/m^2 per day, given over 4 days) followed by systemic 5-FU/leucovorin [36]. No complete responses were reported, and among patients that received at least one dose of HAI FUDR, the response rate was 46%. Five patients were subsequently able to undergo liver resection. Median time to progression and overall survival were 6 and 13 months, respectively. The authors considered these outcomes similar to historical controls treated with long-term HAI chemotherapy (i.e., delivered via a surgically placed catheter/reservoir system or percutaneously via an attached port system), positing single-dose HAI chemotherapy as an alternative strategy for unresectable hepatic metastases or for adjuvant therapy following liver resection. Two additional prospective trials have tested sequential percutaneous HAI chemotherapy in combination with systemic chemotherapy. In a French, multi-institutional phase II trial of HAI pirarubicin (60 mg/m^2 administered at 16-day cycles) given concurrently with systemic irinotecan and 5-FU/leucovorin [30], the overall response rate was 48%, with 11 of 31 patients ultimately undergoing liver resection. Median progression-free and overall survival were 9.1 and 20.5 months, respectively. Finally, a Chinese, single-institutional trial tested trimodal HAI chemotherapy with FUDR (500 mg/m^2), oxaliplatin (100 mg/m^2), and irinotecan (120 mg/m^2) given every 4–8 weeks in combination with systemic FUDR/leucovorin [31]. The overall response rate was 61.3%, and median progression-free and overall survival were 10.1 and 24.8 months, respectively.

In pretreated patients with colorectal cancer liver metastases, the majority of the existing data come from phase I dose-finding studies [33–35]. Two dose-finding studies of HAI irinotecan have been reported in predominantly patients with metastatic colorectal cancer, one with HAI irinotecan utilized as a single-agent [35] and the other

Table 32.3 Nonrandomized prospective studies in treatment-naïve colorectal cancer liver metastases

Trial site(s)	Patient population	Study design	Treatment group(s)	Outcomes
University of Nebraska	Treatment-naïve[a] unresectable CRCLM	Phase II, single-arm ($n = 43$, 5 patients did not receive indicated treatment)	• HAI FUDR (60 mg/m^2) followed by systemic 5-FU/leucovorin	• Response rate: 41% • Conversion to resection: 13% • Median OS: 13 months • Median PFS: 6 months
France, 3 centers	Treatment-naïve[a] CRCLM (resectability status not indicated)	Phase II, single-arm ($n = 31$)	• HAI pirarubicin (60 mg/m^2) with systemic irinotecan and 5-FU/leucovorin	• Response rate: 48% • Conversion to resection: 35% • Median OS: 21 months • Median PFS: 9 months
Fudan University (China)	Treatment-naïve[a] unresectable CRCLM	Single-arm ($n = 31$)	• HAI irinotecan (120 mg/m^2), oxaliplatin (100 mg/m^2), and FUDR (500 mg/m^2) followed by systemic 5-FU/LV	• Response rate: 61% • Median OS: 25 months • Median PFS: 10 months

[a] Not including adjuvant therapy after resection of primary tumor

with concurrent systemic therapy (bevacizumab, cetuximab, or oxaliplatin) [33]. The maximum tolerated dose of HAI irinotecan alone (administered every 2 weeks) was 240 mg/m^2, with dose-limiting toxicities including granulocytopenia, diarrhea, and pain. The majority of patients treated for planned ≥4 cycles demonstrated stable disease. Median time-to-progression was 4.7 months, and median overall survival was 15.6 months. When HAI irinotecan was utilized in combination with targeted therapy or oxaliplatin, the maximum tolerated dose was expectedly lower (45–75 mg/m^2 dosed every 4 weeks). At this dose, in combination with other systemic agents, only two patients demonstrated a partial response, and stable disease at 6 months was rare (11 of 63 evaluable patients). Similarly, HAI oxaliplatin was tested in a dose-finding study of concurrent escalating doses of HAI 5-FU with systemic bevacizumab (in *KRAS* wild-type patients) or escalating doses of systemic 5-FU/leucovorin and cetuximab with bevacizumab (in *KRAS*-mutant patients). The only dose-limiting toxicity in either group was diarrhea, and the maximum dose utilized in the escalation phase (1750 mg/m^2 of HAI 5-FU, 400 mg/m^2 of systemic 5-FU, and 500 mg/m^2 of systemic cetuximab) was ultimately utilized in the expansion phase. In *KRAS* wild-type patients, the response rate was 21%, median time to treatment failure was 3.1 months, and median overall survival was 6.8 months. In *KRAS*-mutant patients, the response rate was 40%, median time to treatment failure was 3.8 months, and median overall survival was 11.5 months. While larger trials are needed in this patient population, these studies suggest that a strategy including totally percutaneous HAI chemotherapy can provide a treatment response in select patients who have been previously treated—and in many cases heavily pretreated—for colorectal cancer liver metastases.

Notably, percutaneous HAI chemotherapy has also been tested in patients with localized colorectal cancer in order to prevent hepatic metastasis. Two randomized trials, both led by the same group from Fudan University in Shanghai, have evaluated totally percutaneous HAI chemotherapy in the neoadjuvant setting (Table 32.4) [37, 38].

The first was a single-institution trial that randomized 222 patients with stage II and III colorectal cancer to either preoperative hepatic and regional arterial chemotherapy or surgery alone, with both groups planned to receive adjuvant systemic chemotherapy (FOLFOX4) after

Table 32.4 Randomized controlled trials in patients with localized (nonmetastatic) colorectal cancer

Trial site(s)	Patient population	Treatment group(s)	Outcomes
Fudan University (China)	Stage II/III colorectal cancer undergoing resection of primary followed by adjuvant FOLFOX4	• Experimental arm: Preoperative hepatic and regional FUDR (500 mg) and oxaliplatin (50 mg) ($n = 110$) • Control arm: No preoperative treatment ($n = 112$)	• 3-year OS: 91% (experimental arm) vs. 83% (control arm), ($p = 0.03$) • 3-year PFS: 81% (experimental arm) vs. 69% (control arm) ($p = 0.04$) • 3-year liver-metastasis-free survival: 86% (experimental arm) vs. 80% (control arm) ($p = 0.04$)
China, multicenter	Stage II/III colorectal cancer undergoing resection of primary followed by adjuvant mFOLFOX6	• Experimental arm: Preoperative hepatic and regional FUDR (375 mg) and oxaliplatin (37.5 mg) ($n = 341$) • Control arm: No preoperative treatment ($n = 347$)	• 3-year OS: 84% (experimental arm) vs. 76% (control arm) ($p = 0.005$) • 5-year PFS: 77% (experimental arm) vs. 65% (control arm) ($p = 0.001$) • 5-year liver-metastasis-free survival: 93% (experimental arm) vs. 84% (control arm) ($p < 0.001$)

surgery [37]. Percutaneous hepatic and regional arterial chemotherapy consisted of FUDR (500 mg) and oxaliplatin (50 mg), which was administered separately to the common hepatic artery and the main artery supplying the primary colorectal tumor. Surgery to remove the primary colorectal tumor was then performed 1 week later. Postoperative outcomes were equivalent between groups, and while hepatic toxicity was not described in detail, grade 3 events were reported in only 2% of patients treated with hepatic artery chemotherapy. The primary outcome was 3-year disease-free survival, which was significantly longer in patients treated with percutaneous hepatic and regional arterial chemotherapy (80.9% vs. 68.7%, $p = 0.04$), translating to an improvement in 3-year overall survival (91.3% vs. 83.3%, $p = 0.03$). Improvements in outcome were most pronounced in patients with stage III primary tumors, including disease-free (74.6 vs. 58.1, $p < 0.001$) and overall survival (87.7% vs. 75.7%, $p = 0.02$). The risk ratio for developing liver metastases was also significantly reduced in stage III patients treated with percutaneous hepatic and regional arterial therapy (0.73, $p = 0.02$), and the time to development of liver metastases after surgery was prolonged (16 vs. 8 months, $p = 0.01$).

A subsequent, multicenter trial of 688 patients with stage II or III colorectal cancer similarly randomized patients to percutaneous hepatic and regional arterial chemotherapy versus surgery alone, with all patients planned to receive adjuvant systemic chemotherapy (mFOLFOX6) [38]. In this trial, percutaneous hepatic and regional arterial consisted of FUDR (650 mg/m^2) and oxaliplatin (75 mg/m^2), with half the dose provided via the common hepatic artery and the other half administered to the main primary tumor-feeding artery. Results from this trial largely corroborated the prior study, including improvements associated with percutaneous hepatic and regional arterial chemotherapy in 3- and 5-year disease-free survival, liver-metastasis-free survival, and overall survival. Again, improvements in outcomes were most pronounced in patients with stage III disease, where 5-year disease-free survival (68% vs. 53%, $p = 0.011$), liver-metastasis-free survival (90% vs. 76%, $p < 0.001$), and overall survival (77% vs. 66%, $p = 0.025$) were all markedly improved in patients receiving percutaneous hepatic and regional arterial chemotherapy. Perioperative morbidity was reported with greater granularity in this larger trial, and again no differences were reported in short-term outcomes. No catheter-related complications requiring intervention were reported, and no 30-day postoperative morality was reported in either group.

In summary, totally percutaneous HAI chemotherapy has demonstrated response rates in approximately half of treatment-naïve colorectal cancer liver metastases, and in select patients with heavily pretreated colorectal cancer liver metastases, although randomized data in the metastatic setting is currently lacking. Alternatively, two randomized controlled trials have demonstrated that single-dose HAI chemotherapy (with concurrent regional arterial chemotherapy to the primary tumor) can reduce liver recurrence after primary resection, translating to an improvement in survival outcomes.

Other Primary and Metastatic Liver Cancers

Over the past two decades, MD Anderson Cancer Center has led a series of tumor agnostic phase I trials testing various HAI chemotherapy regimens, some in isolation and others with concomitant systemic chemotherapy or targeted therapy [33, 39–43]. In general, these studies have utilized a "3 + 3" escalation and expansion study design to determine dose-limiting toxicities and maximum tolerated doses. In some cases, response rates have been reported, although these are difficult to interpret given that studies enrolled patients with diverse primary liver cancers and hepatic metastases from various primary sites, including colorectal, gastroesophageal, lung, cutaneous, and breast cancers. In each study, sequential hepatic artery catheterization was achieved via femoral access, with the catheter removed between treatment cycles. Among these studies, HAI oxaliplatin [34, 39], irinotecan [33], and nab-paclitaxel [40–42] have each been tested across diverse tumor types. In these studies, partial response rates have generally been low (5–20%), although higher rates of disease stability have been reported (up to 39% at 4 months in one study testing HAI oxaliplatin in combination with systemic capecitabine and bevacizumab [39]).

More focused studies have been performed in patients with liver metastases originating from breast cancer [44, 45]. Small studies have also been performed in patients with metastatic biliary tract cancers [46, 47].

An early study in 34 breast cancer patients with hepatic metastases who had failed prior systemic chemotherapy tested HAI cisplatin (100 mg/m^2 over 2 h) and vinblastine (1.7 mg/m^2 over 5 days) at 4-week intervals. Partial response rates were observed in 33%, and 24% of patients had what was described as a "minor" response. Progression occurred at a median 7.2 months, and median overall survival was 11 months. Two decades later, two phase II trials were performed testing systemic capecitabine (1300–2000 mg/m^2) with concurrent oxaliplatin, the latter dosed every 2 weeks alternating between an intravenous and HAI route (70–85 mg/m^2). The pooled results demonstrated a response rate of 42%, median progression-free survival of 10.8 months, and median overall survival of 27.6 months. Notably, pharmacokinetic studies found no difference in plasma concentration of oxaliplatin when it was administered via the intravenous versus HAI route.

Finally, two studies have been performed testing totally percutaneous HAI chemotherapy in patients with metastatic biliary tract malignancies. The first tested HAI epirubicin (50 mg/m^2), cisplatin (60 mg/m^2) followed by systemic 5-FU (200 mg/m^2) in patients with metastatic cholangiocarcinoma repeated at 3-week intervals [46]. Among 10 patients, the time to treatment failure was 10 months, and 2-year survival was 55%. A subsequent study in 20 patients with metastatic biliary tract cancer tested the same HAI regimen of epirubicin and cisplatin in combination with capecitabine (1000 mg/m^2), also repeated at 3-week intervals [47]. The partial response rate was 31.5%, with stable disease observed in 47.5%. Median progression-free survival was 11.6 months, and 1-year survival was 74%. While these data require validation in larger, prospective trials, they do support potential activity associated with various HAI chemotherapy regimens across hepatic metastases from diverse primary tumors.

Concluding Remarks

In summary, totally percutaneous HAI is an alternative delivery strategy for intra-arterial chemotherapeutics that has been extensively studied in Europe and more recently in Asia. A wide variety of agents have been tested but fluoropyrimidine analogues (5-FU and FUDR) and oxaliplatin are the best studied. Patients with locally advanced HCC secondary to chronic hepatitis B infection and patients with stage III colon cancer seem to have the greatest survival benefit. Sequential percutaneous access has been shown to be safe and well-tolerated with low complication rates, but outcomes have never been compared to implantable pump systems. Larger, prospective trials are needed in Western populations.

References

1. Bierman HR, Miller ER, Byron RL, Dod KS, Kelly KH, Black DH. Intra-arterial catheterization of viscera in man. Am J Roentgenol Radium Ther. 1951;66:555–68.
2. Byron RL, Perez FM, Yonemoto RH, Bierman HR, Gildenhorn HL, Kelly KH. Left brachial arterial catheterization for chemotherapy in advanced intra-abdominal malignant neoplasms. Surg Gynecol Obstet. 1961;112:689–96.
3. Clarkson B, Young C, Dierick W, Kuehn P, Kim M, Berrett A, Clapp P, Lawrence W. Effects of continuous hepatic artery infusion of antimetabolites on primary and metastatic cancer of the liver. Cancer. 1962;15:472–88.
4. Reed ML, Kuipers FM, Vaitkevicius VK, Clark MD, Drake EH, Eyler WR. Treatment of disseminated carcinoid tumors including hepatic-artery catheterization. N Engl J Med. 1963;269:1005–10.
5. Stewart JD, Drake EH, Gale HH. Hepatic artery catheterization for local organ perfusion in malignant disease. Henry Ford Hos Med J. 1965;13:251–63.

6. Fortuny IE, Theologides A, Kennedy BJ. Hepatic arterial infusion for liver metastases from colon cancer: comparison of mitomycin C(NSC-26980) and 5-fluorouracil (NSC-19893). Cancer Chemoth Rep. 1975;59:401–4.
7. Geddes EW, Falkson G. Malignant hepatoma in the Bantu. Cancer. 1970;25:1271–8.
8. Cady B, Oberfield RA. Arterial infusion chemotherapy of hepatoma. Surg Gynecol Obstet. 1974;138:381–4.
9. Bern MM, McDermott W, Cady B, Oberfield RA, Trey C, Clouse ME, Tullis JL, Parker LM. Intraarterial hepatic infusion and intravenous adriamycin for treatment of hepatocellular carcinoma. A clinical and pharmacology report. Cancer. 1978;42:399–405.
10. Weiss GR, Hersh M, Kuhn JG, Ludden TM, von Hoff DD, Kisner DL, Pirtle TE. A phase I and pharmacokinetic comparison of hepatic arterial and peripheral vein infusions of bisantrene for liver cancer. Cancer Chemother Pharmacol. 1985;15:144–8.
11. Fujimoto S, Miyazaki M, Endoh F, Takahashi O, Okui K, Morimoto Y. Biodegradable mitomycin C microspheres given intra-arterially for inoperable hepatic cancer. With particular reference to a comparison with continuous infusion of mitomycin C and 5-fluorouracil. Cancer. 1985;56:2404–10.
12. Carcinoma ESG for H. Intra-arterial administration of epirubicin in the treatment of nonresectable hepatocellular carcinoma. Cancer Chemother Pharmacol. 1987;19:183–9.
13. Shepherd FA, Evans WK, Blackstein ME, Fine S, Heathcote J, Langer B, Taylor B, Habal F, Kutas G, Pritchard KI. Hepatic arterial infusion of mitoxantrone in the treatment of primary hepatocellular carcinoma. J Clin Oncol. 1987;5:635–40.
14. Harada A, Nonami T, Kishimoto W, Nakao A, Takagi H. Results of hepatic resection and postoperative arterial chemotherapy for hepatocellular carcinoma. Cancer Chemother Pharmacol. 1992;31:S35–7.
15. Jones DV, Patt YZ, Ajani JA, Abbruzzese J, Levin B, Carrasco CH, Charnsangavej C, Wallace S. A phase I-II trial of mitoxantrone by hepatic arterial infusion in patients with hepatocellular carcinoma or colorectal carcinoma metastatic to the liver. Cancer. 1993;72:2560–3.
16. Oka M, Hazama S, Yoshino S, Shimoda K, Suzuki M, Shimizu R, Yano K, Nishida M, Suzuki T. Intraarterial combined immunochemotherapy for unresectable hepatocellular carcinoma: preliminary results. Cancer Immunol Immunother. 1994;38:194–200.
17. Patt YZ, Charnsangavej C, Yoffe B, Smith R, Lawrence D, Chuang V, Carrasco H, Roh M, Chase J, Fischer H. Hepatic arterial infusion of floxuridine, leucovorin, doxorubicin, and cisplatin for hepatocellular carcinoma: effects of hepatitis B and C viral infection on drug toxicity and patient survival. J Clin Oncol. 1994;12:1204–11.
18. Lygidakis NJ, Pothoulakis J, Konstantinidou AE, Spanos H. Hepatocellular carcinoma: surgical resection versus surgical resection combined with pre- and post-operative locoregional immunotherapy-chemotherapy. A prospective randomized study. Anticancer Res. 1995;15:543–50.
19. Malik IA, Khan WA, Haq S, Sabih M. A prospective phase II trial to evaluate the efficacy and toxicity of hepatic arterial infusion of ifosfamide in patients with inoperable localized hepatocellular carcinoma. Am J Clin Oncol. 1997;20:289–92.
20. Urabe T, Kaneko S, Matsushita E, Unoura M, Kobayashi K. Clinical pilot study of intrahepatic arterial chemotherapy with methotrexate, 5-fluorouracil, cisplatin and subcutaneous interferon-alpha-2b for patients with locally advanced hepatocellular carcinoma. Oncology. 1998;55:39–47.
21. Chung YH, Song IH, Song BC, Lee GC, Koh MS, Yoon HK, Lee YS, Sung KB, Suh DJ. Combined therapy consisting of intraarterial cisplatin infusion and systemic interferon-alpha for hepatocellular carcinoma patients with major portal vein thrombosis or distant metastasis. Cancer. 2000;88:1986–91.
22. Oyama A, Nouso K, Yoshimura K, et al. Randomized controlled study to examine the efficacy of hepatic arterial infusion chemotherapy with cisplatin before radiofrequency ablation for hepatocellular carcinoma. Hepatol Res. 2021;51:694–701.
23. Nishikawa H, Osaki Y, Kita R, et al. Transcatheter arterial infusion chemotherapy prior to radiofrequency thermal ablation for single hepatocellular carcinoma reduces the risk of intrahepatic distant recurrence. Int J Oncol. 2012;41:903–9.
24. Feng M, Tang C, Feng W, Bao Y, Zheng Y, Shen J. Hepatic artery-infusion chemotherapy improved survival of hepatocellular carcinoma after radical hepatectomy. Onco Targets Ther. 2017;10:3001–5.
25. Hsiao J-H, Tsai C-C, Liang T-J, Chiang C-L, Liang H-L, Chen I-S, Chen Y-C, Chang P-M, Chou N-H, Wang B-W. Adjuvant hepatic arterial infusion chemotherapy is beneficial for selective patients with hepatocellular carcinoma undergoing surgical treatment. Int J Surg. 2017;45:35–41.
26. Hamada T, Yano K, Wada T, Imamura N, Hiyoshi M, Kondo K, Nanashima A. Increased survival benefit of adjuvant intra-arterial infusion chemotherapy in HCC patients with portal vein infiltration after hepatectomy. World J Surg. 2020;44:2770–6.
27. Lyu N, Wang X, Li J-B, Lai J-F, Chen Q-F, Li S-L, Deng H-J, He M, Mu L-W, Zhao M. Arterial chemotherapy of oxaliplatin plus fluorouracil versus sorafenib in advanced hepatocellular carcinoma: a biomolecular exploratory, randomized, phase III trial (FOHAIC-1). J Clin Oncol. 2022;40:468–80.
28. Li Q-J, He M-K, Chen H-W, et al. Hepatic arterial infusion of oxaliplatin, fluorouracil, and leucovorin versus transarterial chemoembolization for large hepatocellular carcinoma: a randomized phase III trial. J Clin Oncol. 2022;40:150–60.
29. He M, Li Q, Zou R, et al. Sorafenib plus hepatic arterial infusion of oxaliplatin, fluorouracil, and leucovorin vs sorafenib alone for hepatocellular carcinoma with portal vein invasion. JAMA Oncol. 2019;5:953–60.

30. Zelek L, Bugat R, Cherqui D, et al. Multimodal therapy with intravenous biweekly leucovorin, 5-fluorouracil and irinotecan combined with hepatic arterial infusion pirarubicin in non-resectable hepatic metastases from colorectal cancer (a European Association for Research in Oncology trial). Ann Oncol. 2003;14:1537–42.
31. Chen Y, Wang X, Yan Z, Wang J, Luo J, Liu Q. Hepatic arterial infusion with irinotecan, oxaliplatin, and floxuridine plus systemic chemotherapy as first-line treatment of unresectable liver metastases from colorectal cancer. Oncol Res Treat. 2012;35:480–4.
32. Guadagni S, Clementi M, Mackay AR, et al. Real-life multidisciplinary treatment for unresectable colorectal cancer liver metastases including hepatic artery infusion with chemo-filtration and liquid biopsy precision oncotherapy: observational cohort study. J Cancer Res Clin. 2020;146:1273–90.
33. Said R, Kurzrock R, Naing A, et al. Dose-finding study of hepatic arterial infusion of irinotecan-based treatment in patients with advanced cancers metastatic to the liver. Invest New Drugs. 2015;33:911–20.
34. Tsimberidou AM, Leick MB, Lim J, et al. Dose-finding study of hepatic arterial infusion of oxaliplatin-based treatment in patients with advanced solid tumors metastatic to the liver. Cancer Chemother Pharmacol. 2013;71:389–97.
35. Eichler K, Dufas T, Hammerstingl R, Gruber-Rouh T, Vogl TJ, Zangos S. Hepatic arterial infusion with irinotecan in patients with liver metastases of colorectal cancer: results of an extended phase I study. Chemotherapy. 2013;59:66–73.
36. Copur MS, Capadano M, Lynch J, Goertzen T, McCowan T, Brand R, Tempero M. Alternating hepatic arterial infusion and systemic chemotherapy for liver metastases from colorectal cancer: a phase II trial using intermittent percutaneous hepatic arterial access. J Clin Oncol. 2001;19:2404–12.
37. Xu J, Zhong Y, Weixin N, Xinyu Q, Yanhan L, Li R, Jianhua W, Zhiping Y, Jiemin C. Preoperative hepatic and regional arterial chemotherapy in the prevention of liver metastasis after colorectal cancer surgery. Ann Surg. 2007;245:583–90.
38. Zhu D, Xia J, Gu Y, et al. Preoperative hepatic and regional arterial chemotherapy in patients who underwent curative colorectal cancer resection. Ann Surg. 2021;273:1066–75.
39. Fountzilas E, Krishnan E, Janku F, et al. A phase I clinical trial of hepatic arterial infusion of oxaliplatin and oral capecitabine, with or without intravenous bevacizumab, in patients with advanced cancer and predominant liver involvement. Cancer Chemother Pharmacol. 2018;82:877–85.
40. Tsimberidou AM, Ye Y, Wheler J, Naing A, Hong D, Nwosu U, Hess KR, Wolff RA. A phase I study of hepatic arterial infusion of nab-paclitaxel in combination with intravenous gemcitabine and bevacizumab for patients with advanced cancers and predominant liver metastases. Cancer Chemother Pharmacol. 2013;71:955–63.
41. Siqing F, Culotta KS, Falchook GS, Hong DS, Myers AL, Zhang Y-P, Naing A, Janku F, Hou M-M, Kurzrock R. Pharmacokinetic evaluation of nanoparticle albumin-bound paclitaxel delivered via hepatic arterial infusion in patients with predominantly hepatic metastases. Cancer Chemother Pharmacol. 2016;77:357–64.
42. Fu S, Naing A, Moulder SL, Culotta KS, Madoff DC, Ng CS, Madden TL, Falchook GS, Hong DS, Kurzrock R. Phase I trial of hepatic arterial infusion of nanoparticle albumin–bound paclitaxel: toxicity, pharmacokinetics, and activity. Mol Cancer Ther. 2011;10:1300–7.
43. Tsimberidou AM, Fu S, Ng C, et al. A phase 1 study of hepatic arterial infusion of oxaliplatin in combination with systemic 5-fluorouracil, leucovorin, and bevacizumab in patients with advanced solid tumors metastatic to the liver. Cancer. 2010;116:4086–94.
44. Lindgaard SC, Brinch CM, Jensen BK, et al. Hepatic arterial therapy with oxaliplatin and systemic capecitabine for patients with liver metastases from breast cancer. Breast. 2019;43:113–9.
45. Fraschini G, Charnsangavej C, Carrasco CH, Buzdar AU, Jabboury KW, Hortobagyi GN. Percutaneous hepatic arterial infusion of cisplatin-vinblastine for refractory breast carcinoma metastatic to the liver. Am J Clin Oncol. 1988;11:34–8.
46. Cantore M, Rabbi C, Guadagni S, Zamagni D, Aitini E. Intra-arterial hepatic chemotherapy combined with continuous infusion of 5-fluorouracil in patients with metastatic cholangiocarcinoma. Ann Oncol. 2002;13:1687–8.
47. Mambrini A, Guglielmi A, Pacetti P, et al. Capecitabine plus hepatic intra-arterial epirubicin and cisplatin in unresectable biliary cancer: a phase II study. Anticancer Res. 2007;27:3009–13.

33 Reservoir-Less Ports for Hepatic Arterial Infusion

Yael Berger, Gali Perl, and Eran Sadot

Introduction

The liver, with its rich vascular supply, constitutes one of the most common sites for cancer metastasis, with the most prominent source for the above being of colorectal origin [1]. Liver metastases, which occur in more than half of colorectal cancer (CRC) patients, are the most common cause of disease-specific mortality in these patients, and appear either as a synchronous or metachronous finding over the course of disease [2]. Treatment options have been rapidly evolving, with a movement toward a multimodality approach.

Hepatic arterial infusion (HAI) is a liver-directed treatment strategy to deliver high-dose chemotherapy directly to the liver by way of the hepatic arterial system. In the modern era, HAI is most commonly performed by an implantable subcutaneous pump with a reservoir and intra-arterial catheter. The current body of HAI literature primarily originates from surgeons and medical oncologists that have trained at Memorial Sloan Kettering Cancer Center (MSKCC), where the majority of research and practice of this therapy has originated. Recently, the implementation of new HAI programs has taken place at more than 70 new centers in the past 5 years in the United States and Europe [3].

In this chapter, we will focus on reservoir-less ports for HAI. This approach utilizes different chemotherapeutic agents and is practiced mainly in Europe and Asia.

Rationale for HAI

Several anatomic and pharmacologic principles support the rationale for HAI as a locoregional treatment for liver tumors:

1. Unlike normal hepatocytes that receive their blood supply from both the portal vein and hepatic artery, the blood supply to hepatic tumors, including colorectal liver metastases (CRLM), intrahepatic cholangiocarcinoma (ICC), and hepatocellular carcinoma (HCC) [4] is predominantly arterial [5].
2. High local concentrations with minimal systemic toxicity may be achieved with arterially delivered drugs that are largely extracted by the liver during first-pass metabolism. The liver extraction ratio of oxaliplatin, the drug most commonly delivered via reservoir-less ports, is 0.47, which means that approximately

Y. Berger · E. Sadot (✉)
Department of Surgery, Hepatobiliary and Pancreatic Surgery Unit, Beilinson Hospital, Rabin Medical Center, Petah-tikva, Israel

Tel Aviv University, Faculty of Medical & Health Sciences, Tel Aviv, Israel

G. Perl
Department of Oncology, Petah-tikva, Israel

Tel Aviv University, Faculty of Medical & Health Sciences, Tel Aviv, Israel

M. D'Angelica, M. Lidsky (eds.), *Hepatic Arterial Infusion for Malignancy*,
https://doi.org/10.1007/978-3-031-74935-3_33

only half of the administered drug reaches systemic circulation, resulting in less systemic toxicity, including cumulative peripheral neuropathy, and increasing its safety profile through HAI administration [6].

3. Drugs with a steep dose–response curve are more useful when given by the intrahepatic route because small increases in the concentration of administered drug result in a large improvement in response. Oxaliplatin demonstrates a relatively linear dose–response relationship [7].
4. Hepatic infusion is more useful when utilizing drugs with a high total-body clearance, and their concentration is affected by hepatic arterial blood flow as well. The high regional exchange rate of hepatic arterial flow (100–1500 mL/min) requires drugs with a high clearance rate [8]. If a drug is not cleared rapidly, recirculation through the systemic circulation mitigates the advantage of intra-arterial therapy versus systemic therapy [9]. Oxaliplatin demonstrates a relatively high clearance rate [10].
5. The possibility of stepwise progression of tumor metastases from the colon via the portal vein to the liver and later to the lungs and other sites [11] may indicate that direct treatment of hepatic metastases would prevent tumor dissemination to other sites, and thus yield prolonged survival for some patients.

Chemotherapy Drugs for HAI

Various chemotherapeutic agents (Table 33.1) have been utilized via HAI administration for the treatment of hepatic tumors. Fluorodeoxyuridine (FUDR) has been extensively studied and is mainly used in North America. Its advantages are the high hepatic arterial exposure (100–400 fold), short half-life (<10 min), and extensive first-pass hepatic extraction (94–99%) [12]. However, FUDR has not gained foothold across the world because of a few hurdles that limit its dissemination. First, it is associated with a relatively high rate of biliary toxicity, which limits its administration. Concomitant intra-arterial steroids are therefore added to improve tolerance. A second hurdle, the HAI pumps that have been used in North America (i.e., Codman and Intera pumps), contains Freon gas that is banned from the EU for environmental reasons. As a result, FUDR is not registered in the EU [13]. Consequently, alternative chemotherapeutic agents have been utilized in the EU and Asia.

Oxaliplatin is an alternative drug administered via HAI that is mostly used with reservoir-less ports and it offers several advantages. First, it has been shown to accumulate preferentially in liver tumors (4.3 ratio of tumor/normal liver parenchyma concentration) compared to normal hepatocytes [14]. Furthermore, it exhibits a liver extraction ratio of 0.47, which translates into a significant decrease in total platinum and filterable platinum. Therefore, it may hold potential benefit in terms of tolerance when used via the HAI route (e.g., decrease in peripheral neuropathy) [15]. These benefits have been established in multiple studies. For example, a multicenter phase II trial by Ducreux et al. [16] demonstrated that HAI oxaliplatin and systemic 5-FU-folinic acid (LV5FU2 regimen) was associated with a 64% response rate and a median overall survival (OS) of 27 months in 28 patients with unresectable CRLM. The main toxicities were grade 3 or 4 neutropenia in ten patients (35%) and severe pain during administration in six patients (21%). Overall, this regimen was felt to be well tolerated. In another study, Goere et al. [17] demonstrated that HAI oxaliplatin combined with systemic chemotherapy succeeded in converting CRLM to complete resection in 24% of patients. Furthermore, 19% of patients who underwent surgery had a complete pathological response. Similar drug efficacy and safety were shown in the OPTILIV trial, a European multicenter phase II prospective trial that included 64 patients with unresectable CRLM. Complete hepatic resection was achieved in 30% of the patients and the response rate was 41% [18]. Another important aspect that played a pivotal role in the dissemination of HAI oxaliplatin is that it is more affordable in most of the world (i.e., US$ 17 a vial). It

Table 33.1 Chemotherapeutic agents commonly used in hepatic artery infusion

Drugs	Mechanism of action [21]	Hepatic arterial exposure (x compared with intravenous delivery)	Half-life (min)	Extraction	Toxicity [21]
FUDR (floxuridine)	Pyrimidine nucleotide analog, antimetabolite; cell cycle-dependent	100–400 [22]	10 [23]	94–99% [24]	Myelosuppression (dose-limiting as bolos); diarrhea and stomatitis (dose-limiting at protracted infusions); other GI toxicities (e.g., nausea, vomiting, anorexia, gastritis, cramping, enteritis, and duodenal ulcers—All rare); liver toxicity (usually cholestatic, dose limiting with HAI); serious neurologic adverse effects (e.g., ataxia and visual changes—Rare) and fever (rare)
Pirarubicin	Anthracycline; inhibits nucleic acids synthesis trough cell cycle cessation at the G2 phase, causing cell death [25]	20 [26]	<10 [27]	80% [25]	Neutropenia (dose-limiting), cardiotoxicity, loss of hair, GI toxicity, hepatic toxicity [25]
5-FU	Pyrimidine antimetabolite; inhibits thymidylate synthase; partial cell cycle-dependency	10 [28]	10–20 [29]	<50% [30]	GI toxicities (primarily mucositis and diarrhea, dose-limiting; patients with dihydropyrimidine dehydrogenase deficiency experience excessive toxicity—Rare); myelosuppression (less when continuously infused); mild nausea and vomiting (uncommon); dermatitis and other cutaneous toxicities (e.g., hand–foot syndrome); cerebellar ataxia and myocardial ischemia (rare)
Mitomycin C	Antitumor antibiotic; inhibits DNA and RNA synthesis	6–8 [31]	10 [23]	22%	Vesicant; myelosuppression (dose-limiting); mild nausea and vomiting; anorexia; fatigue; diarrhea; stomatitis; rash; fever; renal insufficiency; veno-occlusive liver disease; hemolytic–uremic syndrome; interstitial pneumonitis (rare)
Cisplatin	Atypical alkylator; produces intra- and interstrand DNA cross-links via association with platinum molecule, leads to DNA strand breakage during replication	4–7 [24]	20–30 [23]	24% [32]	Nephrotoxicity and painful peripheral neuropathy (both dose-limiting); neurotoxicity; mild myelosuppression; nausea and vomiting; anorexia and diarrhea; cumulative ototoxicity; chronic renal Mg^+ and K^+ wasting; ↑ liver transaminases; alopecia and cardiac conduction abnormalities (rare)
Oxaliplatin	Platinating agent; DNA disruption via intra- and interstrand cross-links with strong platinum association bonds, induces apoptosis in malignant cells	5 [14]	10–25 [33]	47% [15]	Neurotoxicity (dose-limiting); mild myelosuppression; mild fatigue and nausea; diarrhea; stomatitis; edema; cough; hypersensitivity reactions; extravasation injury (rare)

is also notable that this therapy is administered via a cheaper device (reservoir-less port costs about 150 eu while the pump device costs approximately US$ 10,000).

The above-mentioned properties of reservoir-less HAI ports motivated various groups around the globe to apply this treatment approach with additional chemotherapeutic agents. Pernot et al. demonstrated that HAI of 5-FU or mitomycin C is an alternative option in patients with CRLM who have progressed or are intolerant of HAI oxaliplatin [13]. Levi et al. [18] published an international (France, Belgium, Portugal, and Italy) prospective phase II trial in which they administered triplet HAI (irinotecan, oxaliplatin, and 5-FU) in patients with unresectable CRLM. They reported promising results that they feel justify a randomized controlled trial (RCT). In Japan, cisplatin-based hepatic arterial infusion chemotherapy has been widely employed as an alternative therapy to sorafenib for hepatocellular carcinoma patients with portal vein invasion [19]. Recently, a large RCT from China described the application of HAI fluorouracil, leucovorin, and oxaliplatin (FOLFOX) in patients with HCC and portal vein invasion and they demonstrated improved OS with acceptable toxicity compared with sorafenib [20].

Table 33.1 presents common chemotherapeutic agents used in HAI.

Techniques and Considerations

Reservoir-less HAI catheters can be placed either surgically or percutaneously by interventional radiology. Deschamps et al. [34] evaluated the safety and efficacy of the surgical and percutaneous techniques in 126 patients treated for CRLM. They showed that catheter implantation success rates and complication rates were similar.

Anatomic Considerations

Conventional hepatic vascular anatomy is present in approximately two-thirds of patients [35]. Careful review of arterial imaging is imperative prior to HAI-catheter placement in order to ensure adequate access and anticipate aberrant anatomy. Table 33.2 details the common anatomic variations.

The gastroduodenal artery (GDA) remains the preferred site of cannulation in cases of abnormal hepatic anatomy, as long as it connects with a proper hepatic artery that perfuses at least one liver segment. Ligation or embolization of all accessory and replaced hepatic arteries will assure perfusion of all liver segments in these patients through intrahepatic shunts [36].

Table 33.2 Anatomical variations in hepatic arterial supply

Variant	Incidence (%)	Anatomy
Aberrant origin of GDA [35]	6–11	Arises from the right or left hepatic artery, or as a trifurcation with the right hepatic and left hepatic arteries, all arising simultaneously from the common hepatic artery
Accessory left hepatic artery [37]	2–10	Arises from the left gastric artery crosses the gastrohepatic ligament and enters the liver at the base of the umbilical fissure. It typically supplies segments II and III, while the native left hepatic artery, arising from the proper hepatic artery, supplies the left liver as well, typically segment IV
Accessory right hepatic arteries [37]	1–7	Arises from the superior mesenteric artery (SMA), runs through the portacaval space and supplies a portion of the right liver
Replaced left hepatic artery [38]	4–16	Arises from the left gastric artery and supplies the left liver
Replaced right hepatic artery [38]	6–16	Originates from the SMA, runs through the portacaval space, supplying the whole right liver, with no branches to the right liver originating from the proper hepatic artery

Surgical Technique

During the surgical procedure for HAI placement, the GDA and the hepatic artery are dissected to facilitate insertion of the catheter and to avoid inadvertent perfusion of the pancreas, stomach, or duodenum. Branches to the retroperitoneum arising from the right or left hepatic artery are common and should be ligated. The HAI port is then placed over the ribcage. A popular reservoir-less HAI device used in Europe is the Celsite® Arterial access port (Celsite T302 catheter, BBraun, Velizy, France) [18]. Next, the GDA is ligated distally and the catheter is inserted up to the junction with the hepatic artery. If the catheter protrudes into the common hepatic artery, turbulence of blood flow can lead to increased risk of thrombosis of the hepatic artery. Failure to pass the catheter to the junction leaves a short segment of the GDA exposed to full concentrations of chemotherapy without the diluting effect of blood flow, potentially resulting in arterial injury. Perfusion of both lobes of the liver and lack of extrahepatic perfusion is confirmed by an injection of indocyanine green or methylene blue. Cholecystectomy is performed as well in order to avoid chemotherapy-induced cholecystitis. Recently, robotic and laparoscopic HAI catheter placement were shown to be safe and in addition to offer the advantages of minimally invasive approach [39].

Interventional Radiology Technique

Percutaneous implantation of specific port-a-cath systems without laparotomy or general anesthesia represent an additional mode of HAI catheter insertion. Several percutaneous techniques of port-a-cath system implantation are described to date [40–42]. The Seldinger technique is normally used through the left sublclavian and femoral arteries for percutaneous placement of infusion catheters to reach the hepatic artery. The precise placement of the catheter tip is essential in order to perfuse the liver and to avoid extrahepatic drug infusion [43]. Possible anatomical causes for procedure failure include multiple hepatic arterial variants, median arcuate ligament compression causing celiac artery stenosis, target artery invasion by tumor, and previous femoral–femoral bypass surgery [44]. The final position of the infusion catheter tip is usually based on the vascular anatomy of each patient and location of hepatic tumor lesions. With the "fixed-catheter tip" technique [45], the distal tip of the catheter is fixed to the GDA, while the drugs flow through a side hole to the common hepatic artery. Another technique is the "long tapered catheter placement" [46] in which the catheter is positioned distally into the common hepatic artery with the side hole placed at the origin of the proper hepatic artery. Externally, the reservoir-less HAI port is fixed to the fascia in a subcutaneous pocket.

Notably, Asian groups have described HAI chemotherapy without an implanted port/catheter system. In each chemotherapy cycle, they puncture the femoral artery and advance a microcatheter into the hepatic artery. After infusion is complete, the catheter is removed. Repetitive femoral artery punctures and catheterization are performed for each additional cycle [47].

Technical Complications

Despite the similar success rate of surgical and percutaneous HAI port placement, both approaches harbor risk for complications [34].

Extrahepatic drug perfusion occurs at about 2–9% of the patients. Infusion of chemotherapeutic agents into small gastric and duodenal branches of the hepatic artery may occur, causing mucosal irritation and ulceration. Severe pancreatitis may ensue if a pancreatic branch is perfused. As these complications may be lethal, this should be identified and corrected before starting chemotherapy. A 99m-Technetium-labeled macroaggregated albumin scan and subsequent angiogram can be used to demonstrate and identify vessels responsible for the extrahepatic perfusion. If angiography is unsuccessful, a trans-femoral celiac or superior mesenteric artery study may be utilized to both locate and treat the problem [35, 48].

Incomplete hepatic perfusion was reported to take place in 2–6% of the cases. Incomplete perfusion may be caused by failure to ligate or occlude an aberrant hepatic artery in which case the anatomic problem can be identified by CT angiogram and treated by trans-femoral embolization of the accessory vessel. An additional cause is failure to achieve cross-perfusion; in these cases, collateral flow to the remaining liver typically develops over time [49].

Gastroduodenal ulcers are a dangerous complication that were described at a rate of 5%. The most frequent anomaly causing this complication is a small branch arising of the hepatic artery to the lesser curvature of the stomach. This complication is manifested by severe epigastric pain developing during the course of chemotherapy. Endoscopic evaluation shows large gastric or duodenal ulcers, which are nonresponsive to standard anti-ulcer therapy. Surgical ligation or angiographic embolization of the vessel should be performed to treat this condition [50].

HAI port pocket infections are relatively infrequent and occur at a rate of approximately 2–5% [34, 49–51]. Sterile measures must be employed, including using aseptic techniques when inserting or accessing the implantable port system, along with early antibiotic use in case of any sign of local erythema or systemic infection. In comparison to standard pump systems, the reservoir-less port is of smaller size (2 cm diameter vs. 6 cm, respectively), and therefore may be less prone to pocket site infection. Infection rates have been previously shown to be as high as 7% when concomitant bowel resection is performed [51]. However, other data suggests there is no difference in infection rate with and without colonic resection [52], and a combined procedure can be considered safe as long as incision for the subcutaneous devise is away from laparotomy incision or trocar sites, and the skin is closed and sealed off before bowel transection occurs [53].

Arterial thrombosis occurs at a rate of 4–17% [32] and is associated with the chronicity of catheter within the artery, the caliber of the catheter compared to the target vessel lumen, as well as chemotherapeutic toxicity [54–57]. Tissue plasminogen activators may be used as lytic therapy for acute thrombosis; however, prophylactic anticoagulation provides little advantage in reducing this complication and is not generally considered. The occurrence of cerebral vascular events is associated with the use of brachial, axillary, and subclavian arteries as primary accesses in percutaneous placement [58, 59].

Hemorrhagic complications can result from either inadequately ligated vessels (rate <1%), from local hematoma near the port device (<1% for both) [49, 60] or bleeding at the puncture site (4%) [61].

HAI Chemotherapy for CRLM

Treatment Options for CRLM

Complete resection of hepatic metastases is the only therapy that has ever resulted in cure of patients with metastatic colorectal cancer limited to the liver. Over three decades of follow-up has documented that, in well-selected patients who had undergone resection, 5-year survival ranges from 25% to nearly 50% and 10-year survival is approximately 20% [62, 63]. However, only 20% of patients with CRLM are deemed resectable at the time of presentation [64]. Suitability for resection of metastatic disease is based on the likelihood of achieving complete resection with negative surgical margins and maintaining adequate liver reserve. Resectability depends mainly on remaining liver function, which typically necessitates preservation of at least two contiguous hepatic segments with adequate biliary drainage and blood flow in and out of the future liver remnant (FLR) [65, 66]. When the remnant liver is insufficient in size based on cross-sectional imaging volumetrics, preoperative portal vein embolization of the involved liver can be done to expand the future liver remnant. Combined hepatic vein and portal vein embolization has recently shown promising results in inducing accelerated liver hypertrophy [67]. In cases where metastases are deemed unresectable or when patients are ineligible for major surgery (either due to patient comorbidities or insufficient liver reserve), radiofrequency or microwave ablation may be applied [68].

Systemic Therapy

Combined with surgery, systemic chemotherapy has been the mainstay of treatment for patients with CRLM and tumor response rates have been previously demonstrated to correlate with resectability in patients with liver-only colorectal metastases [69]. Since the addition of irinotecan and oxaliplatin to the arsenal of systemic therapy, outcomes have improved significantly, and dual regimen chemotherapy with these drugs in combination with 5-fluorouracil (FOLFIRI or FOLFOX) is frequently used [68]. In patients with initially unresectable disease, oxaliplatin and irinotecan-based regimens aimed at tumor downsizing have achieved response rates of approximately 50% [70] and approximately 12% of these patients were converted to resection [71, 72]. A triplet combination of folinic acid 5-FU, oxaliplatin, and irinotecan has also been studied, and randomized trials comparing fluorouracil, leucovorin, oxaliplatin, and irinotecan (FOLFOXIRI) to fluorouracil, leucovorin, and irinotecan (FOLFIRI) [73] and leucovorin, fluorouracil, irinotecan hydrochloride, and oxaliplatin (FOLFIRINOX) to FOLFOX or FOLFIRI [74] demonstrated the triplet combinations to be associated with improved response rates, progression-free survival (PFS) and OS rates, and increased resection rates, but at an expense of increased toxicity. Molecular tumor biomarker analysis has allowed for further tailoring of systemic therapy according to underlying tumor genotype. RAS wild-type patients have been shown to have improved conversion to resectability and R0 rates when an epidermal growth factor (EGFR) blocker is added to systemic chemotherapy [75]. EGFR blockade in addition to triplet chemotherapy has demonstrated improved response and resection rates as well [76]. Antiangiogenic therapies have been studied for tumor size reduction as well. Conversion rate to resection has been reported to increase with the addition of bevacizumab to XELOX [77]. Similarly, the OLIVIA trial demonstrated increased resection and R0 rates and PFS with the addition of Bevacizumab to triplet chemotherapy [78].

The choice of drug regimen depends on hepatotoxicity and safety profiles [70], whether metastases are synchronous/metachronous and their resectability, tumor biomarkers, and even the side of colonic primary [79], as well as on drug availability, and patient preference.

Immunotherapy represents another treatment option for CRLM patients, which has been proven to be effective specifically in those with microsatellite instability high with deficient DNA mismatch repair (MSI-H/dMMR). The KEYNOTE-177 phase III trial showed that patients with MSI-H/dMMR metastatic colorectal cancer treated with pembrolizumab as first-line therapy have demonstrated significantly longer PFS when compared to chemotherapy (median, 16.5 vs. 8.2 months), and with fewer treatment-related adverse events (22% vs. 66% of grade 3 or higher) [80]. In the CheckMate 142 phase II trial, it was demonstrated that Nivolumab provided durable response rates and disease control in pretreated patients with MSI-H/dMMR metastatic colorectal cancer [81]. However, despite encouraging results of immunotherapy, only about 15% of CRCs have deficient DNA mismatch repair (dMMR), which results in microsatellite instability (MSI) [82]. The rate is even lower in rectal adenocarcinoma, in which about 5–10% are dMMR [83].

HAI for Unresectable CRLM

The majority (80%) of patients with CRLM are diagnosed with unresectable disease [64]. Patients are considered unresectable for technical reasons in which there is no technical way to resect the tumors with a negative margin and leave sufficient liver remnant. Patients are also considered unresectable for oncological reasons in which the number and size of their tumors confer such a poor prognosis that resection is not considered efficacious.

With the markedly improved response rates seen with chemotherapy for metastatic colorectal cancer, many groups have evaluated the role of HAI chemotherapy in converting unresectable CRLM to resectable disease. It is noteworthy that conversion to complete hepatic resection has been repeatedly demonstrated as the strongest prognostic factor associated with long-term survival and cure [72, 84]. The outcomes of the HAI chemotherapy should be interpreted in the context of the outcomes for systemic chemotherapy alone. Modern combination systemic chemotherapy for metastatic colorectal cancer has a response rate of approximately 50% and median survival of at least 20 months. Long-term survival beyond 5 years is uncommon and cure is exceedingly rare. For instance, the TRIBE trial [85] randomized patients with unresectable metastatic colorectal cancer to receive FOLFIRI plus bevacizumab (control) vs. FOLFOXIRI plus bevacizumab (experimental). The rate of complete hepatic resection of metastases was not significantly different in treatment groups (12% in the control group vs. 15% in the experimental group, $P = 0.33$). The 5-year-OS (5Y-OS) was less than 10%.

HAI with oxaliplatin for CRLM has been developed for more than 15 years, mostly in Europe. The major studies are presented in Table 33.3. Recent studies have investigated the combination of doublet or triplet HAI chemotherapy regimens [4, 5]. A recent international multicenter, prospective, phase II trial (OPTILIV) investigated a triplet chemotherapy by HAI (oxaliplatin/5-FU/irinotecan) combined with systemic cetuximab in 64 patients with unresectable RAS-wild-type CRLM, after first-line systemic treatment. Up to three extrahepatic lesions (less than 1 cm) were allowed and were present in 41% of the patients. The objective response rate was 41% and the conversion to resection rate was 30%. The median OS was 26 months. OS was two-fold longer in patients who underwent resection compared with those without resection (35.2 months vs. 18.7 months, respectively). Forty-five percent of resected patients were still alive after 4 years, compared to none in the non-resected group [7].

Table 33.3 Clinical trials on reservoir-less HAI for unresectable CRLM

Reference, year	HAI (+SYS) treatment	Number of patients	Response rate (%)	Conversion (%)	Median PFS (months)	Median OS (months)	Study design
Link 2001 [86]	Folinic acid, 5-FU, mitoxantrone, mitomycin C	63	54	14	12.7	25.7	Prospective, single center
Boige 2007 [87]	Oxaliplatin (+5-FU/leucovorin)	39	62	18	7	16	Prospective, single center
Ducreux 2005 [16]	Oxaliplatin (+5-FU/leucovorin)	28	64	18	27	27	Prospective, multicenter
Del Freo 2006 [88]	Oxaliplatin and 5-FU/leucovorin	21	24	10	5.9	36.1	Prospective, multicenter
Melichar 2006 [89]	Irinotecan, 5-FU/ leucovorin	36	14	10	11	23	Prospective, multicenter
Idelevich 2009 [90]	Irinotecan, 5-FU/ leucovorin (leucovorin)	35	65	29	12	36	Prospective, single center
Goéré 2010 [17]	Oxaliplatin, 5-FU/ leucovorin	87	55	26	NA	42	Prospectively collected, single center
Lévi 2016 [18]	Oxaliplatin, irinotecan, and 5-FU (+ cetuximab)	64	41	30	9.3	25.5	Prospective, multicenter

Of note, a recent single arm phase II trial was published by the MSKCC group that included 64 patients with unresectable CRLM treated with HAI FUDR and systemic therapy, of which 67% were previously treated. Extrahepatic disease was not allowed. The median number of metastases was 13, the objective response rate was 73%, and the conversion to resection rate was 52%. The median OS was 38 months (5Y-OS = 36%), 14% (9 pts) were with no evidence of disease (NED) at a median follow-up of 7 years, and the conversion to resection was the only factor associated with survival (resected patients 5Y-OS = 63%, unresected 5Y-OS = 12%). It is apparent that the patient's characteristics of this trial are somewhat different from the OPTILIV trial and may account for the differences in outcomes. However, it can be appreciated that both HAI oxaliplatin and HAI FUDR treatments are associated with substantial conversion to resection rates in patients who present with initially unresectable CRLM.

To date, no randomized trial has compared reservoir-less HAI combined with systemic therapy (SYS) vs. SYS only [7, 8]. The SULTAN trial (PRODIGE 53) is an ongoing trial planned to answer this question. It is a multicenter, randomized, comparative phase II trial, which includes patients with unresectable CRLM after at least 2 months of first-line induction systemic chemotherapy. Patients are randomly assigned in a 1:1 ratio to receive HAI oxaliplatin combined with systemic FOLFIRI plus targeted therapy (experimental arm) or the best systemic chemotherapy plus targeted therapy. It is designed to evaluate the efficacy of HAI oxaliplatin and the primary outcome is conversion to resection rate.

HAI for Resectable CRLM

The rationale for adjuvant therapy in CRLM derives from the fact that although some patients have long-term disease-free survival after resection, many patients' disease recurs. The liver is the only site of initial recurrence in 50% of patients [91, 92]. Therefore, adjuvant treatment and its impact on recurrence and survival have been evaluated. The EORTC 40983 [93] was an RCT that compared adjuvant (perioperative) systemic FOLFOX versus surgery alone, and demonstrated PFS improvement but no OS benefit.

The MSKCC group published their extensive experience in adjuvant HAI treatment [94]. Out of 2368 patients who had underwent resection of CRLM, the HAI group included 785 patients who were characterized by a more advanced disease (higher rates of synchronous disease, two-stage hepatectomy, ablations, and node positive disease) compared to the no-HAI group (n = 1583). The median OS was 68 versus 46 months (i.e., absolute difference of 2 years) and the 10-year-OS (10Y-OS) was 38% versus 24% for HAI versus no-HAI, respectively. These results remained statistically significant after propensity score matching. Interestingly, greater benefit in median OS was observed in patients with low clinical risk score (absolute difference of 3 years) and patients with node negative primary cancers (absolute difference of 6 years). The authors concluded that adjuvant HAI is associated with a benefit of 2 years in median OS, and that patients with a low clinical risk score or node negative primary may benefit the most from adjuvant HAI. These results led to the development of the PUMP trial [36], which is an ongoing multicenter randomized trial that is designed to focus on adjuvant HAI treatment of patients with low-risk CRLM. Patients randomized to arm A undergo complete CRLM resection without any adjuvant treatment, which is the standard of care in the Netherlands. Patients in arm B receive an implantable HAI pump at the time of CRLM resection and start adjuvant HAI chemotherapy after surgery, with floxuridine. The primary endpoint is PFS.

An alternative adjuvant HAI treatment was mainly developed in France with administration of HAI oxaliplatin. The French group from Gustave Roussy [95] believes that adjuvant HAI treatment should be investigated in oncologically high-risk patients (defined as greater than 4 CRLM) because HAI chemotherapy is technically more demanding than systemic chemotherapy. This is based on their retrospective analysis of 98 high-risk patients who were treated postoperatively with either HAI oxaliplatin plus systemic 5-FU (n = 44) compared to systemic FOLFOX/FOLFIRI ("modern" systemic chemotherapy) (n = 54) [96]). Feasibility was demonstrated for adjuvant oxaliplatin-based HAI chemotherapy, with 84% of patients receiving more than four cycles. The HAI group demonstrated both significantly longer 3-year hepatic DFS and longer 3-year DFS rates when compared to systemic therapy. On multivariate analysis, the only independent prognostic factors for prolonged DFS were adjuvant HAI chemotherapy and R0 resection margin status. Based on these results, mainly the observed DFS benefit, they initiated the PACHA trial [95]. The investigators of this trial mentioned the potential advantages of adjuvant HAI oxaliplatin. First, HAI oxaliplatin is administered by 2-h infusion every 2 weeks (similarly to the systemic administration of oxaliplatin) compared to a 14-day infusion with FUDR. Second, HAI oxaliplatin rarely causes biliary toxicity, unlike FUDR. This study is an ongoing trial designed as a multicenter, randomized phase II/III trial. The main objective is to assess the efficacy of HAI oxaliplatin plus systemic fluoropyrimidine (LV5FU2 regimen) after curative-intent surgery (resection and/or thermal ablation) of at least 4 CRLM compared to adjuvant systemic therapy alone.

HAI Chemotherapy for HCC

Hepatic arterial infusion chemotherapy (HAIC) has been widely employed as an optional therapy for HCC patients with portal vein invasion in Japan [97]. Recently, growing evidence, mostly from Asia, has indicated that HAI with FOLFOX provides a significant survival benefit for patients with advanced HCC.

In 2018, He et al. [20] demonstrated the advantage of HAI in multicenter randomized trial that included 247 patients with HCC and portal vein invasion. Patients were randomized to receive either sorafenib or sorafenib plus HAI FOLFOX. The HAI FOLFOX regimen significantly increased the response rates (41% vs. 2%) and the median OS (13 months compared to 7 months with sorafenib alone).

A recent 2019 meta-analysis by Zhuang et al. [98] of 14 clinical trials, evaluating efficacy and safety of HAI chemotherapy versus sorafenib (1006 and 773 patients, respectively) for advanced HCC, reported that HAI chemotherapy demonstrated improved disease control rate, overall response rate, PFS, and OS when compared to sorafenib. Moreover, sorafenib was associated with a higher adverse event frequency, including hypertension, fatigue, dermatological, and gastrointestinal disorders.

Another recent randomized trial from China was published in 2021 and randomized 315 patients with unresectable HCC to receive either HAI FOLFOX or TACE [47]. Compared to the TACE group, HAI FOLFOX significantly increased median OS (23 vs. 16 months) and response rate (46% vs. 18%). Of note, the incidence of serious adverse events was significantly higher in the TACE group. These promising outcomes support the safety and efficacy of HAI chemotherapy for advanced HCC.

Concluding Remarks

Reservoir-less ports for HAI chemotherapy offer several potential advantages. It is a cheaper device compared to the implantable reservoir HAI pump and therefore may be more affordable for various patients around the world. The safety profile of the chemotherapeutic agents utilized in this approach (lower biliary toxicity rate compared to FUDR) makes it easier to apply in different healthcare systems worldwide. Notably, it was shown to provide similar oncological outcomes compared to the pump. Reservoir-less port HAI of oxaliplatin for unresectable CRLM demonstrated similar outcomes to pump HAI FUDR treatment in two similar prospective trials [18, 99, 100].

Furthermore, reservoir-less port HAI chemotherapy has been widely employed not only in Europe but also in Asia [97] and in recent years, level 1 data [20, 47] has accumulated to support its important role as part of the treatment armamentarium of HCC.

Therefore, reservoir-less port HAI chemotherapy is applicable to selected patients and may prove to be the ideal therapy accessible for them.

References

1. de Ridder J, de Wilt JHW, Simmer F, Overbeek L, Lemmens V, Nagtegaal I. Incidence and origin of histologically confirmed liver metastases: an explorative case-study of 23,154 patients. Oncotarget. 2016;7:55368–76.
2. Boilève A, De Cuyper A, Larive A, et al. Hepatic arterial infusion of oxaliplatin plus systemic chemotherapy and targeted therapy for unresectable colorectal liver metastases. Eur J Cancer. 2020;138:89–98.
3. Sharib JM, Creasy JM, Wildman-Tobriner B, et al. Hepatic artery infusion pumps. Ann Surg. 2022;276:943. https://doi.org/10.1097/SLA.0000000000005434.
4. Rossi S, Garbagnati F, Lencioni R, et al. Percutaneous radio-frequency thermal ablation of nonresectable hepatocellular carcinoma after occlusion of tumor blood supply. Radiology. 2000;217:119–26. https://doi.org/10.1148/radiology2171.r00se02119.
5. Kemeny NE, Fong Y. Hepatic arterial chemotherapy. In: Holland-Frei cancer medicine. 6th ed. BC Decker; 2003.
6. Ranieri G, Laforgia M, Nardulli P, Ferraiuolo S, Molinari P, Marech I, Gadaleta CD. Oxaliplatin-based intra-arterial chemotherapy in colo-rectal cancer liver metastases: a review from pharmacology to clinical application. Cancers (Basel). 2019;11:141. https://doi.org/10.3390/CANCERS11020141.
7. Fohlen A, Bordji K, Assenat E, et al. Anticancer drugs for intra-arterial treatment of colorectal cancer liver metastases: in-vitro screening after short exposure time. Pharmaceuticals. 2021;14:639. https://doi.org/10.3390/PH14070639/S1.
8. Collins JM. Pharmacologic rationale for regional drug delivery. J Clin Oncol. 1984;2:498–504.
9. Collins JM. Pharmacologic rationale for hepatic arterial therapy. Recent Results Cancer Res. 1986;100:140–7.
10. Qin Z, Ren G, Yuan J, Chen H, Lu Y, Li N, Zhang Y, Chen X, Zhao D. Systemic evaluation on the pharmacokinetics of platinum-based anticancer drugs from animal to cell level: based on total platinum and intact drugs. Front Pharmacol. 2019;10:1485.
11. Rahbari NN, Bork U, Kircher A, et al. Compartmental differences of circulating tumor cells in colorectal cancer. Oncologia. 2012;19:2195–202.
12. Kelly RJ, Kemeny NE, Leonard GD. Current strategies using hepatic arterial infusion chemotherapy for the treatment of colorectal cancer. Clin Colorectal Cancer. 2005;5:166–74.
13. Pernot S, Velut G, Kourie RH, et al. 5-FU or mitomycin C hepatic arterial infusion after failure of arterial oxaliplatin in patients with colorectal cancer unresectable liver metastases. Clin Res Hepatol Gastroenterol. 2018;42:255–60.
14. Dzodic R, Gomez-Abuin G, Rougier P, Bonnay M, Ardouin P, Gouyette A, Rixe O, Ducreux M, Munck JN. Pharmacokinetic advantage of intra-arterial hepatic oxaliplatin administration: comparative results with cisplatin using a rabbit VX2 tumor model. Anti-Cancer Drugs. 2004;15:647–50.
15. Guthoff I, Lotspeich E, Fester C, Wallin I, Schatz M, Ehrsson H, Kornmann M. Hepatic artery infusion using oxaliplatin in combination with 5-fluorouracil, folinic acid and mitomycin C: oxaliplatin pharmacokinetics and feasibility. Anticancer Res. 2003;23:5203–8.
16. Ducreux M, Ychou M, Laplanche A, et al. Hepatic arterial oxaliplatin infusion plus intravenous chemotherapy in colorectal cancer with inoperable hepatic metastases: a trial of the gastrointestinal group of the Federation Nationale des Centres de Lutte Contre le Cancer. J Clin Oncol. 2005;23:4881–7.
17. Goéré D, Deshaies I, De Baere T, Boige V, Malka D, Dumont F, Dromain C, Ducreux M, Elias D. Prolonged survival of initially unresectable hepatic colorectal cancer patients treated with hepatic arterial infusion of oxaliplatin followed by radical surgery of metastases. Ann Surg. 2010;251:686–91.
18. Lévi FA, Boige V, Hebbar M, et al. Conversion to resection of liver metastases from colorectal cancer with hepatic artery infusion of combined chemotherapy and systemic cetuximab in multicenter trial OPTILIV. Ann Oncol. 2016;27:267–74.
19. Kudo M, Matsui O, Izumi N, et al. JSH consensus-based clinical practice guidelines for the management of hepatocellular carcinoma: 2014 update by the Liver Cancer Study Group of Japan. Liver Cancer. 2014;3:458–68.
20. He M, Li Q, Zou R, et al. Sorafenib plus hepatic arterial infusion of oxaliplatin, fluorouracil, and leucovorin vs sorafenib alone for hepatocellular carcinoma with portal vein invasion: a randomized clinical trial. JAMA Oncol. 2019;5:953–60.
21. Doroshow JH. Approach to the patient with cancer. In: Goldman L, Schafer AI, editors. Goldman-Cecil med. 26th ed. Elsevier; 2019. p. 1166–95.
22. Aldrighetti L, Arru M, Ronzoni M, Salvioni M, Villa E, Ferla G. Extrahepatic biliary stenoses after hepatic arterial infusion (HAI) of floxuridine (FUdR) for liver metastases from colorectal cancer. Hepatogastroenterology. 2001;48(41):1302–7.
23. Ensminger WD, Gyves JW. Clinical pharmacology of hepatic arterial chemotherapy. Semin Oncol. 1983;10:176–82.

24. Chapelle N, Matysiak-Budnik T, Douane F, Metairie S, Rougier P, Touchefeu Y. Hepatic arterial infusion in the management of colorectal cancer liver metastasis: current and future perspectives. Dig Liver Dis. 2018;50:220–5.
25. Fallik D, Ychou M, Jacob J, et al. Hepatic arterial infusion using pirarubicin combined with systemic chemotherapy: a phase II study in patients with non-resectable liver metastases from colorectal cancer. Ann Oncol. 2003;14:856–63.
26. Munck J-N, Riggi M, Rougier P, Chabot GG, Ramirez LH, Zhao Z, Bognel C, Ardouin P, Herait P, Gouyette A. Pharmacokinetic and pharmacodynamic advantages of pirarubicin over adriamycin after intraarterial hepatic administration in the rabbit VX2 tumor model. Cancer Res. 1993;53:1550–4.
27. Kanat O, Gewirtz A, Kemeny N. What is the potential role of hepatic arterial infusion chemotherapy in the current armamentorium against colorectal cancer. J Gastrointest Oncol. 2012;3:130–8.
28. Ensminger WD, Rosowsky A, Raso V, Levin DC, Glode M, Come S, Steele G, Frei E. A clinical-pharmacological evaluation of hepatic arterial infusions of 5-fluoro-2′-deoxyuridine and 5-fluorouracil. Cancer Res. 1978;38:3784–92.
29. Blaschke M, Blumberg J, Wegner U, et al. Measurements of 5-FU plasma concentrations in patients with gastrointestinal cancer: 5-FU levels reflect the 5-FU dose applied. J Cancer Ther. 2012;3:28–36.
30. Mocellin S, Pilati P, Lise M, Nitti D. Meta-analysis of hepatic arterial infusion for unresectable liver metastases from colorectal cancer: the end of an era? J Clin Oncol. 2007;25:5649–54.
31. Baggiani A, Ierardi AM, Caspani B, et al. Hypoxic liver perfusion with mitomycin-C for treating multifocal metastases and unresectable primary tumours: a single-centre series of 42 patients. La Radiol Med. 2011;116(8):1239–49.
32. Laface C, Laforgia M, Molinari P, Ugenti I, Gadaleta CD, Porta C, Ranieri G. Hepatic arterial infusion of chemotherapy for advanced hepatobiliary cancers: state of the art. Cancers (Basel). 2021;13:3091. https://doi.org/10.3390/cancers13123091.
33. Ehrsson H, Wallin I, Yachnin J. Pharmacokinetics of oxaliplatin in humans. Med Oncol. 2001;194(19):261–5.
34. Deschamps F, Elias D, Goere D, Malka D, Ducreux M, Boige V, Auperin A, De Baere T. Intra-arterial hepatic chemotherapy: a comparison of percutaneous versus surgical implantation of port-catheters. Cardiovasc Interv Radiol. 2010;34(5):973–9.
35. Allen PJ, Stojadinovic A, Ben-Porat L, Gonen M, Kooby D, Blumgart L, Paty P, Fong Y. The management of variant arterial anatomy during hepatic arterial infusion pump placement. Ann Surg Oncol. 2002;9(9):875–80.
36. Buisman FE, Homs MYV, Grünhagen DJ, et al. Adjuvant hepatic arterial infusion pump chemotherapy and resection versus resection alone in patients with low-risk resectable colorectal liver metastases—the multicenter randomized controlled PUMP trial. BMC Cancer. 2019;19:327. https://doi.org/10.1186/S12885-019-5515-6.
37. Qadan M, Kemeny NE. Regional chemotherapy for liver tumors. In: Blumgart's surg liver, biliary tract pancreas, vol. 2–2. 6th ed; 2017. p. 1470–87.e3.
38. Thiels CA, D'Angelica MI. Hepatic artery infusion pumps. J Surg Oncol. 2020;122:70–7.
39. Qadan M, D'Angelica MI, Kemeny NE, Cercek A, Kingham TP. Robotic hepatic arterial infusion pump placement. HPB. 2017;19:429–35.
40. Deschamps F, Rao P, Teriitehau C, Hakime A, Malka D, Boige V, Ducreux M, Elias D, Goere D, De Baere T. Percutaneous femoral implantation of an arterial port catheter for intraarterial chemotherapy: feasibility and predictive factors of long-term functionality. J Vasc Interv Radiol. 2010;21:1681–8.
41. Herrmann KA, Waggershauser T, Sittek H, Reiser MF. Liver intraarterial chemotherapy: use of the femoral artery for percutaneous implantation of catheter-port systems. Radiology. 2000; 215:294–9. https://doi.org/10.1148/radiology2151.r00ap14294.
42. Tanaka T, Arai Y, Inaba Y, Matsueda K, Aramaki T, Takeuchi Y, Kichikawa K. Radiologic placement of side-hole catheter with tip fixation for hepatic arterial infusion chemotherapy. J Vasc Interv Radiol. 2003;14:63–8.
43. Chuang VP, Wallace S. Hepatic arterial redistribution for intraarterial infusion of hepatic neoplasms. Radiology. 1980;135:295–9. https://doi.org/10.1148/radiology13527367615.
44. Ganeshan A, Upponi S, Hon LQ, Warakaulle D, Uberoi R. Hepatic arterial infusion of chemotherapy: the role of diagnostic and interventional radiology. Ann Oncol. 2008;19:847–51.
45. Yamagami T, Iida S, Kato T, Tanaka O, Hirota T, Nakamura T, Nishimura T. Using n-butyl cyanoacrylate and the fixed-catheter-tip technique in percutaneous implantation of a port-catheter system in patients undergoing repeated hepatic arterial. Chemotherapy. 2012;179:1611–7. https://doi.org/10.2214/ajr17961791611.
46. Seki H, Shiina M. Placement of a long tapered side-hole catheter in the hepatic artery: technical advantages, catheter stability, and arterial patency. Am J Roentgenol. 2006;187:1312–20.
47. Li QJ, He MK, Chen HW, et al. Hepatic arterial infusion of oxaliplatin, fluorouracil, and leucovorin versus transarterial chemoembolization for large hepatocellular carcinoma: a randomized phase III trial. J Clin Oncol. 2022;40:150–60.
48. Perez DR, Kemeny NE, Brown KT, Gewirtz AN, Paty PB, Jarnagin WR, D'Angelica MI. Angiographic identification of extrahepatic perfusion after hepatic arterial pump placement: implications for surgical prevention. HPB (Oxford). 2014;16:744.

49. Doussot A, Kemeny NE, D'Angelica MI. Hepatic arterial infusional chemotherapy in the management of colorectal cancer liver metastases. Hepat Oncol. 2015;2:275–90.
50. Chevallier O, Mvouama S, Pellegrinelli J, Guillen K, Manfredi S, Ghiringhelli F, Falvo N, Midulla M, Loffroy R. Percutaneous implantation of a microcatheter-port system for hepatic arterial infusion chemotherapy of unresectable liver tumors: technical feasibility, functionality, and complications. Diagnostics (Basel). 2021;11(3):399. https://doi.org/10.3390/diagnostics11030399.
51. Huk I, Entscheff P, Prager M, Schulz F, Polterauer P, Funovics J. Patency rate of implantable devices during long-term intraaterial. Chemotherapy. 2016;41:936–41. https://doi.org/10.1177/000331979004101107.
52. Turley MC, Moore C, Creasy JM, et al. Combined primary resection with hepatic artery infusion pump implantation is safe for unresectable colorectal liver metastases. J Gastrointest Surg. 2022;26:764–71.
53. Groot Koerkamp B, Grunhagen DJ, Verhoef C. A colon resection and pump implantation in the same surgical procedure: is it safe? Ann Surg Oncol. 2022;29(5):2754–5.
54. Wacker FK, Boese-Landgraf J, Wagner A, Albrecht D, Wolf KJ, Fobbe F. Minimally invasive catheter implantation for regional chemotherapy of the liver: a new percutaneous transsubclavian approach. Cardiovasc Intervent Radiol. 1997;20:128–32.
55. Okuyama K, Tohnosu N, Koide Y, et al. [Complications and their management in intraarterial infusion chemotherapy]. Gan To Kagaku Ryoho. 1992;19:1007–13.
56. Strum S, McDermed J, Korn A, Joseph C. Improved methods for venous access: the Port-A-Cath, a totally implanted catheter system. J Clin Oncol. 1986;4:596–603.
57. Habbe TG, McCowan TC, Goertzen TC, Leveen RF, Culp WC, Tempero MA. Complications and technical limitations of hepatic arterial infusion catheter placement for chemotherapy. J Vasc Interv Radiol. 1998;2:233–9.
58. Hirota T, Yamagami T, Tanaka O, Iida S, Kato T, Nishimura T. Catheter redundancy in the aortic arch increases the risk of stroke in left subclavian arterial port-catheter systems. J Vasc Interv Radiol. 2005;16:471–6.
59. Seki H, Kimura M, Yoshimura N, Yamamoto S, Ozaki T, Sakai K. Hepatic arterial infusion chemotherapy using percutaneous catheter placement with an implantable port: assessment of factors affecting patency of the hepatic artery. Clin Radiol. 1999;4:221–7.
60. Allen PJ, Nissan A, Picon AI, et al. Technical complications and durability of hepatic artery infusion pumps for unresectable colorectal liver metastases: an institutional experience of 544 consecutive cases. J Am Coll Surg. 2005;201(1):57–65. https://doi.org/10.1016/j.jamcollsurg.2005.03.019.
61. Matsumoto T, Yamagami T, Yoshimatsu R, Morishita H, Kitamura N, Sato O, Hasebe T. Hepatic arterial infusion chemotherapy by the fixed-catheter-tip method: retrospective comparison of percutaneous left subclavian and femoral port-catheter system implantation. Am J Roentgenol. 2013;202:211–5. https://doi.org/10.2214/AJR1210502.
62. Fong Y, Fortner J, Sun RL, Brennan MF, Blumgart LH. Clinical score for predicting recurrence after hepatic resection for metastatic colorectal cancer: analysis of 1001 consecutive cases. Ann Surg. 1999;230:309.
63. Tomlinson JS, Jarnagin WR, DeMatteo RP, Fong Y, Kornprat P, Gonen M, Kemeny N, Brennan MF, Blumgart LH, D'Angelica M. Actual 10-year survival after resection of colorectal liver metastases defines cure. J Clin Oncol. 2007;25:4575–80.
64. Padmanabhan C, Nussbaum DP, D'Angelica M. Surgical management of colorectal cancer liver metastases. Surg Oncol Clin N Am. 2021;30:1–25.
65. Lee HY, Woo IS. Perioperative systemic chemotherapy for colorectal liver metastasis: recent updates. Cancers. 2021;13:4590.
66. Xu F, Tang B, Jin TQ, Dai CL. Current status of surgical treatment of colorectal liver metastases. World J Clin Cases. 2018;6:716–34.
67. Heil J, Schadde E. Simultaneous portal and hepatic vein embolization before major liver resection. Langenbeck's Arch Surg. 2021;406:1295–305.
68. Oki E, Ando K, Nakanishi R, et al. Recent advances in treatment for colorectal liver metastasis. Ann Gastroenterol Surg. 2018;2:167–75.
69. Folprecht G, Grothey A, Alberts S, Raab HR, Köhne CH. Neoadjuvant treatment of unresectable colorectal liver metastases: correlation between tumour response and resection rates. Ann Oncol. 2005;16:1311–9.
70. Martin J, Petrillo A, Smyth EC, et al. Colorectal liver metastases: current management and future perspectives. World J Clin Oncol. 2020;11:761–808.
71. Heinemann V, von Weikersthal LF, Decker T, et al. FOLFIRI plus cetuximab versus FOLFIRI plus bevacizumab as first-line treatment for patients with metastatic colorectal cancer (FIRE-3): a randomised, open-label, phase 3 trial. Lancet Oncol. 2014;15:1065–75.
72. Adam R, Delvart V, Pascal G, et al. Rescue surgery for unresectable colorectal liver metastases downstaged by chemotherapy: a model to predict long-term survival. Ann Surg. 2004;240:644.
73. Falcone A, Ricci S, Brunetti I, et al. Phase III trial of infusional fluorouracil, leucovorin, oxaliplatin, and irinotecan (FOLFOXIRI) compared with infusional fluorouracil, leucovorin, and irinotecan (FOLFIRI) as first-line treatment for metastatic colorectal cancer: the gruppo oncologico nord ovest. J Clin Oncol. 2007;25:1670–6.

74. Ychou M, Rivoire M, Thezenas S, et al. A randomized phase II trial of three intensified chemotherapy regimens in first-line treatment of colorectal cancer patients with initially unresectable or not optimally resectable liver metastases. The METHEP trial. Ann Surg Oncol. 2013;20:4289–97.
75. Van Cutsem E, Köhne C-H, Hitre E, et al. Cetuximab and chemotherapy as initial treatment for metastatic colorectal cancer. N Engl J Med. 2009;360:1408–17.
76. Modest DP, Martens UM, Riera-Knorrenschild J, et al. FOLFOXIRI plus panitumumab as first-line treatment of RAS wild-type metastatic colorectal cancer: the randomized, open-label, phase II VOLFI study (AIO KRK0109). J Clin Oncol. 2019;37:3401–11.
77. Wong R, Cunningham D, Barbachano Y, et al. A multicentre study of capecitabine, oxaliplatin plus bevacizumab as perioperative treatment of patients with poor-risk colorectal liver-only metastases not selected for upfront resection. Ann Oncol. 2011;22:2042–8.
78. Gruenberger T, Bridgewater J, Chau I, García Alfonso P, Rivoire M, Mudan S, Lasserre S, Hermann F, Waterkamp D, Adam R. Bevacizumab plus mFOLFOX-6 or FOLFOXIRI in patients with initially unresectable liver metastases from colorectal cancer: the OLIVIA multinational randomised phase II trial. Ann Oncol. 2015;26:702–8.
79. Benson AB, Venook AP, Al-Hawary MM, et al. NCCN clinical practice guidelines in oncology (NCCN Guidelines®) colon cancer version 1.2022—February 25, 2022. In: Natl. Compr. Cancer Netw. 2022. https://www.nccn.org/professionals/physician_gls/pdf/colon.pdf.
80. André T, Shiu K-K, Kim TW, et al. Pembrolizumab in microsatellite-instability-high advanced colorectal cancer. N Engl J Med. 2020;383:2207–18.
81. Overman MJ, McDermott R, Leach JL, et al. Nivolumab in patients with metastatic DNA mismatch repair-deficient or microsatellite instability-high colorectal cancer (CheckMate 142): an open-label, multicentre, phase 2 study. Lancet Oncol. 2017;18:1182–91.
82. Jin Z, Sinicrope FA. Mismatch repair-deficient colorectal cancer: building on checkpoint blockade. J Clin Oncol. 2022;40:2735. https://doi.org/10.1200/JCO.21.02691.
83. Cercek A, Lumish M, Sinopoli J, et al. PD-1 blockade in mismatch repair-deficient, locally advanced rectal cancer. N Engl J Med. 2022;386:2363–76.
84. Pozzo C, Basso M, Cassano A, Quirino M, Schinzari G, Trigila N, Vellone M, Guiliante F, Nuzzo C, Barone C. Neoadjuvant treatment of unresectable liver disease with irinotecan and 5-fluorouracil plus folinic acid in colorectal cancer patients. Ann Oncol. 2004;15:933–9.
85. Loupakis F, Cremolini C, Masi G, et al. Initial therapy with FOLFOXIRI and bevacizumab for metastatic colorectal cancer. N Engl J Med. 2014;371:1609–18.
86. Link KH, Sunelaitis E, Kornmann M, Schatz M, Gansauge F, Leder G, Formentini A, Staib L, Pillasch J, Beger HG. Regional chemotherapy of nonresectable colorectal liver metastases with mitoxantrone, 5-fluorouracil, folinic acid, and mitomycin C may prolong survival. Cancer. 2001;92:2746–53.
87. Boige V, Malka D, Elias D, Castaing M, De Baere T, Goere D, Dromain C, Pocard M, Ducreux M. Hepatic arterial infusion of oxaliplatin and intravenous LV5FU2 in unresectable liver metastases from colorectal cancer after systemic chemotherapy failure. Ann Surg Oncol. 2007;151(15):219–26.
88. Del Freo A, Fiorentini G, Sanguinetti F, et al. Hepatic arterial chemotherapy with oxaliplatin, folinic acid and 5-fluorouracil in pre-treated patients with liver metastases from colorectal cancer. In Vivo. 2006;20:743–6.
89. Melichar B, Vobořil Z, Krajina A, Malířová E, Weiner P, Nová M, Ryška A, Dvořák J. Hepatic arterial infusion of irinotecan, 5-fluorouracil and leucovorin in patients with liver metastases from colorectal carcinoma. Anticancer Res. 2012;32(12):5487–93.
90. Idelevich E, Greif F, Mavor E, et al. Phase II study of UFT with leucovorin plus hepatic arterial infusion with irinotecan, 5-fluorouracil and leucovorin for non-resectable liver metastases of colorectal cancer. Liver Trauma View project analysis of results after sleeve gastrectomy taking care. Chemotherapy. 2009;55(2):76–82. https://doi.org/10.1159/000183732.
91. D'Angelica M, Kornprat P, Gonen M, DeMatteo RP, Fong Y, Blumgart LH, Jarnagin WR. Effect on outcome of recurrence patterns after hepatectomy for colorectal metastases. Ann Surg Oncol. 2011;18:1096–103.
92. Chan KM, Wu TH, Cheng CH, Lee WC, Chiang JM, Chen JS, Wang JY. Prognostic significance of the number of tumors and aggressive surgical approach in colorectal cancer hepatic metastasis. World J Surg Oncol. 2014;12:1–8.
93. Nordlinger B, Sorbye H, Glimelius B, et al. Perioperative FOLFOX4 chemotherapy and surgery versus surgery alone for resectable liver metastases from colorectal cancer (EORTC 40983): long-term results of a randomised, controlled, phase 3 trial. Lancet Oncol. 2013;14:1208–15.
94. Koerkamp BG, Sadot E, Kemeny NE, et al. Perioperative hepatic arterial infusion pump chemotherapy is associated with longer survival after resection of colorectal liver metastases: a propensity score analysis. J Clin Oncol. 2017;35:1938–44.
95. Goéré D, Pignon JP, Gelli M, et al. Postoperative hepatic arterial chemotherapy in high-risk patients as adjuvant treatment after resection of colorectal liver metastases—a randomized phase II/III trial—PACHA-01 (NCT02494973). BMC Cancer. 2018;18:1–8.
96. Goéré D, Benhaim L, Bonnet S, et al. Adjuvant chemotherapy after resection of colorectal liver metas-

tases in patients at high risk of hepatic recurrence: a comparative study between hepatic arterial infusion of oxaliplatin and modern systemic chemotherapy. Ann Surg. 2013;257:114–20.

97. Ueshima K, Komemushi A, Aramaki T, et al. Clinical practice guidelines for hepatic arterial infusion chemotherapy with a port system proposed by the Japanese Society of Interventional Radiology and Japanese Society of Implantable Port Assisted Treatment. Liver Cancer. 2022;11:407–25.
98. Zhuang BW, Li W, Xie XH, Hu HT, De Lu M, Xie XY. Sorafenib versus hepatic arterial infusion chemotherapy for advanced hepatocellular carcinoma: a systematic review and meta-analysis. Jpn J Clin Oncol. 2019;49:845–55.
99. Pak L, D'Angelica M, MSKCC. Prospective phase II trial of combination. Hepática artery infusión and systemic chemotherapy. Physiol Behav. 2019;176:139–48.
100. D'Angelica MI, Correa-Gallego C, Paty PB, Cercek A, Gewirtz AN, Chou JF, Capanu M, Jarnagin WR, Kemeny N. Phase II trial of hepatic artery infusional and systemic chemotherapy for patients with unresectable hepatic metastases from colorectal cancer: conversion to resection and long-term outcomes. Ann Surg. 2016;261:353–60.

Index

M. D'Angelica, M. Lidsky (eds.), *Hepatic Arterial Infusion for Malignancy*,
https://doi.org/10.1007/978-3-031-74935-3

D

E

I

MIX
Papier aus verantwortungsvollen Quellen
Paper from responsible sources
FSC® C105338

If you have any concerns about our products,
you can contact us on
ProductSafety@springernature.com

In case Publisher is established outside the EU,
the EU authorized representative is:
Springer Nature Customer Service Center GmbH
Europaplatz 3, 69115 Heidelberg, Germany

Printed by Libri Plureos GmbH
in Hamburg, Germany